INJURIES AND DISORDERS OF THE HEAD AND BRAIN

LORNE S. LABEL, M.D.

Editor–In–Chief

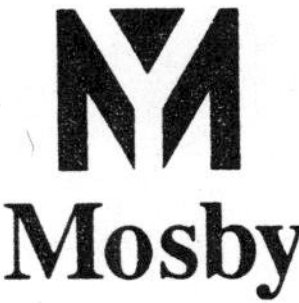

Mosby

MATTHEW BENDER

QUESTIONS ABOUT THIS PUBLICATION?

For questions about the **Editorial Content** appearing in these volumes or reprint permission, please call:

Beverly Lieberman .... 1–800–252–9257 (ext. 2629)
Rina Cascone .... 1–800–252–9257 (ext. 2858)
Outside the United States and Canada please call .... (212) 448-2000

For assistance with shipments, billing or other customer service matters, refer to book code 31925. Please call:

Customer Services Department at .... (800) 426-4545
Outside the United States and Canada, please call   .... (314) 872-8370
Fax number .... (800) 535-9935
Outside the United States and Canada, please fax .... (314) 453-4379

This publication is designed to provide accurate and authoritative information in regard to the subject matter covered. It is sold with the understanding that the publisher is not engaged in rendering professional services. If expert assistance is required, the services of a competent professional should be sought.

Copyright © 1997 by Matthew Bender & Company Incorporated.
All Rights Reserved. Published 1997. Printed in United States of America.
Permission to copy material exceeding fair use, 17 U.S.C. §107, may be licensed for a fee of $1 per page per copy from the Copyright Clearance Center, 222 Rosewood Drive, Danvers, MA 01923, telephone (508) 750-8400.

MATTHEW ◆ BENDER

MATTHEW BENDER & CO., INC.
Editorial Offices
2 Park Avenue, New York, NY 10016-5675 (212) 448-2000
201 Mission St., San Francisco, CA 94105-1831 (415) 908-3200

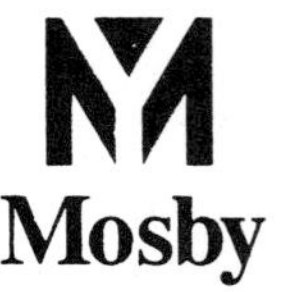

Mosby

MOSBY-YEAR BOOK, INC.
11830 Westline Industrial Drive
St. Louis, MO 63146
(800) 325-4177; (314) 872-8370

Table of Contents

A COMPLETE SYNOPSIS FOR EACH CHAPTER APPEARS
AT THE BEGINNING OF THE CHAPTER

Table of Contents

Table of Contents

Table of Contents

Table of Contents

Preface

Head injury is the fourth leading cause of death in the United States, with mortality rates approximately 22 per 100,000 and frequency averaging 130 per 100,000. Vascular injuries such as stroke and brain hemorrhage account for at least 152 deaths per 100,000 individuals. This "silent epidemic" is becoming less quiet as it changes the lives of increasing numbers of people.

Injuries and Disorders of the Head and Brain explains the most common and important neurologic occurrences. The informative chapters distill complex information into easy-to-understand facts, with every subject treated in sufficient depth for the book to serve as a reference text.

Common disorders such as headache, stroke, brain cancer and Parkinson's disease are covered in depth. So, too, are less common diseases of increasing importance, such as AIDS dementia. A review of diagnostic techniques and treatments in each chapter explains the continuing advance of medical technology, detailing improved imaging of the brain as well as accurate measurements of essential brain functions, such as electrical activity, intracranial pressure and cerebral blood flow.

The perspective and the straightforward explanation of the subject matter in this book will meet the needs of a variety of readers, including therapists, nurses and psychologists as well as other personnel involved in patient care and rehabilitation. The text provides a solid overview of the most important aspects of head and brain trauma and disease, using both the symptom and the disease approach and focusing on the clinical aspects of these disorders. A clear understanding can assist in providing the best possible care for the affected individual.

The 1990s were proclaimed the Decade of the Brain, with the formal goal of obtaining research funding for illnesses affecting the nervous system. In the first half of the decade, major advances were made in the recognition, genetics and treatment of a wide variety of neurologic and neurosurgical disorders, such as the etiology of certain inherited diseases, epilepsy drug treatment and surgery, tumor treatments and immunotherapies. In light of such important advances, it is appropriate and timely to issue *Injuries and Disorders of the Head and Brain.*

Lorne S. Label, M.D.

Publisher's Editorial Staff

Beverly R. Lieberman
Managing Editor

Rina Cascone
Project Editor

Victor Ortiz
Manager of Publishing Operations

About the Editor-In-Chief

LORNE S. LABEL, M.D.

A board-certified neurologist and diplomate of the American Board of Psychiatry and Neurology and the American Academy of Pain Management, Lorne S. Label, M.D., is Associate Clinical Professor of Neurology at UCLA School of Medicine. He is also currently in private practice with California Neurological Specialists as well as Director of the Attention Deficit Disorder Clinic of Southern California. In 1990, California Governor George Deukmejian appointed Dr. Label to the Medical Quality Review Committee of the Medical Board of that state; he is also a hospital survey member of the California Medical Association and the Joint Commission on Accreditation of Hospitals. Previously Dr. Label served as Director of the Traumatic Brain Service at Columbia Los Robles Medical Center and on the Board of Directors of the Ventura County Medical Society, as well as a variety of other hospital and community leadership positions. A Phi Beta Kappa graduate of the University of Texas at Austin, Dr. Label completed a clinical neuromuscular fellowship at the University of Southern California School of Medicine.

CHAPTER 1

Overview: Injuries and Disorders of the Head and Brain

SCOPE

Although the immediate effects of head trauma are the most life threatening, late-appearing disorders have the potential to severely disable the survivor. Mild head injuries can produce significant disability, but the potential for complications and delayed syndromes tends to correlate with the severity of the injury. Mild injury may produce persistent headache, dizziness and memory problems. Delayed complications of major injury include enlarging hematomas, hydrocephalus, loss of brain tissue and sensory deficits in organs supplied by the cranial nerves. Because the brain regulates all the body's organ systems, neurologic damage can affect functioning of organs outside the central nervous system, disrupt hormonal balance and severely compromise motor ability. Cognitive and emotional status are often adversely affected; pre-existing psychological disorders may be aggravated and further complicate rehabilitation. A variety of imaging techniques is available to facilitate diagnosis of existing lesions and secondary pathology that occurs as a result of those lesions. Treatment includes surgical intervention and physical and cognitive rehabilitation.

SYNOPSIS

1.00 INTRODUCTION

Head injury accounts for at least half of the trauma-related deaths in the United States (Goldstein, 1990; Kraus, 1993). About 70 percent of these deaths occur before admission to the hospital. The number of head-injury patients who survive to be evaluated in the emergency room exceeds 2 million annually, and about 25 percent of these patients are hospitalized (White and Likavec, 1992).

Most medical literature uses the terms head injury and brain injury interchangeably. Early, often immediate, effects of brain injury include loss of consciousness, impaired motor (movement) responsiveness and mental confusion in conscious persons. Other injuries may not be evident at the time of injury but may appear days or months later.

Disability from brain injury often is permanent. Of head trauma patients who survive, nearly 100,000 annually suffer lifelong loss of function. Recovery is not well defined, and improvements are generally so gradual that it is difficult to estimate the duration of effects of brain injury (Brown and Nell, 1992).[1]

1.01 Primary and Secondary Injuries of the Head and Brain

Brain injuries may be primary, that is, occurring at the time of impact, or secondary, developing after the initial injury (Gean, 1994). *Primary injuries* are a result of the immediate insult to the brain.

Secondary injury refers to injury arising from the trauma that becomes clinically evident some time after the initial event. The term encompasses both acute and chronic neurologic injury. Much secondary injury is probably due to complex physiologic and biochemical changes taking place in the tissue as part of the body's homeostatic (referring to maintenance of the internal environment) efforts.

1.02 Epidemiology of Head and Brain Injury

Traumatic head injury is most common in males in the 15-to-24 age group; the incidence is higher in lower socioeconomic groups and among single persons (Wrigley, 1994). More than 100,000 children are hospitalized annually for brain injury in the United States (Rivara, et al., 1992).

---

[1] *See* 1.90 *infra* for further discussion of the prognosis for recovery from brain injury.

Causes of head injury include motor vehicle accidents (accounting for nearly 50 percent, with a disproportionate number from motorcycle accidents), accidental falls (nearly 30 percent), gunshot wounds and blows to the head (Jennett and Frankowski, 1990).

Estimates of the incidence of disability from brain injury vary, but one set of figures (Kraus, 1993) estimated the occurrence of 500,000 new cases in 1990, of which 80 percent were mild, with 100 percent discharged alive; 10 percent were moderate, with 93 percent discharged alive; and 10 percent were severe, of which 42 percent were discharged alive. It is difficult to obtain good data because of differences in definition, disagreements about follow-up criteria and inconsistencies among reports from various sources.

1.10 ANATOMY OF HEAD AND BRAIN INJURY

The brain has the most complex anatomy of any organ. Although it is well protected within the skull, it is vulnerable in many respects. An injury to one region can rapidly affect other regions of the brain and lead to disorders elsewhere in the body.

1.11 Anatomy of the Head and Brain

The brain consists of that part of the central nervous system encased by the skull. (The spinal cord within the spinal column is the extension of the brain stem.) The skull, composed of a number of fused bones, provides a rigid protective container for the brain. It is unyielding, even when swelling of the brain takes place as a consequence of injury or disease (White and Likavec, 1992). When an external force causes brain movement, neural tissue may be bruised against its hard inner surface.

The base of the skull has ridges and depressions that can increase injury of brain tissue striking it. Brain areas likely to be affected in this way are the brain stem and the anterior (toward the front) temporal lobe.

Beneath the skull bones, the brain is surrounded by three connective tissue membranes called the meninges. The outermost meningeal covering, the dura mater, consists of two layers that are fused in most regions. Folds of the dura extending into the cranial cavity form barriers between the two cerebral hemispheres, and between these hemispheres and the posterior fossa (back compartment). The latter fold is the tentorium cerebelli, an important demarcation in descriptions of brain anatomy. The next layer, the arachnoid, is a delicate membrane lying loosely on the surface of the brain. The arachnoid has villi, or fine projections, that participate in the absorption of cerebrospinal fluid into the bloodstream. The innermost layer, the pia mater, adheres closely to the brain surface. (*See Figure 1-1.*)

The cerebrum, or cerebral cortex, is composed of two hemispheres, each divided into four lobes: frontal, parietal, occipital and temporal. The two hemispheres are connected by a thick bundle of myelinated axons (white matter) called the corpus callosum. The ventricles comprise a systems of canals within the brain for the synthesis and circulation of cerebrospinal fluid.

Near the center of the brain, beneath the cerebral cortex and above the brain stem, is a group of important regulatory structures. These include the thalamus, an important relay area; the basal ganglia, which are an important part of the motor system; the preoptic area and the hypothalamus, which maintain homeostasis (constancy of the internal environment); and the pituitary gland, or hypophysis, which is the source of many important hormones.

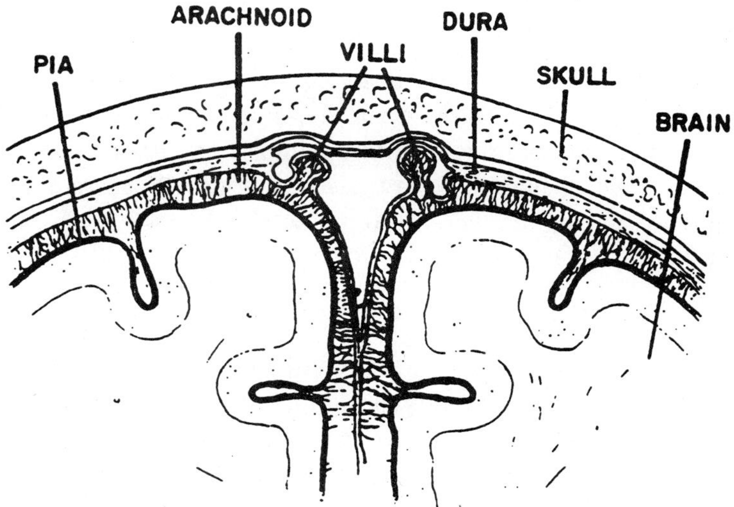

Fig. 1-1. Cross section of the skull and brain, showing the relationship of the meninges to underlying structures. The dura is the outermost meningeal layer; the arachnoid and its projecting villi form the middle layer; and the pia is the innermost layer.

The brain stem is composed of the medulla, pons and midbrain and is the source of cranial nerves III to XII, which control sensation and movement of the head. Cranial nerves I and II lie above the tentorium. All nerve tracts between the brain and the rest of the body pass within the brain stem. In addition, the brain stem contains the centers that control sleep and consciousness, and integrate complex motor activities. (*See Figure 1-2.*)

1.12   Extra-Axial Injuries

Primary brain injuries are classified as extra-axial (outside the brain proper and involving the meninges and meningeal spaces) or axial (comprising the areas of the brain itself). Extra-axial injuries are named by their relation to the dura. They usually are hemorrhagic (bleeding) in character.

Epidural (extradural) hemorrhage refers to rupture of a blood vessel, usually an artery, between the outer surface of the dura and the skull. Typically this results from a severe closed head injury (White and Likavec, 1992). In other cases, the cause is fracture of the temporal bone (located on the side of the head) of the skull. The underlying brain may be uninjured, but secondary brain injury occurs rapidly if the hematoma is not evacuated promptly.[2]

Subdural hemorrhage results from rupture of the blood vessels, usually venous, between the brain and the dura. Immediate mortality from these injuries is high, related to the underlying brain injury and to the mass effect of blood. However, a less extensive laceration can result in slow leakage of blood into the subdural space.[3]

1.13   Axial Injuries

Direct injury can occur within the brain matter itself. Intracerebral injuries include axonal shearing (tearing of nerve processes), hematomas (pooling of blood outside the vessels as a result of vessel leakage or rupture) and contusions (bruises). Injuries may occur at the point of impact (coup) or directly opposite that point (contrecoup).

---

[2] *See also* ch. 4 for further discussion of hemorrhage and hematoma within the brain.

[3] *See also* ch. 3 for further discussion of brain laceration and its consequences.

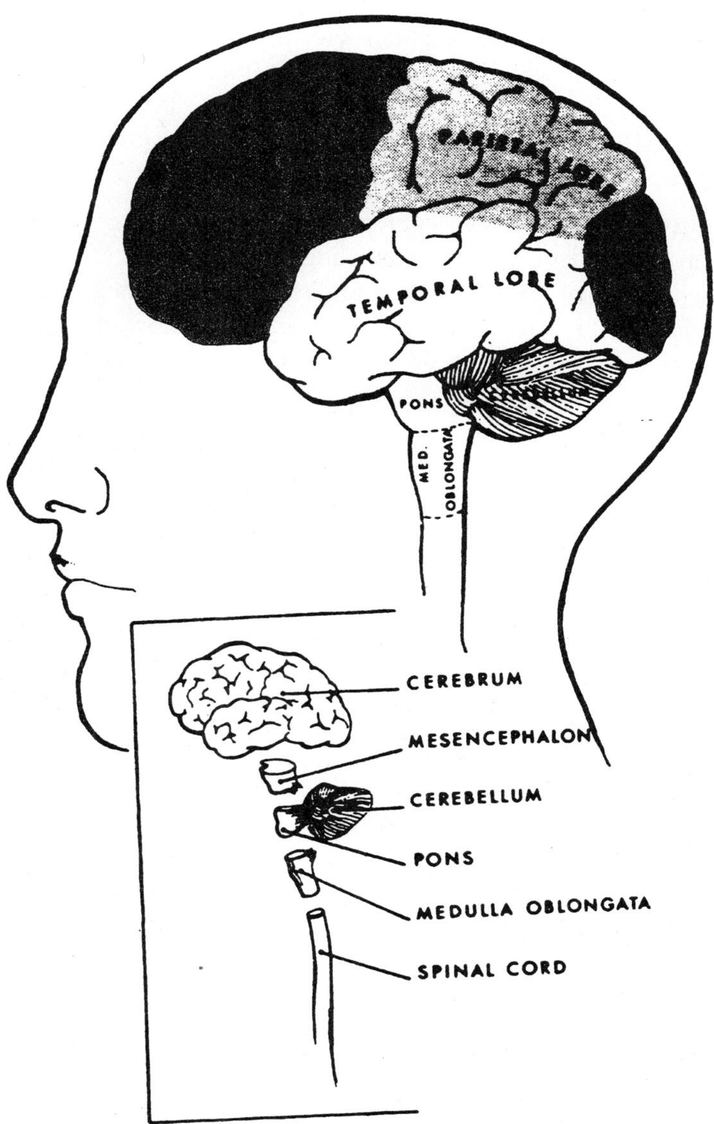

Fig. 1-2. Lateral view of the central nervous system. The brain is divided into two hemispheres, each of which is subdivided into four lobes: the frontal lobe (front shaded section), the temporal lobe, the parietal lobe and the occipital lobe (rear shaded portion). The pons, cerebellum and medulla oblongata are parts of the brain stem, which connects the brain to the spinal cord.

1.20   MECHANISMS AND TYPES OF INJURIES

Head injuries are classified in a variety of ways. They may be closed, with the skull intact, or open, with the skull fractured. They may be mild or severe. Statistics indicate that injury is mild in 80 to 90 percent of persons with brain trauma (Kraus, 1993). Another method of classification separates brain injuries into categories of focal (localized) or diffuse.

Most closed head injuries occur as a result of an acceleration-deceleration mechanism, typically resulting from a blow to the head. They may consist of focal damage at the site of impact, usually hematoma formation; diffuse axonal injury, in which flow of material and impulses within the nerve process is interrupted; hypoxia (lack of oxygen supply); and microvascular (small blood vessel) injury (Salazar, 1989).

Open head injuries may be due to compound skull fracture, possibly with a fragment impinging on or driven into the brain (depressed fracture), or to missile penetration. A bullet crushes tissue along its path; in addition, it creates high pressures at right angles to its path and causes a spherical, outward-moving shock wave. The subsequent inward displacement of tissue into the missile tract creates further damage (Carey, 1989). The resulting wounds usually are fatal. Wounds that are tangential rather than straight through the brain, or that are made by low-velocity bullets, may be survivable.

1.30   DIAGNOSIS OF NEUROLOGIC DISORDERS—
IMMEDIATE AND DELAYED

The analysis of head injuries is a complex process involving clinical assessment and laboratory investigations as well as the use of high-technology tools. The interpretation of symptoms that develop both immediately following and some time after a head injury can be difficult. The patient may be comatose or otherwise incapacitated and unable to give an adequate account of the occurrence, and witnesses may not be available; the patient may have other injuries besides the head trauma, making it difficult to distinguish cause and effect. The situation can be especially complicated if symptoms develop at a time beyond the acute phase, particularly if the patient did not seek medical care for the original injury. If, as frequently happens, there is a lapse between apparent recovery from a head injury and a delayed problem, the patient may not connect the injury to the current symptoms. Diagnosis of new neurologic symptoms in the acute care setting is often complicated by a multiplicity of injuries.

1.31 Clinical History

The patient history can be vital for evaluating delayed complications of head trauma. It is important to ascertain the circumstances, extent and treatment of the original injury. The possibility of more than one previous head injury must also be considered.

1.32 Clinical Signs and Symptoms

The clinical examination includes assessment of reflexes, motor activity, eye movements, auditory status, balance and other aspects of neurologic function. The Glasgow Coma Scale, used in the initial assessment of head trauma, is also helpful in evaluating delayed symptoms. This assigns a score of 3 to 15, based on a combination of eye opening, motor movement and verbal performance: 3 means no response, and 15 signifies no abnormality. A score of less than 8 is predictive of a poor outcome (Kraus, 1989).

Laboratory studies should include tests of renal function, coagulation studies and glucose measurements, in addition to the usual blood tests.

1.33 Mental Status Evaluation

Evaluation of mental status is an important part of the examination when symptoms suggest brain damage. Often it is the awareness of cognitive or emotional changes that prompts the patient to seek medical advice. Testing of mental status can range from simple questions to determine time and place orientation, to complex specialized neuropsychological tests to determine numerical memory, language skills, two- and three-dimensional perception and integration, manual dexterity, attention and concentration, judgment and problem-solving ability (Capruso and Levin, 1992; Dacey, et al., 1993).

Neurobehavioral impairment is also assessed, often using the Rancho Los Amigos Levels of Cognitive Function behavioral scale (Gill-Body and Giorgetti, 1995; Sullivan, 1995). This aids in evaluating the appropriateness of the patient's responses to a variety of stimuli.

1.34 Imaging Studies

Sophisticated imaging techniques are available for the precise localization of most gross brain injuries (Gean, 1994). These include computed tomography (CT), magnetic resonance imaging (MRI), angiography and skull radiographs (x-rays). The newest techniques—positron emission tomography (PET) and single photon emission computed tomography (SPECT)—are used less frequently, because of their expense and limited availability. Although CT scanning is the preferred method for assessing acute head injuries, due to its reliability and ease of use (Hughes and Cohen, 1993; White and Likavec, 1992), delayed syndromes are often best diagnosed by MRI or PET scans (Evans, 1992; McIntosh and Morgan, 1992).

[1]   Computed Tomography (CT)

Computed tomography (CT), which uses a computer to integrate multiple x-ray views and produce a cross-sectional "slice" of the body, is the primary imaging technique for brain injuries. It is particularly effective in detecting the presence of hemorrhage and can distinguish between fresh blood and chronic hematoma (Hughes and Cohen, 1993).

[2]   Magnetic Resonance Imaging (MRI)

Magnetic resonance imaging (MRI) uses strong magnets and radio waves to generate images based on the hydrogen (proton) or carbon content of the tissues. It is particularly useful for imaging extra-axial hematomas and nonhemorrhagic areas of injury (Hughes and Cohen, 1993). MRI is superior to CT for visualizing changes in hydrocephalus[4] and for finding obstructing lesions (Gean, 1994). The severity of shear injuries, arising from tearing of axons and/or small blood vessels, often can be evaluated using MRI. In cases of mild head injury, MRI seems to have some utility for showing lesions that correlate with later impairment in cognition (Evans, 1992). It is used as a complement to CT.

---

[4] *See* 1.52 *infra* for further discussion of hydrocephalus.

[3] Positron Emission Tomography (PET) and Single Photon Emission Computed Tomography (SPECT)

Positron emission tomography (PET) registers the decay of injected radioactive drugs that have excess positive charge (they decay by positron emission). Because the positrons travel only a few millimeters before combining with electrons to produce gamma rays, precise localization is possible. The technique is valuable for examining brain glucose metabolism, receptor distribution and cerebral blood flow. Its use is limited by its high cost, however.

Single photon emission computed tomography (SPECT), a modification of PET scanning, is a relatively new technique, and data about its usefulness in head trauma is sparse. Early reports indicate that SPECT promises to be a sensitive method for evaluating patients with mild to moderate head injury. It can be performed with conventional nuclear medicine cameras and seems to be reliable in helping to make a prognosis for stroke victims. Thus, its use may expand (McIntosh and Morgan, 1992).

[4] Angiography

Angiography—the outlining of blood vessels on radiographic film by injection of a contrast medium—is used mainly for evaluating vascular injuries. It can show some vascular abnormalities with finer detail than CT (Hughes and Cohen, 1993).

[5] Skull Radiographs (X-rays)

The use of skull radiographs is declining as newer methods become available. CT scans generally show more detail and are preferred when possible. Skull images may, however, be beneficial for detecting old injuries in instances of suspected child abuse.

1.35 Neurophysiologic Studies

The use of electroencephalography (EEG) and brain stem auditory evoked responses (BAER) may be helpful in evaluating post-traumatic neurologic symptoms. In addition, appropriate specialized testing may be appropriate for auditory, visual and balance problems. EEG studies have low specificity in cases of mild head injury (Evans, 1992) and thus are limited in usefulness except for seizure disorders.

Intracranial (within the skull) pressure is measured when symptoms suggest elevated pressure or inadequate cerebral perfusion. This is done by a catheter that is screwed into the subdural space. It is useful for monitoring trends in intracranial pressure in the first days after injury, to detect the beginnings of edema (swelling due to accumulation of fluid) (Miller, 1993).

1.40 COMPLICATIONS OF MILD INJURIES

Approximately 75 to 80 percent of all brain injuries are classified as mild (Kraus and Nourjah, 1988). Definitions of mild head injury vary, but suggested criteria include being dazed without losing consciousness or losing consciousness for 5 minutes or less, a Glasgow Coma Scale score of 13 to 15 (a score lower than 8 indicates coma) and absence of localized neurologic pathology (such as intracranial hematomas) (Dacey, et al., 1993; Evans, 1992). (Other criteria use 15 or 30 minutes as the maximum time for loss of consciousness.)

Even minor injuries can lead to problems with balance or memory. Disability can stem from psychological as well as physical complications. The most common complication of mild head injury is post-concussion syndrome (also called post-traumatic syndrome), which occurs in about 50 percent of patients (Mandel, 1989). Symptoms include headaches, dizziness, sensory (vision, hearing, taste, smell) problems, cognitive impairment and psychological changes. The time from injury to symptom appearance can vary from a few hours to several weeks (Evans, 1992). The probability of postconcussion syndrome occurring does not seem affected by whether the patient experiences brief (one hour or less) loss of consciousness or amnesia.[5]

Symptoms may persist for a few months or several years. In general, patients with mild head trauma improve gradually over several months or years (Brown and Nell, 1992). However, problems persist for many years in a significant percentage of patients. The reported incidence of various symptoms include headaches persisting after four years (24 percent), dizziness after two years (18 percent) and psychological complaints after three years (15 percent).

Less common aftereffects of mild head injury include delayed intracranial hematoma,[6] tremor and retrograde amnesia (forgetfulness for events immediately before and including the trauma).

---

[5] *See also* ch. 2 for further discussion of postconcussion syndrome.

[6] *See* 1.51[3] *infra* for further discussion of intracranial hematoma.

Treatment for the sequelae of mild head injury is usually symptomatic and includes analgesics, muscle relaxants, antidepressants, psychological support, physical therapy and education of both patient and family. Any worsening of symptoms mandates use of CT or MRI to determine whether an enlarging chronic hematoma or intracerebral hemorrhage might be present (Andrews and Pitts, 1991).

Repetitive head injuries, even though they may be mild, seem to have a cumulative effect. This is most commonly seen in the syndrome known as dementia pugilistica in boxers (Gean, 1994; Jordan, 1993).

1.50   COMPLICATIONS OF MAJOR INJURIES

The long-term and delayed effects of traumatic brain injury are varied and may include physical, cognitive and psychosocial deficits (Brown and Nell, 1992). Physical symptoms that may persist for years after injury include headaches, dizziness, visual problems, dysarthria (sensory-motor speech difficulty), hyperacusis (abnormal hearing acuteness due to irritability of sensory-neural input) and difficulties in limb use (Evans, 1992). Cognitive problems include memory deficits in at least 50 percent of cases. Moodiness and emotional lability (changeability) contribute to both patient unhappiness and family problems.

Major brain damage is often prompt and instantaneous. A patient who emerges from coma after hemorrhage and/or diffuse axonal injury is likely to suffer long-term, if not permanent, disability.

Complications from head trauma include vascular complications, hydrocephalus, cerebral swelling, epilepsy, tissue loss and herniation (protrusion of part of an organ through an opening in the tissue that contains it). Any injury that breaks the integrity of the dura risks infection, which can lead to additional neurologic damage or death. Increasing amounts of evidence indicate that head trauma may predispose a person to a degenerative neurologic disease, such as Alz–heimer's disease and Parkinson's disease.[7]

1.51   Vascular Complications

Vascular complications typically arise from an undetected bleeding site. A slowly enlarging pool of blood may collect and clot, causing

---

[7] *See also* ch. 12.

it to exert increasing pressure on the brain. Neurologic symptoms typically result from this pressure. Such hematomas (space-occupying collections of blood) include extradural hematoma, subdural hematoma and intracerebral hematoma. Other vascular lesions include thrombosis (clotting within a vessel), aneurysm (dilation or bulging of vessel wall), arteriovenous fistula (abnormal communication between artery and vein) and vasospasm (abnormal contraction of vessel wall).

[1]   Extradural Hematoma

Extradural hematomas, which occur between the skull and the dura, have a relatively low incidence in general but are more common in patients with severe head injuries (Cooper, 1993). They result not from brain injury but from damage to the meningeal vessels and the skull. Normally this type of bleeding is evident within six hours of injury, but it may have a delayed course of several days due to slow bleeding. In the latter case, often the only symptoms are nausea and/or vomiting, but dilation of the pupils and hemiparesis (slight paralysis on one side) may also be present. Prompt diagnosis and evacuation of slowly expanding hematomas generally result in good recovery. (*See Figure 1-3.*)

[2]   Subdural Hematoma

A subdural hematoma, in which blood collects between the dura and the underlying arachnoid membrane, may occur after mild as well as severe injury (Cooper, 1993). This characteristic, coupled with a wide range of symptoms, often leads to misdiagnosis. Recurrent capillary hemorrhage into the hematoma results in increasing pressure on the brain, so that symptoms are delayed or chronic (Graham, et al., 1993).

Symptoms include headache, confusion, paralysis and loss of consciousness. As with all late appearing hematomas, CT scanning will confirm its presence; sometimes MRI is needed to differentiate a chronic hematoma from other lesions (Mendelow, 1993). An expanding subdural hematoma requires prompt attention. It is sometimes treated nonsurgically by control of brain edema with corticosteroids and diuretics, but surgical evacuation is usually preferred. Outcome depends on the patient's neurologic state at the time of treatment. Possible residual effects and complications include seizures, amnesia, attention difficulties, anxiety and headache. (*See Figure 1-4.*)

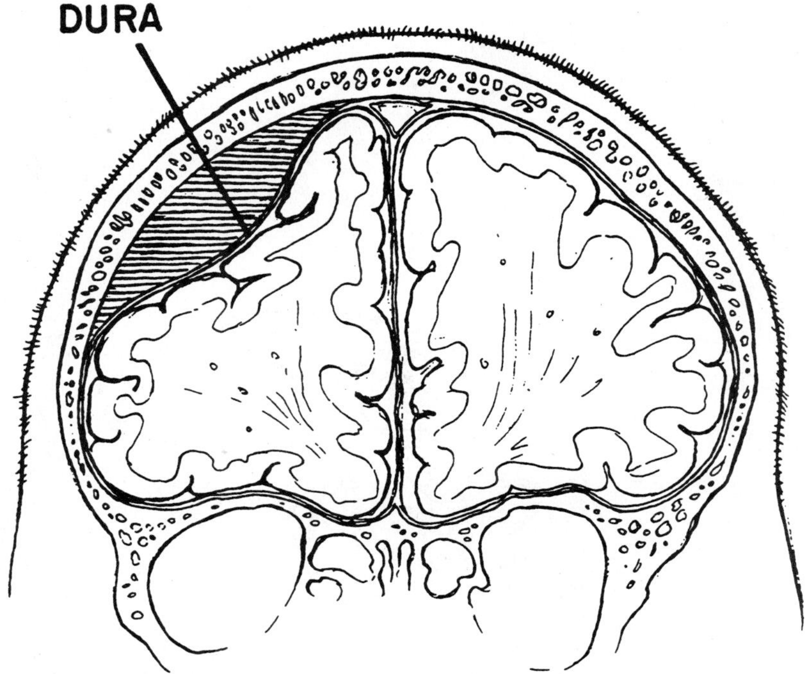

Fig. 1-3. Classic presentation of an epidural (extradural) hematoma, which occurs between the skull and the dura mater.

[3] Intracerebral Hematoma

Although hemorrhage within the tissue of the brain usually produces symptoms in a period as short as minutes or hours after head trauma, in some cases, neurologic deterioration does not occur for several days (Cooper, 1993). Reduction of blood flow (ischemia) occurs around the hemorrhage, extending the damage zone (Mendelow, 1993).

Delayed traumatic intracerebral hemorrhages may develop within a few hours of injury or many days (or even weeks) later (Andrews and Pitts, 1991; Cooper, 1993). The late beginning of such hemorrhages has been confirmed by CT scans. They result in focal (localized) deficits and sometimes in depression of consciousness. Because of this possibility, a patient who fails to improve (or deteriorates) despite a normal scan on admission should have a repeat CT scan.

1.52 Post-traumatic Hydrocephalus

Post-traumatic hydrocephalus has been reported to occur in a significant proportion (estimates range up to 44 percent) of patients

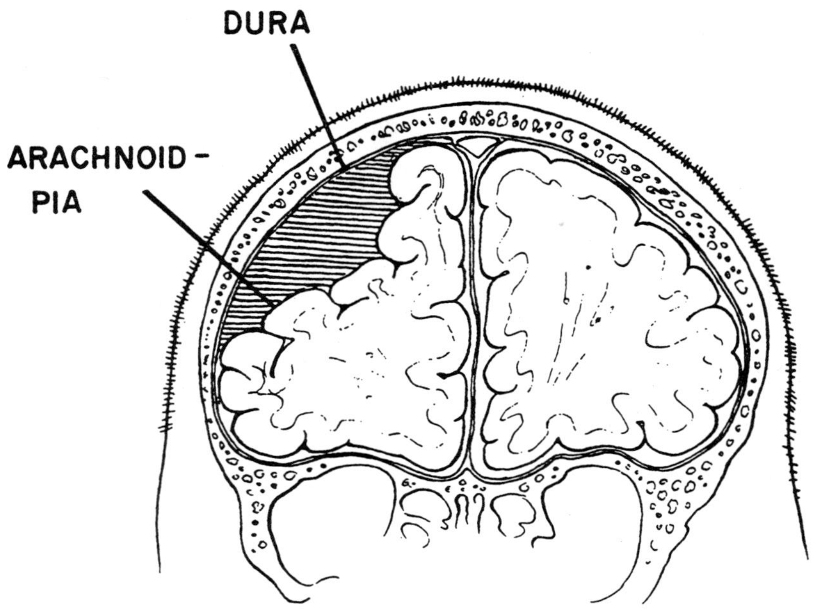

Fig. 1-4. Classic presentation of a subdural hematoma, which occurs between the dura mater and arachnoid.

with brain injury (Sheffler, et al., 1994). Blood breakdown products may interrupt the normal resorption (absorption by the body) of cerebrospinal fluid. Abnormal accumulation of the fluid leads to enlargement of the ventricles of the brain and an increase in intracerebral pressure. This compromises perfusion of the brain and leads to a gradual and often subtle decline in cognitive and motor functioning, frequently accompanied by headache and vomiting. The condition normally occurs within three months after injury.

A very late appearing hydrocephalus, known as normal-pressure hydrocephalus, may become symptomatic several years after the initial trauma (Gean, 1994). In this condition, connective tissue proliferation blocks the arachnoid villi, so that cerebrospinal fluid accumulates. Symptoms include progressive dementia, gait disturbance and urinary incontinence.

If this condition is detected in time, by correlating symptoms with MRI scan results, further deterioration can be averted. Ventriculoperitoneal shunting (placement of a tube from the brain ventricle to the abdominal cavity, in order to drain excess spinal fluid from the brain) can lead to functional gains, particularly if the procedure is performed within six months (Sheffler, et al., 1994). If it remains uncorrected, hydrocephalus leads to irreparable damage, including visual and cognitive deficits. The possibility for correction of functional deficits decreases with time. However, a greater time lapse before shunting does not preclude partial recovery.[8]

1.53 Delayed Effects of Contusions

A contusion is a bruise that, unlike a hematoma (a homogeneous pool of blood), is a mixture of blood and swollen brain tissue. The damage from a contusion (bruise) is focal (Graham, et al., 1993). Contusions are classified by depth (surface versus gliding), lobe and relation to site of impact (*coup,* at the impact site, versus *contrecoup,* on the opposite side). Symptoms depend on contusion location and severity, and on the character of other lesions.

Small contusions usually resolve without treatment, although they may leave a deficit. Larger contusions may increase in size by hemorrhaging, and dying tissue within the contusion may lead to edema (swelling). The patient can deteriorate quickly as a result of increased pressure or mass effect from the edema (Cooper, 1993).

Contusions may also become necrotic (pertaining to death of tissue), followed by development of a cyst (an encapsulated, fluid-filled cavity). These cysts may enlarge by osmotic (involving passage of fluid from a less concentrated to a more concentrated solution) engorgement with fluid.

Cerebral contusions have a high mortality. Some surgeons remove large contusions during treatment for the acute injury.[9]

---

[8] *See also* ch. 5 and ch. 8 for further discussion of hydrocephalus.

[9] *See also* ch. 3 for further discussion of cerebral contusion.

1.54　Post-traumatic Tissue Loss: Cerebral Atrophy and Encephalomalacia

As the brain heals after trauma, it attempts to shed necrotic tissue and isolate the injured from the intact tissue (Gean, 1994). The loss of tissue from the affected areas is referred to as hydrocephalus ex vacuo. When the loss is diffuse, the result is cerebral atrophy (wasting). When the loss is focal, it is termed post-traumatic encephalomalacia.

Cerebral atrophy (shrinking of the brain tissue) has been reported in up to 86 percent of patients who were comatose for at least six hours after injury. This can result from diffuse axonal tearing, ischemia (decreased blood flow) or prolonged cerebral swelling (Gean, 1994). The diffuse loss of cerebral tissue may or may not be accompanied by a reduction in intellectual function.

Encephalomalacia usually follows resorption of a cerebral hematoma that resulted from either closed or penetrating trauma. One or more cystlike cavities result, sometimes with only small bridges of tissue between them.

1.55　Cranial Nerve Injuries

Injury to the nerves supplying the head can result from trauma-induced compression, stretching or transection (being cut through). Generally this occurs at or shortly after the initial trauma, but subsequent brain swelling can result in later damage. The most frequently injured cranial nerves are the olfactory (I), facial (VII) and audiovestibular (VIII) (Keane and Baloh, 1992).

Damage to the olfactory nerve can result from trauma to any part of the head and leads to loss of the sense of smell. The deficit reverses spontaneously in about half the cases (Gean, 1994).

Injury to the facial nerve, resulting in facial paralysis, usually occurs at the time of trauma. However, a delayed nerve trauma may occur as late as two weeks after the original accident; this is probably due to nerve swelling, vascular damage or external compression from an expanding hematoma (Rovit and Murali, 1993).

Results of injury to the audiovestibular nerve, which can occur with temporal bone fracture, include deafness and vertigo (feeling of whirling in space). However, the attacks of vertigo that are common after head injury are frequently due to dislodging of crystals in the inner ear.

Damage to the optic nerve generally results in immediate loss of vision. In a few cases, progressive edema, hematoma formation or enlargement of a post-traumatic aneurysm can lead to delayed visual compromise. Such loss may be reversible, but more commonly, the loss of vision is permanent.

Damage to cranial nerves can result in speech difficulties. Other communication difficulties may stem from cognitive impairment.

1.56　Motor Impairments

Traumatic brain injury can injure any of several motor areas of the brain, leading to hypertonia (extreme muscle tension), rigidity and spasticity (velocity-dependent increase in muscle resistance to passive stretch). Associated motor deficits can include weakness, loss of dexterity and impaired timing of muscle recruitment (Whyte, et al., 1989). Other possible physical impairments include tremor, flaccid (without tone) paralysis and contractures (permanent muscle contractions due to spasms).

Movement disorders, of which there are several types, can develop months or years after trauma. The time span can make it difficult to determine whether the disorder is in fact due to the head injury. Motor dysfunctions include parkinsonism (characterized by muscle tremor and palsy), tremor, dystonia (abnormal muscle tone), chorea (rapid, unpredictable body movement spreading from one muscle group to another) and myoclonus (twitching of muscle).

Tremors (rhythmic to-and-fro oscillations of a part of the body) have been reported after brain stem or cerebellar injury (Goetz and Pappert, 1992). They may be postural (developing when the patient maintains a particular posture) or kinetic (developing when the patient carries out an action).

Dystonias (slow, twisting muscle contortions), often accompanied by pain, can occur after severe trauma. The areas of the brain showing involvement on CT scan are usually the subcortical gray matter structures known collectively as the basal ganglia, typically on the side opposite the affected side.

Chorea may develop days to months after blunt head trauma (Goetz and Pappert, 1992). Frequently a CT scan shows lesions on the basal ganglia.

Myoclonus consists of brief, swift, involuntary jerks that are sufficiently large to move the limbs. Several cases have been attributed to injury to the cortex or brain stem (Goetz and Pappert, 1992).

Possible therapies for such deficits include physical therapy, medication and nerve block.

In addition to motor impairment stemming from a neurologic or neuromuscular (referring to nerve activation of muscle) deficit, movement difficulties can arise from changes in the muscles. For example, immobility after head injury leads to muscle atrophy (wasting) and proliferation of surrounding connective tissue (Anderson, 1995).

1.60 HYPOTHALAMIC-PITUITARY DYSFUNCTIONS

The hypothalamic-pituitary system is responsible for the control and integration of many endocrine, metabolic and neural responses of the body. Dysfunction of this system can begin within the first hours after trauma and complicate the management of the patient, particularly with regard to water and electrolyte balance (Cooper, 1993; Gean, 1994).

Blunt trauma to the head may result in delayed hypothalamic dysfunction. Frequently this is due to compression from cerebral edema, but it can also arise from laceration that leads to hemorrhage or infarction (Gean, 1994). Damage to the hypothalamus can lead to dysfunction of factors that control circadian (day-night) rhythms, temperature regulation, food intake and metabolism, water balance and release of pituitary hormones (Whyte, et al., 1989).

Hormones secreted by the pituitary gland include growth hormone, prolactin (responsible for breast development and milk secretion), gonadotropin-releasing hormone (important in sexual maturation and sex steroid production, and other reproductive functions), thyrotropin-releasing hormone (responsible for thyroid gland function) and corticotropin-releasing hormone (which controls adrenal cortex function). Late-appearing symptoms thus can include alterations in appetite and metabolism, temperature control, sexual interest or behavior, water balance or emotional status. One of the most common of these effects is post-traumatic diabetes insipidus, in which insufficient secretion of antidiuretic hormone leads to excessive excretion of dilute urine (Gean, 1994).

1.70 EXTRACRANIAL COMPLICATIONS OF HEAD INJURY

Because the brain plays a role in the control of all body functions, neurologic damage can adversely affect other systems. Many of these effects take place within the first few minutes or hours of trauma. Other effects are delayed or result from the initial effects. Head injury can interrupt the neural pathways by which the brain monitors and responds to changes in the body. It can also result in an increase or a decrease in the hormones and neurotransmitters that regulate all other body functions. One effect is called a catecholamine storm, which is an outpouring of the neurotransmitters epinephrine and norepineph-rine. Among many other effects, norepinephrine acts to increase heart rate and constrict blood vessels.

1.71 Respiratory Complications

Most respiratory complications of head injury occur early. In particular, brain stem injury can result in fatal derangement of the centers that control vital functions. However, some serious complica-tions can be delayed.

Hypoxia (inadequate oxygenation of body tissues) is a common occurrence in the early period after head injury but symtptoms can develop up to two weeks after trauma (Frost, 1989). Most frequently this condition requires prompt intervention in an acute care setting. Impaired control over breathing can lead to hypoventilation (reduced breathing) or hyperventilation (rapid, shallow breathing). Such events require assisted ventilation. Injury-caused suppression of the cough reflex requires suctioning of bronchial secretions. Early intubation to support ventilation can prevent many problems but must be done carefully to avoid increasing the intracerebral pressure in a semicon-scious person who may struggle against it.

Brain stem injury can result in loss of the protective reflexes that prevent aspiration of mouth or stomach contents. This can lead to development of aspiration pneumonia. In addition, such therapeutic measures as intubation, head elevation and administration of drugs to protect against gastrointestinal bleeding can increase the risk of the patient acquiring pneumonia in the hospital (Chesnut, 1993).

Delayed neurogenic pulmonary edema is an accumulation of water in the lungs that may occur from 12 hours to several days after injury. The mechanism is not understood, but it is thought that the massive release of catecholamines (compounds whose action mimics that of the sympathetic nervous system, e.g., epinephrine) after head injury plays a role (Chesnut, 1993).

Pulmonary embolism, in which a clot causes obstruction of the pulmonary arteries and can lead to pulmonary or cardiac failure, is a risk in any prolonged surgical procedure (Chesnut, 1993). The risk is increased in patients with head injury for several reasons, including release of the clotting factor thromboplastin from the brain. This can lead to intravascular coagulation. Clots may travel to the lungs, resulting in pulmonary distress. The drugs that are frequently given to prevent clots in other circumstances cannot be administered to most patients with head injury because of their increased risk of hemorrhage.

1.72   Cardiac Complications

Severe head injury can result in impairment of cardiac regulation. Arrhythmias (abnormal beating rhythms), tachycardia (rapid heartbeat) and hypertension (elevated blood pressure) may follow (Chesnut, 1993; Frost, 1989). These usually occur in the period immediately after the injury. Because nearly every aspect of major trauma will tend to produce cardiac abnormalities, it is difficult to distinguish which are caused by the neurologic injuries. Many effects of brain injury, such as elevated intracranial pressure, indirectly increase the workload of the heart.

1.73   Disseminated Intravascular Coagulation (DIC)

Disseminated intravascular coagulation (clotting) results from activation of the blood coagulation system. The injured brain's release of large amounts of thromboplastin (a clotting agent) into the circulation leads to widespread clotting of blood in small vessels throughout the body (Chesnut, 1993). Affected organs may become ischemic (lacking blood). The process can affect the brain, resulting in further damage; this is one of the causes of delayed and recurrent hematomas resulting from head injury. The incidence of DIC is unknown, due in part to the usual presence of other trauma induced coagulation disorders.

1.74 Renal (Kidney) Complications

Renal system ischemia (inadequate blood flow) due to disseminated intravascular coagulation can lead to renal failure. In addition, massive disturbances in electrolyte balance occur, due in part to inappropriate secretion of antidiuretic hormone (Chesnut, 1993). There is also an increased breakdown of body protein after any trauma, so that the kidneys have an extra load of nitrogen excretion.

1.80 COGNITIVE AND PSYCHOSOCIAL IMPAIRMENTS

Severe brain injury leads to cognitive impairment in as many as two thirds of patients (Kaplan and Corrigan, 1994). Deficits include reduced attention span and impaired ability to concentrate, slowed reaction time, fatigability and memory disturbances (Jane, 1989). Both retrograde (pertaining to events before the injury) and post-traumatic amnesia may occur. Aspects of mental function such as goal setting and problem solving are often impaired. Orientation to time is recovered later than that to person or place and is an indicator of progress (Kaplan and Corrigan, 1994).

Numerous studies have attempted to correlate injury site with type of personality or cognitive alteration. There is a significant correlation between cognitive deficit and inability to resume self-care activities and motor functioning. Thus cognitive and behavioral impairment following brain injury can impede efforts at rehabilitation.

It is thought that many of the personality changes and motivational defects in a person with brain injury are due not to any psychiatric disturbance but to injury-related deficits in perception and self-awareness (Whyte, et al., 1989). Even mild closed head injury can lead to persistent mood changes in a significant proportion of patients (Grafman, 1989).

Among common behavioral consequences of cerebral damage are emotional instability, depression or euphoria, agitation and aggressive behavior (Galski, et al., 1994). Aggression seems to be correlated with disorientation and with use of anticonvulsant medication. Social inhibitions may be decreased or absent in some patients, while others may suffer from depression and lack of initiative. The emotional effects depend on the location and severity of the injury and on the stage of recovery (Macartney-Filgate, 1990).

In the years following traumatic brain injury, individuals tend to experience difficulty maintaining employment and to need greater social support than they did previously (Kwasnica and Heinemann, 1994). Pretraumatic neurotic tendencies may be exaggerated. In general, psychological problems from major trauma tend to worsen over time.

1.90   RECOVERY FROM BRAIN INJURY

Recovery after head injury varies greatly, even among patients with an apparently similar degree of initial damage. The brain suffers injury in a continuum, and a blow to the head may just miss a vital area for memory—or severely harm it. The brain's plasticity (ability to change in response to environmental circumstances) varies with the individual's age, history and biochemistry. The brain is the body's most individualized organ, and psychosocial factors play more of a role in its healing than they do in other types of injuries (Jane, 1989).

1.91   Importance of Initial Management of Injury

Prompt diagnosis and aggressive treatment of traumatic brain injury are key factors in optimizing the patient's recovery (White and Likavec, 1992). Surgical intervention is frequently needed to relieve brain compression, whether from swelling or from structure displacement, or to stop intracranial bleeding. When needed, the sooner surgery is performed, the better the patient's prognosis (Escobedo, 1989).

When injury is severe, effects such as loss of consciousness, confusion, dizziness and motor impairment are usually obvious immediately or within hours after injury. More subtle injuries may be overlooked, particularly if there is massive trauma to other body systems. Observation of the progression of neurologic symptoms is extremely important.

1.92   Uncomplicated Recovery

Recovery may take place over days or months, until a plateau is reached. The degree of recovery depends on the type, location and extent of injury, the immediacy of treatment and the type and intensity of rehabilitative therapy. Any residual impairment at plateau is considered to be due to the original injury. In uncomplicated recovery, a stable level of functioning is reached some time after the injury and persists.

However, brain injury can lead to delayed consequences that may appear weeks or even years after the initial trauma. Such complications can cause physical, emotional or cognitive (thinking) disability.

1.93 Prognosis in Head and Brain Trauma

Predicting the long-term outcome of traumatic brain injury is important for rehabilitation and discharge planning. Many prognostic studies have attempted to evaluate the likelihood of delayed or chronic effects of various types of head trauma (Evans, 1992; Vollmer, 1993). The prognosis becomes more specific as the patient recovers, with prediction being least specific and accurate in the emergency room and most accurate at discharge from a rehabilitation unit. Factors influencing outcome include initial Glasgow Coma Score,[10] duration of coma and post-traumatic amnesia, age, education, employment and presence of other physical or psychological deficits (Fleming and Maas, 1994). The patient's preinjury personality and alcohol use are significant predictors of the extent of recovery (Evans, 1992). Prior head injury is a risk factor.

Prolonged post-traumatic amnesia is an unfavorable sign, as is the presence of cognitive impairment on discharge from acute care (Fleming and Maas, 1994). An instrument called the Disability Rating Scale (DRS) has been proposed to monitor recovery of physical, cognitive and psychosocial function on a continuum comprising 30 points.

However, the complexity of the nervous system and the degree to which it controls every aspect of human function make accurate prediction difficult. A patient may appear to have made a good recovery, only to develop epilepsy more than a year later (Willmore, 1992). Another patient may slowly regain much more ability than was originally predicted.

---

[10] *See also* 1.32 *supra.*

1.94 Rehabilitation

It is estimated that only about 1 in 20 patients with a brain injury receives formal rehabilitation after release from acute care (Wrigley, et al., 1994). Factors influencing referral to a rehabilitation unit include the severity and characteristics of the injury, the managing physician's specialty (physiatrists are more likely to make such referrals) and affiliation of a rehabilitation unit with the acute care hospital. Older, unmarried patients are more likely to be referred for rehabilitation. Younger patients, however, are likely to derive the most benefit. The shorter the length of time between injury and admission to a rehabilitation unit, the more complete and quick the recovery (Mackay, et al., 1992).

In fact, when trauma rehabilitation is initiated in the acute care hospital, the lengths of coma and of rehabilitation are shorter than when patients do not receive such structured therapy until after release (Mackay, et al., 1992). Such therapy begins while the patient is in a coma and includes multisensory stimulation, positioning, exercise and orientation; the several disciplines involved are physiatry and physical, occupational and speech therapy. This approach has been shown to improve both physical and cognitive skills.

1.100 BIBLIOGRAPHY

Text References

Anderson, D.: Management of Decreased ROM from Overactive Musculature or Heterotopic Ossification. Clin. Phys. Ther. 33:79–97, 1995.

Andrews, B. T. and Pitts, L. H.: Traumatic Transtentorial Herniation and Its Management. Mt. Kisco, N.Y.: Futura Publishing, 1991.

Brown, D. S. O. and Nell, V.: Recovery from Diffuse Traumatic Brain Injury in Johannesburg: A Concurrent Prospective Study. Arch. Phys. Med. Rehab. 73:758–770, 1992.

Capruso, D. X. and Levin, H. S.: Cognitive Impairment Following Closed Head Injury. Neurol. Clin. North Am. 10:879–893, 1992.

Carey, M.: Therapeutic Management. In: Frost, E. (Ed.): Head Injury: Clinical Management and Research. New Issues in Neurosciences, Vol. II, No. 2, 1990.

Chesnut, R. M.: Medical Complications of the Head-Injured Patient. In: Cooper, P.R. (Ed.): Head Injury, 3rd ed. Baltimore: Williams & Wilkins, 1993.

Cooper, P. R.: Post-Traumatic Intracranial Mass Lesions. In: Cooper, P. R. (Ed.): Head Injury, 3d ed. Baltimore: Williams & Wilkins, 1993.

Dacey, R. G., Jr., et al.: Mild Head Injury. In: Cooper, P. R. (Ed.): Head Injury, 3d ed. Baltimore: Williams & Wilkins, 1993.

Escobedo, F.: Severe Closed Head Injuries. In: Frost, E. (Ed.): Head Injury: Clinical Management and Research. New Issues in Neurosciences, Vol. II, No. 2, 1990.

Evans, R. W.: The Postconcussion Syndrome and the Sequelae of Mild Head Injury. Neurol. Clin. North Am. 10:815–847, 1992.

Fleming, J. M. and Maas, F.: Prognosis of Rehabilitation Outcome in Head Injury Using the Disability Rating Scale. Arch. Phys. Med. Rehab. 75:156–163, 1994.

Frost, E. (Ed.): Cardio-Respiratory Effects. In: Frost, E. (Ed.): Head Injury: Clinical Management and Research. New Issues in Neurosciences, Vol. II, No. 2, 1990.

Galski, T., et al.: Predicting Physical and Verbal Aggression on a Brain Trauma Unit. Arch. Phys. Med. Rehab. 75:380–383, 1994.

Gean, A. D.: Imaging of Head Trauma. New York: Raven Press, 1994.

Gill-Body, K. M. and Giorgetti, M. M.: Acute Care and Prognostic Outcome. Clin. Phys. Ther. 33:1–31, 1995.

Goldstein, M.: Traumatic Brain Injury: A Silent Epidemic. Ann. Neurol. 27:327, 1990.

Goetz, C. G. and Pappert, E. J.: Trauma and Movement Disorders. Neurol. Clin. North Am. 10:907–919, 1992.

Grafman, J.: Cognitive and Behavioral Sequelae of Head Injury. In: Frost, E. (Ed.): Head Injury: Clinical Management and Research. New Issues in Neurosciences, Vol. II, No. 2, 1990.

Graham, D. I., et al.: Pathology of Brain Damage in Head Injury. In: Cooper, P. R. (Ed.): Head Injury, 3d ed. Baltimore: Williams & Wilkins, 1993.

Hughes, M. and Cohen, W. A.: Radiographic Evaluation. In: Cooper, P. R. (Ed.): Head Injury, 3d ed. Baltimore: Williams & Wilkins, 1993.

Jane, J.: Mild and Moderate Closed Head Injury. In: Frost, E. (Ed.): Head Injury: Clinical Management and Research. New Issues in Neurosciences, Vol. II, No. 2, 1990.

Jennett, B. and Frankowski, R. F.: The Epidemiology of Head Injury. In: Braakman, R. (Ed.): Handbook of Clinical Neurology, Vol. 13. New York: Elsevier, 1990.

Jordan, B. D.: Chronic Neurologic Injuries in Boxing. In: Jordan, B. D. (Ed.): Medical Aspects of Boxing. Boca Raton: CRC Press, 1993.

Kaplan, C. P. and Corrigan, J. D.: The Relationship Between Cognition and Functional Independence in Adults with Traumatic Brain Injury. Arch. Phys. Med. Rehab. 75:643–647, 1994.

Keane, J. R. and Baloh, R. W.: Posttraumatic Cranial Neuropathies. Neurol. Clin. North Am. 10:849–867, 1992.

Kraus, J. F.: Epidemiology. In: Frost, E. (Ed.): Head Injury: Clinical Management and Research. New Issues in Neurosciences, Vol. II, No. 2, 1990.

Kraus, J. F.: Epidemiology of Head Injury. In: Cooper, P. R. (Ed.): Head Injury, 3d ed. Baltimore: Williams & Wilkins, 1993.

Kraus, J. F. and Nourjah P.: The Epidemiology of Mild Uncomplicated Brain Injury. J. Trauma 28:1637–1643, 1988.

Kwasnica, C. M. and Heinemann, A.: Coping with Traumatic Brain Injury: Representative Case Studies. Arch. Phys. Med. Rehab. 75:384–389, 1994.

Macartney-Filgate, M. S.: Neuropsychological Sequelae of Major Physical Trauma. In: McMurtry, R. Y. and McLellan, B. A. (Eds.): Management of Blunt Trauma. Baltimore: Williams & Wilkins, 1990.

Mackay, L. E., et al.: Early Intervention in Severe Head Injury: Long-Term Benefits of a Formalized Program. Arch. Phys. Med. Rehab. 73:635–641, 1992.

Mandel, S.: Minor Head Injury May Not Be "Minor." Postgrad. Med. 85(6):213–225, 1989.

McIntosh, T. K. and Morgan, A. S.: New Trends in Neurodiagnostics and Therapeutics. Trauma Quart. 8(2):58–73, 1992.

Mendelow, A. D.: Head Injury. In: Walton, J. (Ed.): Brain's Diseases of the Nervous System, 10th ed. New York: Oxford University Press, 1993.

Rivara, J. B., et al.: Predictors of Family Functioning One Year Following Traumatic Brain Injury in Children. Arch. Phys. Med. Rehab. 73:899–910, 1992.

Rovit, R. L. and Murali, R.: Injuries of the Cranial Nerves. In: Cooper, P. R. (Ed.): Head Injury, 3d ed. Baltimore: Williams & Wilkins, 1993.

Salazar, A. M.: Pathophysiology. In: Frost, E. (Ed.): Head Injury: Clinical Management and Research. New Issues in Neurosciences, Vol. II, No. 2, 1990.

Sheffler, L. R., et al.: Shunting in Chronic Post-Traumatic Hydrocephalus: Demonstration of Neurophysiologic Improvement. Arch. Phys. Med. Rehab. 75:338–341, 1994.

Sullivan, K.: Cognitive Rehabilitation. Clin. Phys. Ther. 33:33–54, 1995.

Vollmer, D. G: Prognosis and Outcome of Severe Head Injury. In: Cooper, P. R. (Ed.): Head Injury, 3d ed. Baltimore: Williams & Wilkins, 1993.

White, R. J. and Likavec, M. J.: Review Article: Current Concepts: The Diagnosis and Initial Management of Head Injury. N. Engl. J. Med. 327:1507–1511, 1992.

Whyte, J., et al.: Rehabilitation. In: Frost, E. (Ed.): Head Injury: Clinical Management and Research. New Issues in Neurosciences, Vol. II, No. 2, 1990.

Willmore, L. J.: Posttraumatic Epilepsy. Neurol. Clin. North Am. 10:869–878, 1992.

Wrigley J. M., et al.: Social and Physical Factors in the Referral of People with Traumatic Brain Injuries to Rehabilitation. Arch. Phys. Med. Rehab. 75:149–155, 1994.

Additional References

Bartley, J.: Delayed Cerebrospinal Rhinorrhoea. Aust. N.Z. J. Surg. 63(5):418, May 1993.

Cucciniello, B., et al.: Conservative Management of Extradural Haematomas. Acta Neurochir. (Wien) 120(1–2):47–52, 1993.

Levy, M. L., et al.: The Significance of Subarachnoid Hemorrhage after Penetrating Craniocerebral Injury: Correlations with Angiography and Outcome in a Civilian Population. Neurosurgery 32(4):532–540, Apr. 1993.

Lim, T. C.: Retrobulbar Haematoma (Letter). Br. J. Oral Maxillofac. Surg. 31(2):131, Apr. 1993.

Lui, T. N., et al.: Epidural Hematomas in the Posterior Cranial Fossa. J. Trauma 34(2):211–215, Feb. 1993.

Mathew, P., et al.: Acute Subdural Haematoma in the Conscious Patient: Outcome with Initial Non-Operative Management. Acta Neurochir. (Wien) 121(3–4): 100–108, 1993.

Mayfrank, L., et al.: Bilateral Chronic Subdural Haematomas following Traumatic Cerebrospinal Fluid Leakage Into the Thoracic Epidural Space. Acta Neurochir. (Wien) 120(1–2):92–94, 1993.

Proceedings of the 4th International Symposium on Mechanisms of Secondary Brain Damage—An Update. Abstracts. Acta Neurochir. 120(3–4):193–207, 1993.

Shults, W. T., et al.: Neuro-Ophthalmic Complications of Intracranial Catheters. Neurosurgery 33(1):135–138, July 1993.

Stewart, C. R., et al.: Proptosis as a Presenting Sign of Extradural Haematoma. Br. J. Ophthalmol. 77(3):179–180, March 1993.

Sugar, A., et al.: Retrobulbar Haematoma (Letter). Br. J. Oral Maxillofac. Surg. 31(2):130–131, Apr. 1993.

Takahara, T., et al.: Fatal Traumatic Subarachnoid Hemorrhage Due to Rupture of the Vertebral Artery. Intensive Care Med. 19(3):172–173, 1993.

Toro, V. E., et al.: Posttraumatic Pseudoaneurysm of the Posterior Meningeal Artery Associated with Intraventricular Hemorrhage. A.J.N.R. Am. J. Neuroradiol. 14(1):264–266, Jan.-Feb. 1993.

Tseng, S. H.: Acute Epidural Hematoma Appearing as a Side-By-Side Isodensity and Hyperdensity on Computed Tomographic Scan: Case Report. J. Trauma 34(4):602–603, Apr. 1993.

Tuncer, R., et al.: Conservative Management of Epidural Haematomas. Prospective Study of 15 Cases. Acta Neurochir. 121(1–2):48–52, 1993.

Warburton, R.: Case Report: Chronic Subdural Hematoma Following High-Speed Ejection. Aviat. Space Environ. Med. 64(6):534–537, June 1993.

CHAPTER 2

Concussion

SCOPE

Cerebral concussion is a very common form of closed head injury, caused by violent jarring or shaking that can affect victims of traffic accidents and child abuse as well as participants of contact sports. Commonly referred to as brain concussion or simply concussion, this injury usually manifests as a brief loss of consciousness followed, upon awakening, by headache, amnesia, dizziness or disequilibrium. Although different degrees of severity are recognized, most persons who sustain concussion and are seen by medical personnel are either sent home with a friend or family member or observed overnight. Most have an uncomplicated recovery.

SYNOPSIS

2.00 INTRODUCTION

An estimated 10 million cases of head injuries of varying degrees of severity occur annually in the United States. About 45 percent of these injuries result from motor vehicle accidents, 30 percent from falls, 10 percent from occupational accidents, 10 percent from recreational accidents and 5 percent from assaults (Goldstein, 1991). About half of all head injuries occur in children.

Blunt head injuries (those that do not involve penetration of the skull) often result in cerebral concussion. Usually a concussion, which is generally characterized by a brief loss of consciousness and amnesia, is of little medical consequence. However, sometimes concussion is accompanied by serious brain damage or symptoms such as headache, dizziness and irritability that may persist for weeks, months or even longer.

Although many of the complicating problems associated with cerebral concussion clearly have an organic basis, for some conditions, a scientifically proven organic basis has not been definitely established. Another controversy regarding this injury is that although relatively standardized procedures have been developed for evaluating and managing severe head injuries at the emergency department, in contrast, there is widespread disagreement about what procedures to follow for patients with the more common problem of mild head injury.

2.10   DEFINITION AND MECHANISMS OF INJURY

Cerebral concussion may be defined as traumatic paralysis of nervous system function that occurs as an immediate reaction to an accelerative or decelerative blunt head injury. The effects of a concussion are generally considered to be reversible, although there may be exceptions.

Sometimes a brief loss of consciousness is also included in the definition of concussion, in order to distinguish this injury from traumatic brain lesions, such as contusions.[1] However, objections have been raised to defining concussion on the basis of the length of time of unconsciousness, on the grounds that such a distinction is quantitative rather than qualitative.

The most likely condition for producing a cerebral concussion is a situation in which the momentum of the head is altered. This can occur by either a blow to the head or sudden deceleration of the head as it hits an immovable object, such as a wall or the sidewalk pavement. The blow to the head causes what is known as an acceleration injury, and the head striking the unyielding object causes a deceleration injury.

---

[1] *See also* ch. 3.

A concussion occurs when the brain is subjected to shearing stresses that result from rotational forces. However, the mechanism that produces concussion has still not been determined at a more fundamental level. Speculation often involves various types of damage to neurons, but none of the hypotheses that has been put forth has been proved (Adams and Victor, 1993).

2.20 PATHOPHYSIOLOGY

A concussion is accompanied by amnesia about events immediately before (retrograde) and after (anterograde) the head injury. The length of time for which memory is lost is related to the degree of severity of the concussion. In cases in which unconsciousness persists for 24 hours or more, diffuse brain injury usually occurs (Hardman, 1991).

According to one hypothesis, concussion causes an imbalance between the energy that cells demand and the energy that can be supplied. Mitochondria (organelles) are specialized structures present in all cells. A rapid loss of mitochondrial adenosine triphosphate (a molecule with stored energy that is produced through metabolism) has been observed following head injury, along with an increase in levels of lactic acid. These findings support the notion that the mitochondria, which supply energy to the cells, undergo functional changes. Electron microscope studies of mitochondria following experimental concussion also demonstrate irregularities. At the same time that the mitochondria appear to be unable to supply the cell with normal amounts of energy, the substrates for energy production may also be diminished because of vascular spasm and a rise in intracranial pressure. It is believed that this imbalance in energy triggers numerous biochemical changes, including the release of excitatory neurotransmitter molecules (Menkes and Till, 1990). In addition, experimental studies show that in some instances, the blood-brain barrier (a functional barrier between the brain capillaries and brain tissue that permits some substances to enter the brain but blocks others) near the point of impact is disrupted.

In the individual who has sustained a concussion, other types of brain injuries may also be present. Indeed, a variety of types of brain damage can be attributed to these other forms of injury.

Chronic damage to the brain, as is often seen in boxers, may lead to a specific disorder called the punch-drunk syndrome (dementia pugilistica). An estimated 20 percent of professional boxers eventually experience this condition. The symptoms include problems with speech, clumsiness, loss of equilibrium, spasticity and the Parkinsonian syndrome.[2] Among the pathologic findings in these boxers are neurofibrillary tangles in the brain that appear to be the same as those found in patients with Alzheimer's disease (Hardman, 1991). However, the neuritic plaques characteristically seen in the brain of Alzheimer's disease patients are not present or at least not very evident in the brain of former boxers. That boxers can have permanent damage after repeated concussive injuries suggests that damage from concussion may not actually be reversible.

2.30 CLINICAL MANIFESTATIONS

The immediate clinical results of a concussion include:

- loss of consciousness;
- inhibition of reflexes;
- brief respiratory arrest;
- a short period of bradycardia (slow heartbeat); and
- a decline in blood pressure that follows a very brief rise in blood pressure at the moment of impact.

(See Figure 2-1.) If the impact is strong enough, this initial phase of concussion can be fatal, with death probably resulting from the cessation of breathing.

Recovery usually begins within a few seconds. First, the vital signs quickly return to normal. Then, after a variable period of time, the patient begins to move and opens his or her eyes (although at this point, there is no vision). There is also a return of reflexes. In the next stage of recovery, the patient gradually begins to interact with the surrounding environment. Although the patient may respond slowly to simple commands and questions, no memories are yet being formed.

Full recovery from concussion is considered to occur when memory formation actually begins. There will be a loss of memory for events both immediately before the injury and after the recovery of consciousness. The entire recovery phase varies and can take from minutes to days.

---

[2] *See also* ch. 12 for complete discussion of Parkinson's disease.

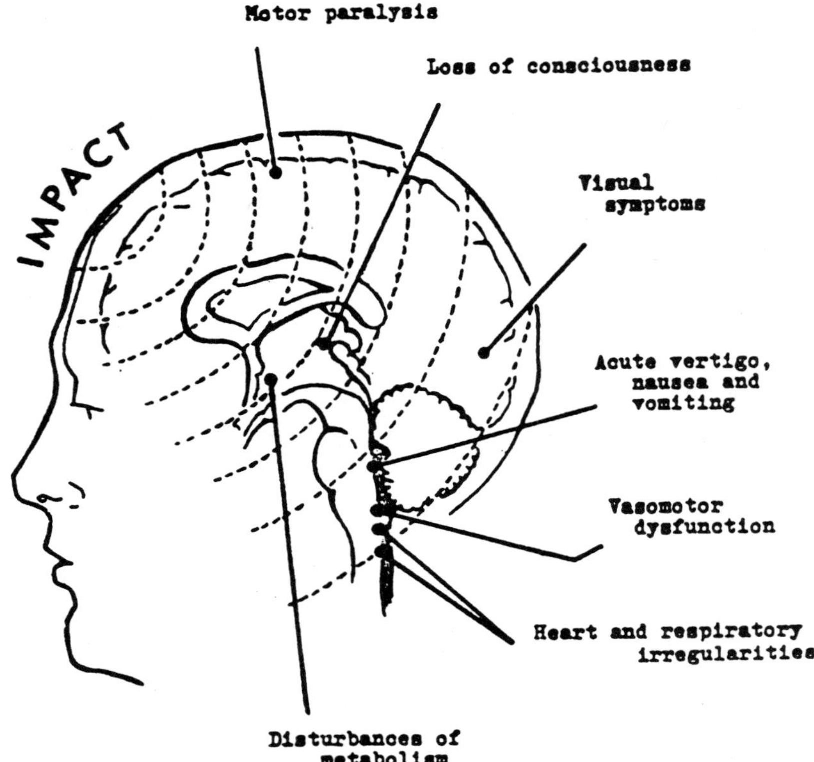

Fig. 2-1. Progressive effect of impact on nerve centers after head injury. The immediate effect of concussion following a forceful injury to the head is marked by an impairment of consciousness. Various effects on the centers of the brain occur, as shown, the degree and nature of which vary considerably from one person to another.

2.40   INITIAL ASSESSMENT

The physician who first encounters a patient with a closed head injury will generally find that the patient is in one of three basic conditions: (1) conscious or quickly regaining consciousness; (2) unconscious since the time of the injury; or (3) unconscious but reportedly was conscious for a while after initially regaining consciousness following the injury (Adams and Victor, 1993).

2.41   The Conscious Patient

The first type of situation is the most common and is generally symptomatic of a mild head injury. Some patients in this category are merely stunned and do not actually lose consciousness, whereas others are briefly unconscious. In either case, the injury is probably of no clinical significance. However, there is the slight possibility of a skull fracture[3] or hematoma (collection of bloody fluid)[4] developing subsequent to the injury. Another possibility is that the patient will go on to have symptoms of the postconcussion syndrome, characterized by headache, dizziness, irritability and other symptoms. Patients who do briefly lose consciousness may not remember what occurred before and after the injury.[5]

Occasionally patients with seemingly mild head injuries will have serious brain damage, such as contusion (bruise on the surface of the brain),[6] hemorrhage or cerebral swelling. Usually such patients remain unconscious for more than one hour, and their normal clarity of consciousness fails to return. Such patients should be regarded as having a serious head injury.

Sometimes following a head injury from which an individual rapidly regained consciousness, the person will suddenly become pale and collapse, and then quickly recover. Called a *vasopressor syncopal attack,* this is not attributable to the head injury per se but, rather, is a response to being frightened about the injury. In other words, it is literally fainting from fright.

2.42   The Patient Who Is Unconscious Since the Injury

It may difficult to determine whether patients in this second category are unconscious because of a concussion or because of contusion. Some of these patients have head injuries or other injuries so severe that they cannot survive. Other patients will begin to show signs of recovering within days or a week or two, but they will not totally recover. Finally, some patients will either remain unconscious, in a stuporous state or have severe loss of cerebral function.

---

[3] *See also* ch. 6.

[4] *See also* ch. 4 for a discussion of hematoma and hemorrhage of the brain.

[5] *See* 2.70 *infra* for a discussion of postconcussion syndrome.

[6] *See also* ch. 3 for a discussion of contusions and lacerations of the brain.

2.43   The Patient Who Is Conscious After Injury, Then Loses Consciousness

The third category of patients—those who are unconscious but reportedly were conscious for a while after the injury (they had a *lucid interval*)—includes a great number of patients who can benefit from rapid surgical intervention. It is important, therefore, that these patients be quickly identified as needing surgery. Of particular concern is the presence of a hematoma (localized collection of blood).

2.50   DIAGNOSIS

Arriving at a diagnosis of cerebral concussion involves a combination of physical examination, ruling out other possible causes of symptoms and use of diagnostic imaging.

2.51   Clinical Examination

Head injuries are classified in terms of their severity. (Often the term *brain injury* is used instead of head injury.) Typically the categories are *mild* or *minor, moderate* and *severe.* These categories lack standardized definitions, and a comparison of various studies will show that the same term may be defined in many different ways. Usually the degree of injury is to a considerable extent defined by the patient's score on the Glasgow Coma Scale. (*See Table 2-1.*)

Total scores range from 3 to 15. The lower the total score on the Glasgow Coma Scale, the more severe the head injury.

A definition of a mild traumatic brain injury has been formulated by a committee of the American Congress of Rehabilitation Medicine (Berrol, 1992). According to this definition, a patient with mild traumatic brain injury (TBI) is someone who has had a traumatically induced physiologic disruption of brain function, as manifested by at least one of the following:

- any period of loss of consciousness;
- any loss of memory for events immediately before or after the accident;
- any alteration in mental state at the time of the accident (for example, feeling dazed, disoriented or confused);

Table 2-1
Glasgow Coma Scale

ACTIVITY	SCORE
Eye Opening	
None	1
To pain	2
To speech	3
Spontaneously	4
Verbal Response	
None	1
Incomprehensible sounds	2
Inappropriate words	3
Confused	4
Oriented	5
Motor Response	
None	1
Extension abnormal	2
Flexion abnormal	3
Flexion withdrawal	4
Localizes pain	5
Obeys	6

- focal neurologic deficits that may or may not be transient but in which severity does not exceed the following:

  1. loss of consciousness of approximately 30 minutes or less;

  2. after 30 minutes, an initial Glasgow Coma Scale total score of 13 to 15; and

  3. post-traumatic amnesia lasting not longer than 24 hours.

Grading systems have been devised to evaluate mild concussion (Vollmer and Dacey, 1991). In such types of grading systems, the emphasis is on duration of cognitive impairment, as opposed to the degree of impairment. Grading systems for mild concussion have particularly been used as an aid for the initial management of sports-related head injuries.

Although the Glasgow Coma Scale plays an important role in assessing the severity of a head injury, the scale is not useful for evaluating infants and younger children, patients in shock or patients who are intoxicated or hypoxic (with inadequate supply of oxygen). Also, certain complicating injuries, such as those affecting the spine, can render the scores invalid.

In addition to the value of the Glasgow Coma Scale, other neurologic assessments should be made. It is important to assess eye movements, oculovestibular reflexes and the condition of the pupils. Signs of decorticate rigidity, such as flexion of the arms or extension of the legs, and signs of decerebrate rigidity, such as extension of both arms and legs, should be looked for.

During the neurologic examination, the patient's head should be examined for scalp lesions as well as lesions of the skull.

2.52　Differential Diagnosis

The fact that a head injury has occurred in most instances is clearly evident. However, the possibility that a condition that was present before the head injury may have led to the accident should be kept in mind. One such condition is a cerebrovascular lesion, commonly known as a stroke.[7]

For patients who are still in a state of unconsciousness hours or days after sustaining a head injury, it may be very difficult to determine whether their condition is a result of a concussion or a contusion. The effects of a concussion are generally considered to be reversible, whereas those of a contusion are not. However, there are patients who have sustained head injuries and remained in a comatose state for a long period of time who have eventually recovered to the point that their neurologic status was normal.

In patients with severe head injury who remain comatose for a prolonged period, it is believed by some authorities that both concussion and contusion are present (Adams and Victor, 1993).

2.53　Computed Tomography (CT)

Computed tomography (CT) has assumed the role as the most important imaging technique in the emergency setting. It is particularly useful for identifying large hematomas, which are of concern even

---

[7] *See also* ch. 9.

in patients with mild head injury. However, considerable disagreement exists over exactly which patients should undergo CT. On one side, there is the view that only patients at high risk of having focal brain damage should undergo CT scanning (Katz and Deluca, 1992), while on the other side of the controversy is the opinion that CT scans should be done on a routine basis, and immediately on all patients with head injuries who have lost consciousness or who have amnesia (Stein and Ross, 1992). Those with the latter opinion claim that CT can identify literally all patients with intracranial lesions and thereby virtually eliminate the risk of subsequent deterioration in patients without identified brain abnormalities (with the possible exception of elderly patients, in whom a brain abnormality may develop at a later time).

In addition to being very useful for identifying large, acute hematomas, CT scans are useful for identifying late ventricular enlargements, cortical atrophy, skull fractures, cerebral swelling and cerebral contusion. It is not a good technique for identifying diffuse axonal injury (a nonfocal type of brain injury in which damage occurs to the portion of neurons that transmits the impulse away from the nerve).

2.54 Magnetic Resonance Imaging (MRI)

Since its introduction as an imaging technique for head injuries, magnetic resonance imaging (MRI) has gained an increasingly important role in diagnosis. In the acute situation, it may be used when CT scanning fails to identify a brain abnormality. For identifying several types of brain abnormalities, magnetic resonance imaging has been shown to be superior to CT.

Two weeks or more after a head injury, MRI can detect intracerebral edema (excessive accumulation of fluid within the tissue spaces) and hemorrhage better than CT. MRI can also detect small intracranial hematomas and effusions (accumulations of fluid in a body cavity or tissue space) that CT fails to reveal. This latter capability of MRI has been useful in confirming the theory that in severe injuries, shearing forces at impact can cause extensive microscopic damage to the brain (Goldstein, 1991).

Magnetic resonance imaging has also been found to be superior to CT in detecting lesions in the white matter of the frontal and temporal regions of the brain after head injuries. Such lesions have been found to closely correspond with deficits in mental abilities that have been revealed through neuropsychological testing (Rosenthal, 1993).

Focal brain contusions that have escaped detection by CT have been detected by MRI. In addition, MRI is superior to CT in detecting injury to the subcortical gray matter, brain stem and corpus collosum (the brain structure connecting the left and right cerebral hemispheres). However, CT is better at detecting subarachnoid (beneath the arachnoid membrane, the middle of three membranes covering the brain) hemorrhage and skull fractures as well as potentially reversible intracranial hematomas (Doezema, et al., 1991). *(See Figure 2-2.)*

2.55   X-ray Examination

X-ray studies can show whether a patient has a fractured skull. Mild head injury patients with skull fractures have a higher risk of having an intracranial lesion. However, some authorities believe that there is little value in determining if a patient's skull is fractured. For example, in one study of 13 patients with mild head injuries who had abnormal results of computed tomography scans, all but 2 had normal skull x-rays (Livingston, 1991). In all, only about 5 percent of patients with mild head injuries have skull fractures.

Disagreement exists over whether routine skull radiographs should be obtained after patients with mild head injury arrive at the emergency department (Stein and Ross, 1993). However, there is onsensus that a normal skull radiograph and a normal neurologic examination do not exclude the possibility of an intracranial lesion.

2.56   Cerebrospinal Fluid Examination

Lumbar puncture involves retrieving a small amount of cerebrospinal fluid (CSF) from the L4-L5 interspace for the purpose of examination. Cerebrospinal fluid examination has for the most part been replaced by CT and MRI and by intracerebral monitoring. Following a simple concussion, the CSF usually appears normal. Following severe head injury, the levels of acetylcholine (a neurotransmitter molecule) and lactate are generally raised for three to four days because of leakage from the damaged brain.

2.57   Single Photon Emission Computed Tomography (SPECT)

Single photon emission computed tomography (SPECT) is an imaging technique that measures regional blood flow in the cerebrum,

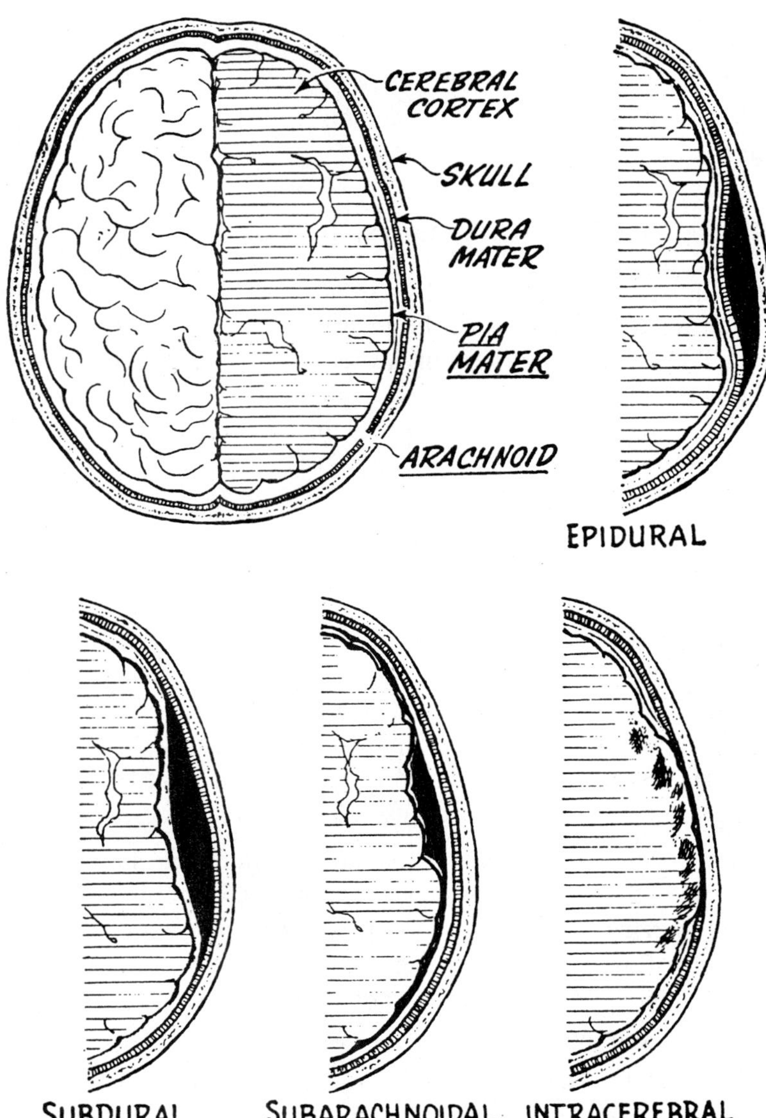

Fig. 2-2. The three meninges surrounding the brain (top left) and the types of hemorrhage that can develop in and around them (top right and bottom). Subarachnoid hemorrhage is one of the more common types.

thereby providing a direct measure of regional brain function. *(See Figure 2-3.)* In patients with severe head injuries, SPECT can detect more areas of contusion and ischemia in the cerebrum than either CT or MRI. In patients with mild head injuries, SPECT may be able to detect brain damage in areas where such damage has so far not been detected (Rosenthal, 1993). SPECT may also play a role in predicting late deterioration in head injury patients who have an intracerebral hematoma (Katz and Deluca, 1992).

2.58 Positron Emission Tomography (PET)

Positron emission tomography (PET) provides superior spatial resolution, in comparison with the image provided by SPECT. However, PET is a much more expensive technique and is frequently not available. Positron emission tomography can be used to measure metabolism and blood flow in the brain, as well as various other physiologic variables.

2.59 Other Diagnostic Modalities

The electroencephalogram (EEG) is a recording of electrical potentials of the brain derived from electrodes attached to the scalp. *(See Figure 2-4.)* The EEG findings in a patient following a simple concussion will be normal. As a result, EEG is not useful as a diagnostic tool in the initial evaluation of patients with mild head injuries. However, a newer, related technique, quantitative electroencephalography, may prove to be useful.

Electroencephalography does have an important role in evaluating patients with the postconcussion syndrome (a condition in which headache, dizziness, irritability and lack of concentration persist for more than a few weeks following a concussion).[8] In patients with postconcussion syndrome, various abnormalities are detected on the electroencephalogram (Zasler, 1992).

Evoked potentials may be useful in evaluating patients with the postconcussion syndrome. Somatosensory, auditory and visual evoked potentials have all been studied in such patients (Goldstein, 1991). Abnormalities in evoked potentials have been found in head injury patients who did and did not lose consciousness.

---

[8] *See* 2.70 *infra.*

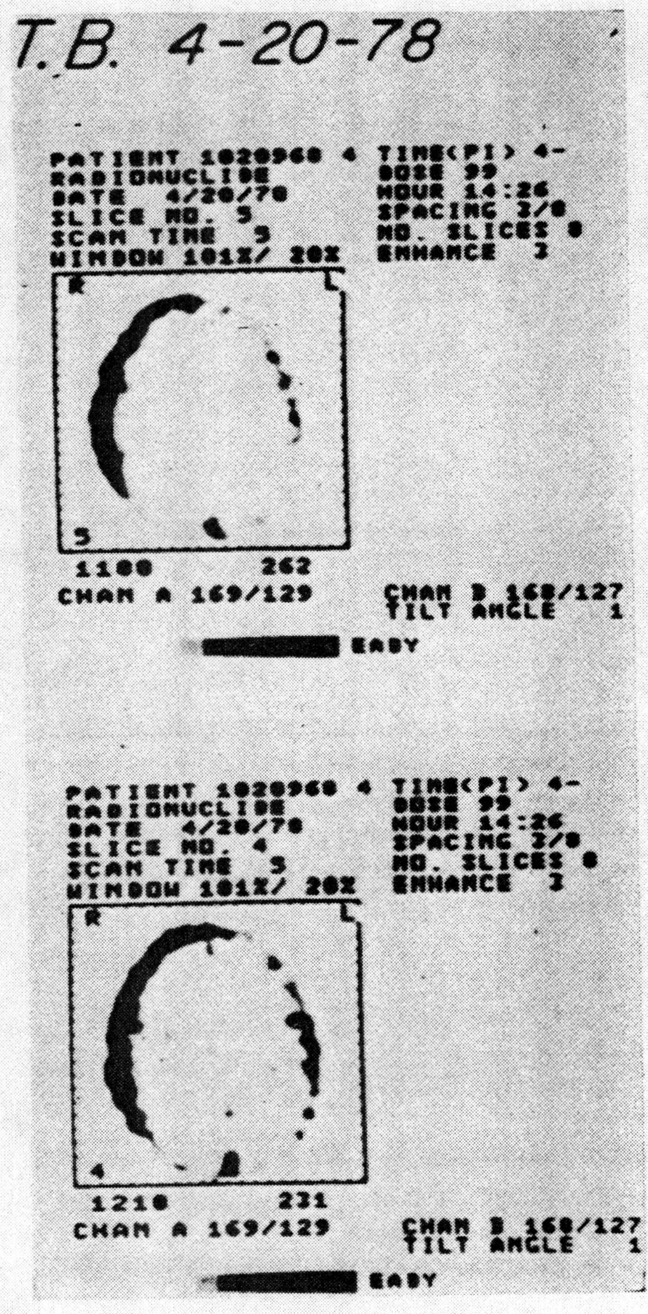

Fig. 2-3. A single photon emission computed tomography (SPECT) scan of a patient with subdural hematoma.

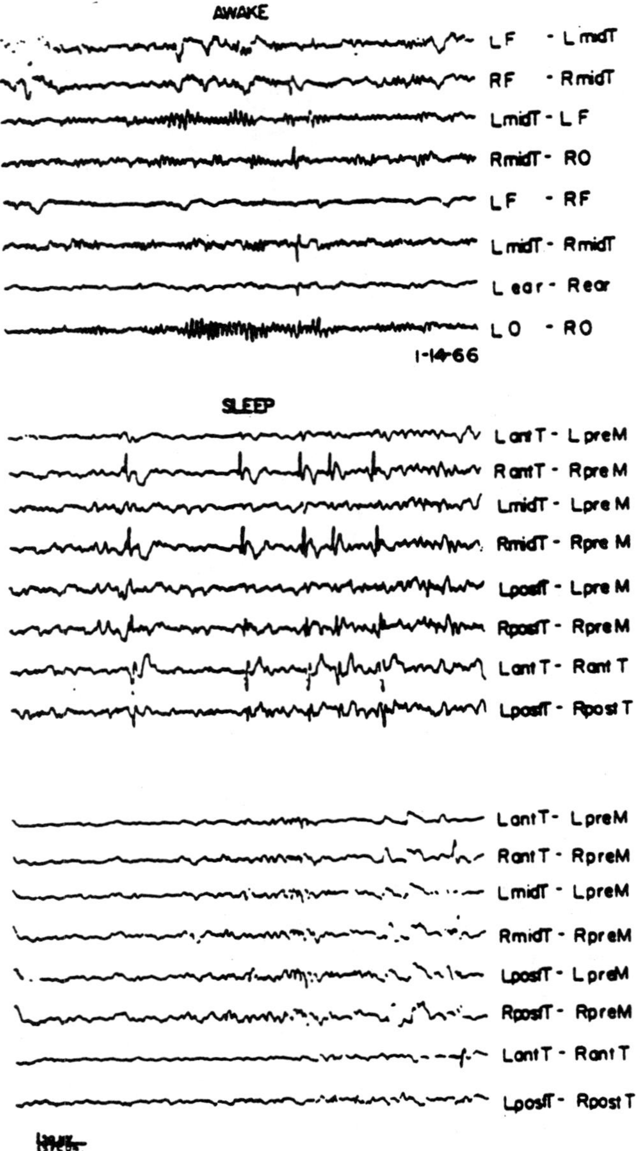

Fig. 2-4. An electroencephalogram measures brain function in wave patterns.

Neurologic impairment following a mild head injury can be identified in the patient by administering a neuropsychological examination. Usually this examination focuses on postconcussion symptoms as ascertained through an interview, efficiency in processing information and memory. The revised Paced Auditory Serial Addition Test (PASAT-R), which requires the patient to sequentially add numbers presented orally at increasing speeds, has been shown to be especially good in revealing minor traumatic brain injury (Katz and Deluca, 1992).

2.60   COMPLICATIONS

Most head injuries are classified as mild and usually result in nothing worse than a slight concussion. However, in some instances, the situation is complicated by a more serious injury, such as a hematoma or contusion. In moderate and severe head injuries, the likelihood of complicating brain injuries is much greater.

2.61   Acute Epidural Hematoma

Acute epidural hematomas usually occur in patients who are only briefly unconscious after a mild head injury. These patients usually have a lucid interval before the symptoms of the hematoma begin to appear. Bleeding into the space between the dura mater (the outer of the three membranes covering the brain) and the skull is a direct cause of acute epidural hematoma. *(See Figure 2-5.)*

The hemorrhage usually results from rupture of the middle meningeal artery. Less often, the bleeding comes from a tear in the dural venous sinus. Usually this type of hematoma occurs only on one side of the brain. If the source of blood is from the middle meningeal artery, the hematoma will enlarge rapidly, and symptoms will appear within a few hours or up to a day after the injury. If, on the other hand, the origin of bleeding is the dural venous sinus, the hematoma will enlarge more slowly, and symptoms may not appear for days or even a week.

Acute epidural hematomas can cause a life-threatening situation by compressing the temporal lobe of the brain and causing herniation of part of the temporal lobe through the tentorium (the membrane separating the cerebrum from the cerebellum). This leads to crushing of the midbrain and inevitable death.

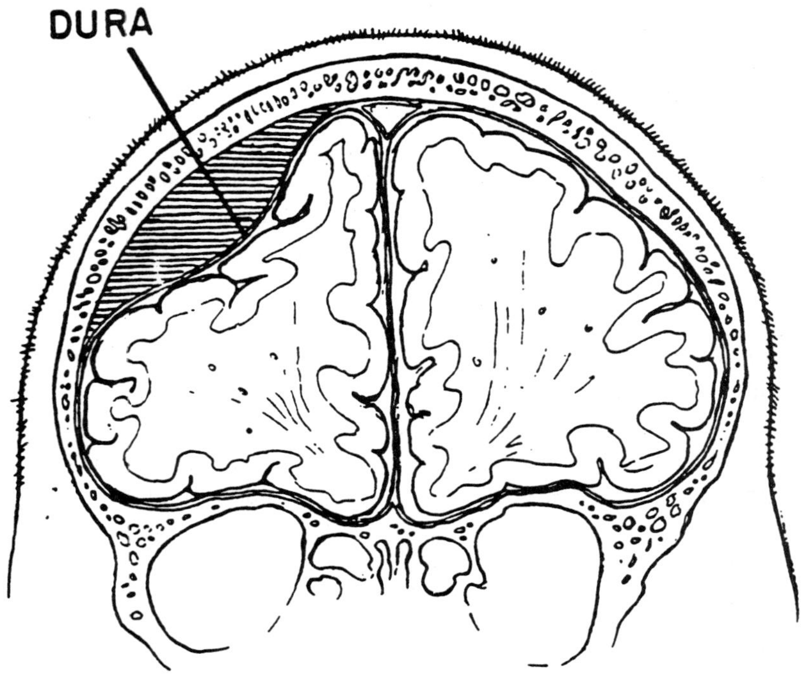

Fig. 2-5. Classic presentation of an epidural hematoma.

The symptoms of temporal lobe compression include headache of increasing intensity, vomiting, confusion, drowsiness and seizures. Muscle weakness may occur on one side of the body (hemiparesis). Neurologic examination may reveal a slight increase of tendon reflexes and Babinski signs (abnormal reflex characterized by extension of the large toe and fanning of the other toes upon stimulation of the lateral aspect of the sole of the foot). *(See Figure 2-6.)* The patient will gradually lapse into a coma. Without proper treatment, respiration will become more and more abnormal and will eventually stop.

The most commonly used diagnostic method for detecting an acute epidural hematoma is CT scanning. On the CT scan, the clotted blood of the hematoma will appear biconcave (shaped like a lens). Computed tomography can be used to distinguish an epidural hematoma from a subdural hematoma on the basis of the shape of the clot. Magnetic resonance imaging can also be useful for detecting an epidural hematoma.

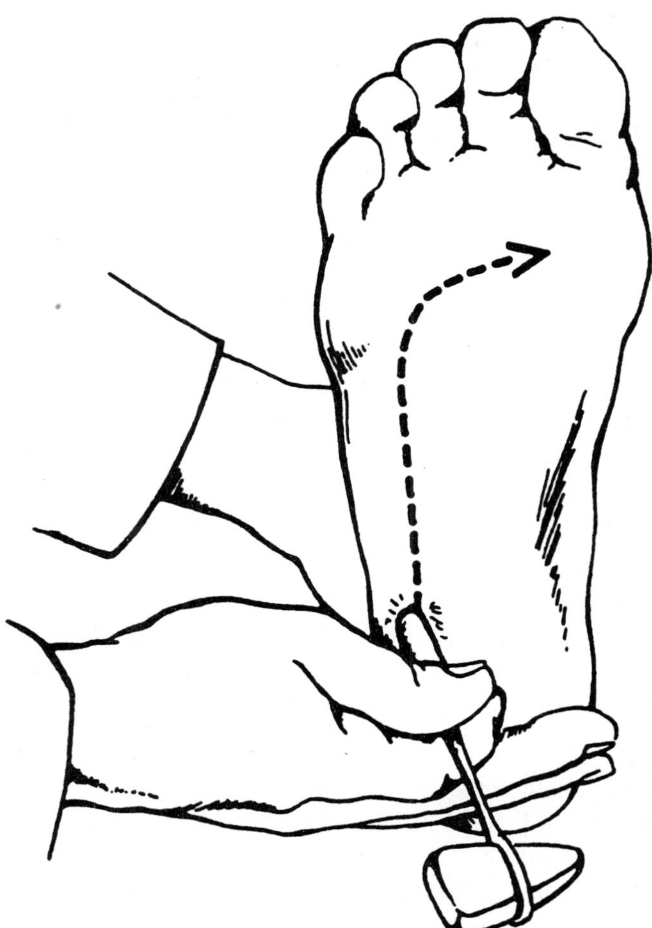

Fig. 2-6. The Babinski, or plantar, reflex test is performed by stroking the foot in the direction indicated with a dull instrument, such as the end of the reflex hammer. A positive sign is extension of the big toe upward, with downward flexion and sometimes spreading of the other toes.

Treatment for an epidural hematoma is surgical. The procedure consists of drainage, identifying the bleeding vessel and tying it off.

In cases in which the epidural hematoma is detected quickly and neurosurgical intervention is prompt, the prognosis is excellent. However, in cases in which treatment is delayed or there is additional severe brain injury, there is a considerable probability of death.

2.62   Acute Subdural Hematoma

A subdural hematoma results from bleeding into the space between the dura mater and the brain. *(See Figure 2-7.)* The bleeding occurs from the rupturing of the bridging veins that drain blood from the cerebral cortex. The bleeding may occur on one side of the brain (unilateral) or on both sides (bilateral).

Generally the patient with an acute subdural hematoma is unconscious from the time of injury and will progressively fall into a deeper coma. There are patients, however, who experience a brief lucid interval.

The symptoms of an acute subdural hematoma are attributable to the brain being compressed by an enlarging blood clot. In contrast to an epidural hematoma caused by rupture of an artery in which bleeding continues, in a subdural hematoma, the bleeding from the veins is often stopped by a rise in intracranial pressure. Often a patient with an acute subdural hematoma will have other brain lesions, making correlation of symptoms with a specific lesion a difficult task.

The best techniques for confirming a diagnosis of acute subdural hematoma are CT and MRI. In most cases, the clot can be visualized on a CT scan alone. An acute subdural hematoma can usually be differentiated on CT scans from an epidural hematoma because the former is likely to be crescent shaped, as opposed to the biconcave shape of the latter.

Treatment for an acute subdural hematoma consists of a craniotomy (making a wide opening in the skull) in order to permit control of bleeding and removal of the blood clot.

2.63   Chronic Subdural Hematoma

A chronic subdural hematoma tends to develop over a period of weeks. This type of lesion can occur in the elderly as a result of a

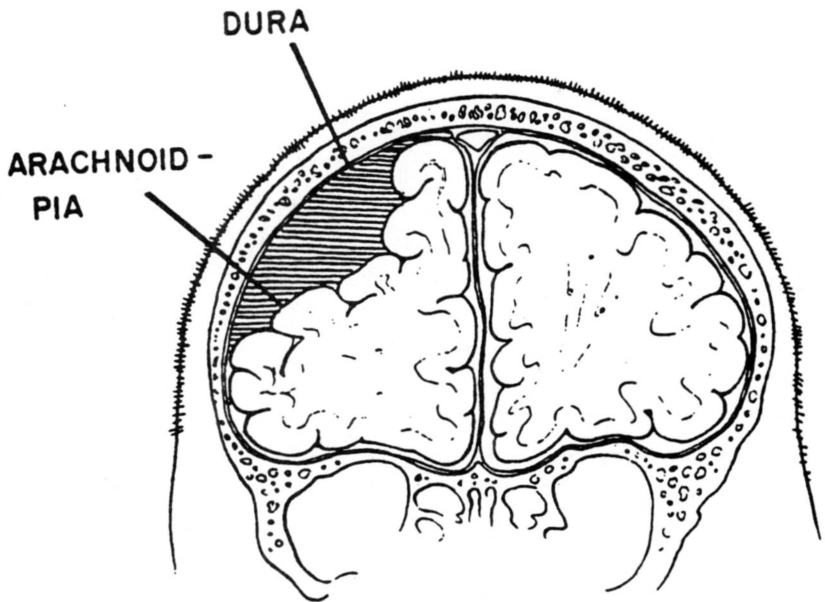

Fig. 2-7. Classic presentation of a subdural hematoma.

head injury that seemed so insignificant at the time that it was forgotten. The main symptoms include headache, confusion, apathy and sleepiness. Eventually the patient will become comatose, but during this progressive course, there will often be periods of greater awareness.

Computed tomography and MRI are the best diagnostic tools for confirming the presence of a chronic subdural hematoma. On the CT scan, these lesions appear less dense than the surrounding tissue. After a period of time subsequent to the injury, a membrane begins to grow from the dura and encapsulates the collection of blood.

A chronic subdural hematoma that results from a relatively small amount of bleeding may be resorbed (absorbed by the body). On the other hand, some may continue to enlarge.The reason these hematomas gradually enlarge was originally thought to be that the protein albumin was in high concentration within the hematoma and therefore drew water across the encapsulating membrane by osmotic pressure. However, this explanation has been disproved by subsequent research.

Treatment for a chronic subdural hematoma consists of removing the blood clot through burr holes placed in the skull. This must be performed before the patient reaches a deep comatose state. The blood may be drained through a catheter placed through the burr holes. *(See Figure 2-8.)*

2.64   Cortical Contusion

A cortical contusion is a bruise on the surface of the brain.[9] In most cases, the dura mater remains undamaged. If the lesion is at the site of impact to the head, it is called a *coup* contusion. If the lesion is on the opposite side of the brain from the impact, it is called a *contrecoup* contusion. The type that occurs is dependent on whether the person's head is moving at the moment of impact. If the head is stationary at impact, a coup injury will result, whereas free movement of the head at the moment of impact will result in a contrecoup injury. Usually contusions occur on either the frontal or temporal lobes of the brain.

Focal neurologic signs, including seizures, are useful for making a diagnosis of contusion based on clinical findings. The diagnosis can often be confirmed by the results of CT scans. Differentiating a cerebral contusion from a concussion can be difficult under certain circumstances.[10]

The prognosis for recovery from a cortical contusion is quite good, provided there is no diffuse axonal injury, swelling of the brain or additional bleeding. Autopsy results have revealed that healed contusions are not necessarily associated with clinical evidence of permanent brain damage.

2.65   Diffuse Axonal Injury

Diffuse axonal injury occurs most often as a result of head injuries sustained in vehicular accidents. Patients are usually unconscious after the injury and remain in a comatose state. In about half of the cases, CT scans will not show any mass lesion in the brain. The brain of patients who have died will often appear almost normal to the naked eye. However, microscopic examination will reveal abnormalities,

---

[9] *See also* ch. 3.

[10] *See* 2.52 *supra.*

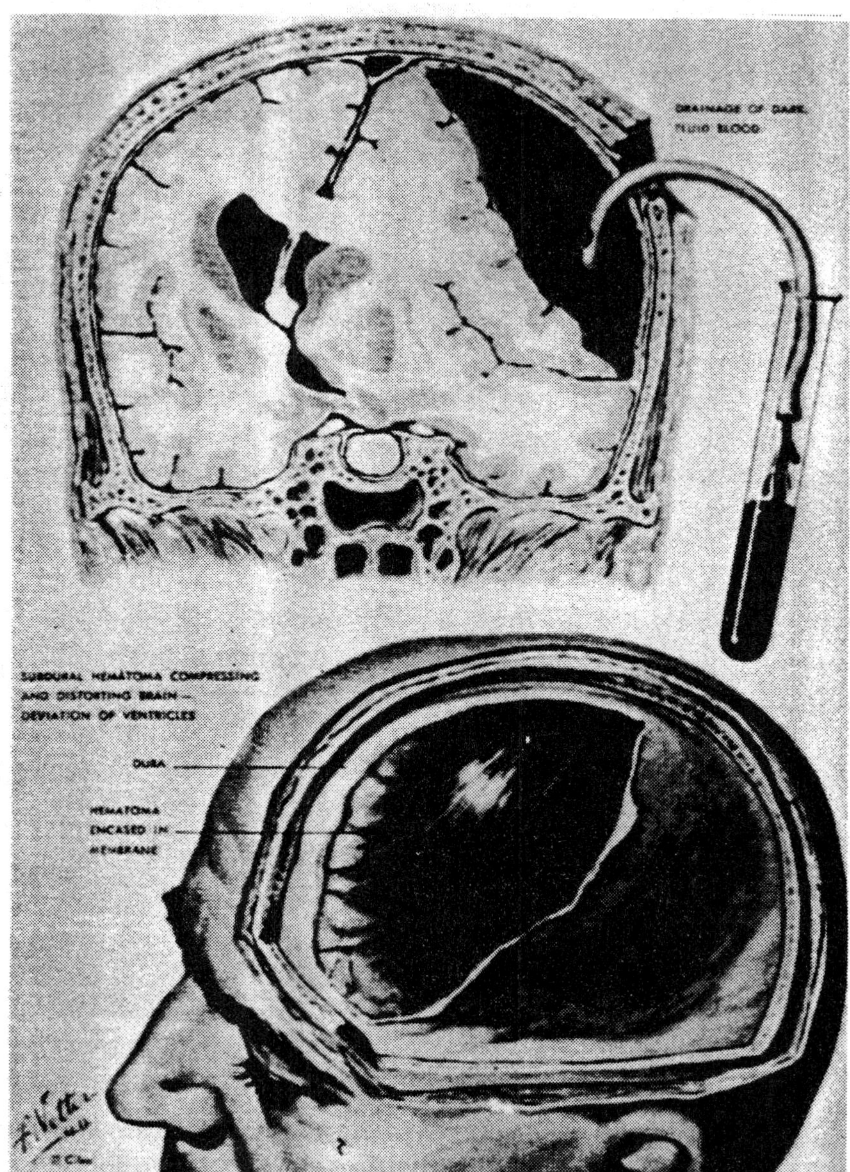

Fig. 2-8. A chronic subdural hematoma. Drainage of the blood may be performed through a catheter placed through the skull.

particularly swelling of the nerve axons in the cerebral white matter, corpus collosum and upper portion of the brain stem.

The mechanism producing diffuse axonal injury seems to be sudden, angular rotation of the head. Such motion is believed to result in strain on the axons in the areas of the brain where the diffuse injury appears.

2.70 POSTCONCUSSION SYNDROME

Following a concussion, some patients experience persistent symptoms that, together, are known as postconcussion syndrome. This consequence of head injury is also referred to as post-traumatic syndrome and post-traumatic headache syndrome.

2.71 Symptoms

Postconcussion syndrome can include numerous symptoms, but headache is the most prominent. The headache can be generalized in nature or focused on the site of head injury. Descriptions of this type of headache vary widely among patients. The pain is usually intensified by strain and alleviated by rest.

The second most prominent symptom is dizziness, which is usually described as lightheadedness rather than actual vertigo (sensation of whirling in space). However, some patients do seem to have true vertigo.

Other reported symptoms include nausea; weakness and fatigue; numbness; intolerance of noise, crowds and emotional excitement; lack of attention and concentration; ringing in the ears (tinnitus); oversensitivity to light and inability to tolerate alcohol in amounts usually consumed. There also may be problems with memory and information processing ability.

Psychological and psychiatric sequelae are also included as part of the postconcussion syndrome. Although there are doubts whether these sequelae are really related in any way to headache and other neurologic postconcussion symptoms, in general, this relationship is considered to exist (Goldstein, 1991).

Post-traumatic neurosis consists of a number of psychiatric symptoms. The most frequently seen neurotic symptom is anxiety. The patient's personality before the head injury appears to play a large role in the development of post-traumatic neurosis. Other factors such as stress and the environment may also play a role.

More severe head injuries can lead to *post-traumatic psychosis*. The type of psychoses that have been noted following severe head injuries include schizophrenic, manic depressive or bipolar, and severe personality disorders.

The symptoms of the postconcussion syndrome may last for months or even years, although after a minor head injury, the symptoms usually do not persist longer than three months.

2.72 Pathogenesis

There is lack of agreement about whether the symptoms of postconcussion syndrome have an organic basis or are attributable to purely psychological factors, although evidence demonstrating an organic basis is accumulating. Alternatively, the symptoms may be attributable to a combination of organic and psychological factors.

The symptoms following mild head injuries have been ascribed to both focal and diffuse damage of the brain. Magnetic resonance imaging studies have demonstrated focal lesions in the frontal and temporal brain regions that are believed to correlate with behavior abnormalities seen after mild head injuries. Such focal lesions are believed to result from blood-brain barrier changes, inducing release of neurotransmitters, thereby facilitating abnormal interactions at neuronal receptor sites (Hayes, et al., 1992). The diffuse damage observed in the brain following mild head injury is believed to be attributable to swollen axons in the white matter of the cerebrum. Such swelling can lead to disconnection and degeneration of axons.

The argument for a purely psychological basis for the postconcussion syndrome is supported by several observations. There is a lack of good correlation between the severity of the head injury and the length of time symptoms persist. Also, following a head injury, patients often experience strong emotions, such as fear, which could be blamed for postconcussion symptoms. Factors such as a neurotic personality may also play a role.

Another view of the pathogenesis of the postconcussion syndrome is known as the interaction concept. The basis of this concept is actually a combination of the organic and psychological viewpoints regarding causation. The interaction concept stresses the interplay of organic and psychological factors; this theory has gained wide support, because of the inability of either the purely organic or purely psychological views to explain the observations associated with the postconcussion syndrome. For example, the organic view does not seem to explain how it is possible for symptoms to first develop weeks or even months subsequent to a mild head injury, while the psychological view seems to be at odds with the accumulating evidence of organic brain damage (Bohnen and Jolles, 1992).

Finally, there is another explanation for postconcussion syndrome, which is known as the coping hypothesis. This hypothesis states that the attempts of patients to compensate for cognitive defects on a long-term basis are responsible for the symptoms of postconcussion syndrome.

2.73 Diagnostic Considerations

In patients with mild head injury, neuropsychological testing provides the most useful diagnostic information (Katz and Deluca, 1992). However, it is essential that the patient not only be given neuropsychological tests but also be interviewed. The interview is extremely important, because it is possible to fake neuropsychological test results. A trained and experienced neuropsychologist can detect patients engaged in such faking.

The diagnosis of brain damage is made on the basis of the interpretation of the interview, an extensive evaluation of the patient's mental status and the data obtained from neuropsychological testing. Symptoms are assessed for the most part through the interview, and information processing efficiency and memory function through the mental status examination and neuropsychological tests.

The most sensitive neuropsychological test for detecting brain damage in patients with mild head injury is the PASAT-R.[11] Memory tests have shown that patients with mild head injury who have brain damage do more poorly than control subjects on verbal testing when a month has elapsed following the injury. The difference between the two groups narrows as more time elapses. A test called the revised Wechsler Memory Scale, which measures delayed memory, is more sensitive in detecting brain damage in patients with mild head injury

---

[11] *See* 2.59 *supra.*

than the revised Wechsler Adult Intelligence Scale (WAIS-R), which measures intelligence.

In making the diagnosis of postconcussion syndrome, the most important condition to exclude is a neurotic reaction to head injury, which is a maladjustment to head injury characterized by anxiety and depression (Bohnen and Jolles, 1992). It is also important to differentiate the postconcussion syndrome from post-traumatic stress disorder (PTSD). The latter condition involves emotional symptoms in response to an event that is particularly distressing. Consideration should also be given to the possibility that the patient is malingering.

One other possibility that may be considered is postwhiplash syndrome. As in the case of head injury, a whiplash injury may produce subjective symptoms, such as headache and fatigue. However, the whiplash syndrome is associated with dizziness, neck pain and cervical paresthesias (abnormal sensations such as burning) more often than the postconcussion syndrome. There is growing evidence that cervical (neck) injuries can indirectly result in damage to subcortical brain structures. Such injuries can damage the same brain structures that are damaged in a concussion.

2.80 INDICATIONS FOR HOSPITAL ADMISSION OR RELEASE

Whereas it is standard procedure to admit all patients with severe head injuries, the procedure for admission of patients with mild head injuries varies from hospital to hospital. Although patients who have mild head injury have a much lower risk of complications than those with severe head injury, an estimated 3 percent of mild head injury patients will deteriorate. Some of these patients are not identified as being in serious jeopardy, because the results of their neurologic examinations are normal.

2.81 Role of Computed Tomography

The central question regarding the use of CT in evaluating patients with mild head injury who have lost consciousness or have had amnesia is whether all such patients should undergo CT scanning. There are strong advocates on both sides of the controversy.

The main argument for routine CT scanning of all patients who fall into this category is that this technique is very accurate for identifying patients with focal intracranial injuries, such as hematomas. In one study of 1,538 patients with mild head injury (brief loss of consciousness or amnesia, a Glasgow Coma Scale total score of 13 to 15 and normal or near-normal neurologic examinations on admission), CT scanning identified 265 patients with either skull fractures or intracranial injuries. Of 1,339 patients without evidence of intracranial injury on CT scanning, none deteriorated (Stein and Ross, 1992). The authors believe that a patient with a normal CT scan and no other indications for admission can be safely discharged from the emergency department.

The usefulness of CT scanning for deciding which patients to admit was also confirmed in a study of 111 patients with mild head injury (transient loss of consciousness or significant post-traumatic amnesia, Glasgow Coma Scale total score of 14 or 15 and a normal neurologic examination) (Livingston, et al., 1991). The authors concluded that CT scanning is an accurate technique for identifying patients with mild head injury who are at risk for subsequent deterioration, and that patients with a negative CT scan and normal neurologic examination can be safely discharged without being admitted to the hospital.

Discharge under these conditions is recommended even in instances in which there is no reliable person at the patient's home to serve as an observer. According to the authors, CT scanning of patients with mild head injuries would permit more than 80 percent of these patients to be discharged from the emergency room.

Another opinion about the role of CT in the initial evaluation of patients with mild head injury advocates its use only on a selective basis. Instead of using CT routinely, an alternative strategy (Pitts, 1991) separates patients with a total score of 13 on the Glasgow Coma Scale into "good" and "bad" patients, based on their level of function. The "good" patients would not be required to undergo CT scanning initially but instead could be observed and required to undergo CT scanning if there was deterioration or no improvement over the subsequent six to eight hours. The "bad" patients would undergo initial imaging studies. Patients with a total score of 14 or 15 on the Glasgow Coma Scale would not undergo CT scanning unless there was suspicion of a depressed skull fracture or penetrating skull injury, or some sort of focal abnormality had been detected on the neurologic examination. If these patients deteriorated or failed to improve, then CT scanning would be indicated. The great majority of these patients do not have intracranial abnormalities that would require treatment and could be discharged from the emergency room or hospital ward without undergoing imaging studies.

There is also opposition to routine CT scanning on the basis of cost factors. However, this objection has been countered by arguments demonstrating that routine imaging studies are cost effective as well as resource effective (Stein, et al., 1993).

2.82   Potential Role of Magnetic Resonance Imaging

Magnetic resonance imaging is generally not used to assess patients with mild head injury when they arrive at the emergency room. The reasons include the fact that MRI scanners are usually located in an area of the hospital that is far from the emergency department, thereby creating a logistic problem, and the need for the patient to be placed inside a large magnetic ring to obtain images makes it difficult to manage patients with acute head injuries. Nevertheless, there is interest in MRI as an early assessment tool, because it is reported to be more sensitive than CT for detecting a number of brain abnormalities, such as diffuse axonal injury and subcortical contusion.

In one study, it was found that about 10 percent of patients with mild head injury who were discharged from the emergency room had brain abnormalities detected by MRI (Doezema, et al., 1991). Although it was possible that these abnormalities had no clinical significance, it was also possible that detection of such abnormalities may permit prediction of which patients will go on to have persistent symptoms or cognitive dysfunction. If the abnormalities were found to have predictive clinical value, then patients could be referred for neuropsychological testing or, in some instances, could be provided with information to help them adapt.

2.83   In-Hospital Observation

A major reason for admitting patients with mild head injury to the hospital is to permit them to be carefully observed for signs of deterioration. However, whether adequate observation is really provided has been questioned. One study on this subject found that in some hospitals, observation did not prevent mortality in patients with head injuries who were considered to be at low risk (Klauber, et al., 1989).

It has also been argued that if patients with mild head injury were routinely admitted to the hospital (as is sometimes advocated), many beds would be filled with patients who really do not need to be closely observed, while patients who did need close observation would find a lack of beds and attention (Stein and Ross, 1992).

2.84 Observation at Home

One common criterion for discharging a patient with mild head injury from the emergency room is the presence of a reliable person at home to observe the patient in case his or her condition begins to deteriorate. However, many patients do not have a reliable person at home to observe them, which means many patients with normal CT and neurologic examinations would be admitted, even though such patients almost invariably will not deteriorate neurologically (Livingston, et al., 1991). Moreover, many persons who are responsible for observation do not follow instructions given at discharge, and a sizable number deny ever receiving such instructions.

2.85 Age Factor

Another factor in deciding whether patients with mild head injury should be admitted to the hospital is age. Infants and the elderly are reported to be at increased risk of intracranial hematomas following initial evaluation, even in cases in which the results of neurologic examination are normal and CT scans are negative. Therefore, such patients should probably be routinely admitted to the hospital for observation and follow-up CT studies (Stein and Ross, 1993). Also, although vomiting following a minimal head injury is not connected with increased risk of intracranial complications, repeated vomiting by children can best be managed in the hospital.

2.90 TREATMENT AND REHABILITATION

Most patients who have sustained a simple concussion do not require treatment. After being evaluated in the emergency department, they are either discharged or admitted to the hospital for observation. Their symptoms generally begin to improve after a short period of time and continue to improve until they are totally resolved, usually within four weeks. In such cases, no follow-up is required. On the other hand, in some patients, postconcussion symptoms will persist beyond four weeks.

There are two main categories of persistent symptoms: neurologic sequelae, such as headache and dizziness, and cognitive and neurobehavioral sequelae.

Headache is the most common symptom that persists after a concussion. Treatment depends on whether the headache is a vascular type or related to muscle contraction (Goldstein, 1991). Drugs given for the vascular type of headache include beta-adrenergic blocking agents, calcium-channel blocking agents, nonsteroidal anti-inflammatory drugs (NSAIDs) and sometimes phenothiazines (a class of antipsychotic drugs). For headaches related to muscle contraction, patients are usually given NSAIDs or muscle relaxants.

If psychotropic drugs are given, they should be selected in accordance with the needs of the individual patient. Success in treating post-traumatic headache has been reported after giving the drug amitriptyline (a tricyclic antidepressant) and providing a counseling program. Administering phenelzine (a monoamine oxidase inhibitor antidepressant) is useful for treating depression following head injury initially and subsequently for treating headache. Behavioral techniques such as biofeedback therapy may also be useful.

Treatment of the various other types of neurologic symptoms, such as dizziness and ringing in the ears, that occur after cerebral concussion depends on the specific symptom (Zasler, 1992).

The recognition of cognitive and neurobehavioral sequelae following mild head injury has occurred relatively recently. With this awareness has come the establishment of special treatment programs to deal with these sequelae. Such treatment is generally done on an outpatient basis and consists of a multidisciplinary program that may continue for up to six months. Among the types of treatment offered are biofeedback therapy, stress management training, relaxation techniques, psychotherapy and counseling (Rosenthal, 1993). Whether such programs are really beneficial has not been adequately determined.

Rehabilitation programs for patients who have had a minor head injury include four components: reassurance, education, support and monitoring of progress (Katz and Deluca, 1992). Reassurance helps the patient realize that her or his symptoms are common and almost invariably will eventually disappear. Education is important because the patient as well as the patient's family require knowledge about what generally happens after a head injury. The importance of support is that it helps the patient deal with stresses that may seem overwhelming. With regard to monitoring, a series of neuropsychological tests can be given to guide, among other factors, the pace at which the patient resumes previous activities.

2.100   PROGNOSIS

Most patients who have a simple concussion recover fully after a few weeks and often sooner. The most lasting effect is probably a memory loss for events immediately before and after the head injury. Some patients do have persistent symptoms, called the postconcussion syndrome, that may last for months or even longer.[12] In most cases, these symptoms will eventually disappear.

If patients have undergone CT scanning and the results are negative, it is almost certain that they do not have an intracranial hematoma. If patients have not undergone CT scanning, there a slight possibility of a missed hematoma. Except among the elderly and infants, delayed-onset intracranial hematomas following a mild head injury do not occur. There is no known method for determining exactly which patients will develop delayed-onset hematoma.

2.110   CONCUSSION IN CHILDREN

Of the approximately 5 million children who have head injuries each year in the United States, about 200,000 of them are admitted to hospitals, and about 4,000 of them die. Although the vast majority of children fully recover, some end up with physical disabilities, learning problems, behavior and emotional disorders, and seizures.

2.111   Clinical Picture

Mild head injuries generally produce a brief period of initial unconsciousness. When consciousness is regained, the child is usually confused, sleepy and listless. The patient may also exhibit vomiting and irritability; infants are particularly prone to these symptoms following head injuries that do not even cause a loss of consciousness.

---

[12] *See* 2.70 *supra.*

Linear fractures of the skull occur relatively often in children with mild head injuries. However, such fractures do not seem to have an effect on the patient's clinical course.

Children who have severe head injuries are generally unconscious for longer periods of time than those with mild head injuries. There is also a much greater likelihood of finding focal neurologic signs, indicating the presence of a brain contusion.[13]

Usually the initial phase of a severe head injury will be accompanied by the greatest degree of neurologic deficit. If additional, nonlocalized neurologic signs begin to appear, this may indicate brain swelling; if localized neurologic signs develop, a secondary complication, such as a hemorrhage,[14] may be present. The lucid interval often experienced by adults after a loss of consciousness usually does not occur in children.

Infants and younger children are particularly prone to massive brain swelling as a result of severe head injury. Brain injury in general can lead to circulation problems and abnormal shifting of water and ions among neurons, glia (supporting cells in the brain) and spaces between cells. The shifting of calcium ions from the spaces between the brain cells into the neurons can lead to cerebral swelling as cellular membranes begin to break down. In the most serious situations, a vicious cycle can develop in which brain injury produces more cerebral swelling, and the increase of cerebral swelling exaggerates the effects of brain injury. If this cycle reaches the point that the intracerebral pressure is equal to the arterial pressure, the patient will not recover. In cases in which cerebral swelling cannot be easily controlled, surgery may be indicated.

Following a concussion, the child may seem drowsy, complain of a headache, act confused and sometimes vomit (this can also occur in adults). These symptoms are similar to those caused by an epidural hemorrhage; however, after a few hours, the symptoms disappear.

2.112   Diagnosis

The neurologic examination should emphasize ascertaining the state of consciousness, size and similarity of the pupils and their response

---

[13] *See also* ch. 3 for a discussion of brain contusion.

[14] *See also* ch. 4 for a discussion of hemorrhage and hematoma.

to light, extent of spontaneous movements and their symmetry, and reflex status. The patient's blood pressure, pulse and respiratory rate should be recorded during the examination. It is often valuable to examine the patient at close intervals, such as every five minutes, in order to detect whether the patient is progressing toward normal responses or the condition is deteriorating.

The Glasgow Coma Scale,[15] which is used to assess the status of adult patients with head injuries, is not useful for infants and younger children. Modifications of the Glasgow Coma Scale have been proposed. In one such proposal, the patient is rated from 4 to 1 on the basis of whether he or she open the eyes spontaneously, to speech, to pain or not at all; from 5 to 1 on the basis of whether his or her best verbal response is oriented, words, vocal sounds, cries or none at all; and from 5 to 1 on the basis of whether the child's best motor response is to obey commands, localize pain, flex to pain, extend to pain or no response. Normal total scores are based on age, with normal scores as follows (Menkes and Till, 1990):

- children 6 months old or younger—9;
- children ages 6 to 12 months—11;
- children ages one to two years—12;
- children ages two to five years—13; and
- children five years or older—14.

Since the length of memory loss for events before and after the accident is a useful indicator of the severity of the head injury, the extent of memory loss should be acertained, if possible.

As is the case for adults with head injuries, computed tomography scanning is the most useful diagnostic imaging technique for assessing whether there are intracranial complications in children with head injuries.[16] The value of magnetic resonance imaging in children appears to be similar to that in adults.[17]

Since most children with mild head injuries fully recover, it may be difficult to decide which children should be hospitalized. Generally it is thought that a child who has had only a brief loss of consciousness can be sent home and the parents instructed on watching for potential

---

[15] *See* 2.73 *supra.*

[16] *See* 2.53 *supra.*

[17] *See* 2.54 *supra.*

problems. Some reasons to admit children with mild head injury are a deterioration in the level of consciousness, persistent confusion and lethargy, excessive vomiting, uncertainty about the history of trauma, focal neurologic signs, seizures, a confirmed skull fracture (this is a matter of controversy, with some experts believing that children with skull fractures can be sent home), age less than two and a suspicion of child abuse.

2.113 Complications

There is an age difference in the incidence of acute subdural and epidural hematomas. Acute subdural hematomas are usually seen in infants at approximately six months of age. Acute epidural hematomas usually occur in children older than two years. This difference in incidence occurs because in older children, the dura is not as firmly attached to the skull, thereby permitting bleeding between the dura and skull to occur more readily. Physically abused infants who are repeatedly shaken with excessive force are particularly prone to developing a subdural hematoma.

Although a child's chance of death from an acute subdural hematoma is lower than that for an acute epidural hematoma, there is a greater chance of functional problems, such as motor deficits and cognitive impairment, due to the increased risk of brain injury.

2.114 Sequelae

The most prominent symptom of postconcussion syndrome in adults is headache, a condition that occurs only occasionally in children. Likewise dizziness, another prominent symptom in adults, occurs only infrequently in children. In general, there is much less consistency of post-traumatic symptoms in children than in adults, which makes it difficult to prove that this syndrome actually occurs in children. The most common symptoms that are believed to be manifestations of the postconcussion syndrome in children include hyperactivity, shortened attention span, outbursts of temper, sleep problems, moodiness and lack of discipline.

The child who exhibits the symptoms of postconcussion syndrome should be carefully evaluated to rule out the presence of some other condition. Support and reassurance should be given. In most cases, the symptoms will improve without intervention.

2.115 Prognosis

For children who have had a mild head injury with a brief loss of consciousness and no neurologic symptoms, full recovery can be expected in almost all cases. In one study of 53 children with mild head injury, no significant long-term deficits were found in intellectual, neuropsychological, academic or daily routine functioning, in comparison with a control group (Fay, et al., 1993). However, although a group as a whole may not show any deficits, certain individuals within the group may.

In children with more severe head injuries, the prognosis is more complicated. In general, children have a better prognosis than either infants or adults. For children under two years of age, the prognosis is poor.

One major difference between children and adults with regard to neurologic recovery from head injury is that children may demonstrate continued progression for more than three years, while in adults, recovery stops much sooner.

Approximately 25 percent of children who have an acute epidural hematoma will die. For the 75 percent of children who survive, the probability is high that they will not have neurologic problems (Roseman, 1990).

In general, if a child has only behavioral abnormalities during the period shortly following a head injury, full recovery should be anticipated. In some children who have had head injuries, sleepiness during the daytime has been found to persist for months and even years.

2.120 SPORTS-RELATED CONCUSSIVE INJURIES

Concussions are a relatively commonplace occurrence among individuals engaged in contact sports such as football. Nearly one in five high school football players will sustain a concussion in a single year.

For a number of reasons, concussions that occur during competitive sports can be considered a special type of mild head injury. In most instances, these injuries are less severe than head injuries occurring under other circumstances, such as vehicular accidents. In addition, they are often not related to any other injuries. Also, in almost all cases, sports-related head injuries are witnessed by players and spectators, so there is no question about the history of the incident. And uniquely, the management of an athlete with a head injury is often subject to the desire expressed by the athlete to return to competition.

Recommendations have been made about managing sports-related concussive injuries (Vollmer and Dacey, 1991). In the case of a mild injury in which any mental state of confusion lasts for less than one minute, the individual may return to playing again within 5 days, provided there are no post-traumatic symptoms. If the injury is severe enough to cause disorientation or confusion lasting for several minutes, the injured person should not play again until at least 10 days have elapsed. Injuries that are more severe should be managed in the same way as any other similar head injury that was not sports-related.

2.130 AMA EVALUATION OF PERMANENT IMPAIRMENT

Criteria for the evaluation of permanent impairment resulting from dysfunction of the brain have been developed by the American Medical Association in its *Guides to the Evaluation of Permanent Impairment* (AMA, 1993). These criteria are based on the limitations that the impairments impose on the patient with regard to carrying out the activities of daily living. Because neurologic impairment is closely related to mental and emotional functioning, behavioral disorders, mental disorders and pain should be considered when a neurologic evaluation is performed. Although it is rare for a cerebral concussion to result in any permanent damage, the failure to recognize and treat potential complications may, indeed, lead to permanent deficits.

2.200 BIBLIOGRAPHY

Text References

Adams, R. D. and Victor, M.: Principles of Neurology, 5th ed. New York: McGraw-Hill, 1993.

American Medical Association: Guides to the Evaluation of Permanent Impairment, 4th ed. Chicago: American Medical Association, 1993.

Berrol, S.: Terminology of Post-concussive Syndrome. State Art Rev. Phys. Med. Rehabil. 6:1-8, 1992.

Bohnen, N. and Jolles, J.: Neurobehavioral Aspects of Postconcussive Symptoms after Mild Head Injury. J. Nerv. Ment. Dis. 180:683-692, 1992.

Doezema, D., et al.: Magnetic Resonance Imaging in Minor Head Injury. Ann. Emerg. Med. 20:1281-1285, 1991.

Fay, G. C., et al.: Mild Pediatric Traumatic Brain Injury: A Cohort Study. Arch. Phys. Med. Rehabil. 74:895-901, 1993.

Goldstein, J.: Posttraumatic Headache and the Postconcussion Syndrome. Med. Clin. N. Amer. 75:641-651, 1991.

Hardman, J.M.: Cerebralspinal Trauma. In: Davis R. L. and Robertson D. M. (Eds.): Textbook of Neuropathology, 2nd ed. Philadelphia: Lea & Febiger, 1989.

Hayes, A. L., et al.: Pathophysiology of Mild Head Injury. State Art Rev. Phys. Med. Rehabil. 6:9-20, 1992.

Katz, R. T. and Deluca, J.: Sequelae of Minor Traumatic Brain Injury. Am. Fam. Physician 46:191-198, 1992.

Klauber, M. R., et al.: Determinants of Head Injury Mortality: Importance of the Low Risk Patient. Neurosurgery 24:31-36, 1989.

Livingston, D. H., et al.: The Use of CT Scanning to Triage Patients Requiring Admission Following Minimal Head Injury. J. Trauma 31:483-487, 1991.

Livingston, D. H.: Minimal Head Injury: Is Admission Necessary? Am. Surg. 57:14-17, 1991.

Menkes, J. H. and Till, K.: Postnatal Trauma and Injuries. In: Menkes J. H. (Ed.): Textbook of Child Neurology. Philadelphia: Lea & Febiger, 1990.

Pitts, L. H. The Role of Neuroimaging in Minor Head Injury (editorial). Ann. Emerg. Med. 20:1387-1388, 1991.

Roseman, N. P.: Acute Head Trauma. In: Oski, F. A., et al. (Eds.): Principles and Practice of Pediatrics. Philadelphia: J. B. Lippincott, 1990.

Rosenthal, M.: Mild Traumatic Brain Injury Syndrome. Ann. Emerg. Med. 22:1048-1051, 1993.

Stein, S. C. and Ross, S. E.: Minor Head Injury: A Proposed Strategy for Emergency Management (editorial). Ann Emerg. Med. 22:1193-1196, 1993.

Stein, S. C. and Ross, S. E.: Mild Head Injury: A Plea for Routine Early CT Scanning. J. Trauma 33:11-13, 1992.

Stein, S. C., et al.: Is Routine Computed Tomography Scanning Too Expensive for Mild Head Injury? Ann. Emerg. Med. 20:1286-1289, 1991.

Vollmer, D. G. and Dacey, R. G. Jr.: The Management of Mild and Moderate Head Injuries. Neurosurg. Clin. N. Am. 2:437-455, 1991.

Zasler, N.: Neuromedical Diagnosis and Management of Postconcussive Disorders. State Art Rev. Phys. Med. Rehabil. 6:33-68, 1992.

Additional References

Bohnen, N., et al.: Water Metabolism and Postconcussional Symptoms 5 Weeks After Mild Head Injury. Eur. Neurol. 33(1):77-79, 1993.

Strugar, J., et al.: Long-term Consequences of Minimal Brain Injury: Loss of Consciousness Does Not Predict Memory Impairment. J. Trauma 34:555-558, 1993.

Zwil, A. S., et al.: Organic and Psychological Sequelae of Traumatic Brain Injury: The Postconcussional Syndrome in Clinical Practice. New Dir. Ment. Health Serv. (57):109–115, Spring 1993.

CHAPTER 3

Contusions and Lacerations of the Brain

SCOPE

Contusions and lacerations are among the most serious effects of head trauma. Secondary events, such as brain swelling and herniation, can result in more extensive brain damage following the initial injury. Infants and young children sustain brain injuries less often and less severe than adults subjected to the same trauma. Quick and accurate diagnosis and treatment of surgically correctable lesions as well as management of the secondary consequences of brain injury help decrease the high mortality and disability that can be experienced. Because neurologic impairment is closely related to mental and emotional functioning, behavioral disorders, mental disorders and pain should be considered when a neurologic evaluation is performed.

SYNOPSIS

3.00   DEFINITION AND MECHANISMS OF INJURY

A head injury, particularly if it is severe, can result in a bruise of the brain tissue of the cerebral hemispheres, an injury called a cerebral contusion. This common type of cerebral injury differs from one in which the brain tissue is actually torn (a laceration). Although the initial impact of a head injury resulting in a contusion may lead to irreversible damage to brain cells in the bruised area, secondary events that are potentially reversible, such as brain swelling, may occur and result in even more extensive brain damage during the period following the initial injury.

It has not yet been determined exactly what mechanism causes a cerebral contusion. Usually it results from a blunt rather than a penetrating head injury. There is agreement that a contusion is usually related to the sudden acceleration/deceleration movement of the brain within the skull. Rotary forces of shear strain resulting from angular movements, as opposed to linear ones, are believed to play an important role.

There are two main types of cerebral contusions: coup and contrecoup. The latter type is the more common. A coup contusion occurs at the site of impact and results from an injury in which, at the moment of impact, the head is motionless. The impact causes accelerated motion of the brain. An example of the type of head injury is one resulting from a punch in a boxing match.

A contrecoup contusion occurs opposite the site of impact. The type of injury that produces a contrecoup contusion is one in which the head is moving and strikes an unyielding surface, such as occurs in a fall or hitting the dashboard in an automobile accident. In this type of injury, the skull stops first while the brain continues moving forward until it hits the skull. This is considered a deceleration injury.

Other types of contusions are herniation and fracture contusions (Hardman, 1989). In a *herniation contusion,* the brain has been forced through openings in the tentorium, the membrane separating the cerebrum from the cerebellum. A *fracture contusion* occurs along the edges of a depressed fracture of the skull. Since fracture contusions occur at the site of impact, they can be considered to be a form of coup contusion. The term contusion may also be used to refer to a bruise located deep within the brain, as opposed to the more typical contusion affecting the cerebral cortex. *(See Figure 3-1.)*

It is common for cerebral contusions to involve either the inferior surface of the frontal lobes or the anterior or frontal aspects of the temporal lobes. These portions of the brain are most often bruised because of the anatomic characteristics of the inside of the skull. The base of the skull contains a number of bony ridges and protuberances, including the sphenoid ridge and clinoid processes on the sphenoid bone, the petrous ridge on the temporal bone and the cribriform plate of the ethmoid bone. A contusion is much more likely to occur when the brain contacts these bony prominences than when contact is made with a much smoother surface, such as the inside of the superior aspects of the skull.

When infants and small children are subjected to the same head trauma as adults, they sustain brain injuries less often, and the injuries that do occur are comparatively less severe. Infants in particular are less prone to brain injury from a blow to the head, partly because the bones of the skull are not yet completely fused. In effect, in an infant's

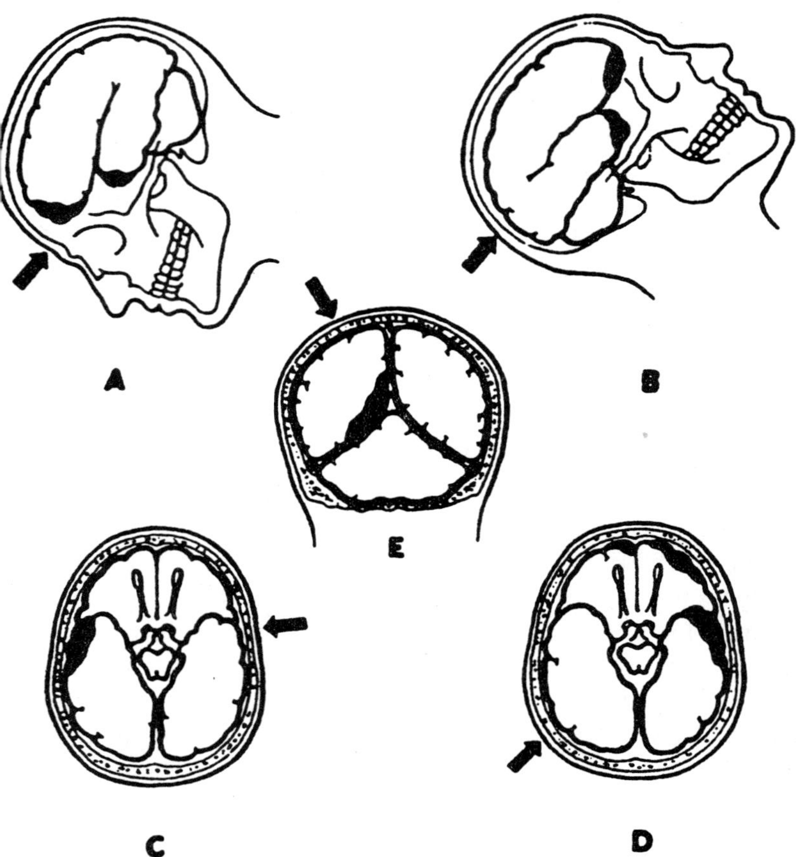

Fig. 3-1. Mechanisms of cerebral contusion. Arrows indicate point of application and direction of force; black area indicates location of contusion: (A) frontotemporal contusion secondary to frontal injury (coup); (B) frontotemporal contusion following occipital injury (contrecoup); (C) contusion of temporal lobe due to contralateral injury (contrecoup); (D) frontotemporal contusion due to injury to opposite temporo-occipital region (contrecoup); (E) diffuse medial temporo-occipital contusion due to blow on vertex.

skull, the unfused cranial sutures—the lines of union between adjoining bones—act as joints, providing some flexibility in response to mechanical force. To a lesser extent, small children also have an increased ability to absorb head blows (Ghajar and Hariri, 1992).

3.10 PATHOPHYSIOLOGY

The initial pathology of a contusion is similar to that of other bruises. Gross examination at this stage reveals a softening and discoloration of the brain tissue in the contused area. This configuration, known as pulping, first becomes evident about 12 hours after the injury. The damaged area swells and softens and reaches its greatest volume within 5 to 7 days.

3.11 Primary Event

In a cerebral contusion, tiny hemorrhages called petechiae appear; these result from torn capillaries. Blood from the bruised tissue may reach the surface of the brain and enter the cerebrospinal fluid (CSF). The severity of brain damage resulting from a contusion is related to the extent of vascular damage.

A cerebral contusion most often involves damage to the cerebral cortex (outer layers) of the brain. Microscopic studies show that although a contusion may cause neuronal death throughout the entire thickness of the cortex, most of the damage usually occurs in the more superficial layers.

When viewed under a microscope, the neurons within the area of the lesion have an ischemic appearance. (Ischemia is a reduction of blood flow due to constriction or blockage of blood vessels.) In a contusion, the lesion generally involves the crowns of the gyri, the convoluted ridges between anatomic grooves or *sulci* of the cerebrum.

Petechiae can also appear within the white matter of the cerebrum, below the cortex or gray matter. Such hemorrhages are usually diffuse and are also a result of damaged capillaries. In addition, a contusion within the white matter involves nerve fibers that can be severed or badly damaged.

The evolution of changes seen at a microscopic level in a cerebral contusion can be divided into three separate phases: acute damage, clearing and repair (Okazaki, 1989).

In the *acute damage* phase, cell death occurs in association with the small hemorrhages. In the *clearing phase,* phagocytic cells become active and engage in the removal of the damaged tissue. Finally, in the *repair phase,* there are large numbers of fibrillary astrocytes (highly branched neuroglial cells) along the outer margin of the lesion;

there is evidence of a repair process involving collagen (a fibrous protein that is abundant in connective tissue); and proliferation of fibroblasts (undifferentiated cells that give rise to connective tissue). The repair process often results in the healed area of brain adhering to the dura mater (the tough outer membrane that covers the brain). As a result, there may also be so-called fibroglial scars, which are believed to be responsible for seizure activity.

3.12 Secondary Events

During the period following a severe head injury resulting in cerebral contusion, swelling of the brain may develop. Such swelling can cause more brain damage than the initial impact and in many instances is potentially fatal.

Secondary brain damage probably occurs because once the brain has been traumatized, its cells are rendered more vulnerable to alterations in the extracellular environment. This enhanced vulnerability may be attributable to metabolic and ultrastructural derangements that occur within the traumatized cells.

Several pathophysiologic factors are associated with high morbidity and mortality following a severe brain injury (Ghajar and Hariri, 1992). These factors are:

- high intracranial pressure that does not readily respond to treatment;
- a lack of blood reaching the brain cells due to blood vessels being constricted or blocked (cerebral ischemia); and
- a decrease of blood flowing to the brain (secondary cerebral hypoperfusion).

Although both high intracranial pressure and dysfunction of the cerebral blood vessels are related to high morbidity and mortality, the relationship between these factors has not been clarified.

The propensity for swelling to occur following an injury to the brain is partly attributable to the anatomy of the skull and brain.

3.20 CLINICAL MANIFESTATIONS

In a severe head injury, the clinical findings vary according to the site of injury, the type of injury and the degree of cerebral edema (increase in amount of fluid in the brain outside the blood vessels) that develops.

Severe head injury usually results in loss of consciousness that lasts a considerable length of time. If there is a localized contusion of the brain, focal neurologic signs, such as weakness in the limbs, speech disorders, memory deficits or emotional dysfunction, may be evident. Continued development of neurologic signs indicates that the brain is progressively swelling.

Certain signs are associated with a poor prognosis. These signs include pupils that are fixed and dilated, cessation of breathing, decorticate posture (flexion of the arms or extension of the legs) and a score on the Glasgow Coma Scale (evaluation system for patients with brain injury, using indications such as eye opening and motor and verbal response) of less than 8.[1]

Patients who have had a moderately severe head injury may develop acute contusional swelling (Adams and Victor, 1993). Usually such patients are initially unconscious for five minutes to approximately one hour. After this period of unconsciousness, the patient starts to recover, but soon a relapse occurs, and the patient goes into a light coma or stupor. In cases in which there is a contusion but no other serious brain damage, relapse can be reversed by giving the patient dehydrating drugs. The effectiveness of dehydrating drugs in this situation appears to indicate that the relapse is attributable to brain swelling. In these patients, the plantar reflexes, which are elicited by stroking the sole of the foot, may be abnormal. (*See Figure 3-2.*) Such patients may have an increase in pulse rate and above normal temperatures over the course of several days. Usually their cerebrospinal fluid (CSF) contains blood, and the pressure is raised.

For a number of days after the head injury, the patient remains in jeopardy of having the temporal lobe of the brain herniate through the tentorium, an event of extreme seriousness resulting in compression of the vital brain stem and eventual death.

3.21 Temporal Lobe Contusion

The anterior and inferior portions of the temporal lobe are common sites of cerebral contusion. As is generally the case with lesions

---

[1] *See* 3.31 *infra.*

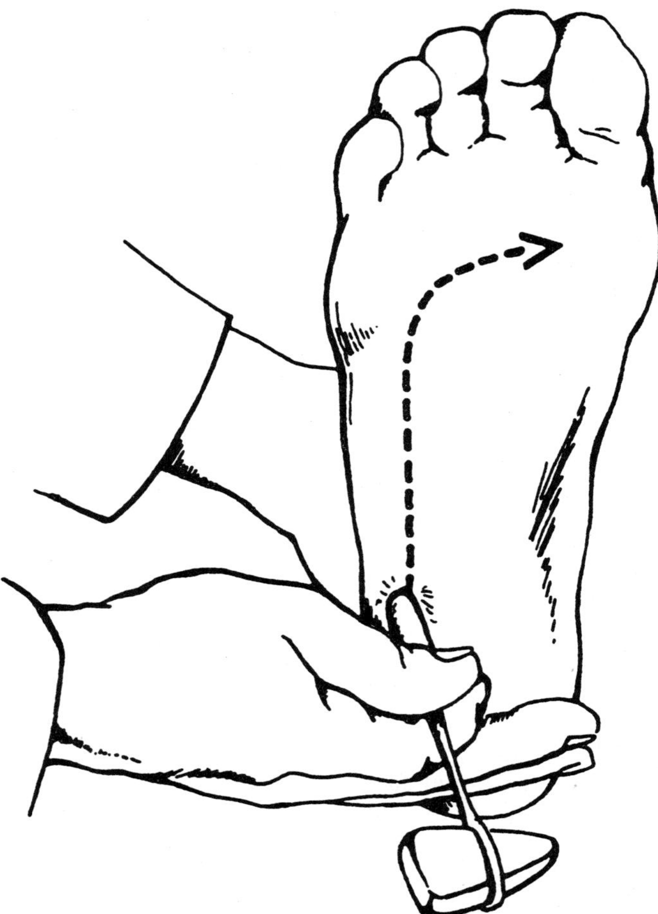

Fig. 3-2. The plantar or Babinski reflex is performed by stroking the foot in the direction indicated with a dull instrument, such as the end of the reflex hammer. A positive sign is extension of the big toe upward with downward flexion, and sometimes spreading of the other toes.

involving the cerebral cortex, the clinical manifestations depend on the extent of the injury, the type of injury and exact site. The temporal lobe is regarded as having an important role in such functions as visual recognition, perception of sounds, memory formation and emotion.

The left cerebral hemisphere, often referred to as the dominant hemisphere, usually plays the major role in language function, and left temporal lobe lesions have a detrimental impact on various functions involving language. *(See Figure 3-3.)* Lesions of the non-dominant right temporal lobe have been associated with loss of nonverbal memory. Some functions are affected regardless of which temporal lobe is damaged. These effects include emotional and behavioral changes.

The posterior superior region of the left temporal lobe is particularly important for language function. This critical part of the brain for language also involves adjacent areas of the parietal lobe and the inferolateral frontal lobe. A lesion in this area can result in *Wernicke's*

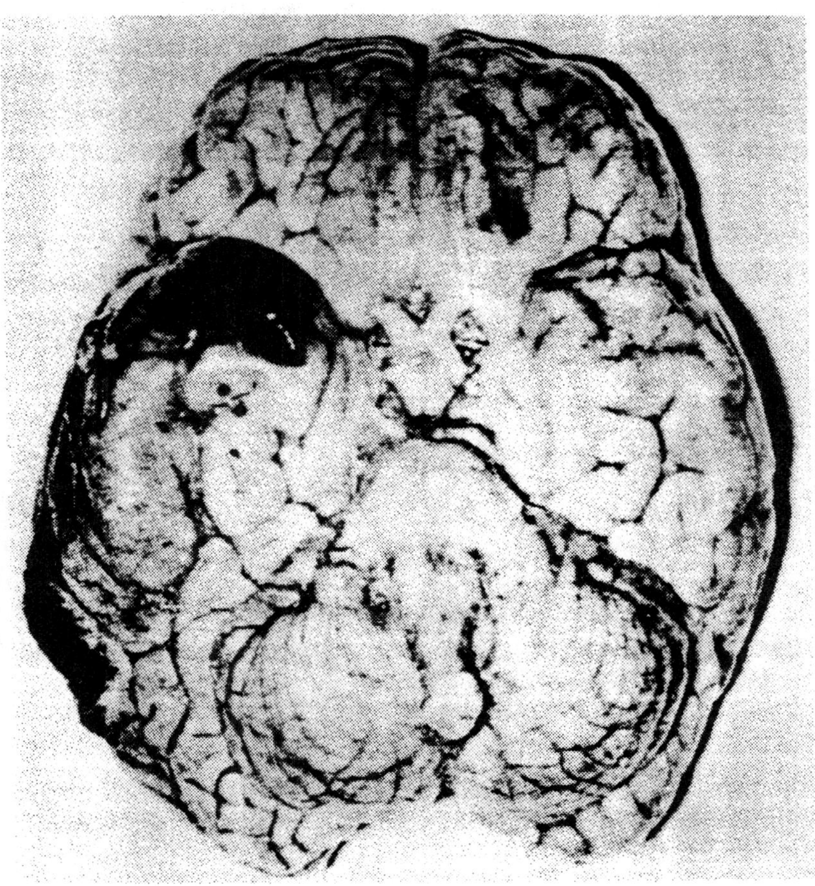

Fig. 3-3. Brain of a patient who died of cerebral contusion and intracerebral hematoma. The contusion is located in the left frontal lobe of the cerebrum.

aphasia, a condition in which the affected individual has problems with comprehending words, although the motor ability for speech remains intact. A patient with Wernicke's aphasia may speak and gesture freely while appearing to be unaware of any language problem. Although speech is fluid and accompanied by intonation and gestures, the words lack meaning. There are also patients with Wernicke's aphasia whose speech is not fluent. In these patients, speech is hesitant, and the individual may frequently appear to be trying to find the right word.

In the more severe cases of Wernicke's aphasia, patients may have a complete loss of social functioning, since they are unable to communicate. Reading and writing abilities are affected as well.

In one study of patients with brain contusions, it was found that in comparison with patients who had concussions, a contusion of the right temporal lobe was associated with an increased risk of impaired memory, impaired concentration, speech problems and sleep problems. A contusion of the left temporal lobe was associated with speech problems (Eide and Tysnes, 1992). Other symptoms were not found to be associated with a contusion specifically of the left or right temporal lobes.

3.22　Frontal Lobe Contusion

One of the most common sites of cerebral contusion is the inferior surface of the frontal lobe. The frontal lobe was the most recent portion of the brain to evolve, and it remains the least understood. The frontal lobes are the part of the brain most associated with the so-called higher functions, such as personality, abstract thinking, introspection, thinking ahead and so forth. These types of concepts are extremely difficult to define and study in a quantitative manner. Indeed, the relation between structure and function for most areas of the frontal lobes are continuing to be searched with positron emissin tomography (PET) scans and other techniques.

Smaller lesions of the frontal lobes often result in no discernible abnormalities. However, other lesions may cause clinical effects. These effects include:

- motor abnormalities;
- cognitive functional impairment, especially with regard to attention, concentration and the ability to sustain action;

- impairment of voluntary movement and diminished initiative and spontaneity; and

- personality changes with regard to such aspects of the personality as mood and self-control.

3.23 Parietal Lobe Contusion

Contusions of the parietal lobes are much less common than those of the frontal and temporal lobes, because the parietal lobes are adjacent to relatively smooth areas of the inner skull. The parietal lobes play a major role in somatosensory perception. The perception of the body and its relationship to the external world depends to a large extent on the functioning of the parietal lobes, particularly an area known as the postcentral gyrus. Small lesions of the postcentral gyrus can result in a loss of a patient's ability to recognize objects by using the sense of touch, a condition known as *astereognosis*. Lesions of either parietal lobe, but more often lesions of the right lobe, can result in a patient not paying attention to one side of the body, a condition referred to as *anosognosia*. Various other types of deficits have also been associated with parietal lobe lesions.

3.24 Occipital Lobe Contusion

Like the parietal lobes, the occipital lobes are adjacent to relatively smooth areas of the inner surface of the skull and therefore are not often bruised in head injuries. The occipital lobes, which are situated in the posterior part of the brain, are critical for visual perception and recognition. Lesions of the occipital lobes can cause a loss of vision and deficits of visual perception called *visual agnosia*. Disorders of visual perception include the lack of ability to identify and recognize faces, pictures, spatial arrangements, words, objects and colors.

3.25 Hypothalamus Contusion

The hypothalamus is a part of the brain that modulates the function of the pituitary gland, which releases hormones that control many functions of the body. Hypothalamic function is influenced by nerve pathways originating from many parts of the brain.

Six neurohormones are secreted by the hypothalamus. These neurohormones are dopamine, somatostatin, thyrotropin-releasing hormone, gonadotropin-releasing hormone, corticotropin-releasing hormone and growth-hormone-releasing hormone. The neurohormones secreted by the hypothalamus modulate the release by the pituitary of hormones affecting the endocrine glands such as the thyroid and those involved in reproduction.

Lesions of the hypothalamus may alter neurohormone secretion and therefore result in changes of pituitary gland function. Depending on the lesion, secretion of one, several or all the hypothalamic neurohormones may be decreased. Also, some lesions may result in an excessive increase of hypothalamic neurohormone secretion.

3.30   DIAGNOSIS

Rapid diagnosis of patients who have sustained head wounds is critical in lowering mortality. An estimated 60 percent of fatalities occur before patients can be admitted to a hospital—40 percent at the accident scene and 20 percent in the emergency room (Rowland, et al., 1989).

3.31   Neurologic Examination

The neurologic examination should emphasize evaluating the level of consciousness, the size of the pupils and how they react to light, the degree of spontaneous movement and whether such movements are symmetric, and reflexes.

The level of consciousness is evaluated by determining the score on the Glasgow Coma Scale. This scale ranges from a score of 3 to 15. The higher the score, the more alert the patient is believed to be. Quantitative scores are given for motor responses, verbal responses and eye opening. *(See Table 3-1.)*

Assessing the level of consciousness in infants and toddlers is a problem if they are too young to speak or respond to commands, since the Glasgow Coma Scale assumes these abilities. To overcome this problem, a children's Coma Scale may be used. This scale is based on ocular, verbal and motor responses, and total scores range from a maximum of 11 to a minimum of 3.

During the initial evaluation, the patient's vital signs, blood pressure, pulse and respiration should be recorded. Often, recordings are also made of the arterial blood gases.

Table 3-1
Glasgow Coma Scale
Level of Response

	Scale Value
Verbal Response	
Oriented	5
Confused	4
Inappropriate words	3
Incomprehensible	2
None	1
Eye Opening	
Spontaneously	4
To speech	3
To pain	2
None	1
Motor Response	
Obeys commands	6
Localizes pain	5
Withdraws	4
Abnormal flexion	3
Abnormal extension	2
None	1

It is extremely important that vital signs and neurologic status be checked repeatedly in order to determine if the patient's condition is deteriorating.

3.32 Computed Tomography (CT)

After the neurologic evaluation is completed, the patient generally undergoes computed tomography (CT) scanning. CT scanning records relative densities of intracranial tissues by transmission of x-ray photons through the cranium from a rotating source. A three-dimensional image of the brain and its surrounding bones is obtained.

CT scanning is often chosen over magnetic resonance imaging (MRI), a more sensitive and accurate technique, because CT is faster and involves less confinement and distress for the patient.

A small contusion located in the outer portion of the cerebral cortex may escape detection on an initial CT scan. A small area of atrophy may be detected by MRI about one month after injury (Kirkwood, 1990).

More severe contusions are much more easily detected on initial CT scanning. The lesion will be characterized by heterogeneous areas of high density that are surrounded by low-density areas with irregular margins. The high-density areas represent petechial hemorrhages, and the low-density areas represent necrotic tissue and edema (Olshaker, et al., 1993).

On a CT scan taken two weeks to six months after the injury, a contusion will have a different appearance. The high-density areas representing hemorrhage will be gone. The areas representing necrotic tissue will increase in density until they have a density that is similar to that of cerebrospinal fluid (CSF).

Five days after the injury, granulation tissue begins to proliferate around the edges of injured tissue. New small blood vessels form, but these new vessels do not have the property of a blood-brain barrier. The lack of a blood-brain barrier can be a source of diagnostic confusion if CT scanning with contrast material is carried out months later and it is not known that the patient had a head injury. In such cases, the contrast material can form ring-shaped areas of enhancement around the areas where the new blood vessels have developed. This type of pattern can be mistaken for a tumor, an infarction or an infection (Kirkwood, 1990).

3.33   Magnetic Resonance Imaging (MRI)

Contusions are demonstrated with great accuracy on MRI, and this diagnostic method may be used as the next step following initial CT scanning (Bernardi, et al., 1993). MRI employs proton resonance induced by a magnetic field to produce an image of tissue. Very low intensity signal areas representing hemorrhage are surrounded by high-intensity areas representing edema. The areas representing hemorrhage become brighter over the period of three to ten days following the head injury, during which time the hemorrhage is resorbed. The appearance of a contusion on MRI weeks or months after the injury is dependent on the amount of hemorrhage that was initially present.

There is evidence that MRI used in conjunction with single photon emission computed tomography (SPECT), a technique that permits direct measurement of regional brain function by measuring regional blood flow in the cerebrum, may provide improvements in evaluating patients with contusions. Like MRI, SPECT appears to be more sensitive than CT for detecting contusions. In a study of 18 patients with severe head injuries who had normal CT scans, both SPECT and MRI demonstrated brain damage in every patient (Prayer, et al., 1993). For 65 percent of the detected lesions, there did not seem to be any correlation between the brain structure that was damaged and loss of function. However, a complementary injury pattern suggesting a poor outcome was found. On MRI, 8 of 12 patients who had a poor outcome had cortical contusions and diffuse axonal injury. On SPECT, these same patients had cortical and thalamic hypoperfusion. It was concluded that by synthesizing the anatomic information obtained from MRI and the functional information obtained from SPECT, it was possible to better assess post-traumatic brain damage and to improve the accuracy of predictions of outcome (Prayer, et al., 1993).

3.40   TREATMENT

If patients with severe head injuries are resuscitated quickly and treated aggressively in a specialized medical setting, their functional prognosis can be improved. Without the advantages of such trauma centers, many patients are saved but are left with severe debilitation (Shackford, et al., 1989).

Once a contusion is diagnosed, the central concern becomes trying to prevent the potentially damaging effects of secondary processes, such as intracranial hypertension and cerebral hypoxia (lack of oxygen to the brain). Usually measures are taken immediately to control the intracranial pressure.

3.41   Cerebral Perfusion Considerations

Therapeutic intervention to prevent damage from secondary processes is related to the mechanisms of cerebral perfusion (the flow of blood to the brain).

In order to function, the brain requires a constant supply of oxygen from the blood. Under most circumstances, the brain maintains a constant cerebral blood flow through regulation of the smooth muscles of the cerebral vessels. This regulation is based on a linkage between metabolism and blood flow (Ghajar and Hariri, 1992).

The most important factor in regulating the smooth muscle tone is arterial carbon dioxide pressure, which affects the muscles through changes in hydrogen ion concentration in the blood. An increase in arterial carbon dioxide pressure and hydrogen ion concentration, and a decrease in arterial oxygen pressure, all cause the cerebral arterioles to dilate, which results in an increase in cerebral blood volume and intracranial pressure.

3.42 Intracranial Pressure Monitoring

In order to control the intracranial pressure, which should not exceed 15 to 20 mm Hg, monitoring is necessary. Usually the intracranial pressure is measured with a strain gauge or fiberoptic device attached to a catheter.

The measurements can be taken in the cerebral ventricles (a system of open spaces in the brain that have continuity with the central canal of the spinal cord), or they can be obtained epidurally (in spaces between the skull and dura mater), subdurally (in spaces between the dura mater and arachnoid) or in subarachnoid areas (in spaces between the arachnoid and the brain).

Although it is more difficult to go through the brain into the ventricles to measure the intracranial pressure, obtaining the measurements from the ventricles has advantages. For example, readings from the ventricles are global pressure values, which are important with regard to the administration of pressure-lowering drugs. Because of the way the brain is compartmentalized by the tentorium and falx cerebri, pressure readings obtained from places other than the ventricles may not reflect global values. Also, the CSF can be drained directly from the ventricles, which may reduce the intracranial pressure.

The procedure used to place a catheter in the ventricles, called a *ventriculostomy,* can be performed at the patient's bedside as well as in more specialized settings. In this procedure, a hole is drilled in the skull, and an opening is made in the dura mater using a special needle. A ventricular catheter is then passed through the hole in the skull, the opening in the dura mater and the brain, until the ventricle is reached. A loss of resistance to the catheter is felt when the ventricle has been entered.

In some patients who have diffuse cerebral edema, the ventricles are greatly reduced in size, resulting in so-called slit ventricles. For such patients, the decision may be made to monitor the intracranial pressure from an area other than the ventricles. However, even under such difficult conditions, by altering the ventriculostomy technique, it is still possible to achieve ventricular monitoring (Ghajar and Hariri, 1992).

One drawback of measuring the intracranial pressure with a ventricular catheter is the risk of infection, which is reported to be about 8 percent. Because of this risk, samples of CSF fluid are generally taken on a daily basis in order to monitor for infection. These samples are used to measure protein and glucose levels and obtain cell counts, and to do bacterial culture tests.

3.43 Reduction of Intracranial Pressure

The main objective of therapeutic intervention is to reduce intracranial pressure. Even if the patient's intracranial pressure is not elevated, prophylactic measures may be taken to prevent pressure elevation. Therapy is directed at keeping the pressure below 15 mm Hg.

Several types of therapeutic measures, both pharmacologic and nonpharmacologic, can be administered to lower intracranial pressure. These measures are often done in a stepwise manner, so that the ones that are usually most effective are performed initially, and the others are only done if the earlier measures fail.

[1] Hyperventilation

The first step in reducing elevated intracranial pressure is usually to lower the carbon dioxide level in the blood, that is, inducing hypocarbia, through hyperventilation. Since carbon dioxide is expelled during expiration, excessive respiration reduces the amount of carbon dioxide dissolved in the blood. The goal of this maneuver is to maintain the carbon dioxide pressure at 28 to 33 mm Hg (Adams and Victor, 1993). Since increased carbon dioxide pressure causes arteriolar dilation of the cerebral blood vessels and increased cerebral blood volume, keeping the carbon dioxide pressure at a low level should result in arteriolar vasoconstriction and therefore a decrease in cerebral blood volume. These events should lead to a decrease in intracranial pressure and an increase in cerebral perfusion.

Although hyperventilation is used routinely to reduce intracranial pressure, evidence indicates that in some cases, hyperventilation may actually result in a decrease in cerebral perfusion and therefore may be harmful (Ghajar and Hariri, 1992). The arteriolar vasoconstrictive effect of hyperventilation usually begins to decrease within two days, due to compensatory mechanisms of the kidneys that respond to changes in the acid-base relationship in the blood. Therefore, maintaining the vasoconstrictive effect requires additional hyperventilation. Patients may have to be hyperventilated for several days, with the carbon dioxide pressure maintained below 25 mm Hg, in order to overcome the effects of the kidneys' influence on blood volume. In these circumstances, when hyperventilation is finally stopped, there may be a rapid rise in intracranial pressure, and further hyperventilation may be of no avail. Indeed, prolonged hyperventilation can have an adverse effect (Muizelaar, et al., 1991).

In a study of 186 patients with severe head injuries (Glasgow Coma Scale score 8 or less), it was found that during the initial 12 hours after an injury, cerebral blood flow is significantly reduced and there is an increase in extraction of oxygen from the brain, which is indicative of ischemia (Bouma, et al., 1991). During this early period, hyperventilation to prevent brain edema may reduce blood flow to the brain even further and therefore be detrimental.

[2] Drug Administration

Among the types of pharmacologic steps that can be taken to lower intracranial pressure, the most effective is probably the use of diuretics. The osmotic diuretic agent mannitol is often given. Mannitol is administered as a 20 percent solution, with the dosage generally based on body weight.

Although mannitol is often effective in reducing the intracerebral pressure, it does present some disadvantages. One problem is that under certain circumstances, mannitol can cause increased brain edema. In cases in which the blood-brain barrier has been damaged by injury, mannitol is believed to leak through the damaged areas into the brain and cause local edema (Menkes and Till, 1990). If mannitol is given repeatedly to a patient, it can result in a state of excessive osmolarity (body fluids become more concentrated). It is important to recognize that if mannitol is given to a patient whose body fluid volume is already below normal (e.g., from dehydration or bleeding), he or she can go into shock from even a single dose of mannitol (Ghajar and Hariri, 1992).

Furosemide is a nonosmotic diuretic that is frequently given to lower intracranial pressure. This agent is sometimes considered to be preferable to mannitol because it has beneficial effects on sodium transport into the brain.

If neither of these measures work, barbiturates may be given. Barbiturates are usually not effective in lowering the intracranial pressure, but in some cases, they may work by reducing the metabolic activity of the brain (Adams and Victor, 1993). One danger in using barbiturates is that these drugs can lower the blood pressure and thereby have a detrimental effect.

Sometimes, when all else fails, steroids are administered, but their effectiveness is highly questionable.

[3] Other Measures

One other step used to reduce intracranial pressure is to lower the patient's body temperature, that is, induce a state of hypothermia. This is done by applying ice packs or covering the patient with a cooling blanket. By reducing metabolic demand and lowering the CSF pressure, brain damage may be avoided. However, this method in most cases is not effective.

If measures to lower intracranial pressure fail and the patient's condition starts to deteriorate, the existence of an intracerebral mass such as a hematoma should be ruled out, using CT scanning. It is critical that a mass be found and evacuated before herniation of the brain occurs and the advanced signs of brain stem compression, such as decerebrate or decorticate posture (rigid extension of the limbs), high blood pressure and slow heart rate, become evident.

Infants and young children with severe head injuries are especially prone to experiencing massive brain swelling. Procedures to control intracranial pressure for children are similar to those used in adults.

3.44 Prevention of Post-traumatic Seizures

Epileptic seizures may result from a head injury.[2] Of the estimated 420,000 patients in the United States who are hospitalized because of head injury each year, from 5,000 to 30,000 will develop post-traumatic seizures (Temkin, et al., 1990). Post-traumatic seizures are

---

[2] *See also* ch. 11.

those that develop after the initial injury, as opposed to seizures that may occur temporarily at the time of the injury.

The probability of seizure activity may be increased by scars formed on the surface of the cerebral cortex when contusions heal. Seizures are a special problem during the post-traumatic period, because they greatly increase the metabolic demands of the brain, which leads to an increase in blood volume in the brain and therefore an increase in intracranial pressure.

Post-traumatic seizures can require treatment for the remainder of a patient's life. To prevent such seizures from developing, antiepileptic drugs may be given prophylactically. A commonly prescribed drug for this purpose is phenytoin. To assess whether phenytoin is actually effective when given prophylactically, 208 patients were given the drug and 196 were given placebo in a double-blind study (without the physician or patient knowing which had been given) (Temkin, et al., 1990). It was found that during the first week of therapy, the group that had received phenytoin had a significantly lower incidence of seizures than the control group. However, after one week, the incidence of seizures was similar in both groups. It was concluded that phenytoin has a beneficial effect in preventing seizures in patients with serious head injuries only during the first week after the injury.

It is common for brain-injured children to receive prophylactic treatment for post-traumatic seizures. Usually they are given phenytoin, but if they are hypersensitive to phenytoin, they may be given phenobarbital or carbamazine.

3.50   PROGNOSIS

The level of consciousness is a good prognostic indicator. An estimated 85 percent of patients with a Glasgow Coma Scale score of 3 to 4 will die within the first 24 hours of being injured (Adams and Victor, 1993). The average mortality rate for adults with a Glasgow Coma Scale score of 8 or less is about 40 to 50 percent. Patients with a Glasgow Coma Scale score of greater than 8 have a lower probability of dying as a result of a head injury but may still have temporary or permanent neurologic deficits.

During the first week after the injury, the intracranial pressure may also be useful as a prognostic indicator in patients with a Glasgow Coma Scale score of 8 or less (Ghajar and Hariri, 1992). If the intracranial pressure persists above 40 mm Hg, there is a significant probability that the patient will die or be left with a major neurologic deficit, including the possibility of falling into a continuous vegetative state. If the intracranial pressure is in general less than 20 mm Hg, there is only a low probability of death, although it is possible that the patient will have long-term neurologic deficits.

The early and late outcome of head injury patients with clinical evidence of brain contusions of one or both cerebral hemispheres has been studied (Eide and Tynes, 1992). This study also included an analysis of the outcome of patients with concussion. In the first three months after the head injury, 43 percent of 86 patients who had more than one brain area with contusions either on one or both hemispheres had died. On the other hand, the 57 patients with a contusion of only one brain area and the 117 patients with concussion had made either good recoveries or had moderate disabilities. Late outcome was considered to be one to five years after the head injury.

Among contusion and concussion patients, headache, dizziness and sleep problems occurred with similar frequency. However, the patients with contusions had a greater incidence of impaired memory, impaired concentration, speech problems, weakness in the arms and legs, and seizures with loss of consciousness. The patients with contusions involving both hemispheres had the most difficulty in returning to school or work, in carrying out daily living activities and in social functioning.

In the long term, patients with head injury generally do better if they are given reassurance about their prognosis. In many cases, rehabilitation can begin once the CSF is determined to be clear, which is often within several weeks of the injury (Adams and Victor, 1993). Many rehabilitation centers are available for helping patients recover from head injuries.

The prognosis for children following a head injury is different than that for adults. The average mortality rates for children are about half those reported for adults. However, children under five years of age have higher mortality rates than children above five. For children under two, the outcome of a severe head injury is almost always poor.

Children who awaken from a coma within 14 days of a head injury have a high likelihood of eventually having normal function or close to it (Haslam, 1992). This is because the child's brain, still being in the developmental stage, has a greater ability to adapt to functional loss than does an adult's brain. In general, children have more complete recovery of function than adults and achieve recovery more rapidly. Unlike adults, children can continue to show recovery of neurologic function up to three years after a head injury and recovery of neuropsychologic function as long as five years postinjury.

3.60   AMA EVALUATION OF PERMANENT IMPAIRMENT

Criteria for the evaluation of permanent impairment resulting from dysfunction of the brain have been developed by the American Medical Association and appear in its *Guides to the Evaluation of Permanent Impairment* (AMA, 1993). These criteria are based on the limitations the impairments impose on the patient with regard to carrying out the activities of daily living. Because neurologic impairment is closely related to mental and emotional functioning, behavioral disorders, mental disorders and pain should be considered when a neurologic evaluation is performed.

Nine common categories of impairment are associated with disorders affecting the cerebrum. These categories are as follows:

1. permanent disturbances in the level of consciousness and awareness;
2. aphasia and disturbances of communication;
3. disturbances of mental status and integrative functioning;
4. emotional and behavioral disturbances;
5. special types of preoccupation and obsession;
6. major sensory and motor abnormalities;
7. disorders of movement;
8. episodic neurologic disorders; and
9. sleep and arousal disorders.

The system that has been developed uses percentage impairment of the whole person. Since a patient may have more than one of the nine criteria of impairment for cerebral dysfunction, a method has been developed to obtain the total cerebral impairment. Based on this method, the most severe of the first five categories with regard to percentage impairment is used to represent the cerebral impairment.

To find the total cerebral impairment, any of the percentage impairments from the last four categories are combined with the most severe of the first five categories, using a Combined Values Chart. (This chart permits the combining of any two percentage impairment values to obtain the combined value. Using the chart, any number of impairment values can be combined by combining two values and then combining the result with a third value, and so forth. Values can be combined from different organ systems as well as from the same system.)

3.61   Permanent Disturbances in the Level of Consciousness and Awareness

This category pertains to conditions found in stupor, coma and continuous vegetative state.

Brief repetitive or persistent change in the level of consciousness that limits the patient's ability to carry out ordinary activities is rated at 0 to 14 percent. A prolonged change in the state of consciousness that reduces capability for personal care and other daily activities is rated at 15 to 29 percent. Semicoma with total dependency and subsistence by artificial medical means is rated at 30 to 49 percent. Persistent vegetative state or permanent comatose state requiring total medical support is rated at 50 to 90 percent.

3.62   Aphasia and Disturbances in Communication

This category is concerned with deficits in comprehending and understanding both oral and written language and with deficits in speaking, reading and writing. These deficits are related to the symbolic use of language rather than motor ability.

Minimal disturbance in comprehending and producing language symbols used in daily living is rated at 0 to 9 percent, and moderate disturbance, at 10 to 24 percent. Inability to comprehend language symbols and production of unintelligible or inappropriate language is rated at 25 to 39 percent. A total inability to communicate or comprehend language symbols is rated as a 40 to 60 percent impairment.

3.63 Disturbances of Mental Status and Integrative Functioning

This category includes deficits concerning such general capabilities as being oriented with regard to time, place and personal identity; recent memory; the ability to perform simple calculations, repeat words or a short paragraph, spell, and understand and explain abstract thoughts; and judgment.

A condition in which impairment exists but the ability remains to perform adequately most activities of daily living is rated at 1 to 14 percent impairment. A patient who requires direction and supervision of daily living activities is rated as having a 15 to 29 percent impairment. Someone who equires directed care under continued supervision and confinement to home or other facility is rated at 30 to 49 percent; an individual who requires supervision for personal care and safety in any situation is rated as having a 50 to 70 percent impairment.

3.64 Emotional and Behavioral Disturbances

This category includes disturbances resulting from neurologic impairment and having psychiatric components as well. Examples of such disturbances are depression, manic states, behavior that is socially unacceptable and involuntary laughing or crying.

Mild limitation in daily social and interpersonal functioning is rated at 0 to 14 percent. Moderate limitation in a portion of daily social and interpersonal functioning is rated 15 to 29 percent. Severe limitation in essentially all daily social and interpersonal functioning is rated 30 to 49 percent. Severe limitation in all daily function so that there is a requirement of total dependence on another person is rated a 50 to 70 percent impairment.

3.65 Special Types of Preoccupation and Obsession

This category is related to emotional and behavioral disturbances.

3.66 Major Sensory and Motor Abnormalities

This category includes sensory disturbances that may be fairly typical as well as some that may be difficult to assess on a medical examination. Judgment may be required in order to decide whether such disturbances can be considered to permanently impair a patient's ability to perform daily activities.

This category also includes motor abnormalities, such as involuntary movements, disturbances of tone and posture, disturbances that limit voluntary movements, impairment of movements carried out synergistically, disturbances affecting walking and manual dexterity, and convulsive disorders involving the cerebrum. *(See Figure 3-4.)*

3.67   Disorders of Movement

This category is related to motor abnormalities.

3.68   Episodic Neurologic Disorders

This category includes epilepsy, seizures and convulsive disorders.

A paroxysmal (sudden recurrence) disorder that has predictable characteristics but occurs unpredictably and does not impose limitations on ordinary activity is rated at 0 to 14 percent. A paroxysmal

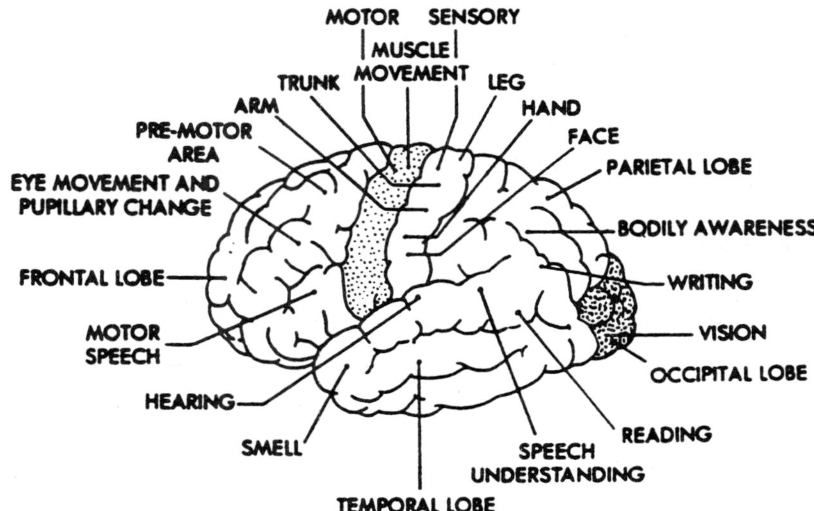

Fig. 3-4. The cerebrum, showing the function of each cortical zone.

disorder interfering with some daily living activities is rated at 15 to 29 percent. A severe paroxysmal disorder that occurs so often that activities must be supervised, protected or restricted is rated at 30 to 49 percent. An uncontrolled paroxysmal disorder that is so severe and occurs so often that a patient's daily activities are completely limited is rated at 50 to 70 percent.

3.69 Sleep and Arousal Disorders

This category concerns disorders related to an inability to fall asleep or to remain sleeping, excessive sleeping, an abnormal sleep-wake schedule and dysfunctions involving the stages of sleep.

Reduced alertness during the day that still permits most daily activities to be carried out is rated at 1 to 9 percent. Reduced alertness during the day to the extent that some supervision is required for carrying out daily activities is rated at 10 to 19 percent. Reduced alertness during the day that greatly limits daily activities and requires supervisory care is rated as a 20 to 39 percent impairment. Severely reduced alertness during the day making it impossible for patients to care for themselves in any way is rated at 40 to 60 percent.

3.100 BIBLIOGRAPHY

Text References

Adams, R. D. and Victor, M.: Principles of Neurology, 5th ed. New York: McGraw-Hill, 1993.

American Medical Association: Guides to the Evaluation of Permanent Impairment, 4th ed. Chicago: American Medical Association, 1993.

Bernardi, B., et al.: Neuroradiologic Evaluation of Pediatric Craniocerebral Trauma. Top. Magn. Reson. Imaging 5:161-173, 1993.

Bouma, G. J., et al.: Cerebral Circulation and Metabolism after Severe Traumatic Brain Injury. The Elusive Role of Ischemia. J. Neurosurg. 75:685-693, 1991.

Eide, P. K. and Tysnes, O. B.: Early and Late Outcome in Head Injury Patients with Radiological Evidence of Brain Damage. Acta Neurol. Scand. 86:194-198, 1992.

Ghajar, J. and Hariri, R. J.: Management of Pediatric Head Injury. Pediatr. Clin. North Am. 39(5):1093-1125, 1992.

Hardman, J. M.: Cerebrospinal Trauma. In: Davis R. L. and Robertson D. M. (Eds.): Textbook of Neuropathology, 2nd ed. Philadelphia: Lea & Febiger, 1989.

Haslam, R. H. M.: Chapter 20: The Nervous System. In: Behrman, R. E., et al. (Eds.): Nelson Textbook of Pediatrics, 14th ed. Philadelphia: W. B. Saunders, 1992.

Kirkwood, R. J.: Essentials of Neuroimaging. New York: Churchill Livingstone, 1990.

Menkes, J. H. and Till, K.: Postnatal Trauma and Injuries. In: Menkes, J. H. (Ed.): Textbook of Child Neurology. Philadelphia: Lea & Febiger, 1990.

Muizelaar, J. P., et al.: Adverse Effects of Prolonged Hyperventilation in Patients with Severe Head Injury: A Randomized Clinical Trial. J. Neurosurg. 75:731-739, 1991.

Okazaki, H.: Fundamentals of Neuropathology: Morphologic Basis of Neurologic Disorders, 2nd ed. New York: Igaku-Shoin, 1989.

Olshaker, J. S., et al.: Head Trauma. Emerg. Med. Clin. North Am. 11:165-186, 1993.

Prayer, L., et al.: Cranial MR Imaging and Cerebral 99mTc HM-PAO-SPECT in Patients with Subacute or Chronic Severe Closed Head Injury and Normal CT Examinations. Acta Radiol. 34:593-599, 1993.

Rowland, L. P., et al.: Merritt's Textbook of Neurology: Trauma. Philadelphia: Lea and Febiger, 1989.

Shackford, S. R., et al.: Epidemiology and Pathology of Traumatic Deaths Occurring at a Level I Trauma Center in a Regionalized System: The Importance of Secondary Brain Injury. J. Trauma 29:1392-1397, 1989.

Temkin, N. R., et al.: A Randomized Double-Blind Study of Phenytoin for the Prevention of Post-traumatic Seizures. N. Engl. J. Med. 323:497-502, 1990.

CHAPTER 4

Traumatic Intracranial Hemorrhage and Hematoma

SCOPE

The clinical consequences of hemorrhages and hematomas depend on the size and location of the vessel and the amount of bleeding. Epidural hematomas can result from head trauma that seems minimal. Favorable outcome is strongly correlated with shorter interval from injury to care. Subdural hemorrhages or hematomas are divided into acute, subacute and chronic stages. Subarachnoid hemorrhages commonly arise from trauma but may also be spontaneous. CT is the diagnostic method of choice, with cerebral angiography no longer part of the routine evaluation. Traumatic aneurysms can develop immediately following injury, or months or years later. Although surgery is not always indicated, when it is undertaken, it should be extensive enough to adequately take care of any problems that are present. The AMA evaluation system describes several categories of impairment resulting from damage to the brain.

SYNOPSIS

4.00 INTRODUCTION

Traumatic intracranial hemorrhages and hematomas result from trauma to the arteries, veins and dural sinuses of the brain. Injury to the brain can cause one or more vessels to rupture and hemorrhage. The clinical consequences of the injury depend on the size and location of the vessel and the amount of bleeding that results.

Traumatic brain injury is a significant health problem. Approximately 7 million traumatic brain injuries occur in the United States each year, and approximately 100,000 of these result in lifelong debilitating loss of function (Gean, 1994). Although most survivors of severe head injuries suffer major cognitive deficits, even minor injuries are associated with an increased incidence of memory deficits, difficulties with balance and psychological symptoms lasting for months following the injury.[1]

Head injuries are traditionally divided into primary and secondary injuries. *Primary* injuries are those that occur at the moment of impact and are directly related to the initial contact or inertial forces occurring during the injury. *Secondary* injuries are those that develop after the initial impact. Although an infinite number of combinations of

---

[1] *See also* ch. 1.

variables can interact to produce different injuries, the location and severity of traumatic brain lesions are often quite predictable.

Primary traumatic lesions can be extra-axial or intra-axial. *Extra-axial* lesions usually result from hemorrhage into the meningeal spaces and include subdural, epidural, subarachnoid and intraventricular hemorrhage. *(See Figure 4-1.)* These lesions are usually produced by shearing of the blood vessels on the surface of the brain or by injuries altering the formation of the skull and brain, causing direct laceration of the meningeal vessels. *Intra-axial* primary lesions include cerebral hematomas, which result from direct laceration of the brain or from shearing strains and pressures generated during impact.

Secondary traumatic brain lesions are usually due to complicating pathologic processes that occur as a result of the brain's response to injury. These injuries may develop within hours to years following the initial trauma. They include infection, hypotension (low blood pressure), hypoxia (insufficient supply of oxygen), anoxia (total lack of oxygen), post-traumatic seizures, elevated intracranial pressure, brain herniation, fluid imbalance, delayed hemorrhage and disorders of cerebrospinal fluid formation, circulation and resorption.

Secondary brain injuries are generally considered to be treatable. The majority of patients who die despite extensive medical treatment and surgery do so because of secondary injuries, usually cerebral edema (swelling due to accumulation of fluid) and brain stem compression. Accurate and expeditious diagnosis of primary and secondary injuries optimizes treatment and helps prevent further secondary damage.

4.01   Classification of Hemorrhage and Hematoma

Intracranial hemorrhages can be classified into extra-axial and intra-axial hemorrhages. *Extra-axial* hemorrhages develop within the spaces surrounding the exterior of the brain. *Intra-axial* hemorrhages develop within the brain matter.

Extra-axial hemorrhages are characterized according to their location in relation to the three meningeal layers surrounding the brain. The pia mater is the deepest layer of the meninges. It completely covers the brain surface, conforming to the cortex, and also covers the cerebral vessels that extend into the brain parenchyma (functional tissue). The arachnoid layer is superficial to the pia mater and is

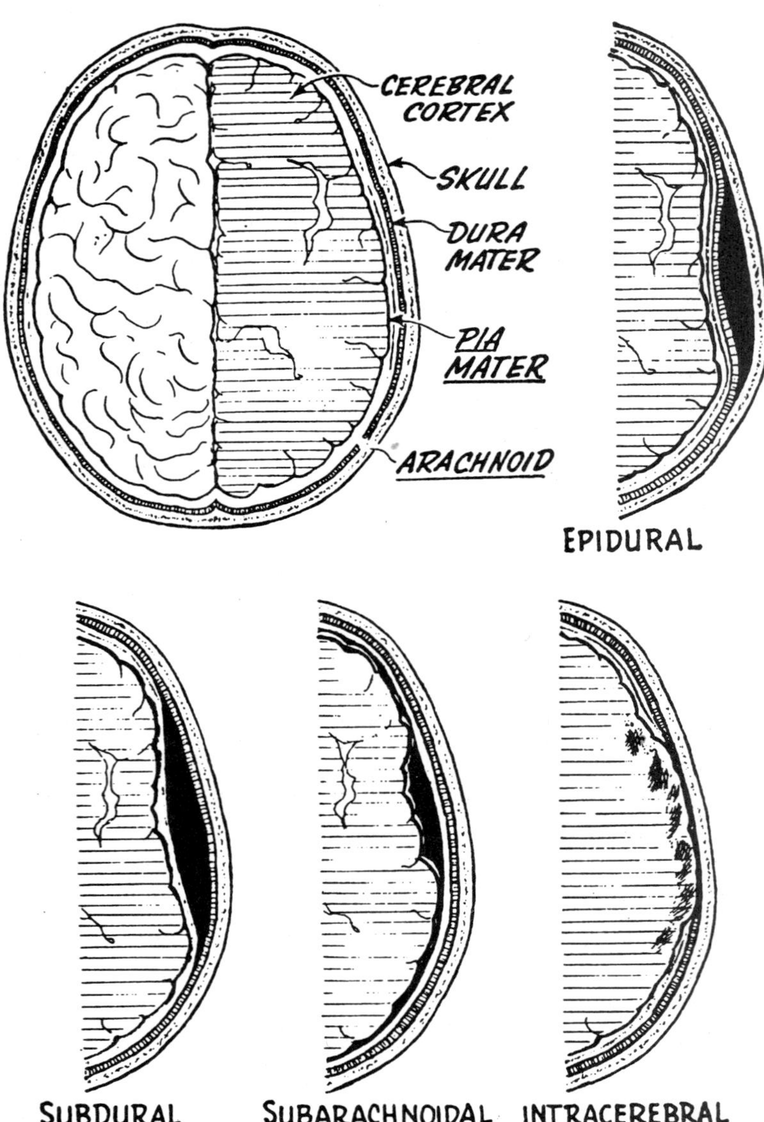

Fig. 4-1. The meninges surrounding the cerebrum (top left), and common types of intracranial hemorrhage.

attached to the pia and, therefore, the brain surface by fine arachnoid trabeculations (bands of tissue). The subarachnoid space is located between the arachnoid and pia; it is normally very thin and contains a small amount of cerebrospinal fluid (CSF). The third layer is the dura mater, a tough fibrous bi-layered membrane overlying the arachnoid. It has an inner meningeal layer and an outer periosteal layer. The major types of meningeal hemorrhages are epidural, subdural and subarachnoid.

[1]　Epidural (Extradural) Hemorrhage (EDH)

Extradural or epidural hemorrhage (EDH) develops between the outer dural layer and the inner table of the skull in the potential space called the epidural space. Blood from ruptured vessels between the dura and skull has no means of exit, causing it to accumulate within the epidural space, thereby forming a hematoma. As the hematoma expands, it acts like a space-occupying mass lesion, which compresses the brain (herniation).

[2]　Subdural Hemorrhage

Subdural hemorrhage occurs between the dural membrane and the underlying arachnoid membrane. This is normally a thin space containing a small amount of fluid. There are few attachments between the dura and arachnoid; therefore, when hemorrhage occurs within the subdural space, a spreading mass lesion may come to occupy a large surface area and cause herniation of the brain.

[3]　Subarachnoid Hemorrhage (SAH)

Subarachnoid hemorrhage (SAH) is the presence of blood in the subarachnoid space (located between the arachnoid and pia membranes). This space normally contains cerebrospinal fluid (CSF). Therefore, when bleeding occurs, the blood mixes with cerebrospinal fluid and usually does not clot or form a space-occupying mass lesion.

[4]　Intraventricular Hemorrhage

Intraventricular hemorrhage is the presence of blood within the ventricles of the brain. Most typically it develops via direct extension from an adjacent intracerebral hematoma. It can also be produced by direct penetrating wounds.

Other types of intra-axial hemorrhage include intracerebral hemorrhage, which may range from small petechial hemorrhages to massive fatal hemorrhages. Intracerebellar hemorrhages are frequently associated with lacerations of the brain. Contusions (injuries to the cerebral cortex) may result in extravasation (seepage) of blood into tissues.[2]

Although the various types of hemorrhage are usually discussed separately because of their distinctive clinical features, it is important to remember that on many occasions, they do not occur alone and that the patient may have two or more of these lesions simultaneously.

4.02   Other Traumatic Vascular Lesions

Primary vascular lesions may remain clinically silent for days to years and then become manifest as a secondary vascular lesion. This is often true for injuries such as vascular dissection, carotid-cavernous sinus fistula and pseudoaneurysm. Post-traumatic infarction may also occur; this can be caused by hypoxia-anoxia, arterial embolic disease, increased intracranial pressure, venous thrombosis and vascular compression due to brain herniation or an overlying extra-axial (within the spaces surrounding the exterior of the brain) collection of blood. It is extremely important to recognize that these lesions may develop after a history of head trauma. Early recognition and treatment significantly improve the prognosis for these conditions, which are often life threatening.

4.10   EPIDURAL HEMATOMAS

Epidural hematomas (EDHs) are usually a result of head trauma. They are often caused by skull fractures;[3] however, they may also result from seemingly minimal trauma. Under normal conditions, there is no intracranial epidural space because of the close attachment of the outer dural layer to the inner table of the skull. An epidural space can be created following trauma if the dura is forcefully stripped away from the skull at the moment of impact. This space can then fill with blood from injured meningeal vessels, diploic veins (vessels of the cranial bones) or dural sinuses, thus creating an epidural hematoma. In addition to the force of impact creating an epidural space, arterial extravasation (leakage) may exert sufficient pressure to strip the dura farther from the skull, resulting in rapid enlargement of the EDH.

---

[2] *See also* ch. 3.

[3] *See also* ch. 6.

The size of the enlarging hematoma is often limited by arterial thrombosis at the site of injury and by a tamponade effect of the underlying brain. This helps explain the fact that not all linear skull fractures result in EDHs. Not all trauma resulting in injury to the dura and meningeal artery results in EDH, probably due to the fact that the epidural space can be spontaneously decompressed if the extravasated blood escapes through either a skull fracture, a tear in the dura or a venous fistula.

4.11 Incidence

Epidural hematomas have been reported to occur in 0.2 to 12 percent of all patients with head trauma (Gean, 1994). The peak incidence is in the second and third decades of life, with less than 6 percent occurring in patients over 60 years of age and less than 3 percent occurring in patients less than 3 years of age.

There are several reasons for the lower incidence of EDHs among children and the elderly. Most significantly, the incidence of severe head trauma is less common in these patients than in young and middle-aged adults. In the elderly, the dura is more adherent to the inner surface of the skull and, therefore, it is less likely to separate to form an epidural space. In children, the skull is more compliant and the meningeal groove is very shallow; therefore, the artery can be more readily displaced without damage.

4.12 Location of Hematoma

Clearly, the location of hematoma is related to the site of injury. The most common region for epidural hematomas is beneath the squamosal region of the temporal bone. This area accounts for approximately 75 percent of all EDHs. The middle meningeal artery running beneath this region is particularly prone to injury.

The high incidence of EDHs in this region is probably due to the fact that this is the thinnest portion of the skull, and the middle meningeal artery in this region is partially embedded in the inner table and therefore is relatively fixed within the skull. Other sites of EDHs include the parietotemporal, frontotemporal, parieto-occipital and frontal regions.

Although subdural hematomas are more common than EDHs in the supratentorial region (the tentorium cerebelli separates the superior surface of the cerebellum from the occipital lobes, defining supratentorial and infratentorial compartments), EDHs are more common in the infratentorial region. Infratentorial EDHs are more likely to be of venous origin than arterial, and venous EDHs are the most common space occupying masses in the posterior fossa. Venous EDHs are due to bleeding from the meningeal and diploic veins or from the dural sinuses into the epidural space.

Several factors account for the predominance of venous-derived EDHs in the infratentorial region. One is that there are more posterior fossa dural veins than dural arteries. These veins include the straight sinus, occipital sinus, transverse sinuses and sigmoid sinuses, which surround a large portion of the cerebellum. In comparison, only three significant meningeal arteries are located in the posterior fossa: the anterior and posterior meningeal arteries and the meningeal branch of the occipital artery.

Another reason for the prevalence of venous EDHs is that the thick wall of the occipital bone and the thick, soft tissues of the neck may serve to buffer the energy of impact in the posterior fossa. Veins are more easily disrupted than arteries, and the force generated within the posterior fossa may often be insufficient to sever arteries but sufficient to disrupt the veins. Most posterior fossa EDHs involve the torcular Herophili (the confluence of the dural sinuses) or the transverse sinus, and they are almost always caused by a linear fracture originating near the inion (a point on the external occipital protuberance at the intersection of the midline) and extending across the posterior fossa to the foramen magnum.

In contrast to the infratentorial dural sinuses, the bridging cortical veins located between the cerebellar hemispheres and the inner layer of the dura are not frequently disrupted. Motion of the cerebellum is less than the cerebrum, because cerebellar mass is considerably less than that of the cerebrum. Therefore, the surface cerebellar veins crossing the subdural space are less often injured. In addition, the cerebellum is surrounded by large spaces containing cerebrospinal fluid, which can absorb a considerable portion of the energy of impact.

Venous EDH should always be suspected whenever a fracture occurs over a major venous sinus. The presence of air within the dural sinus should also suggest laceration of the sinus wall. Venous EDHs in the supratentorial region usually result from an injury to either the superior sagittal sinus or the sphenoparietal sinus. Unlike arterial extravasation, venous extravasation does not usually exert sufficient pressure to cause further stripping of the dura from the inner table. Therefore, venous EDHs rarely expand. If they do expand, it is usually because a large section of dura is stripped from the skull at impact.

Acute life-threatening epidural hemorrhages are usually arterial. Bleeding may be followed by spasm and clot formation. However, if the artery continues to bleed and the dura is stripped away from the skull, the large, egg-shaped hematoma begins to compress the adjacent brain tissue. If hemorrhage is sufficient, it can produce a sizeable mass that causes compression of the underlying brain. This may occur within 24 hours of the injury. Typically the temporal lobe of the cerebrum is then forced downward and medially by the enlarging hematoma, causing herniation of the uncus underneath the tentorium (piece of dura mater that separates the cerebrum from the cerebellum). This brain shift and herniation cause compression of blood vessels, particularly the posterior cerebral artery, which lies beneath the uncus and hippocampus. This circulatory disturbance can cause necrosis (tissue death) of the compressed vessels. Stasis (cessation of function) of cerebral circulation due to decreased venous return and blood sludging will produce sudden death. When herniation results in brain stem compression, death occurs because the centers that regulate cardiorespiratory function located in the brain stem are interfered with and no longer function.

Organization and resorption of EDHs involve essentially the same processes as those occurring in subdural hematomas. Resorption is carried out by perivascular cells, including phagocytes, fibroblasts and an glioblasts, which are derived from the inner dural layer. These proliferate and grow into the blood clot. New blood vessels formed following the injury are less resilient than the original vessels and are, therefore, more vulnerable to minor stresses than the original dural vessels.

4.13   Signs and Symptoms

If the underlying brain is not injured during the initial trauma, the signs and symptoms caused by an EDH are due to the mass effect of the expanding extra-axial collection. Although there is usually a correlation between the size of the mass and the severity of symptoms, there are exceptions to this trend. Brain compression and death may follow in the wake of a small acutely developing hematoma, while a larger clot may be tolerated for weeks if its rate of accumulation is slow.

The larger the accumulated mass, the higher the incidence of preoperative coma. EDHs greater than 150 mL (milliliters) in volume are observed in approximately 25 percent of comatose patients and 3 percent of noncomatose patients. EDHs of less than 90 mL in volume are observed in 56 percent of comatose patients and in 86 percent of noncomatose patients (Rivas, et al., 1988).

The presenting symptoms of an EDH are also determined by the location of the hematoma. EDHs located in the temporal region usually present earlier, due to their displacement of the brain stem. Temporal EDHs often cause uncal herniation, producing anisocoria (a condition in which the two pupils are not of equal size) in approximately 40 percent of patients. In most of these patients, the dilated pupil is ipsilateral (on the same side) to the EDH. Up to 60 percent of patients experience hemiparesis (weakness affecting one side of the body) that, in 90 percent of patients, is contralateral (on the opposite side) to the epidural mass.

Classically EDHs have been associated with a brief initial period of unconsciousness followed by a lucid interval during which the patient's neurologic status returns to normal. Subsequently, as the EDH increases in size, rapid deterioration of consciousness occurs. However, this classic sequence of events occurs in less than 30 percent of patients and can be caused by other brain lesions in addition to EDH.

Approximately half the patients with EDH never experience a loss of consciousness after the injury. Patients with venous hemorrhages tend to have longer lucid intervals than those with arterial hemorrhages. Patients with a rapidly developing EDH located within the posterior fossa rarely have a lucid interval, and signs of acute brain stem compression with respiratory disturbances can occur before any localizing signs.

[1]   Headache

Headache is the most common symptom among conscious patients and is most likely due to stretching of the pain-sensitive meningovasculature as the brain is displaced away from the skull. Convulsive seizures may occur and be generalized or focal.[4]

[2] Pupils

Early in the course of hematoma development, many patients have normal and reactive pupils, although there may be divergent strabismus (cross eyes) or conjugate deviation toward the side of the hematoma. With displacement of the temporal lobe and brain stem compression, oculomotor abnormalities may occur.

Displacement of the oculomotor nerve, the fibers of which constrict the pupils, can cause paralysis of the nerve, producing a dilated, fixed pupil that is unreactive to light on the same side as the hematoma (ipsilateral). Occasionally the ipsilateral pupil is constricted. Further temporal lobe displacement induces compression of the opposite oculomotor nerve, causing the opposite (contralateral) pupil to become fixed and dilated. Ptosis (drooping of the upper eyelid) may occur.

[3] Vision Disorders

With incisural herniation and compression of the posterior cerebral artery, infarction of the occipital lobe can occur, producing a hemi-anopsia (visual field defect) on the contralateral side. This is a disturbance in which the patient sees clearly only a small portion of an object upon which his or her gaze is fixed. Edema or swelling of the optic disc may be observed about six hours following trauma.

[4] Cardiorespiratory Symptoms

Blood pressure may be normal or elevated. The pulse may become rapid and thready. Respiration becomes disturbed as intracranial pressure is elevated. It becomes irregular or may develop the Cheyne-Stokes pattern, consisting of two alternating phases in which breathing first undergoes a gradual increase in depth to a peak and then gradually decreases until it stops for a brief period. Following this period of apnea (cessation of breathing), the first phase resumes with gradual increase in depth.

[5] Venous Thrombosis

In rare cases, venous EDHs involving a major venous sinus, such as the sagittal sinus or dominant transverse sinus, can compromise

---

[4] *See also* ch. 11.

blood flow through that sinus and manifest as elevated intracranial pressure. This can produce papilledema, headache, retinal hemorrhage and cranial nerve findings. An incomplete dural tear involving the superior sagittal and transverse sinuses can result in partial or complete venous thrombosis (clot formation).

The symptoms of venous thrombosis depend on the location. If the thrombosis is limited to the rostral third of the superior sagittal sinus or to one transverse sinus, there may be no major neurologic deficits. If the caudal (toward the tail) two thirds of the superior sagittal sinus or dominant transverse sinus are obstructed, more severe neurologic sequelae develop.

4.14   Diagnosis

Although epidural hematomas are usually readily diagnosed, the mortality associated with EDHs remains high. Acute EDHs are life threatening unless the clot is surgically removed and the bleeding stopped swiftly. Therefore, accurate and efficient diagnosis is essential to survival. Deterioration of consciousness, regardless of how slight, requires evaluation to rule out an epidural hematoma as well as other brain abnormalities. Although there is a classic clinical progression of symptoms, these occur in less than half the patients with EDH. Other signs and symptoms that may be present include weakness or paralysis, headache, vomiting and restlessness, and cold and clammy skin.

The cornerstone to diagnosis of EDH is radiographic examination, specifically computed tomography (CT) scanning or magnetic resonance imaging (MRI). However, the choice of method is usually determined by the resources available. The American College of Surgeons recommends that "all head injured patients will require CT scanning" (American College of Surgeons, 1989). This is possible in most parts of the United States but not in the majority of the rest of the world at present. The alternative to CT scanning is to use the skull x-ray and the level of consciousness as factors for determining the approach to therapy. In some institutions, MRI is replacing CT as the primary investigative tool. Although comparative studies with CT and MRI have demonstrated that MRI reveals more lesions than CT, it is doubtful whether MRI reveals any more lesions that are likely to require surgery, and therefore, CT scanning will remain the diagnostic tool of choice (Mendelow, 1993).

[1]   Roentgenographic (X-ray) Examination

If CT scanning is not available, x-ray of the skull should be performed. The overwhelming majority of epidural hematomas are associated with a linear type fracture, which should be looked for, particularly one crossing the middle meningeal groove or a dural sinus. Evidence of displacement of the pineal gland, if it is calcified, may clearly indicate the presence of a space-occupying hematoma. However, x-rays do not always reveal fracture, and fracture may not be present in EDH, particularly in children. Therefore, physicians must not interpret the absence of a skull fracture as cause for eliminating EDH from the differential diagnosis.

A complete set of skull films takes time to obtain. In the case of a rapidly enlarging EDH, this may place the patient in a critically compromised condition. Therefore, if CT is available, it may be preferable to go directly to CT scanning and bypass obtaining skull x-rays.

[a]   Computed Tomography (CT) Scan

If it is available, the patient suspected of having an EDH, or in the event of any head trauma, for that matter, should undergo CT scanning. The classic CT appearance of an acute EDH is of a well-defined bi-convex high-attenuation extra-axial mass that causes well-defined focal brain compression. If the EDH is located over the vertex, it tends to have less well defined margins, due to the fact that the skull and brain have a steeper curvature as they approach the vertex, and there are no sutural margins to limit the border of the EDH.

Greater than 75 percent of EDHs arise from laceration of the middle meningeal artery, and therefore they are located in the temporoparietal region. Subtemporal EDHs may be more difficult to identify, as they are more likely to be confused with intra-axial processes on CT. Coronal and sagittal MRI has been used to make this distinction more clearly. Other sites for EDH, in order of decreasing incidence, include the posterior fossa (12 percent incidence), the frontal region (8 percent) and the occipital region (5 percent). In very rare instances, an EDH may develop in the region of the clivus (downward sloping surface). Retroclival EDH is characterized by separation of the tentorial membrane and dura over the clivus from the foramen magnum to the dorsal sella.

Determining whether an extra-axial collection of blood is located in the epidural or subdural space is not always possible. In fact, 20 percent of patients with EDH have blood in both the epidural and subdural spaces. However, certain features strongly indicate an epidural location. Because the periosteal layer of the dura is tightly adherent to the cranial sutures, it is rare for an EDH to extend across suture lines. One exception to this rule is in the region of the sagittal suture. The periosteum beneath the sagittal suture does not invest the sutural margins as tightly as it does elsewhere in the skull, and therefore an EDH can cross the midline. This is in contrast to a subdural hematoma, which is limited by the falx.

Another feature that favors an epidural over a subdural mass on CT is the presence of a sharply localized lentiform (lens-shaped) mass. The sharp localization is due to the fact that the dura remains adherent to the skull at the edge of the hematoma. This sharp localization contributes to the classic lentiform shape of an EDH. Conservative management of an EDH often results in a gradually evolving crescent-shaped appearance on CT.

Another distinguishing factor for an EDH is that it can extend both above and below the tentorium, because continuous involvement of the supratentorial and infratentorial space is achieved only via the epidural space. This relationship is more clearly observed with MRI than with CT imaging. A final distinguishing factor is that displacement of the venous sinuses confirms an epidural location, because the venous sinuses are composed of both dural layers.

Epidural hematomas are rarely bilateral, but they frequently occur with a contralateral subdural hematoma (SDH). This is often the case after coup-contrecoup injuries (in which the head is hit hard on one side, forcing the brain violently to the other side of the skull so that it sustains deceleration damage in the area exactly opposite the point of impact). Although SDHs are usually found at the contrecoup location (opposite the site of impact), EDHs are usually located at the coup site and are very rare at the contrecoup location. *(See Figure 4-2.)*

Skull fractures are found in 85 to 95 percent of adults with EDH. The percentage is lower in children because of the elastic properties of the skull before adulthood.

However, many children thought to have an intact skull on CT have been found to have a fracture at surgery. Rare bilateral EDHs are

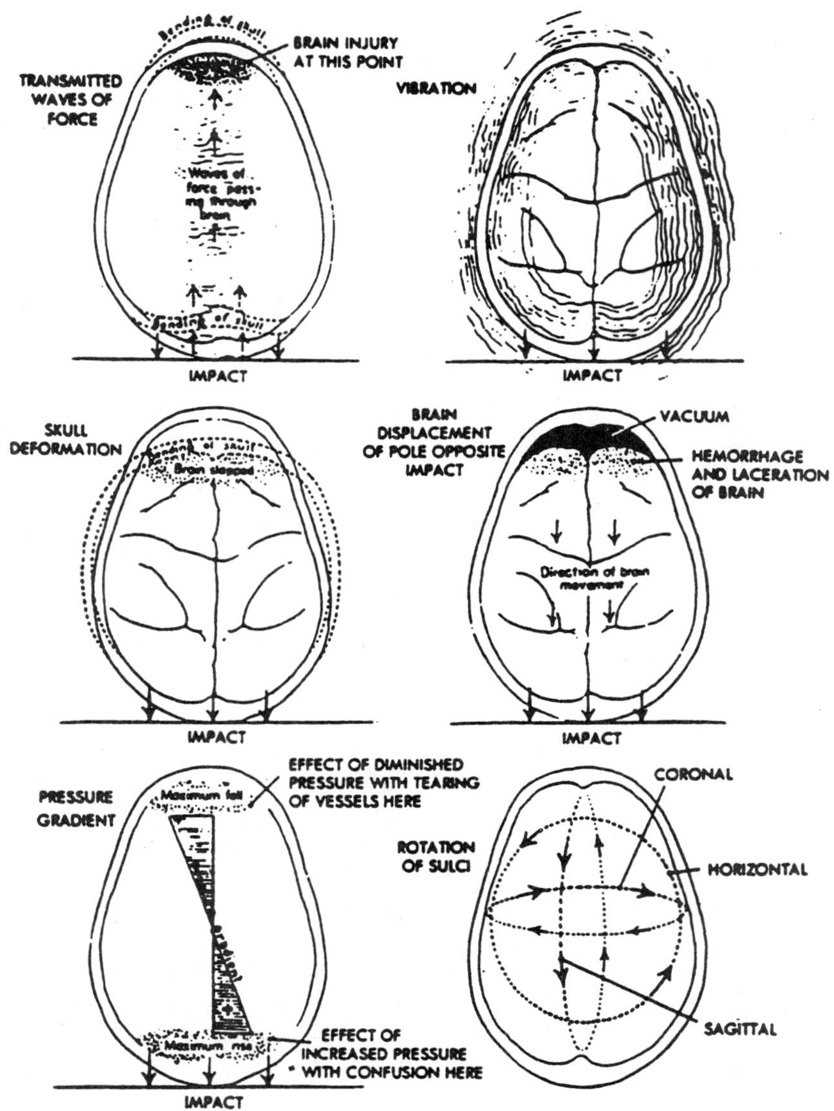

Fig. 4-2. Theories of the mechanism of contrecoup injury of the brain include transmitted waves of force, vibration, skull deformation, brain displacement, pressure gradient and rotation of sulci (furrows of the brain) along various planes.

believed to be caused by vertex fractures that cause midline venous EDHs or by head injury occurring in the anteroposterior direction rather than from a lateral force.

In some cases of acute EDH, the image on CT may appear heterogeneous. Areas of low attenuation within an EDH are a danger sign, because they indicate active bleeding with insufficient time for the blood to clot. Extravasation of contrast material may also be observed in these instances.

Although the majority of epidural hematomas appear on initial imaging, up to 8 percent only appear on follow-up imaging. The delayed appearance has been attributed to several factors, including hypertension, rupture of a traumatic middle meningeal artery pseudoaneurysm, arteriovenous shunting and a loss of the tamponade effect provided by an elevated inctracranial pressure (ICP) that is suddenly normalized.

There may be a minimal increase in size of conservatively managed EDHs one to two weeks following injury. This has been attributed to osmotic factors or slow rebleeding into the collection of blood by the organizing vessels. This expanding stage of an EDH is always associated with a decrease in attenuation. Calcification of EDH may also occur.

[b] Angiography

With the widespread use of CT scanning as well as the availability of MRI, angiography (x-ray study of the blood vessels) is rarely indicated in the diagnosis of EDH.

[2] Lumbar Puncture

Lumbar puncture involves obtaining a sample of cerebrospinal fluid (CSF) through a needle inserted into the space between the fourth and fifth lumbar vertebrae (L4-L5). The CSF is studied for the presence of diagnostic markers. This method of diagnosis is only mentioned because it is considered an entirely useless and dangerous procedure if epidural hematoma is thought to be even a possibility. It cannot be defended as part of the method of coming to a differential diagnosis and can have the dramatically adverse effect of precipitating herniation and therefore deterioration of the patient.

[3]   The Neurologic Examination and Emergency Care

In the diagnosis of epidural hematomas, it is important to emphasize that the possibility of associated hemorrhagic lesions should always be kept in mind. The fact that a patient has an epidural hematoma does not rule out the possibility of the simultaneous existence of two or more types of intracranial bleeding, such as intracerebral, subarachnoid and intraventricular hemorrhages. Multiple lesions are often manifested, particularly in individuals who have been involved in vehicular accidents.

The importance of a careful neurological evaluation cannot be overemphasized, as well as the need for repeated evaluations.

Time is of the essence, and the ability to transport the patient from the site of injury to the hospital and then into a surgical suite has enabled advanced trauma centers to reduce the mortality rate from approximately 50 percent to 30 percent.

4.15   Treatment

Favorable outcome correlates strongly with the time interval from injury to definitive care, with the shorter interval associated with better outcome. Efforts have been made to improve patient management at the scene of an accident, particularly with regard to limiting shock and hypoxia.[5] These conditions are associated with higher morbidity and mortality rates in patients with head injury, probably because they contribute to an increase in intracranial pressure.

A deliberate effort to achieve early diagnosis and intervene before a patient's condition continues to deteriorate further improves outcome. Although the CT is of proven value, it can take 15 to 30 minutes to complete. If the patient is rapidly deteriorating, a single midcranial CT "trauma slice" is obtained and evaluated, which allows for prompt identification of a severe mass effect requiring immediate surgical intervention.

In rare cases, an emergency burr hole exploration (EBHE) without a prior CT scan may be necessary. In a patient with clinical signs of transtentorial herniation and who deteriorates neurologically too quickly for any imaging study to be performed, a low temporal burr hole is made on the same side as the dilated pupil to evacuate a

---

[5] *See also* ch. 1.

potential epidural or subdural hematoma. The rationale for EBHE is that prompt decompression minimizes the secondary brain injury caused by elevated ICP and mechanical displacement of brain tissue. If the EBHE has negative results, a CT scan should be performed immediately.

Nonsurgical conservative management of acute EDHs remains controversial. Spontaneous resolution of an EDH can occur and has been attributed to resorption via the formation of a neomembrane or by external drainage of the hematoma through a skull fracture, dural tear or venous fistula. Generally, spontaneous resorption of a conservatively treated EDH occurs over one to three weeks. Conservative management has been recommended for hematomas that are small (less than 1.5 cm in width, or less than 40 mL in volume), minimally symptomatic and with high convexity, if they are not associated with intradural lesions.

In the setting of transtentorial herniation, it is important to reduce intracranial pressure (ICP); however, in cases without major neurologic symptoms, there may be disadvantages to lowering ICP. Hyperventilation and administration of mannitol assist in lowering ICP by decreasing the volume of residual normal brain tissue. These approaches do not, however, decrease the size of the EDH, and decreasing the volume of normal brain can actually increase epidural bleeding as a result of the loss of a tamponade effect.

Current trends are to operate on all patients with EDH with a corresponding neurologic deficit. If a patient is asymptomatic, surgical evacuation is performed if there is midline shift or if the volume of the collection exceeds 40 mL. Surgical treatment involves removal of the clot.

There are several methods of obtaining surgical exposure of the hematoma. Epidural hematomas can usually be evacuated by means of a limited small craniectomy (removal of a portion of the bony cranium). Hematomas over the convexity of the brain often require a cranial flap. Good hemostasis (control of bleeding) is essential for preventing postoperative complications. Active bleeding from the torn vessel or vessels is controlled by coagulation or occlusion if necessary.

4.16   Prognosis

The prognosis of an epidural hematoma (EDH) depends on the extent of co-existent intracerebral injury, the size of the EDH, the rate of development of the hematoma, the location of the bleed and the promptness of neurosurgical intervention.

With the introduction of CT, the mortality rate of surgically treated patients with acute supratentorial EDH has dropped from approximately 30 percent to 8 percent. This dramatic improvement in survival during the past two decades is predominantly due to more expedient and accurate means of imaging diagnosis. In most cases in which the EDH is promptly evacuated, the brain returns to normal shape and position within 48 hours. In contrast to evacuation of a subdural hematoma (SDH), after which the underlying parenchyma often swells, evacuation of an EDH is usually followed by rapid return of the ventricular system to the midline position and the brain matter to its normal configuration.

Quality of care also plays a role in prognosis. Trauma victims who are not treated in a trauma center have a significantly higher risk of dying than those who are treated in a trauma center. Associated medical injuries can also adversely affect the patient's outcome. Associated systemic injuries are present in more than half of patients with head injury.

4.20 SUBDURAL HEMATOMA

A subdural hemorrhage or subdural hematoma (SDH) is a collection of serosanguinous fluid (a variable mixture of blood and/or cerebrospinal fluid) located above the arachnoid and beneath the inner layer of the dura. This site between the dural membrane and the arachnoid membrane covering the brain and spinal cord is referred to as the subdural space, although it is actually a potential space.

The majority of SDHs are caused by traumatic disruption of the fine superficial cerebral veins and their arachnoid sheaths near the major sinuses. When this occurs, low-pressure venous blood dissects the arachnoid away from the dura. The enlarging hematoma creates the subdural space. Stretching of the remaining intact bridging veins can cause further disruption and additional bleeding, resulting in an even larger hematoma.

Subdural hematomas typically accumulate until the intracranial pressure rises to equal the venous pressure. The SDH may act like a space-occupying lesion, causing compression of the underlying brain and necessitating surgical intervention to remove the hematoma. *(See Figure 4-3.)*

A subdural hygroma, or hydroma, is a subdural collection of cerebrospinal fluid (CSF). It develops following laceration of the arachnoid, allowing CSF to escape from the subarachnoid space into the subdural space. The signs and symptoms of a subdural hygroma are often indistinguishable from those of a subacute SDH.

SDHs are traditionally divided into three stages—acute, subacute and chronic—based on the pathologic, clinical and imaging characteristics. Unfortunately, there is no precise uniform nomenclature, and no experimental model entirely explains the evolution of the SDH. The *acute* phase is considered to last for up to one week following injury; the *subacute* stage occurs between one and three weeks postinjury and is characterized by progressive liquefaction of the clot. The *chronic* stage occurs approximately three weeks following injury.

4.21 Incidence

Acute subdural hematomas are more common than epidural hematomas. In patients undergoing CT following head injury, the incidence is between 5 and 10 percent in children, and between 15 and 20 percent in adults. Acute SDHs may be divided into two types, depending on the presence of associated parenchymal injury. *Simple* SDHs have no underlying parenchymal injury; they have a mortality rate of approximately 20 percent. *Complicated* acute SDHs are more severe and have associated parenchymal injury. They have been associated with a 53 percent rate of mortality (Gean, 1994).

Chronic SDHs are more common in the elderly population and have a peak incidence at age 60. Unlike patients with acute SDH, up to half the adults with a chronic SDH have no history of prior trauma. The mortality rate is low: probably less than 10 percent. For the subacute SDH, mortality is in the 25 to 35 percent range.

4.22 Causes and Mechanisms of Injury

Any type of head trauma may provoke hemorrhage into the subdural space. The most common precipitating trauma is blunt injury or closed head injury. Penetrating trauma, such as stab and bullet wounds, as well as any injury resulting in either simple or compound fractures

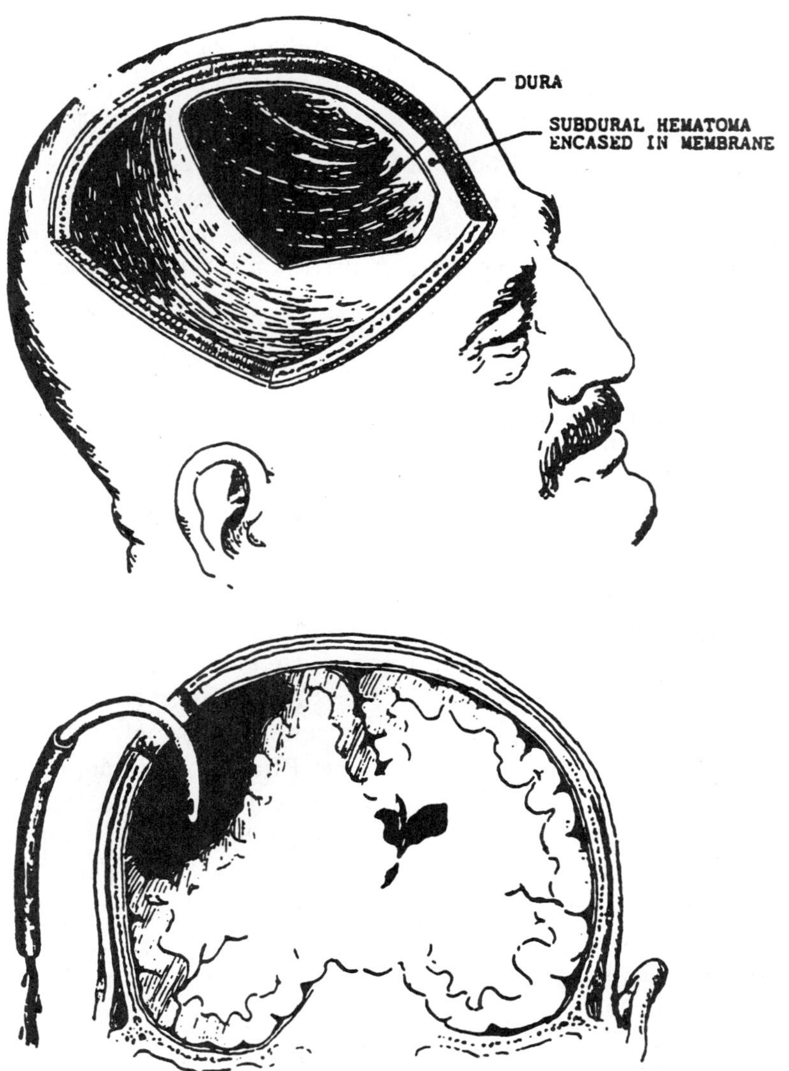

Fig. 4-3. Subdural hematoma. The upper drawing shows the dura pulled back to expose the hematoma encased in a fibrous membrane. The lower drawing shows drainage of the blood from the hematoma, which has compressed and distorted the brain.

of the skull, may result in subdural hemorrhage. Other specific injuries that may result in SDH include blows to the chin, falls on the buttocks, underwater blast concussions, birth injuries and sports injuries.

In football injuries, subdural hematomas constitute an important cause of death. Use of a helmet prevents abrasion, lacerations of the scalp and skull fracture on impact, but the formation of subdural hematoma continues due to relative movements in inertial stress propagation of the brain, with tearing of connecting veins.

Trauma to the head need not be severe to precipitate a subdural hematoma. The degree of disturbance is partially related to the direction of the force and the area of impact, but the actual amount of energy involved may be extremely small in proportion to the severity of the injury.

4.23   Pathophysiology

Most subdural hematomas are a result of traumatic disruption of the superficial cerebral veins near the major venous sinuses over the convexities. The cortical veins bridging the temporal lobe may also be ruptured. Remaining intact bridging veins may be ruptured as the hematoma enlarges, further contributing to the size of the hematoma.

The bridging cortical veins are relatively straight. Therefore, they are particularly vulnerable to rotation, stretching and tearing during excessive movement of the brain. They are also considered to be strain-rate sensitive, meaning that they are sensitive not only to stretching itself but also to the rate of stretching. Bridging veins are especially susceptible to sudden, high strain forces that do not cause deep tissue strains severe enough to produce coma and diffuse brain tissue injury. Therefore, SDHs are more likely to occur after injuries such as falls or assaults than after motor vehicle accidents, which frequently cause deeper tissue shearing injuries. It is important to realize that direct impact to the head is not a prerequisite for development of an SDH.

While SDHs are most commonly due to shearing of the bridging cortical veins, they may also arise from a direct contusion[6] to the underlying cerebral parenchyma that extends through the pia-arachnoid or from the rupture of an expanding hematoma into the subdural space. SDHs can occur in either the coup (same side) or

---

[6] *See also* ch. 3.

contrecoup (opposite side) location, although the contrecoup location is more common.

Another potential cause of SDH is shunting of obstructive hydrocephalus (accumulation of fluid in the brain). This may occur when the cortical veins tear as the ventricles decompress. SDH has been reported in 3 to 28 percent of individuals following ventriculostomy (establishment of an opening in a ventricle to relieve hydrocephalus). This is more common in adults and after shunting of communicating as opposed to noncommunicating hydrocephalus. SDHs that develop following ventricular shunting may be complicated by ventriculitis, shunt malfunction and meningeal fibrosis.

The majority of SDHs are located over the cerebral convexity, especially the parietal region. The next most common location is above the tentorium cerebelli. SDH may also occur beneath the tentorium, such as within the posterior fossa. While this is quite rare in adults, it may occur in the neonate following perinatal injury to the tentorium or vein of Galen.

Subdural blood collecting between the two cerebral hemispheres is called interhemispheric SDH. Blood typically extends along one side of the falx and compresses the medial aspect of the adjacent hemisphere. These lesions are often produced by laceration of the veins that enter the superior or inferior sagittal sinuses.

Interhemispheric collections are more common in children, and they can be an important indicator of child abuse. They are less common in adults, due to acquired adhesions that obliterate the subdural space at the apex of the brain.

Subdural blood accumulating within the two leaves of the falx cerebri is called intrafalcial SDH. This is rare in both children and adults, although it is slightly more common in children. Other unusual locations for SDHs include adjacent to a cortical infarct, around the frontal pole, on the floor of the middle cranial fossa or in the retroclival region.

The persistence of blood in the subdural space initiates a tissue reaction designed to organize and resorb the hematoma. This process produces membranes that may be submitted for pathologic examination; however, it is generally believed that the membranes do not have to be removed. The majority of the organization and resorptive activity in a persistent hematoma occurs on the outer or dural aspect, where proliferating fibroblasts and capillaries permeate the clot. The resulting granulation tissue is thick and somewhat rubbery; it is called the outer membrane. This membrane develops at a relatively predictable rate and is therefore useful in dating the onset of the hematoma.

Along with the maturation of the outer membrane, a reaction occurs on the arachnoidal or inner aspect of the hematoma in which cells construct a delicate inner membrane. This membrane lacks the capillarities that are prevalent in the outer membrane. Formation of the inner membrane is slower than the outer membrane. The two membranes remain distinct and easily separable. Organization of the hematoma begins at 5 to 7 days, and after 10 to 20 days, the process is rapidly advancing. Formation of the membranes is usually complete in 4 to 8 weeks. Once encapsulation is complete, the subdural hematoma may resolve spontaneously if blood is absorbed and bleeding stops. If bleeding continues, enlargement and further symptoms may develop.

Expansion is an important characteristic of subdural hematoma. It is expansion rather than the size of the initial hemorrhage that often brings the lesions to the attention of physicians. Enlargement is usually due to rebleeding from the delicate capillaries of the outer membrane. These new hemorrhages may become encapsulated by another membrane. The continuing cycle of bleeding followed by encapsulation creates multiple membranes (Burger, et al., 1991).

4.24   Acute Subdural Hematoma

Acute subdural hematomas are those that develop within one week of traumatic head injury. Most patients with acute SDH have a history of major cranial trauma within two to three days prior to the onset of clinical signs. The signs and symptoms are derived from increased intracranial pressure, which necessitates immediate surgical evacuation.

The amount of blood and underlying brain injury associated with acute subdural hematomas varies dramatically. They may consist of comparatively small collections of blood over the brain, secondary to extensive contusion of the brain surface, or they may consist of a large subdural collection of blood, often observed in conjunction with free bleeding prompted by laceration of surface vessels, but limited contusive injury.

Extensive contusion is characterized by brain swelling with a concomitant dramatic rise in intracranial pressure. The symptoms are primarily those of rapid and massive brain compression following trauma. Patients with large subdural collections but with limited contusion usually have less brain swelling and thus less increase in intracranial pressure.

The prognosis is very different for these two types of patients. Prognosis is very poor for those with extensive contusion. Those with less contusive injury and large subdural hematomas respond favorably to evacuation of the hematoma and have a better prognosis.

[1] Clinical Considerations

In acute subdural hematoma, the clinical signs and symptoms are usually directly related to the recent traumatic event and are often indistinguishable from those of a cerebral contusion or an epidural hematoma. The majority of SDHs are associated with other brain injuries.

Patients with SDH may or may not suffer an initial loss of consciousness. Approximately a third of those who lose consciousness experience a lucid interval. Patients with relatively minor blows to the head may become merely dazed but then deteriorate over several hours. Patients with rapid and massive brain compression with edema and herniation experience persistent loss of consciousness, and a lucid interval is very rare.

Conscious patients with acute SDH usually complain of increasingly severe headaches that often cannot be localized to a specific area of the head. Patients may experience nausea, vomiting or convulsions, with the development of drowsiness, confusion and disorientation, followed progressively by stupor and coma.

Localizing neurologic signs are present in only about 50 percent of patients at the time of their admission; however, they are of great clinical importance and should be elicited, since these neurologic signs, particularly in the unconscious patient, often suggest the development of an enlarging mass lesion with the threat of herniation. They include ocular manifestations, motor signs, convulsive disorders, other focal signs and changes in vital signs.

[a] Ocular Manifestations

Ocular manifestations consist of abnormalities of the pupil and ocular muscles. The most common abnormality is a dilated, fixed pupil on the same side as the hematoma. However, the pupil may be constricted, or the pupil opposite the side of the lesion may be dilated. An enlarged or dilated pupil on the side of the brain with the hematoma is seen in about 50 to 80 percent of patients. In about 8 percent, the dilated pupil is on the contralateral (opposite) side.

There may be various ocular palsies, usually relevant to the oculomotor nerve (third cranial nerve). Sixth nerve (abducens) paralysis results from increased intracranial pressure. With increased intracranial pressure, the optic fundi (back of the eye) may show evidence of retinal vein engorgement or retinal hemorrhages.

[b] Motor Signs

The most common motor signs are hemiparesis (weakness) or hemiplegia (paralysis) of the limbs on the opposite side of the body. Hematomas that cause bilateral involvement of the lower limbs and possibly triplegia or quadriplegia arise from superior sinus bleeding overlying both motor strip areas of the brain. In the unconscious patient, hemiparesis is indicated by absent motor response to painful stimuli as well as by abnormal reflexes. In about 15 percent of patients, the weakness is on the side of the lesion, while bilateral weakness is observed in about 10 percent of patients, usually in the presence of bilateral hematomas.

Pyramidal motor tract signs may be present, such as absent abdominal reflex, increased deep reflexes or positive toe signs on the contralateral side. There may also be weakness of the face of the central type (having brain or nuclear origin) involving the lower two thirds of the facial muscles.

[c] Convulsive Disorders

Convulsive seizures may or may not develop. These may be generalized or unilateral.

[d] Other Focal Signs

Other neurologic focal signs may develop, depending upon the site and extent of brain compression. These include aphasic speech disturbances due to compression of the dominant hemisphere, and the occurrence of a peculiar catatoniclike state. If the visual pathways or visual cortex are affected, visual field defects, such as homonymous hemianopia (loss of vision in half the visual field in the corresponding lateral halves of the eyes), may be experienced.

[e] Changes in Vital Signs

Changes in vital signs (pulse, respiration and blood pressure) are not reliable signs of rising intracranial pressure, because variations occur ranging from normal to marked disturbances. However, with rapid deterioration of the patient's condition, the following usually occur:

- the pulse becomes fast and thready;

- respiration becomes irregular and labored, and may be Cheyne-Stokes in type;[7] and

- body temperature elevations ranging from 101 degrees to 103 degrees are not uncommon.

Intracranial pressure must be monitored if elevation is to be detected before serious neurologic deterioration occurs.

Decorticate posturing implies early brain herniation, causing damage to the upper brain stem. Decerebrate rigidity (rigid extension of the limbs) occurs from midbrain damage and compression following tentorial herniation. When tentorial herniation is completed, the pupils will be fixed and dilated, with characteristic changes in vital signs as well as decerebrate posturing. In full decerebrate posturing, all four limbs are extended. The arms are adducted (in a position of inner rotation), and the feet are in plantar flexion (arched downward). With very rare exceptions, such posturing indicates deep coma, and approximately 80 percent of patients in this condition die.

[2] Diagnosis

In most cases, CT (computed tomography) scanning provides the cornerstone for diagnosing and planning management of subdural hematomas. In situations in which CT scanning or MRI (magnetic resonance imaging) is unavailable, other methods, such as skull x-rays, isotope scanning or angiography, may be employed.

[a] Skull X-rays

The role of skull radiography in evaluating head injury is a matter of controversy. Some experts (Gean, 1994) do not believe that skull radiographs significantly affect the management of head trauma patients, as there is little correlation between skull injury and intracranial injury.

---

[7] *See* 4.13[4] *supra.*

If films (x-rays) are used in the diagnosis of SDH, they may demonstrate erosion or thinning of the skull over the hematoma, calcification or asymmetry. Skull films may show a shifted, calcified pineal gland shadow, resulting from the hematoma pushing the brain to one side.

[b]   Isotope Brain Scanning

Isotope brain scans are rarely obtained in the diagnosis of acute subdural hematoma.

[c]   Computed Tomography (CT) Scanning

Definitive diagnosis of acute subdural hematoma is accomplished by CT scan. CT scanning provides information regarding the following:

- localization of the hematoma;

- extent of brain displacement;

- existence of concomitant lesions, such as intracerebral or epidural hematoma; and

- presence of cerebral edema (swelling due to accumulation of fluid).

Diagnosis can be made as soon as hemorrhage occurs, due to the fact that it is easy to demarcate extravasated blood from the underlying brain. Acute extravasated blood is hyperdense compared to the normal blood. CT scanning can also distinguish acute from subacute and chronic subdural hematomas, because with time, the blood undergoes liquefaction and its density changes to resemble the underlying brain. It is then referred to as being *isodense,* which is characteristic of the subacute stage.

The typical acute SDH appears as a homogeneous, hyperdense, crescent-shaped mass located between the skull and the brain parenchyma (functional tissue). If it is small, the SDH may blend in with the adjacent skull and be overlooked. In infants and children, there may only be an indication of a thin amount of blood present, despite large amounts evacuated at surgery. If the extent of midline brain shift appears excessive for the size of the SDH, underlying cerebral swelling should be suspected. Conversely, if appropriate midline shift is not identified, a contralateral mass lesion should be suspected.

While the majority of acute SDHs are homogeneous and show high attenuation on CT, they may appear to be the same density as the gray matter of the brain. Situations that may result in this picture include anemia with a hemoglobin level of less than 10 g/dL, the hematoma being mixed with cerebrospinal fluid, and a clotting abnormality known as disseminated intravascular coagulation (DIC).

Another exception to the classic appearance of the SDH is the atypical or hyperacute SDH, which may represent up to a quarter of all acute SDHs. Patients with this type of SDH have a heterogeneous lesion on CT. The majority of the lesion has high attenuation, but scattered areas of low attenuation are also present. Atypical SDHs may also be lentiform (lens-shaped) as opposed to having the classic crescent shape, and they are often associated with enlargement of the ipsilateral (same side) ventricle. Atypical acute SDH appears to exert more mass effect, is often larger and is associated with increased mortality, as compared with a typical acute SDH.

[d]　Cerebral Angiography

Cerebral angiography has been replaced by CT scanning for identifying brain herniation and intracranial mass lesions. Conventional angiography is currently reserved for cases in which the CT or MRI findings are inconsistent with a patient's neurologic status, for cases of suspected vascular injury that necessitate direct visualization of the vessels and for cases requiring neurointerventional therapeutic techniques.

On angiography, the SDH typically appears as an extracerebral mass that is avascular and sandwiched between the inner table of the skull and the cortical branches of the middle cerebral artery.

[e]　Twist-drill Ventriculogram

An alternative emergency diagnostic method is the twist-drill ventriculogram, in which an opaque liquid is instilled through a skull opening directly into the ventricular system. The ventricular system is quickly delineated as well as the location of any mass lesion. This procedure may have a role if CT scanning is unavailable.

[3]　Management

Management of the patient with an acute SDH depends on the patient's neurologic status, the size of the mass, the involvement of the underlying brain, the extent of the mass effect, associated systemic injuries, the patient's age and the overall medical condition.

A general neurosurgical guideline for managing mass lesions is that a lesion that produces a midline shift of 5 mm or greater demonstrated on CT scan or angiography is operable (Narayan, 1991). Most SDHs producing shifts of greater than 5 mm are surgically evacuated. Patients are given mannitol to reduce cerebral swelling and hyperventilated prior to surgery. Time is of the essence, because the sooner the mass lesion is evacuated, the better the possibility of a good recovery.

Surgical evacuation involves a craniotomy (opening into the skull) and removal of the collected blood. After evacuation of the blood, recurrent bleeding of significant volume is rare. However, swelling of the brain into the evacuated cavity may occur.

The intracranial pressure remains elevated postoperatively in about half of all acute SDH cases. This may be due to incomplete evacuation of the mass, reaccumulation or development of a new lesion. Cerebral edema (swelling), vascular engorgement or interference with CSF circulation may also complicate the situation. Management of persistently elevated intracranial pressure includes repeat surgical evacuation and drainage, hyperventilation, administration of osmotically active agents such as mannitol and, occasionally, barbiturates.

[4]   Mortality Rate and Prognosis

The mortality rate associated with an acute SDH is probably higher than with any other type of post-traumatic brain lesion, ranging from 42 to 90 percent. Preoperative neurologic condition is probably the most important factor in determining a patient's prognosis. Early surgical evacuation occurring within four hours of injury has been shown to decrease mortality, in comparison with delayed surgical removal. Underlying cerebral injury accompanying the hematoma appears to be the major cause of the continued high morbidity and mortality that accompany this lesion, despite advances in rapid diagnosis and treatment.

4.25   Subacute Subdural Hematoma

The subacute stage of SDH occurs between one and three weeks after injury and is characterized by progressive liquefaction of the acute clot. The signs and symptoms of subacute SDH are similar to those for acute SDHs, although they tend to be milder and not as rapidly progressing. Drowsiness and disorientation are often observed for several days after the impact, which may have produced immediate loss of consciousness for a brief period. A relatively lucid interval lasting for several days is observed in about 50 percent of patients. This period may be followed by coma if the hematoma is not evacuated.

Diagnosis is made with CT scanning. Subacute SDH is often seen as a lentiform mass, thus mimicking an epidural hematoma. A hematocrit effect can be observed due to layering of high-attenuation cellular elements and low-attenuation serum. Toward the end of the subacute phase, the cellular elements are being removed from the clot and the entire collection becomes isodense and then hypodense on CT scan. During the isodense period, CT diagnosis depends on recognition of displacement of various elements, including distortion of the white matter, ventricle system, cortical veins, a midline shift or abnormal separation of the gray matter–white matter junction from the inner table of the skull. Contrast-enhanced CT scans can aid in the diagnosis of isodense subacute SDH.

Management of subacute SDH is usually carried out by evacuating the liquefied clot through multiple burr holes or a twist-drill craniostomy. Other aspects of management are similar to those for an acute SDH.

Prognosis and the quality of survival are better as a rule for patients with subacute subdural hematoma than for those with an acute SDH.

4.26 Chronic Subdural Hematoma

Chronic and acute SDHs are both part of a spectrum of the same pathologic entity. However, their clinical presentations are often very different. Chronic SDHs appear after approximately three weeks, when the collection begins to organize, and they are rarely associated with underlying brain injury.

One of the most important diagnostic factors is that about half of patients with chronic SDH cannot identify a precipitating traumatic episode. This may be because the trauma appeared trivial to the patient or, alternatively, it may have occurred during a period of altered consciousness, such as after alcohol ingestion, or while waking up from sleep, or it may be a result of memory loss due to the chronic hematoma itself.

Chronic subdural hematoma is more prevalent among elderly patients, due to the fact that atrophy results in diminished brain size and linear displacement of the brain can occur with a comparatively minor head injury. This injury is not restricted to this group, however, and occurs in children and young adults as well.

One or both sides of the fronto-temporo-parietal region is the site of the hematoma in the majority of cases, and multiple hematomas occurring in the same patient at different periods of time are not uncommon, particularly in an alcoholic individual, who may fall many times during the course of his or her life.

While trauma is the primary cause of chronic SDH, it may also occur because of aneurysm rupture or during the course of anticoagulant drug therapy for a thrombotic condition.

[1] Pathophysiology

Cerebral atrophy or shriveling is responsible for the frequency of hematoma accumulation or successive hematomas in the elderly, because an impact will readily stretch and tear the venous tributaries of the sagittal sinus.

The process of organization of the clot begins with thin strands of connective tissue beneath the dura sprouting into the surface of the SDH. Phagocytic and fibroblastic cells extend into the hematoma. Ultimately the organizing vessels form a membrane that completely encapsulates the hematoma. The liquid center gradually resorbs, and the inner and outer membranes fuse. Finally the only residual of an SDH may be a thin, collagenous membrane facing the arachnoid and a thicker membrane attached to the dura. This process takes weeks to months, depending upon the size of the initial collection.

It is unclear why some acute SDHs progress to chronic SDH and others do not. The majority of small acute SDHs resolve completely without progressing. Cases that do progress probably undergo enlargement via osmotic expansion by proteins and other red blood cells, or via blood extravasated from bridging veins, or by recurrent hemorrhage from vessels involved in organizing the clot

[2] Clinical Picture

Chronic SDHs are most common in the elderly, with a peak incidence at age 60. Approximately half of all adults with a chronic

SDH have no history of prior trauma. History and neurologic findings in patients with chronic SDH are more similar to those of a cerebral neoplasm than to those of a traumatic intracranial hemorrhage.

Gradual enlargement of the hematoma may be well tolerated at first, because of accommodation provided by displacement of the brain. This compensatory shift accommodates the hematoma without increasing intracranial pressure or producing symptoms. Neurologic symptoms usually appear once the size of the extra-axial collection exceeds the buffering reserve of a patient's cerebral compliance and underlying atrophic change.

Patients with a chronic SDH often complain of headache, probably due to the stretching and tearing of the pain-sensitive meninges and blood vessels as the brain is displaced from the skull. Mental aberrations or a reduction in the degree of alertness with memory loss occur over a variable period from weeks to months following the injury. Marked personality disorders may surface early, with frequent and extreme emotional lability (mood swing) alternating between restlessness, apathy, lethargy, irritability and explosive temper outbursts. A mistaken diagnosis of neurosis is often made. Signs of elevated intracranial pressure and paresis (partial paralysis) may develop, including swelling of the optic disc (papilledema), rigidity and hemiparesis (paralysis on one side).

Cerebral atrophy and alcoholism predispose to the development of chronic SDH. Diagnosis of SDH in the alcoholic individual may be delayed, however, because symptoms of chronic SDH are similar to those of chronic alcoholism; namely, headaches and memory impairment.

[3]   Diagnosis

It is important to recognize that the signs of a chronic SDH may mimic those of psychiatric conditions as well as alcoholism and dementia. Dulling of consciousness or a change in mental status even after a minor head trauma should arouse suspicion. Progressive deterioration of mental function is an important element in the diagnosis. Because chronic SDHs are usually readily diagnosed on CT, it is the suspicion of diagnosis that must be appropriately aroused.

Chronic SDH is very conspicuous on CT. Typically it appears as a well-defined, low-attenuation or extra-axial collection, with multiple internal septations and fluid levels. If there is no rebleeding within the collection, it appears uniformly low in attenuation. It is bilateral in approximately 25 percent of cases.

[4] Management

Treatment can be surgical or nonsurgical. It is also quite possible for a chronic subdural hematoma to undergo spontaneous resolution. The majority of chronic subdural hematomas are evacuated. Liquefied and more indolent (slowly developing) chronic SDH can usually be evacuated through burr holes or a twist-drill craniostomy. If the hematoma is clotted or multilocular, a craniotomy is indicated in order to obtain adequate exposure to remove the entire lesion. Patients with chronic SDH who are neurologically stable and intact may be managed nonoperatively.

After evacuation, recurrent bleeding may result in a significant space-occupying mass. Management of persistent postoperative increased intracranial pressure follows the same procedures as those discussed for acute SDH. Results of surgical evacuation are usually good, and the most important predictor of outcome is probably the level of consciousness at the time of surgery.

4.30 SUBARACHNOID HEMORRHAGE

Subarachnoid hemorrhage (SAH) occurs when blood leaks into the subarachnoid space, either from a ruptured artery or vein or from an intracerebral hemorrhage that dissects through the parenchyma to the surface of the brain or into the ventricles. It is spontaneous if there is no apparent cause, or traumatic if there has been injury. Traumatic SAH is the most common type.

4.31 Mechanism and Site of Injury

Subarachnoid hemorrhage is the most common form of intracranial bleeding seen following head trauma. It often occurs in conjunction with severe contusion and laceration of the cerebral cortex, with rupture of a corticomeningeal blood vessel causing blood to be extravasated into the spinal fluid space, producing bloody cerebrospinal fluid (CSF) and a subarachnoid hemorrhage. Although blood within the CSF is present to some degree at lumbar puncture in most patients with significant head trauma, in many of these cases, the hemorrhage is clinically insignificant. However, the significance of the head trauma does not always dictate the severity of the hemorrhage, and sudden death may result from hemorrhage precipitated by an apparently minor trauma.

In minor trauma, subarachnoid hemorrhage (SAH) may result from venous blood derived from injury to small cortical veins passing through the subarachnoid space. Although the CSF within the subarachnoid space provides some cushioning, protecting the brain from impact against any prominences, traumatic forces can easily exceed this buffering capacity. SAH is also common underneath a skull fracture due to direct laceration of the surface arteries and veins. SAH can occur via rupture of an intracerebral hematoma into a ventricle and flow of blood through the fourth ventricular outlet. Brain motion can also disrupt surface vessels and adhesions. Patients with an enlarged subarachnoid space, such as the elderly and infants, are particularly susceptible to disruption of surface vessels by brain motion. In closed head trauma, the amount of bleeding is less than with penetrating injuries, which can produce severe bleeding. *(See Figure 4-4.)*

Important sites for contusions and lacerations of the brain are the frontal lobe and anterior portions of the temporal lobes. At these sites, rotational oscillations are thought to account for the production of subarachnoid hemorrhage, since the brain is tethered by bony irregularities particularly at the base of the skull in the anterior and middle fossas and the sharp edge of the sphenoid shelf that separates them.

4.32   Clinical Considerations—Signs and Symptoms

Post-traumatic subarachnoid hemorrhage produces elevation of temperature, restlessness, severe headache, stiff neck (nuchal rigidity) and a positive Kernig's sign, which is elicited by flexing the thigh to a right angle on the abdomen and attempting to extend the leg. *(See Figures 4-5 and 4-6.)* Additional symptoms include lumbar discomfort that develops when blood has seeped down into the lumbar subarachnoid space, and bilateral plantar reflexes (dorsiflexion of the great toe and fanning of the other toes when the sole of the foot is stroked).

Typically there is no dynamic progression of signs and symptoms such as occurs with an expanding hematoma. Signs of progressive deterioration or neurologic deficit are usually indicative of associated injuries or of secondary factors, such as brain edema.

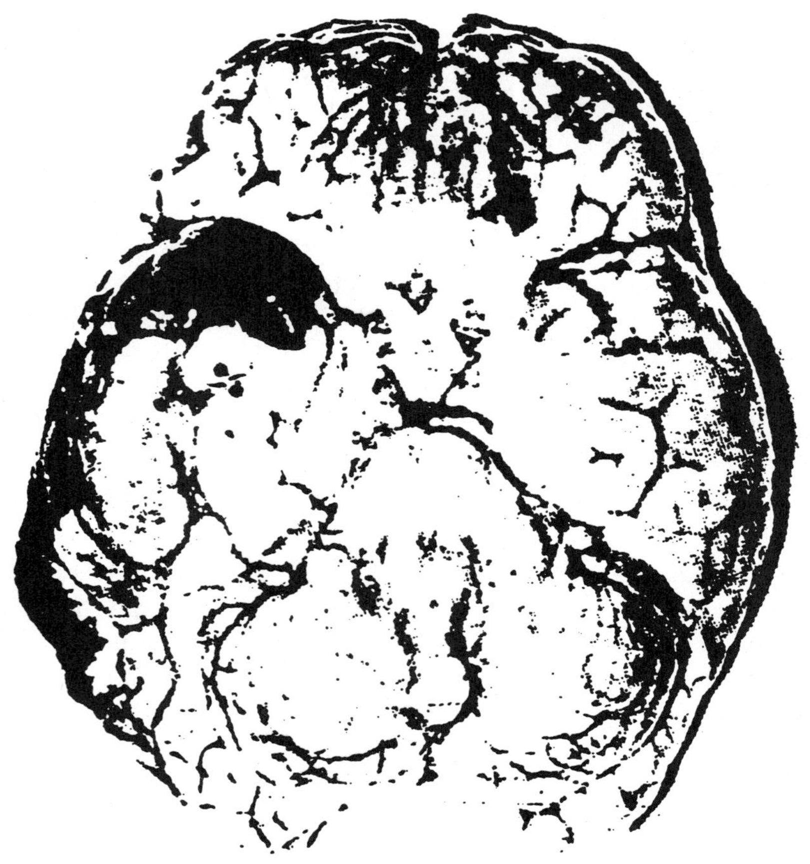

Fig. 4-4. Brain of a patient who died of cerebral contusion and intracerebral hematoma.

4.33   Diagnosis

Cerebrospinal fluid analysis provides the diagnosis of subarachnoid hemorrhage. As long as the lumbar puncture performed to obtain the CSF does not cause bleeding into the CSF, blood-stained CSF signifies subarachnoid hemorrhage or intracerebral hemorrhage that has ruptured into the subarachnoid space. CSF pressure is usually increased.

Other laboratory abnormalities include an elevated white blood cell count (leukocytosis) of 15,000 to 20,000 cells/mm^3. The erythrocyte sedimentation rate is usually mildly to moderately elevated.

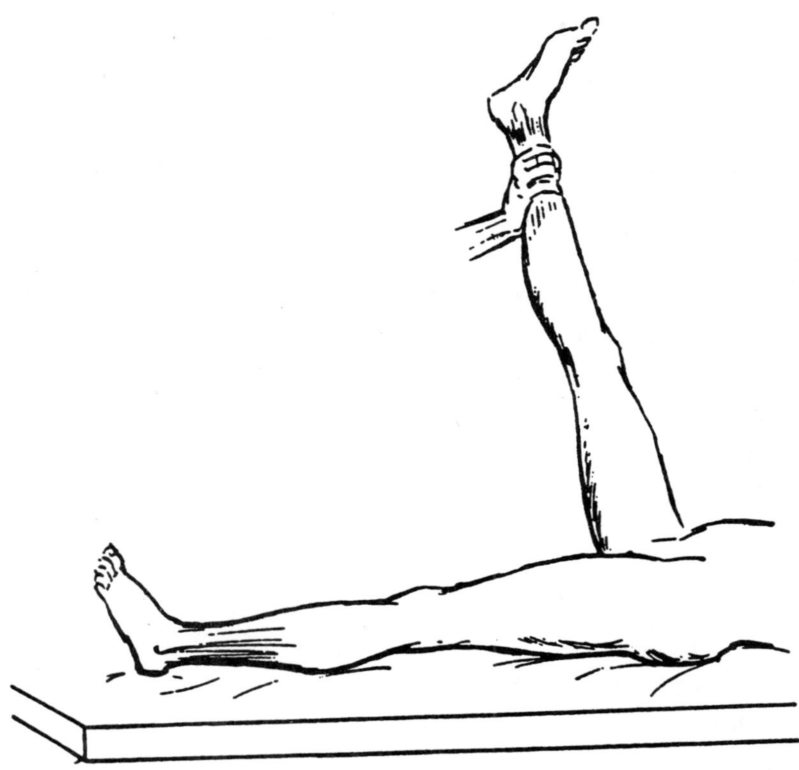

Fig. 4-5. Kernig's test is performed by flexing one of the lower limbs at the hip until the thigh is in a vertical position.

CT scanning is imperative for diagnosis and proper management of SAH. It should be done to determine the presence of blood in the subarachnoid space and confirm the diagnosis, to detect associated bleeding and to determine the source of the bleeding. On CT scans, subarachnoid hemorrhage appears as serpentine, linear areas of high attenuation conforming to the sulcal and cisternal spaces. In some cases, the location of the SAH is not related to either the site or the direction of impact because the blood, diluted by the CSF, tends to spread within the subarachnoid space.

Sensitivity of detecting SAH on CT depends on the volume of extravasated blood, the patient's hematocrit (the number of red blood

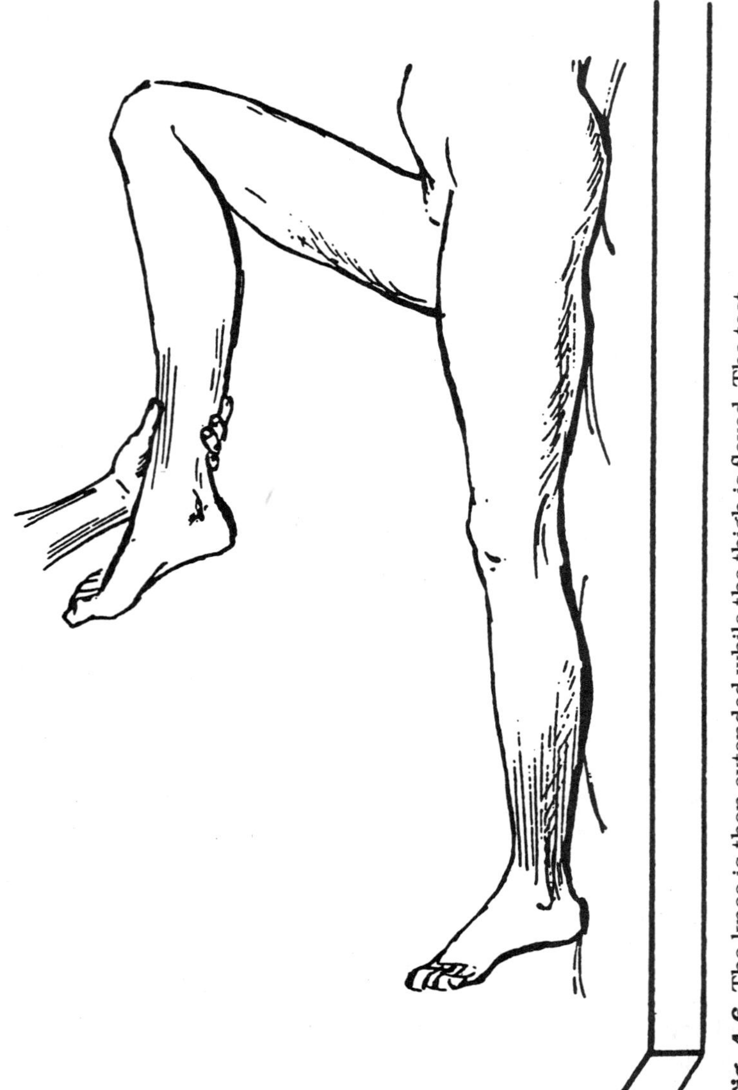

Fig. 4-6. The knee is then extended while the thigh is flexed. The test is positive if this maneuver produces pain.

cells in the blood) and the time interval from injury. If blood is spread very thin, if the hemoglobin concentration is 10 g/dL or less or if injury occurred more than one week previously, SAH may not be visible on CT scan.

Acute SAH cannot be imaged reliably with present magnetic resonance (MR) imaging techniques. MRI is useful later in the course, because as hemoglobin breaks down, it is converted into methemoglobin, which can be demonstrated on MRI. MRI can also detect the residua of prior SAH.

4.34   Treatment

Unlike primary spontaneous subarachnoid hemorrhage, which is a cerebrovascular disease whose most common cause is rupture of an aneurysm, traumatic subarachnoid hemorrhage does not usually require surgical intervention, and treatment is nonspecific. In the acute phase, spinal drainage should not be performed, but if severe headache persists, lumbar puncture may be performed in order to lessen discomfort. Some patients, however, can tolerate large amounts of blood within the subarachnoid space without the necessity of spinal drainage of the bloody fluid.

The most common complication of SAH is obstructive hydrocephalus. The normal flow and resorption of cerebrospinal fluid is disrupted, and the fluid accumulates, producing hydrocephalus. The larger the quantity of extravasated blood, the greater the likelihood of hydrocephalus (accumulation of fluid in the brain). Obstructive hydrocephalus should be suspected whenever a patient reaches a plateau in clinical recovery and then deteriorates. Head trauma may result in secondary brain atrophy or symmetric ventricular dilation, which must be distinguished from obstructive hydrocephalus.

Other complications of SAH may ensue if blood enters the subarachnoid sleeves of the cranial and spinal nerves. Subsequent growth of connective tissue may produce sensorineural deafness, cerebellar ataxia (confusion), dysesthesia (unusual sensations) or pain. Traumatic arachnoiditis can result in the development of an arachnoid cyst. If scarring develops around the optic chiasm, vision loss may occur. SAH may also produce cerebral vasospasm.

4.40 INTRACEREBRAL HEMORRHAGE

Traumatic intracerebral hemorrhage (ICH) consists of bleeding into the brain matter. Invariably when a head injury is severe enough to produce a hematoma within the brain, there are other concomitant brain injuries, and many patients have both extracerebral and intracerebral bleeding. In most cases, intracerebral hemorrhages are multiple and scattered, although single hemorrhages have been observed. The temporal lobe is the most common site for traumatic hematomas.

4.41 Mechanism and Site of Injury

Mass movements resulting in deep contusions of the brain or shearing of blood vessels within the brain matter result in intracerebral hematomas. The location of the hematoma is related to the type and direction of the force involved, as well as to its magnitude.

The most common site for traumatic hematomas is the temporal lobe. The incidence of traumatic ICHs involving the temporal lobe has been reported to be between 70 and 80 percent (Caplan, 1994). Less common sites are the frontal lobes and the parietal and occipital lobes. Favored sites for the development of hematomas are near the basal surfaces within the orbital frontal lobes, the inferomedial temporal lobes and the paramedian frontal lobe above the cingulum or within the corpus callosum.

Parietal lobe hematomas typically result from blunt skull injuries or represent contrecoup injuries.[8] Deep hematomas and basal ganglionic hematomas result from shearing and tearing of lenticulostriate and anterior choroidal arterial penetrating branches. These most commonly occur from motor vehicle accidents.

4.42 Pathophysiology

Most intracerebral hemorrhages begin as liquid hematomas that dissect along fiber tracts, compressing surrounding tissue while tearing traversing venules and capillaries. Vessels ruptured by the accumulating clot add their complement of blood, and the process accelerates. The brain swells, and normal tissue is compressed, leading to secondary infarcts, edema and transtentorial herniation. If bleeding vessels

---

[8] *See* 4.14[1][a] *infra.*

constrict spontaneously or clot, bleeding may stop, and the pathologic process is abated.

Most large intracerebral hemorrhages are fatal. Death is caused by rupture into the ventricular system or by swelling resulting in herniation of the medial portions of the temporal lobes through the tentorium cerebelli. This results in displacement and compression of the midbrain, hemorrhage of the midbrain and pons, and eventually death. In patients who survive, the blood eventually resorbs, leaving a cavity of fibrous tissue.

When the hematoma is of venous origin, or when arterial bleeding ceases soon after onset, tissue separates to accommodate the local hematoma. Its progressive enlargement by surrounding edema can simulate a neoplasm (tumor).

The blood vessels from patients with traumatic ICH undergo considerable change. Smaller veins and capillaries may show extreme distension and engorgement, and luminal (pertaining to the hollow interior of blood vessels) contents show evidence of hemolysis (breakdown) and homogenization of red blood cells, indicating stasis of blood flow. Vessel walls have increased permeability, evidenced by distension of perivascular spaces, with extravasated (leaked) serum and red blood cells. With time, small blood vessels show degenerative changes. Tissue elements of these walls are difficult to define, and they may become necrotic (die).

4.43   Clinical Considerations

Most patients with traumatic intracerebral hematoma (ICH) have other medical problems that complicate the interpretation of clinical signs and symptoms. Hyperventilation may be caused by increased intracranial pressure and stupor or from cardiopulmonary injury. Loss of blood and body fluids from other injuries may cause shock, hypotension (low blood pressure) and reduced cerebral perfusion. Traumatic occlusion or dissection of extracranial vessels can lead to brain infarction. Concomitant hemorrhages, such as epidural and subdural; skull injuries; brain contusions and lacerations can all add to the patient's clinical picture. Findings of headache, vomiting, stiff neck, reduction of consciousness and seizures are common generally in patients with head injuries, whether or not they also harbor brain hematomas.

On presentation, it may not be clear that brain lesions are traumatic. Retrograde amnesia (loss of memory of events that occurred before the event causing the amnesia), clouding of consciousness and cognitive deficits often limit the patient's ability to tell the medical staff what happened. Associated superficial injuries may or may not be present. CT or MR scanning may help in identifying a traumatic etiology.

Temporal lobe hematomas cause shifting of the intracranial contents and herniation of medial temporal lobe structures against the midbrain. Third nerve palsies and coma with decerebration (cutting of nerve fibers between the brain and spinal cord) can result and can be fatal.

The "pulped temporal lobe syndrome" occurs when the anterior temporal lobe is badly injured and hemorrhagic and it swells dramatically, pushing out of the confines of the middle cranial fossa. Smaller lesions may affect the limbic structures, causing a change in behavior and personality. Patients may become uncharacteristically aggressive or hostile, and they also may become physically or verbally abusive. Changes in food preferences or sexual appetites may occur. Memory may be affected. New memory formation may be interfered with, or retrograde amnesia may occur. Aphasia (speech abnormalities) may occur after lesions of the dominant (usually left) temporal lobe occur. Seizures develop more commonly after temporal lobe or frontal lobe hematomas than those at other sites.

Clinical signs due to frontal lobe hematomas depend on the size of the hematoma and its location within the frontal lobe. Hematomas tend to evolve in the orbital, basal surface and to occur just above the corpus callosum. Frontal lobe hemorrhages most typically are accompanied by contralateral hemiparesis (weakness on the side of the body opposite the injury) and bifrontal headache. Focal motor seizures may occur as well as classic frontal lobe release signs, such as sucking and grasping responses, and conjugate eye deviation toward the diseased hemisphere. Orbital frontal hematomas often cause a disinhibited, aggressive state in which patients may be argumentative, uncooperative and physically or sexually aggressive. They may also have difficulty concentrating and have memory disturbances. During the acute stage, patients may be disoriented. Patients with large frontal hematomas are less spontaneous and have decreased speech and motor activity, and an inability to remain with tasks.

Parietal lobe hematomas primarily result in sensorimotor, cognitive and behavioral changes A typical presentation is pain in the ipsilateral (same side) temple, moderate contralateral sensory deficit and mild hemiparesis. The side and size of the hematoma are important determinants of symptoms. Occipital lobe hematomas can cause headache localized to the ipsilateral orbital region. They typically cause visual field abnormalities.

Basal ganglionic, deep hematomas are often large and associated with considerable mass effect. Clinical abnormalities are often motor, cognitive and behavioral. Most patients have hemiparesis when they are initially seen. If lesions involve the posterior limb of the internal capsule, the hemiparesis is usually persistent. Those with more anterior lesions or with hematomas that spare the capsule have better recovery of strength.

Speech deficits are very common after dominant hemisphere basal ganglionic hematomas. Muteness, reduced verbal fluency and naming difficulties may all occur.

4.44   Diagnostic Procedures

Diagnostically, intracerebral hemorrhage may be confused with subarachnoid hemorrhage, infarction, hypertensive encephalopathy and possibly fulminating meningitis or brain abscess. The differentiation of hemorrhage from infarction by history and examination may not be possible; however, CT or MRI scanning make it obvious.

Signs indicating an intracerebral hemorrhage, include papilledema (swelling of the optic disc), retinal hemorrhages and signs of meningeal irritation, such as resistance to neck flexion. Other indications of cerebral hemorrhage as opposed to infarction include an absence of localizing signs in a comatose patient and transient unconsciousness followed by progressive deterioration of the sensorium.

Laboratory findings of an intracerebral hemorrhage include a leukocytosis (elevated white blood cell count) of 15,000 to 20,000/ cubic mm. Elevated levels of albumin and glucose may appear in the urine, and glucose may be increased in the blood.

Lumbar puncture may provide important information: however, it must not be performed prior to CT or MRI. If imaging demonstrates hemorrhage, then lumbar puncture is not necessary and may be contraindicated if brain structures are shifted from their normal positions.

CT scans of intracerebral hemorrhage demonstrate a dense, sharply delineated, homogeneous mass that displaces structures from their normal positions. Surrounding it may be a ring of reduced density caused by interstitial degeneration and edema. Blood usually is visible in CSF unless it has been diluted.

Intracerebral hemorrhage also results in an elevated hematocrit (red blood cell count). This usually occurs within 30 minutes of hemorrhage and lasts for 3 to 10 days, during which time the hemorrhage is clearly visible on CT. Intracerebral hemorrhage disappears from CT scans within 30 days and leaves an area of decreased density, indicating resorption of clot.

If the CT is normal and there are no signs of increased intracranial pressure, lumbar puncture with CSF analysis might provide the answer to a diagnostic dilemma. However, no blood is found in the CSF of between 15 and 25 percent of patients with cerebral hemorrhages, because blood has not yet entered the subarachnoid space.

Acute intracerebral hemorrhage is often better demonstrated by CT than MRI. During the first three to five days, the hematoma may be isodense with the brain and therefore not distinguishable. Within a week of onset, the hematoma is usually visible on MRI.

Several imaging characteristics of CT and MRI scans may help identify a traumatic etiology. Evidence of traumatic etiologies include skull fractures, small collections of blood in the dural spaces and subarachnoid hemorrhages. Traumatic hematomas are often multiple, predominantly temporal and frontal, emphasize the orbital and basal surfaces, often have mixed densities due to edema and ischemic necrosis (tissue death due to lack of blood to a body part) within the contusion, are located in a path that might suggest coup and contrecoup injuries, and are often irregular in shape as compared with the round shape of acute hypertensive intracerebral hemorrhage. MRI is superior for detecting hematomas along the basal surfaces, since these lesions are often obscured on CT by the bony margins.

4.45 Treatment

Once bleeding begins within the brain, there is no effective medical means of stopping it. Therapy is aimed at keeping the patient alive and as quiet as possible in the hope that the hemorrhage will stop spontaneously. General supportive measures include parenteral feeding (obtaining nutrition through means other than the mouth), tracheostomy, anticonvulsant therapy and control of blood pressure. If high blood pressure is thought to be due to elevated intracranial pressure, steroid therapy and surgical decompression should be considered.

Certain patients are candidates for surgical evacuation of blood through a burr hole or evacuation of a clot through a craniotomy. These measures should be confined to patients who are generally healthy, whose hypertension is controllable, who are not comatose and whose lesion lies in the nondominant hemisphere or in the poles of the dominant hemisphere. Evacuation of intracerebral hematoma located in the subcortical white matter may produce dramatic improvement, but those involving the internal capsule or the thalamus should not be touched.

Surgery should be considered for patients in whom an acute deficit is followed by a lucid interval of partial recover, and then by gradually evolving signs of increasing intracranial pressure with cerebral compression, such as bradycardia (slow heart rate), increasing blood pressure, diminishing respiratory rate, deterioration in the level of consciousness and possibly third nerve paralysis. For these patients, immediate evacuation of a clot may be lifesaving.

Patients who have acute cerebral deficit followed by stabilization without recovery may benefit from surgery if a mass is demonstrated on CT. Patients with signs of increased intracranial pressure due to hydrocephalus should be considered for ventricular drainage.

4.46 Prognosis

The prognosis of a patient depends mostly on the size and location of the hematoma. Prior to the advent of CT, the mortality rate was between 50 and 70 percent. Improved detection of small hematomas by CT, as well as improved management, has decreased the mortality rate to between 20 and 25 percent (Toole, 1990). Mortality tends to increase with age and hypertension, and with coma in patients over 60 years of age.

Hemorrhage in the pons carries a particularly poor prognosis. Hemorrhage extending into the ventricles has a worse prognosis (approximately 60 percent mortality rate), as compared with those that remain confined to the cerebral substance (approximately 20 percent mortality rate).

The prognosis for patients with traumatic basal ganglionic hematomas is very poor. More than 60 percent of patients with either single or multiple lesions may die or become vegetative or severely disabled (Caplan, 1994). The worst outcome occurs in those patients with large hematomas and raised intracranial pressure.

Between 35 and 50 percent of surviving patients show adequate functional recovery. Complications include secondary pneumonia, electrolyte disturbance, pulmonary embolism and myocardial infarction (heart attack).

4.50   INTRACEREBELLAR HEMORRHAGE AND HEMATOMA

The literature on traumatic cerebellar hemorrhage and hematoma is very limited, since these lesions were typically identified only after death. Acute cerebellar injuries most often occur after gunshot injuries. Symptoms of cerebellar hematoma in patients with a closed head injury include headache, stiff neck, drowsiness and ataxia (inability to coordinate the muscles) prior to the rapid onset of coma.

Coma and death result from brain stem compression by the enlarging cerebellar hematoma. Detection of cerebellar hematomas by CT and MRI has decreased the likelihood of this chain of events leading to death.

4.51   Clinical Considerations

The characteristic symptoms at onset of cerebellar hemorrhage include headache, vertigo (sensation of whirling in space), vomiting and inability to stand. Headache is experienced by 60 to 70 percent of patients and is typically bilateral occipital or frontal. Inability to stand has been reported by up to 93 percent of patients with cerebellar hemorrhage (Kase, 1994).

Findings on neurologic examination in patients with cerebellar hemorrhage include oculomotor abnormalities, such as ipsilateral horizontal gaze palsy and sixth nerve palsy, limb hemiataxia and gait ataxia in the absence of hemiplegia or hemiparesis. A triad of signs indicating cerebellar hemorrhage has been identified: ipsilateral limb ataxia, horizontal gaze palsy and peripheral facial palsy.

The clinical course of cerebellar hemorrhage is extremely varied. Patients may experience a sudden deterioration in association with cerebellar herniation. Herniation can occur upward through the tentorial notch or downward through the foramen magnum (large opening in the bottom of the skull, through which the spinal cord enters the spine). Herniation rapidly produces coma, with the majority of patients who become comatose doing so within 24 to 48 hours following injury. Once coma has developed, the prognosis is very poor.

In dramatic contrast to patients who develop brain herniation, some patients with cerebellar hemorrhage may have a benign course with clinical recovery achieved without surgical therapy.

4.52 Diagnosis

Before the use of CT scanning, the diagnostic suspicion of cerebellar hemorrhage was generally followed by posterior fossa angiography (x-ray of blood vessels) and ventriculography, which showed an avascular cerebellar mass, frequently associated with hydrocephalus. The sensitivity of radiologic diagnosis of cerebellar hemorrhage was dramatically improved with the introduction of CT scanning, which permits the immediate diagnosis of acute hemorrhage regardless of its size, as well as imaging the secondary effects of the hemorrhage on adjacent structures, including the ventricular system below and above the tentorium.

In very rare cases, an acute cerebellar hematoma may be missed on CT. However, CT is considered virtually 100 percent sensitive for the detection of intracerebellar hemorrhage.

4.53 Treatment

The selection of therapy in cerebellar hemorrhage is primarily dictated by clinical criteria. Level of consciousness and, to a lesser extent, signs of pontine cranial nerve involvement are the most valuable parameters for deciding between conservative and surgical therapy. It is important to maintain close clinical observation of patients who have a stable level of consciousness and small hematomas with or without hydrocephalus. Patients with any new sign of declining level of consciousness or pontine cranial nerve dysfunction should most likely be operated on promptly. Patients who present with an already deteriorating level of consciousness, irrespective of the size and location of hematoma or presence or absence of hydrocephalus, should undergo emergency surgical treatment

The choice of surgical procedure in patients with cerebellar hemorrhage is controversial. Relatively poor results have been obtained with needle aspiration of the hematoma and with ventricular drainage procedures. Better results have been achieved with suboccipital craniotomy with wide exposure of the cerebellar hemisphere for adequate clot evacuation. This must be followed by careful attention to hemostasis and intraoperative and postoperative blood pressure control.

Some physicians report excellent results with ventricular drainage of hydrocephalus alone for the treatment of cerebellar hemorrhage with hydrocephalus. Others believe that the clot must be evacuated along with ventricular drainage. It appears that ventricular drainage alone may be more often performed as a palliative measure in severely compromised patients or those who are poor surgical risks. A new surgical approach is CT-guided stereotactic fibrinolysis of cerebellar hematomas (Mohadjer, et al., 1990). This involves stereotactic puncture (a meticulous surgical procedure for destroying deep-brain structures using three-dimensional lines of reference) of the hematoma, followed by injection of urokinase to dissolve the clot.

4.54 Prognosis

Factors that are known to relate to prognosis include hematoma size and location, presence of hydrocephalus and obliteration of the quadrigeminal cistern (area on the roof of the midbrain). Hematoma size is related to outcome with hematomas of 3 cm or greater that are associated with a progressive course leading to brain stem compression, whereas smaller hematomas are usually benign. Hematoma size is also correlated with the presence of hydrocephalus, which is more common with larger hematomas. Midline hematomas are generally associated with the acute onset of coma, and these are often fatal unless emergency surgery can be performed before the development of coma and signs of bilateral brain stem dysfunction.

4.60 INTRAVENTRICULAR HEMORRHAGE

Blood can enter the ventricles in several ways: by contiguous extension from a cerebral hematoma, through shearing of the subependymal (pertaining to the lining membrane of the ventricles) veins and through retrograde extension of subarachnoid blood via the fourth ventricular outlet foramina. Direct penetrating wounds can also result in intraventricular hemorrhage. The most obvious mode of entry is via direct extension from an adjacent intracerebral hematoma. The ventricular lining is composed of a single epithelial layer and therefore presents no significant barrier.

Blunt forces may result in a cerebrospinal fluid–blood fluid level that layers dependently in the occipital horns. This is usually due to shearing of the subependymal veins.

Intraventricular hemorrhage is gradually diluted by the CSF and washed from the ventricular system into the subarachnoid space. If there is no recurrent hemorrhage, the blood rarely persists within the ventricular system for more than two weeks. Blood may form a cast, however, and remain within the ventricular system for longer periods. If blood remains within the CSF for a relatively long time, it may irritate the ventricular wall, producing an ependymitis (a proliferation of subependymal cells, which break through the ependymal lining of the ventricular system). Ependymitis can result in obstructive hydrocephalus.

Uncomplicated intraventricular hematoma alone generally does not require specific treatment, as the hematoma will usually resolve spontaneously. Particularly large volumes of blood or the onset of hydrocephalus requires drainage in order to enhance recovery and prevent further complications of hydrocephalus.

4.70   TECHNIQUE OF CRANIOTOMY

A basic premise of neurosurgery is that whatever surgery is undertaken, it should be extensive enough to adequately take care of the problems present. To do a less than sufficient procedure in hopes of sparing the patient a more extensive procedure exposes the patient to a much greater risk of neurologic damage in the long run.

4.71   The Scalp Flap

The basic concept of local flap transfer is to move available tissue, with its circulation intact, from an area of excess to an area of deficiency. In order to successfully move a flap, knowledge of the skin circulation is essential. Large flaps are usually successful as long as the circulatory system between the galea (thin layer of tough tissue situated on top of the skull) and the skin is not violated by either poor flap design or by obstruction of venous return by tight closure or by the accumulation of fluid between the galea and the pericranium.

The defect as well as the location and quantity of available excess tissue should be evaluated, and a plan drawn on the scalp. Only when the pattern fits should the flap be incised, through the skin and galea but not through the pericranium. Elevation can then be done easily by blunt dissection to the base or beyond in the areolar plane. Minimal bleeding will be encountered except at the skin edges.

The prevention of fluid accumulation beneath the flap is critical in preventing venous congestion in the flap. Virtually all flap failures relate to venous obstruction rather than poor arterial flow, and if venous congestion is suspected, the prompt removal of tight sutures or a hematoma may restore circulation and save the flap.

4.72 Bone Flaps

There are basically two types of bone flap. The first is a free flap whereby the periosteum is completely separated from the skull and the entire section of bone is lifted off, and then replaced at the conclusion of the procedure. This free flap is quicker and promotes less bleeding.

The second type is an osteoplastic flap hinged on the temporalis muscle. The appropriate piece of bone remains attached to the periosteum and muscle. The advantage of this type of flap is that the blood supply to the bone is not completely disrupted, and this increases the likelihood of having a successful closure and long-term health of the skull following the procedure.

4.73 Unroofing of the Skull

It is essential that the appropriate area of the skull is exposed and that sufficient exposure is obtained to adequately treat the underlying condition. A miscalculation regarding the location or extent of exposure required precludes success of the surgery.

Burr holes are made at the periphery of the area to be exposed. Sufficient burr holes should be used to avoid tearing the dura. This usually means that more burr holes are required in elderly patients. A high-speed craniotome is used to cut the skull between the burr holes. Special attention must be paid to homeostasis (control of bleeding), since bleeding associated with the skull and scalp has contributed to postoperative morbidity in the past.

4.74   Exposure of the Dura Mater

Once the skull has been unroofed, attention is directed to the next exposed layer—the dura mater. This is a tough, thick envelope that completely surrounds the brain. It receives its blood supply from the anterior, middle and posterior meningeal arteries.

The dura is opened across the base, and the blood vessels are cauterized or clipped as the incision is made. The dura is elevated so that it is virtually hinged at the upper level or midline. Some surgeons deliberately cut out a free dural flap in order to decrease postoperative dural bleeding.

4.75   Exposure of the Brain

When the dura has been elevated and the underlying brain exposed, accurate localization of the lesion will permit surgery. Removal of a subdural hematoma is done with cup forceps accompanied by irrigation. Bleeding sites are coagulated. Bleeding in the area of the sagittal sinus must be managed by coagulation or application of Gelfoam ® or muscle along the sinus. Finally a systematic and thorough inspection is performed in each direction— frontally, medially, occipitally and temporally—to determine if there is a clot or any bleeding.

4.76   Dural Closure

After resection of hematoma and necrotic tissue is complete, hemostasis must be meticulous to avoid postoperative hematoma. Once hemostasis is complete, the dura is carefully replaced and sutured. The type of suture employed varies and is left to the discretion of the surgeon. If there is marked brain swelling in spite of removal of the hematoma, then the dura may be loosely replaced and/or an artificial dura may be added. The bone flap, either free or osteoplastic, is wired down in its customary position, or in special circumstances (e.g., severe cerebral edema), it may not be used at all. When the skull is reattached, the procedure is referred to as a craniectomy rather than a craniotomy.

4.77 Surgery of the Brain

Evacuation of the hematoma is accompanied by inspection of the underlying brain for areas of significant contusion or damage. Decisions must then be made regarding how much tissue should be debrided. Only necrotic, nonviable tissue is debrided. This will appear purplish and mottled, and will be quite suctionable in consistency. As long as the surgeon concentrates on removing the necrotic tissue, there should be little chance of increasing neurologic deficit.

Gunshot wounds, gutter fractures of the brain or depressed fractures that have thrust fragments of bone, scalp or other foreign detritus within the brain must be followed along their pathways and cleaned out. These bodies, if they are not removed, will set up a nidus (focal point) for the later formation of a brain abscess or seizure disorder.

4.78 Closure

The scalp flap is now applied over the skull and periosteum, the periosteum and muscle having been previously sutured in place. The scalp clips or clamps are now removed, one at a time, to determine if any blood vessels have begun to leak. Vessels are coagulated as required. The inner layer of the scalp, the galea aponeurotica, is sutured. Scalp closure must carefully approximate the margins, being firm enough to prevent bleeding but not tight enough to exert tension or to produce necrosis of the scalp margins.

4.79 Anesthesia

The major consideration in the selection of an anesthetic agent for patients with head injuries is that the agent or agents do not increase intracranial pressure. Any agent that causes cerebral vasodilation (increase in size of the blood vessels) is likely to cause an increase in intracranial pressure and should be avoided. Ketamine is one the most powerful cerebral vasodilators and, therefore, should be avoided in the head-injured patient.

All inhalation anesthetic agents can increase cerebral blood flow to some degree. Halothane, enflurane and isoflurane all increase cerebral blood flow, but they are probably safe in low concentrations. Nitrous oxide has a slight vasodilatory effect that is probably not clinically significant and is considered to be a good choice for head-injured patients. A commonly used combination is nitrous oxide to oxygen (50 to 70 percent oxygen), an intravenous muscle relaxant and thiopental. The use of hyperventilation and mannitol prior to and during induction can blunt the vasodilatory effect and limit intracranial hypertension to some degree while the cranium is being opened. If, during surgery, malignant brain swelling occurs that is refractory to hyperventilation and mannitol, thiopental in large doses (5 to 10 mg/kg) should be given. As a last resort, brain swelling may be reduced by trimethaphan or nitroprusside.

4.80 TRAUMATIC CEREBRAL THROMBOSIS

Traumatic cerebral thrombosis involves the occlusion of a blood vessel within the brain in the setting of head trauma. Post-traumatic vascular complications can involve both the arterial and venous systems. They may be noted at the time of injury, or they may not become apparent until several days or months following the injury.

The incidence of vascular complications associated with head injury is not known. Because cerebral angiography is no longer part of the routine evaluation of head trauma, the data base is not likely to be expanded significantly. Clinicians, therefore, must maintain a high index of suspicion and obtain angiograms when the clinical picture cannot be explained by CT or MRI scans.

4.81 Site and Mechanism of Injury

The pathogenesis of post-traumatic vascular thrombosis and infarction (lack of blood flow to a region of the body) involves both local and systemic factors. Systemic factors contributing to post-traumatic infarction include any process that reduces the effective oxygenated perfusion of the brain, for example, systemic hypotension, reduced cardiac output, respiratory failure due to muscular or pulmonary trauma and depletion of oxyhemoglobin due to alcohol intoxication. The extent of the injury depends on the duration and intensity of the hypoxia, the presence of underlying anemia and coexisting occlusive vascular disease. Changes in the brain resulting from hypoxia further contribute to cerebral swelling and exacerbate elevated intracranial pressure.

Local factors contributing to traumatic thrombosis and infarction include cerebral edema, brain herniation, mass lesions, underlying arteriosclerosis, inflammatory arterial disease, congenital vascular anomalies, direct vascular injury (for example, laceration, transection or dissection) with subsequent thrombosis, fat embolism, embolization of fractured atheromatous plaque, vasospasm and post-traumatic infection. Injury to cortical cerebral vessels can also occur in association with a skull fracture and result in vascular narrowing or occlusion.

Post-traumatic infarction resulting from extrinsic vascular compression is usually secondary to brain herniation or to direct pressure on the cerebral cortex by an extra-axial mass. In many instances, this type of injury affects the middle cerebral artery as it courses through the sylvian fissure. Cerebral vasospasm is another cause of post-traumatic infarction. Subarachnoid hemorrhage and direct vascular injury predispose to vasospasm. The most common site for post-traumatic vasospasm is the intradural portion of the distal internal carotid artery. Vasospasm generally causes ischemic cortical injury and spares the deep gray nuclei and white matter.

4.82   Signs and Symptoms

The symptoms and course of traumatic thrombosis are dependent upon the size and location of the occluded vessel as well as the amount of brain tissue destroyed by infarction. Infarction typically has a delayed onset, with ischemic deficits developing within minutes to several days.

Venous thrombosis results in a damming of the venous drainage of the brain. Its features and clinical presentations will be related to the amount of blood collected, availability of alternative venous collateral channels and involvement of the particular area of the brain affected.

4.83   Diagnosis

Vascular occlusion can be diagnosed by angiography. Angiography, however, is not able to determine whether the cause of occlusion is thrombosis or vasospasm. The middle cerebral artery is the most susceptible to post-traumatic occlusion.

CT scanning is able to detect infarction that results from vascular occlusion and can help in detecting which vessel may be occluded, but it usually will not indicate the specific site of occlusion. CT findings are generally unremarkable within the first few hours. Earliest CT manifestations include a subtle loss of gray matter–white matter differentiation, mild mass effect and a slight decrease in attenuation values. Within 48 hours, the infarction becomes more defined, further decreases in attenuation value and takes on a wedge-shaped morphology. When an initially bland infarct transforms into a hemorrhagic infarct, an embolic etiology should be suspected.

MR imaging is usually more sensitive to brain infarction than CT. MR imaging has a major advantage over CT in assessing post-traumatic infarction, because it can assess vascular patency by the presence of a flow void. An absent flow void is highly suggestive of a vessel occlusion. A decrease in caliber of a vessel due to vasospasm, dissection or brain herniation is also better demonstrated on MRI. On both the CT and MRI scans, the lesion often takes on a gyriform morphology (convoluted shape), which can help identify a vascular etiology as opposed to a neoplasm.

4.84   Carotid Artery Thrombosis

Carotid artery occlusion secondary to blunt neck trauma occurs rarely. It may follow fracture of the sphenoid bone or fracture of the base of the skull. A crush type injury may cause the damage if the artery is caught between splinters or fragments. Torsion injuries secondary to hyperextension or hyperflexion of the neck may produce partial or complete tearing of the artery.

Occlusion of the carotid artery most commonly occurs at the C2 vertebral level. If occlusion is a result of a dissecting artery, the entire vessel between the carotid bulb and the ophthalmic artery can undergo rapid thrombosis, regardless of the site at which the dissection originates.

Clinical diagnosis is often difficult, and there may be a symptom-free period of up to 24 hours. Patients may experience transient ischemic attacks, develop a neck hematoma or develop Horner's syndrome (lagging of the upper lid of one eye, recession or sinking of the eyeball, constriction of the pupil, narrowing of the palpebral fissure between the margins of the two eyelids, and lack of perspiration on one side of the face). Once the occlusion occurs, a focal neurologic deficit may develop, although this may be hard to separate in the setting of a primary brain injury.

[1] Treatment

Blood flow through the occluded artery can be restored through several mechanisms: Vasospasm may spontaneously resolve, the thrombus may be spontaneously lysed (broken up) or the vessel may be recanalized through instrumentation. The role of anticoagulation therapy is a matter of controversy.

[2] Prognosis

The mortality rate for traumatic carotid thrombosis in the neck is reported to be between 40 and 90 percent (Narayan, 1991). If the patient survives, there is a great probability that he or she will be left with severe and permanent neurologic sequelae, as the internal carotid artery supplies (through its branches: anterior and middle cerebral arteries) a major part of the hemispheres and forward portions of the deep structures of the brain. Thrombosis of this artery tends to be catastrophic, causing extensive infarction and necrosis, with severe neurologic deficits.

4.90 TRAUMATIC ANEURYSMS AND FISTULAS

Head trauma may stretch the arteries, particularly at the base of the brain, sufficiently to rupture their intima (the elastic inner layer of the artery wall). When this occurs, the damaged part of the arterial wall dilates, forming the aneurysm, which is actually a bulge produced by weakness in the wall of the structure. Pseudoaneurysms or false aneurysms are produced following laceration of an arterial wall. Hemorrhage is locally confined by a blood clot or hematoma. This surrounding hematoma, which is partly liquefied and partly solidified, enlarges and communicates with the damaged artery, creating the pseudoaneurysm. *(See Figure 4-7.)*

Traumatic aneurysms may affect either the cerebral arteries on the surface of the brain or those within the brain. More than half of all traumatic intracranial aneurysms develop in the middle cerebral artery and its branches.

4.91 Mechanism of Injury

The majority of traumatic aneurysms are precipitated by closed head injuries. They can be caused by indirect trauma, in which case it is

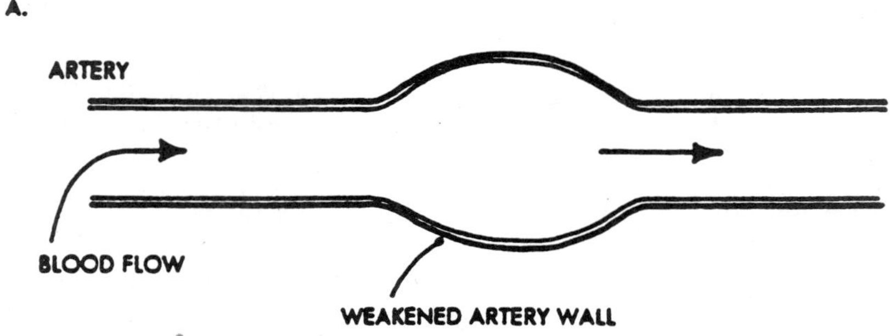

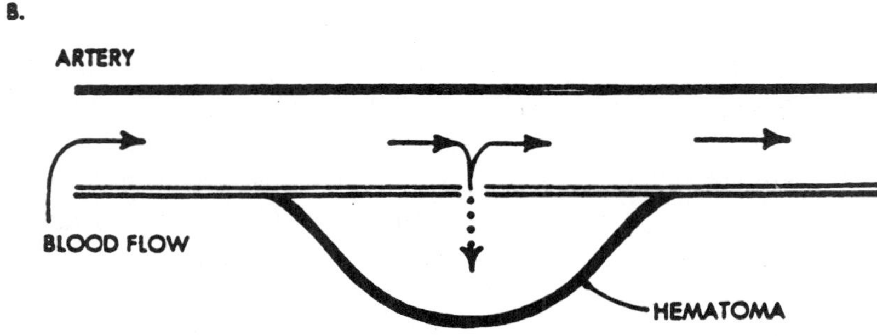

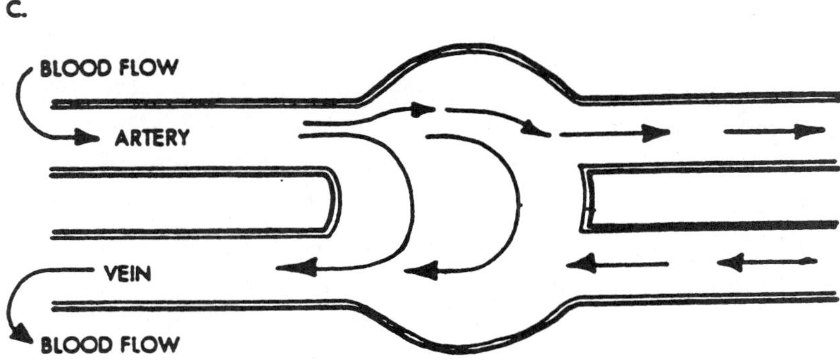

Fig. 4-7. Vascular lesions occurring in cases of head injury: (A) aneurysm; (B) pseudoaneurysm or false aneurysm; and (C) arterio-venous fistula.

theorized that the artery is torn at impact by the movement of the brain within the skull. Causative injuries associated with traumatic aneurysms include lesions such as extradural or intracerebral hematomas, skull fractures and other acute types of head trauma.[9]

Traumatic aneurysms of the middle cerebral artery and its branches are presumably due to skull fractures that lacerate the dura, allowing immediate herniation of cerebral cortical tissue through the site of laceration and fracture. Simultaneously, tissue of the cortex as well as vessels can be trapped by the bony margins of the fracture site. If penetrating trauma is the cause of the aneurysm, clearly the location of the aneurysm is related to the path of penetrating trauma. Traumatic aneurysms carry an increased risk of intraluminal thrombus formation that may subsequently embolize.

4.92 Incidence

The incidence of traumatic aneurysms varies significantly between adults and children following head injury. Intracranial aneurysms are relatively rare following head injury in adults. However, they account for between 10 and 20 percent of all pediatric cases of aneurysms.

4.93 Diagnosis

Aneurysms can develop immediately following head trauma, or they may develop insidiously over a period of months to even years. The most common time for presentation is two to eight weeks following trauma. Clinically, patients present with visual deficits, cranial nerve palsies, neck pain or intermittent ischemic episodes (temporary condition involving insufficient supply of blood to a body part) due to distal embolization of mural thrombi. In rare cases, a traumatic aneurysm may present as a pulsatile mass causing compressive symptoms.

The location of the traumatic aneurysm is related to the location and nature of the precipitating trauma, the vascular suspensory points of the brain and vascular contiguity with the edges of the dura. Traumatic aneurysms occasionally involve the peripheral cortical vessels or the meningeal vessels, secondary to penetrating trauma or an adjacent skull fracture. Aneurysm has also been reported to follow

---

[9] *See also* ch. 6 for a discussion of skull fractures.

needle aspiration of a subdural hematoma. Skull fractures may cause aneurysm of an extracranial vessel, particularly the superficial temporal artery. These injuries typically present with an enlarging pulsatile scalp mass.

On angiography, traumatic aneurysms typically have an irregular contour and a wide or nonexistent aneurysmal neck. The wall of the aneurysm offers little structural support unless it is surrounded by firm structures, such as bone, ligaments or dura. Angiography underestimates the true size of a partially or totally thrombosed aneurysm, because it only visualizes the patent lumen (hollow interior of the vessel).

On MRI, the appearance of an aneurysm depends on its size and the extent of the thrombosis. If there is no turbulence or thrombosis, the lesion appears as a small, rounded area of signal loss, contiguous with its parent artery but projecting outside its normal confines. Pulsation of the aneurysm appears as oscillatory phase artifacts radiating away from the lumen. When partial thrombosis of the aneurysm is present, the lesion presents as a rounded mass with concentric laminated rings of hemorrhage in various stages of evolution.

MR imaging is superior to CT scanning for determining the size of an aneurysm, the degree of patency, the extent of thrombosis and the relationship of the aneurysm to the surrounding hematoma (if ruptured) or brain (if not ruptured). MR imaging is most sensitive in detecting aneurysms around the circle of Willis (at the base of the brain), and more peripherally located traumatic aneurysms may be difficult to identify on MRI. These lesions require conventional angiography.

4.94 Management

Management is aimed at preventing the aneurysm from rupturing and bleeding. This is usually accomplished by obliterating the aneurysm as soon as possible. No single therapeutic regimen fits all groups of patients, and management is affected by age, sex, the clinical condition of the patient, the specific aneurysm site, the time interval since trauma, and the size and configuration of the aneurysm. The experience of the physician in treating aneurysms is also an important factor in determining appropriate management,

The clinical condition at the time therapy is begun is the fundamental determinant in selecting appropriate therapy. In high-risk, comatose patients, little is gained by an immediate operation unless an intra-parenchymal clot (one that is within the function tissue of the brain) is present. Many comatose patients will improve with conservative therapy, allowing a definitive operation to be performed later with less risk.

If the aneurysm is accessible to surgical intervention, various surgical techniques are employed to obliterate the aneurysm: The artery may be ligated (tied off), the aneurysm may be excised (cut out) or trapped between metallic clips, or the artery may be cauterized.

4.95 Prognosis

Mortality is related to factors such as early or late diagnosis, type of surgical treatment and the nature and extent of the trauma that precipitated the aneurysm. Approximately 50 percent of traumatic aneurysms not undergoing spontaneous reduction in size will probably rupture within three weeks of the initial trauma. Surgery has reduced the mortality rate associated with traumatic aneurysms from approximately 50 to 20 percent. Patients who are comatose at the time therapy is begun have the highest mortality rate, and alert patients have the lowest mortality rate.

4.96 Traumatic Aneurysm of the Internal Carotid Artery

Traumatic aneurysm of the internal carotid artery (ICA) usually involves the cavernous segment, although the supraclinoid, intrapetrous and upper cervical segments also may be affected. Aneurysms associated with these less common locations are frequently associated with an anterior basilar skull fracture. When the common carotid artery or the lower cervical portion of the ICA is damaged, the cause is usually a gunshot wound or blunt trauma to the neck.

[1] Clinical Picture

Symptoms and signs of carotid artery aneurysm depend upon the segment involved and whether it is above or below the origin of the ophthalmic artery; the rapidity of development; the availability and adequacy of collateral circulation; and the area of brain affected, whether it is in the distribution of the anterior cerebral artery or the middle cerebral artery. Hoarseness or difficulty swallowing will be present if the aneurysm is large enough to protrude into the pharynx (throat) or to cause compression of vagus and sympathetic nerve chains.

Characteristically a mass can be felt under the lower jaw or in a portion of the pharynx, expanding and contracting like an arterial pulse. Other symptoms include tinnitus (ringing in the ears), vertigo (a sensation of whirling in space), and dyspnea (shortness of breath). If the flow of blood to the brain is compromised and there is inadequate collateral flow to prevent ischemia, other neurologic signs will develop. These can be extremely varied, since the carotid artery and its branches supply a great deal of the brain. Rupture of a traumatic internal carotid artery aneurysm into the sphenoid sinus may cause epistaxis (nosebleed), with profuse and catastrophic hemorrhage.

[2]   Diagnosis

While angiography will usually reveal the exact location of an aneurysm, it should only be performed when the diagnosis is in doubt and surgical reconstruction is being considered. It should only be performed by individuals skilled in the management of patients with cerebrovascular disease, and it should not be done unless facilities for immediate reconstructive vascular surgery are available (Toole, 1990).

On angiography, a traumatic aneurysm often appears as an irregularly contoured vessel with a wide or an absent aneurysmal neck. On MRI, the aneurysm may appear as a small, rounded area of signal loss, contiguous with the parent artery but projecting outside its normal confines.

[3]   Differential Diagnosis

The differential diagnosis of traumatic carotid aneurysm includes peritonsillar or retropharyngeal abscesses. If carotid aneurysms are mistaken for one of these entities and are lanced, the results can be disastrous.

[4]   Management

Carotid aneurysms carry a high probability of death in the event they rupture. Spontaneous rupture into the pharynx can occur, leading to exsanguination (massive loss of blood) or death by aspiration of blood into the lungs. Surgery is imperative, therefore.

[a] Immediate Carotid Ligation

The primary rationale for carotid artery ligation (tieing off) is that it reduces the intravascular pressure above the location that a clamp is placed and within the aneurysm. It also decreases forces on the aneurysm wall and causes flow reduction. This results in a fall in retinal artery pressure, and after carotid ligation, an average reduction of 40 percent in retinal artery pressure can be expected.

It is difficult to compare the efficacy of carotid artery ligation with other therapeutic procedures. In the short term, it appears that carotid ligation is superior to a direct intracranial approach, but it is less effective in preventing long-term, late rebleeding. For middle cerebral aneurysms, intracranial clipping is probably the preferred treatment. However, if patients are elderly or have severely compromised neurologic or medical status, they may not be candidates for an intracranial approach, and carotid ligation may be the only option.

In the presence of vasospasm, carotid ligation exacerbates ischemic complications. Therefore, ligation should be deferred until the patient's condition improves and stabilizes. The clamp may be applied, but total occlusion should be delayed until vasoconstriction subsides.

Patients who are oriented and cooperative should undergo local anesthesia; others should undergo general anesthesia. The carotid artery is exposed at the level of the carotid bifurcation by making an incision over the anterior border of the sternocleidomastoid muscle. A Crutchfield, Selverstone or other clamp is placed about 2 cm beneath the bifurcation, and the screwdriver portion of the clamp is applied. Pressure measurements of the vessel distal to the clamp should be made. If the pressure reduction is less than 50 percent with the clamp closed, total closure can usually be made in three to four days. If the pressure difference exceeds 50 percent, five to seven days may be required. Some surgeons do not believe these pressure indicators have any prognostic value but merely complicate the procedure. Postoperatively, bed rest is maintained until the clamp has been totally closed and the screwdriver portion removed.

[b] Late Complications of Carotid Artery Ligation

Rebleeding has been reported to occur in approximately 3 percent of patients following carotid artery ligation (Smith, et al., 1991). Other complications include ischemia (lack of blood supply) and distal embolization; these occur in less than 57 percent of patients. Complications may arise at any time following surgery: within the perioperative period, within a day or up to many years later. If other vessels become involved with atheromatous plaques, late ischemic complications may develop.

[c] Elective Surgery

Many factors are involved in the choice of surgical techniques, but protection of the intracranial circulation should be considered paramount. Accordingly, surgical planning must be meticulous, with provisions made for maintaining adequate cerebral blood flow.

The type of repair utilized will be contingent not only upon the situation itself but also upon the surgeon's own base of experience and familiarity with the details of fine arterial procedures performed under the operating microscope. A rent in the wall of an artery, running in a straight line, may be closed by primary sutures. An artery that is long, meandering and twisting, in combination with a small aneurysm, will be amenable to aneurysm resection and to end-to-end arterial anastomosis (surgical construction of a connection between two hollow structures).

Synthetic material may be used to bridge the gap created by a large aneurysm.

4.97   Traumatic Carotid-Cavernous Fistula

Rupture of the carotid artery within the cavernous sinus results in a carotid-cavernous fistula. Virtually every case in individuals under 40 years of age is due to trauma.

[1] Etiology

Traumatic disruption of the carotid artery probably occurs secondary to bone fracture and laceration of the artery within the sinus. Nowhere else in the body does a large major artery pass through a venous sinus.

Arterial blood will enter the sinus channel and gain entry into the superior ophthalmic veins. These veins ultimately exit in the superior eyelid, communicating with the facial vein and draining into the jugular system. Flow in the ruptured internal carotid artery escapes through the cavernous sinus, but the fistula may draw blood from all available sources. As such, blood may flow into the sinus from the opposite internal carotid artery, the vertebrobasilar artery and the meningeal vessels.

[2]   Clinical Picture

The most common symptom is a loud, continuous, machinerylike bruit (whooshing sound heard usually with a stethoscope over an area of blood flow) beginning a short time after the injury. Within a few days, proptosis (protrusion of the eyeball) may become pronounced on the side of the fistula. If both cavernous sinuses are affected, there may be bilateral proptosis. Proptosis may be associated with pulsations of the globe.

The bruit can readily be heard with a stethoscope and may be audible with the normal ear. Ocular muscle paralysis may occur, and there is often congestion and thickening of the conjunctiva. The cornea may become neovascularized with new vessels extending almost to the limbus (edge of the eye).

Impaired vision occurs regularly with carotid-cavernous fistulas. Impaired acuity is attributable to loss of retinal circulation. Secondary glaucoma complicates approximately a third of cases. Recurrent severe epistaxis (bleeding from the nose) caused by neovascularity in the nasal mucosa may lead to anemia and death. Some patients may experience transient ischemic episodes because of the stealing of cerebral blood flow in the enormous fistula.

[3]   Diagnosis

Diagnosis is multifaceted and includes a thorough neurologic and ophthalmologic examination. The classic CT scan findings of a carotid-cavernous fistula include a tortuous and dilated superior ophthalmic vein, thickened extraocular muscles, proptosis and a prominent ipsilateral cavernous sinus.

If the superior ophthalmic vein is significantly asymmetric or exceeds 4 mm, a fistula should be suspected. Chronic fistula can cause erosion of the carotid sulcus and canal, due to the increase in size of the internal carotid artery.

The morphology of a fistula on CT scan resembles that seen on MR images. MRI, however, is superior to CT for evaluating the aneurysm lumen, increased flow into the cavernous sinus, secondary venous distension of the draining veins and venous hypertension within the involved cerebral parenchyma. Cerebral angiography may be indicated to assess more accurately the veins, in order to evaluate potential collateral circulation and to rule out anomalous vasculature or to provide access for embolization.

[4] Treatment

The most up to date surgical treatment of carotid-cavernous fistula uses detachable balloons to fill the cavernous sinus and block the fistula. The major benefit of this procedure is that it allows the carotid and retinal circulation to be spared. This technique of detachable balloons should be the primary therapy for carotid-cavernous fistula.

Older techniques, such as carotid artery occlusion, trapping and all other operative techniques are physiologically unacceptable alternatives. However, the detachable balloon technique must be performed by experienced hands in order to prevent complications due to embolization, which may occur frequently.

[5] Complications

The major complications of older procedures for surgically repairing carotid-cavernous fistulas were that the retinal artery pressure and the circulation to the eye were further reduced. Because retinal ischemia is the most common cause of blindness and the primary indication for therapy in the first place, the carotid and ophthalmic artery circulation must be preserved, not further diminished.

The introduction of the detachable balloon technique for repairing the fistula spares the carotid and retinal circulation from being further reduced. The major complication of the balloon procedure is that embolization may occur, producing further complications.

4.100 AMA EVALUATION OF PERMANENT IMPAIRMENT

Traumatic intracranial hematomas can eventually affect any part of the brain. Therefore, they have the potential to cause any type of brain abnormality, from the least conspicuous change to weakness, personality changes, coma and death. The permanent impairment that results depends on the area or areas of the brain that are permanently damaged.

The America Medical Association (AMA, 1993) system for evaluating permanent impairment describes several categories of impairment resulting from damage to the brain. An impairment evaluation includes three components: The medical examination covers history, diagnosis and current clinical status; the analysis of the findings documents the effect of the impairments on the patient's ability to perform activities of daily living; and an overall estimate of the patient's impairment is made as a percent impairment of the whole person.

4.101   Aphasia and Communication Disturbances

Impairment ranges from minimal disturbance in comprehension and production of language symbols (0 to 9 percent impairment of the whole person) to complete inability to communicate or comprehend language symbols (40 to 60 percent).

4.102   Disturbances of Mental Status and Integrative Function

Impairment ranges from mild impairment, in which the patient can perform most activities (1 to 14 percent), to the individual being unable to care for himself or herself, or to be safe without supervision (50 to 70 percent).

4.103   Disturbance in Level of Consciousness and Awareness

Impairment ranges from brief repetitive or persisting alteration of state of consciousness (0 to 14 percent) to persistent vegetative state or irreversible coma requiring total medical support (50 to 90 percent).

4.104   Episodic Neurologic Disorders

Impairment ranges from a paroxysmal disorder with predictable characteristics and unpredictable occurrence that does not limit usual activities but is a risk to the patient or limits performance of daily activities (0 to 14 percent), to uncontrolled paroxysmal disorder of such severity and constancy that it totally limits the individual's daily activities (50 to 70 percent).

4.105   The Cranial Nerves

Complete destruction of both optic nerves is a 100 percent impairment of the visual system and an 85 percent impairment of the whole person. Visual field impairment ranges from 28 to 62 percent impairment. Impairment due to damage of the seventh cranial nerve (facial) ranges from 1 to 45 percent. Impairment due to damage of the eighth cranial nerve (auditory) ranges from 1 to 70 percent.

4.106 Station and Gait

Impairment ranges from ability to rise but difficulty with elevations, grades, stairs and walking long distances (1 to 9 percent), to inability to stand without help from others (40 to 60 percent).

4.107 Use of Upper Extremities

Impairment for one impaired extremity ranges from problems with digital dexterity (1 to 9 percent), to inability to use the involved extremity for self-care and daily activities (30 to 60 percent). If the patient has two impaired extremities, impairment ranges from difficulty with digital dexterity (1 to 19 percent), to inability to use upper extremities (80 percent).

4.108 Respiration

Impairment from respiratory difficulty ranges from difficulty with activities of daily living that require exertion (5 to 9 percent), to no capacity for spontaneous respiration (greater than 90 percent).

4.200 BIBLIOGRAPHY

Text References

American College of Surgeons: Advanced Trauma Life Support Course for Physicians. Chicago: American College of Surgeons, 1989.

American Medical Association: Guides to the Evaluation of Permanent Impairment, 4th ed. Chicago: American Medical Association, 1993.

Burger P. C., et al.: Surgical Pathology of the Nervous System and its Coverings. New York: Churchill Livingstone, 1991.

Caplan L. R.: Head Trauma and Related Intracerebral Hemorrhage. In: Kase, C. S. and Caplan, L. R. (Eds.): Intracerebral Hemorrhage. Boston: Butterworth-Heinemann, 1994.

Gean, A. D.: Imaging of Head Trauma. New York: Raven Press, 1994.

Kase, C. S.: Cerebellar Hemorrhage. In: Kase, C. S. and Caplan, L. R. (Eds.): Intracerebral Hemorrhage. Boston: Butterworth-Heinemann, 1994.

Mendelow, D. A.: Head Injury. In: Walton, J. (Ed.): Brain's Diseases of the Nervous System. Oxford: Oxford University Press, 1993.

Mohadjer, M., et al.: CT-guided Stereotactic Fibrinolyis of Spontaneous and Hypertensive Cerebellar Hemorrhage: Long-term Results. J. Neurosurg. 73:217-222,1990.

Narayan, R. I. Q.: Head Injury. In: Grossman, R. G. (Ed.): Principles of Neurosurgery. New York: Raven Press, 1991.

Rivas, J. J., et al.: Extradural Hematoma: Analysis of Factors Influencing the Courses of 161 Patients. Neurosurgery 23:44-51, 1988.

Smith, R. R. and Miller, J. D.: Aneurysms and Carotid-Cavernous Fistulas. In: Grossman, R. G. (Ed.): Principles of Neurosurgery. New York: Raven Press, 1991.

Toole, J. F.: Cerebrovascular Disorders. New York: Raven Press, 1990.

Yuh, W. T. C., et al.: N-1r Imaging of Cerebral Ischemia: Endings in the First 24 Hours. A.J.R. Am. J. Roentgenol. 157:565-573,1991.

Additional References

Jennett, B. and Lindsay, K. W.: An Introduction to Neurosurgery, 5th ed. Boston: Butterworth-Heinemann, 1994.

Meyer, F. B. (Ed.): Sundt's Occlusive Cerebrovascular Disease, 2nd ed. Philadelphia: Saunders, 1994.

Smith, R. R., et al.: Cerebral Aneurysms. New York: Springer-Verlag, 1994. Smith, R. R., et al.: Cerebral Aneurysms. New York: Springer-Verlag, 1994. Stein, S. C., et al: Delayed and Progressive Brain Injury in Close-Head Trauma—Radiological Demonstration. Neurosurgery 32:25-31, 1993.

CHAPTER 5

Ventricular and Meningeal Injuries

SCOPE

Injuries to the three meningeal tissues covering the brain and spinal cord or to the ventricles that circulate the cerebrospinal fluid increase the risk of infection and metabolic problems that can cause irreversible damage to brain tissue. Subdural hygroma and arachnoid cyst produce space-occupying lesions that can compress vital brain structures. Conditions that result in blockage of the ventricles or abnormal retention of cerebrospinal fluid can cause hydrocephalus, which increases the risk of brain compression and herniation. Penetrating injuries that breach the meninges can result in pneumocephalus and leaking of cerebrospinal fluid from the ears or nose. If a cerebrospinal fluid fistula forms from penetrating injury, pathogens can be conducted to the brain, resulting in potentially fatal meningitis or other central nervous system infection. Most traumatic ventricular and meningeal lesions can be detected with diagnostic imaging. Although some can be treated conservatively, all should be considered serious injuries until the risk of infection and further tissue damage has been controlled.

SYNOPSIS

5.00   INTRODUCTION

Traumatic injuries to the head and neck may result in lesions that damage structures designed to protect and nurture the brain. A breach in these structures—the meninges and the ventricles of the brain—introduces the risk of infection and metabolic disturbances that may lead to irreversible tissue damage. Early detection and treatment are essential to prevent the development of life-threatening conditions. These types of lesions often cannot be detected on gross examination but may be signaled by subtle metabolic and anatomic changes. Monitoring the patient continually for any post-traumatic developments will ensure the best possible therapeutic outcome.

5.01   The Meninges

The brain and spinal cord are surrounded by three membranes known collectively as the meninges. These structures are the dura mater, arachnoid and pia mater. (*See Figure 5–1.*) The dura mater is a tough protective outer membrane of collagenous tissue. The middle layer—the arachnoid—is a delicate membrane enclosing a space filled with cerebrospinal fluid (CSF), called the subarachnoid space. The pia mater is an inner vascular membrane carrying blood vessels into the brain. Together the meninges primarily protect central nervous system tissue from injury, remove toxic substances and maintain normal concentrations of electrolytes, nutrients and fluids.

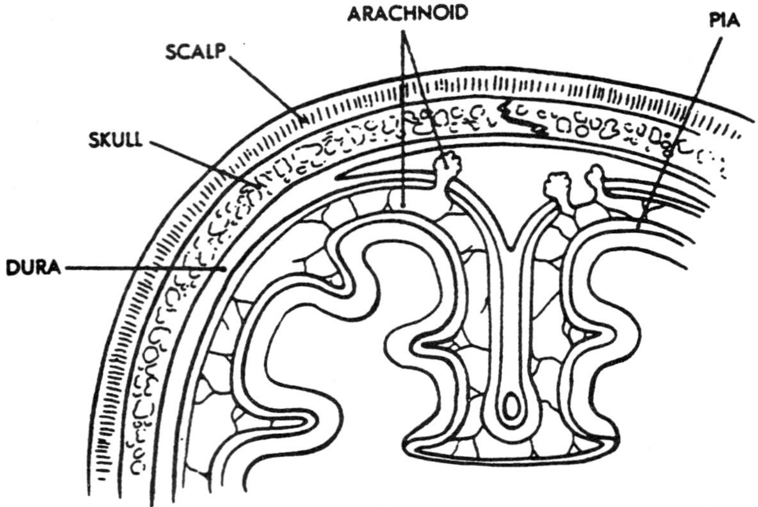

Fig. 5-1. The coverings (meninges) of the brain, from the outermost to the innermost: the scalp, skull, dura mater, arachnoid and pia mater.

5.02   The Ventricles

The central nervous system develops in the embryo from a hollow structure known as the neural tube. The rostral (headward) end develops into three expanded hollow regions, called ventricles. As the embryo matures into a fetus, this primitive three-part forebrain curves and develops into a six-part mature nervous system, consisting of the spinal cord, medulla, pons and cerebellum (two separate structures that develop together and function cooperatively to control involuntary body functions, e.g., respiration), midbrain, diencephalon ("between brain;" the region between the two cerebral hemispheres) and cerebrum. (*See Figure 5-2.*)

Each cerebral hemisphere contains a lateral ventricle that communicates with the third ventricle by way of an intraventricular foramen (opening). The third ventricle is a structure lying between the two halves of the diencephalon. It is narrow, resembling a slit. The fourth ventricle is located in the medulla, and running through the midbrain and pons to the fourth ventricle is a small channel called the cerebral aqueduct. The fourth ventricle contains three openings in its roof: two lateral foramina of Luschka and a single midline foramen of Magendie. (*See Figure 5–3.*) These foramina communicate with the subarachnoid space of the spinal cord and brain.

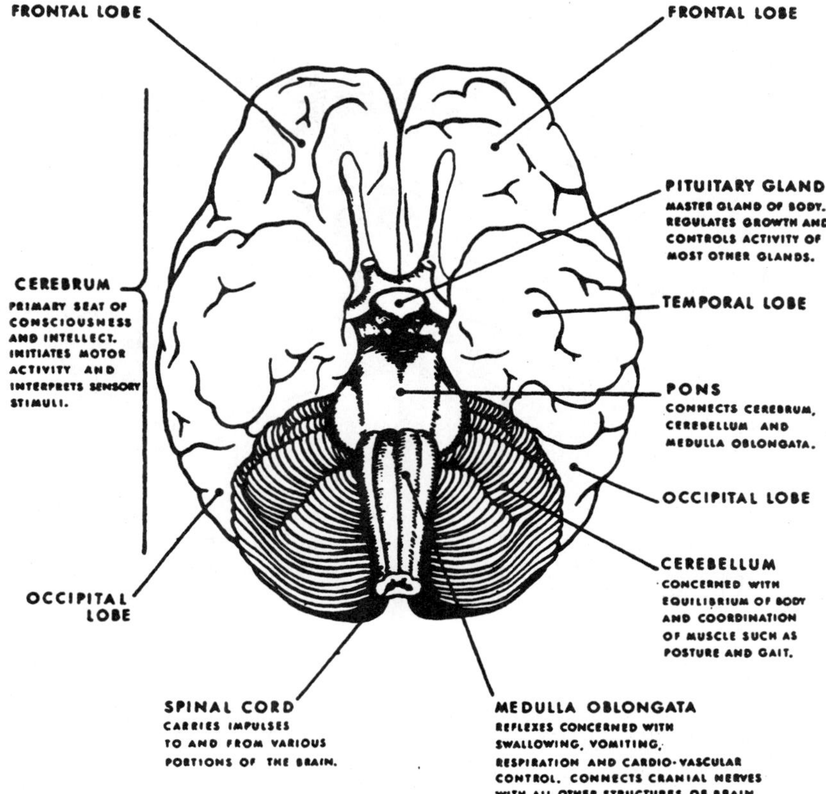

Fig. 5-2. Underside of the brain, showing the relationship of the lobes to the structures of the brain stem. Portions of the mature nervous system include the spinal cord, medulla, pons, cerebellum and cerebrum.

The ventricles serve as passageways for cerebrospinal fluid (CSF), which bathes and cushions the brain and spinal cord. A blockade in any portion of the ventricular pathway can cause an accumulation of fluid and expansion of the blocked ventricle.

5.03   Cerebrospinal Fluid

Cerebrospinal fluid is a clear, colorless fluid that flows in and around brain tissue and helps maintain the concentrations of electrolytes, nutrients and water required for normal neuronal (nerve cell) growth and excitability. CSF also removes many harmful substances from brain tissue and acts as a cushion against mechanical injury. It may play an important role in the transport of hormones as well as substances required to fight infection.

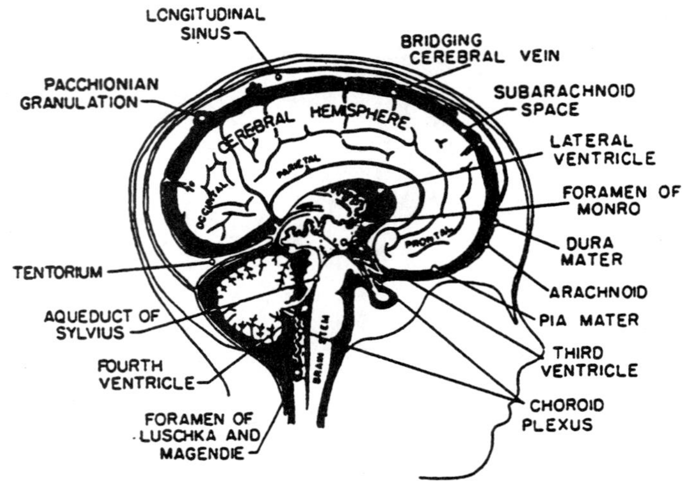

Fig. 5-3. Cerebrospinal fluid (CSF) circulates in a top-to-bottom direction through the ventricles and then into the subarachnoid space through the foramina of Luschka and Magendie.

5.10 SUBDURAL HYGROMA

A subdural hygroma is an accumulation of watery fluid within the subdural space (beneath the dura mater), either as a result of the liquefaction of a chronic subdural hematoma (localized collection of coagulated blood)[1] or seepage of CSF through a tear in the arachnoid layer. An arachnoidal tear can act like a valve, closing after fluid enters the subdural space and preventing its escape. The accumulated fluid has the same effect as any other lesion, in that it may increase total fluid pressure within the skull or act as a mass lesion, putting pressure on underlying brain tissue and causing neurologic damage (McLaurin and Towbin, 1989). As in the case of a chronic subdural hematoma, the pooling of fluid in the subdural space often triggers the formation of a subdural neomembrane (a porous structure that lies just beneath the dura mater and becomes vascularized) (Hasegawa, et al., 1992).

It can be difficult to distinguish between a subdural hematoma and a hygroma, especially when blood seeps through the arachnoid lesion and mixes with the effusion (Lusins and Levy, 1993). In fact, the similarities between the two conditions are so strong that any attempt

---

[1] *See also* ch. 4.

at distinguishing between them is considered artificial by some authorities (McLaurin and Towbin, 1989).

5.11   Diagnosis

Evidence of subdural effusion in hygroma is very similar to that of subdural hematoma. There is usually a history of head trauma, often something as forgettable as a slight bump on the head or a mild contusion (bruising or tear of brain tissue) caused by lurching forward in a vehicle that comes to a sudden stop (Ropper, 1991). A hygroma may also develop as a complication of a ventricular shunt (McLaurin and Towbin, 1989; Milhorat, 1989), such as the kind used to treat hydrocephalus.[2] In infants, the history may include severe shaking, which can cause a rupture in the delicate meningeal membranes. Evidence of shaking severe enough to cause a subdural hematoma or CSF effusion often suggests child abuse.

Signs of a hygroma may not develop for weeks or months. These signs tend to be nonspecific and include confusion, personality changes and slowed thinking. Patients often complain of headaches, which may fluctuate with changes in position (Ropper, 1991).

The condition can be detected radiologically by plain x-rays or, more accurately, by a computed tomography (CT) scan (in which several x-rays taken along a predetermined plane are processed by computer to reconstruct a cross-sectional view of a discrete body region), ultrasonography (use of sound waves to visualize internal body structures) or magnetic resonance imaging (MRI; visualization of internal body structures by placing the body in a magnetic field and measuring energy emitted during transient changes in the orientation of atoms within body tissues).

A skull x-ray is the least reliable diagnostic tool, as it may show only a slight shift in the position of an intracranial structure, typically the pineal gland (a small, rounded, hormone-secreting structure located near the third ventricle).

A CT scan taken without contrast medium may reveal a low-density mass and may also indicate the displacement of structures along the midline of the skull and compression of the lateral ventricles, especially if the condition has existed for two to six weeks (Ropper, 1991).

------

[2] *See* 5.61[2] *infra.*

Ultrasonography has been used successfully in infants, though it may miss smaller accumulations of fluid, especially in the upper convexity of the brain (McLaurin and Towbin, 1989).

MRI remains the most reliable method of detecting subdural effusions (Teasdale and Galbraith, 1989) and is especially important in distinguishing between a hematoma and a hygroma and between a hygroma and normal cerebrospinal fluid (Hasegawa, et al., 1992).

5.12 Treatment

Limited hygromas usually resolve on their own. Persistent hygromas may expand and have the same physical effects as a tumor, including a rise in intracranial pressure (Ropper, 1991) and, in infants and young children, seizures or porencephaly (a condition characterized by the presence of cavities or cysts within a cerebral hemisphere).[3]

The treatment may be similar to that required for persistent hematomas. Drainage is sufficient to relieve symptoms in most patients. This may be accomplished simply by making a burr hole, usually in the frontal or parietal eminence (a bony projection; the frontal eminence projects from the frontal bone above the eyes, and the parietal eminence bulges from the parietal bone near its border with the temporal bone) and through the dura, then releasing the fluid. (*See Figure 5–4.*) Drainage is followed by irrigating the cavity with saline (Teasdale and Galbraith, 1989).

As long as the patient's recovery is adequate, follow-up CT scans are not necessary, since CT findings often do not correlate with patient improvement. If the patient fails to improve within a reasonable length of time, however, a CT scan may be warranted to find the cause of prolonged hygroma, such as the development of hydrocephalus (accumulation of cerebrospinal fluid within the skull) or a cerebral infarction (death of a discrete area of brain tissue due to the blockage of local blood supply). In a small percentage of patients, the drainage procedure has to be repeated. This introduces an additional risk of infection, and careful post-therapeutic patient monitoring is essential (Teasdale and Galbraith, 1989).

Other therapeutic recommendations include glucocorticoid therapy or (at least for patients with subdural hematomas) surgery, especially

---

[3] *See* 5.70 *infra.*

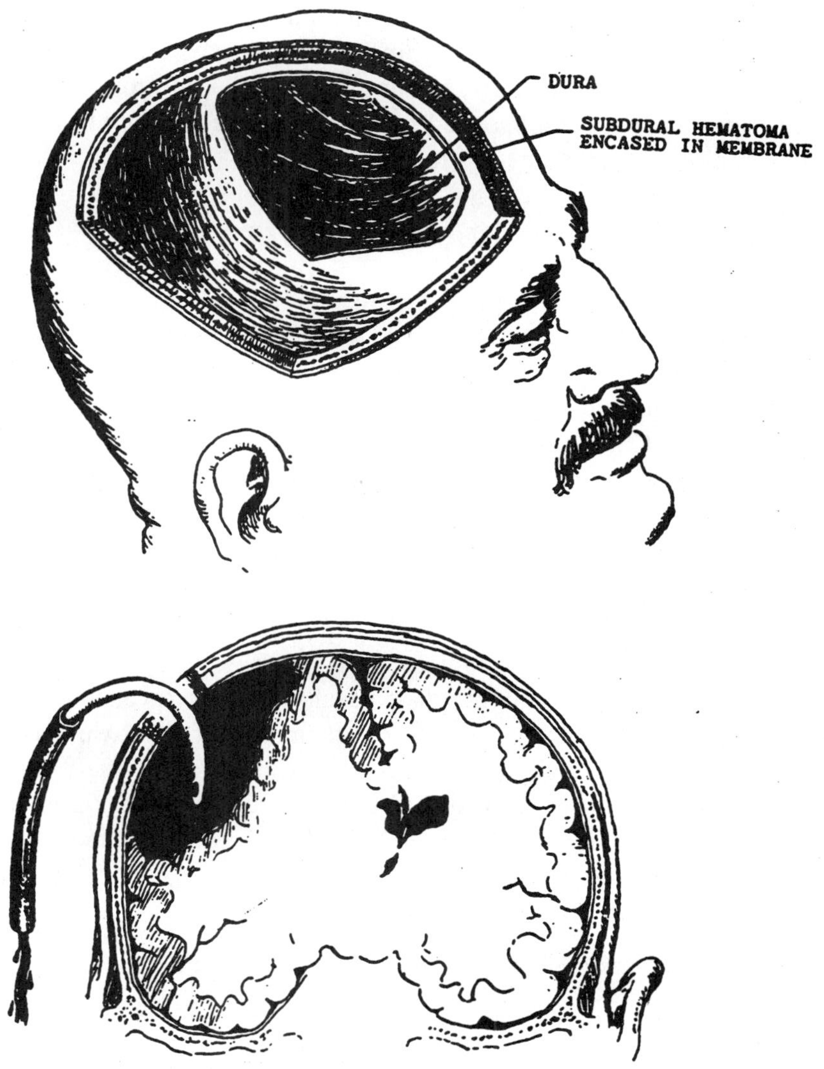

Fig. 5-4. Subdural hematoma. The upper drawing shows the dura pulled back, and exposure of the hematoma encased in a fibrous membrane. The lower drawing shows drainage of blood from the hematoma, which has compressed and distorted the brain.

when intracranial hypertension or recurrence of the hematoma occurs. The surgical procedure involves a craniotomy (surgical opening of the cranium), during which the meningeal membranes may have to be removed. A lumbar puncture (needle aspiration of CSF from the L4-L5 disc space) is not recommended for fluid drainage, because of the risk of additional tissue damage (Ropper, 1991).

5.20　CEREBROSPINAL FLUID FISTULA

Trauma to the cranial bones that results in a disruption of the dura and arachnoid meningeal layers may create an abnormal passageway, called a fistula, between the subarachnoid space and the surface of the body. This may result in CSF leaking out of the body. Rhinorrhea (drainage of CSF from the nose) and otorrhea (drainage of CSF from the ear) are considered evidence of cranial fractures, particularly in the base of the skull.[4] A critical component of accurate diagnosis of a CSF fistula is identifying the fluid as cerebrospinal fluid and not, in the case of rhinorrhea, tears or nasal fluid. These fluids can be differentiated clinically by analyzing their glucose content.

Tears have a maximum glucose concentration of approximately 5 milligrams per deciliter (mg/dL); nasal discharge, even when it is mixed with blood, has a glucose concentration of approximately 10 to 20 mg/dL and usually has a mucoid appearance (Greenfield, 1990). In contrast, normal CSF, which is clear and colorless, has a glucose concentration of approximately 50 to 75 mg/dL (deGroot and Chusid, 1988). (*See Table 5-1.*)

TABLE 5-1

Comparison of Cerebrospinal Fluid and Serum

Component	CSF Content	Serum Content
Water (%)	99	93
Protein (mg/dL)	35	7000
Glucose (mg/dL)	60	90
Sodium (Na+) (mEq/l)	138	138
Potassium (K+) (mEq/l)	2.8	4.5
Calcium (Ca++) (mEq/l)	2.1	4.8
Chlorine (Cl-) (mEq/l)	119	102

[4] *See also* ch. 6 for a discussion of skull fractures.

The difference is so striking that a negative Dextrostix ® test, which is not sensitive to low glucose concentrations, can be used to rule out a CSF leak (Greenfield, 1990). Other factors have been studied for their potential use in distinguishing between CSF levels and leaks consisting of other body fluids. A protein called beta–2 transferrin has been found to be highly specific to CSF. Tests involving the use of antibodies to this protein are being evaluated for their ability to detect its presence in rhinorrhea and otorrhea fluids, which would also be positive proof of the presence of CSF (Fransen, et al., 1991).

5.21   Rhinorrhea

Rhinorrhea (drainage of CSF from the nose) occurs most frequently in trauma cases; less than 4 percent of cases occur as a result of surgery. It usually stops within one to two weeks after injury; most cases resolve within four weeks. For this reason, the condition is usually treated conservatively, with the patient undergoing CSF drainage for a few days, either by means of multiple lumbar punctures or a continuous closed-circuit drainage system created by inserting an in-dwelling catheter into the subarachnoid space in the lumbar region of the spine (Greenfield, 1990; Shapiro and Scully, 1992).

Both drainage methods are relatively simple and safe. For example, an eight-year study of patients treated for various conditions by closed continuous CSF drainage revealed only the following (relatively minor) complications (Shapiro and Scully, 1992):

- low frequency of infections (2 percent);
- overdrainage resulting in temporary neurologic problems (3 percent);
- occlusion (blockage) requiring catheter replacement when silicone catheters were used (5 percent) and when Teflon ® catheters (33 percent) were used; and
- transient lumbar nerve root irritation (14 percent).

[1]   Antibiotic Therapy

The use of antibiotics is considered controversial because of the general threat of bacterial resistance (the ability of a pathogen to lose its sensitivity to a specific antimicrobial agent over several generations, as a result of repeated exposure to the drug). However, in some settings, the threat of meningitis and other infections of the central nervous system outweighs the need for such caution. For example, patients with craniofacial fractures—who are prone to CSF fistula formation—often require nasal intubation after surgery. Although a 1992 study suggested that nasal intubation following this kind of surgery is not contraindicated in patients with CSF fistulae and fractures at the base of the skull, in other centers, nasal intubation is believed to increase the risk of meningitis among these patients (Bahr and Stoll, 1992; Bannister, et al., 1993).

Whenever there is a threat of CNS infection, prophylactic antibiotic therapy may be warranted, in which case a culture should be taken of the nasopharyngeal region (the nasal cavity and throat) in order to identify specific pathogens. The therapeutic plan should be altered to include drugs that are effective specifically against those pathogens.

Patients with rhinorrhea resulting from a fracture in a bone at the base of the skull, such as a trans-sphenoidal fracture, may require antibiotic therapy (Greenfield, 1990). Such trauma results in the disruption of the sphenoid bone (an irregularly shaped bone that lies at the base of the brain and forms the floor of the cranial fossa, a trenchlike depression in the base of the skull). (*See Figure 5-5.*) A break in this particular bone would create a passageway to brain tissue, including the pituitary gland, which secretes hormones that enable the body to react to changes in its external and internal environment (Kupfermann, 1991).

Patients who experience this kind of trauma should be treated prophylactically for organisms common to the nasopharynx. If a specific pathogen is identified, then antibiotic therapy should be modified to control the growth of that organism. During antibiotic therapy, the patient's head should be elevated to an angle of approximately 45 degrees to facilitate drainage of potentially contaminated fluid away from the fracture (Greenfield, 1990).

[2]   Surgery

Not all cases of rhinorrhea are self-limiting. When a CSF fistula fails to stop leaking within a period of 10 days (Vrankovic and Glavina, 1989), a craniotomy (surgically made opening in the skull) may have to be performed to find the fistula and close it. Other indications for surgery include recurrent meningitis and pneumocephalus (intracranial accumulation of air).[5] Precise location of the dural

---

[5] *See* 5.30 and 5.40 *infra.*

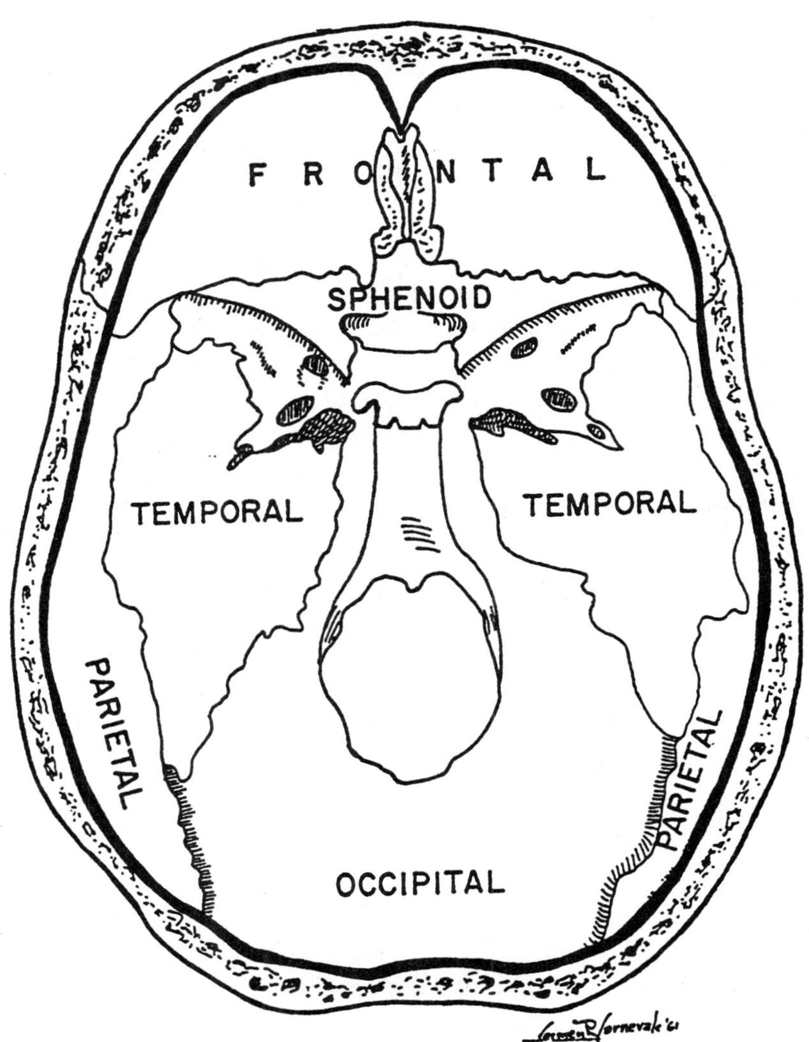

Fig. 5-5. View from above of the base of the skull, showing the sphenoid bone. Patients with rhinorrhea resulting from a fracture in a bone at the base of the skull, such as a trans-sphenoid fracture, may require antibiotic therapy.

defect is crucial for the success of this procedure. The "gold standard" for locating such defects is computed tomographic cisternography (CTC) (Creamer, et al., 1992)—a radiograph (x-ray) obtained by taking several views along different planes and processing them by computer to produce a cross-sectional representation of the basal cisterns (dilated regions within the subarachnoid space overlying the cerebral peduncles, two large masses of nerve fibers that form the front of the midbrain).

Noninvasive diagnostic methods are also available. Some experts recommend MRI for the detection of CSF fistula in severe cases of rhinorrhea, since this method can locate soft tissue injuries (including shearing injuries) deep within the cerebral cortex (Miner and Wagner, 1989). Other noninvasive methods include immunoelectrophoresis of rhinorrhea and the use of isotope tracers. In immunoelectrophoresis, proteins in rhinorrheal fluid are separated by being passed through an electric field, then allowed to flow through a gel along with known antibodies. The proteins that interact with these antibodies precipitate near the antibody in a characteristic pattern and are identified by the co-precipitating antibody.

Another noninvasive technique is isotope tracing. An isotope (an element with an altered number of neutrons) is added to the compound being studied. Instruments capable of measuring energy emitted by isotopes, such as the liquid scintillation counter, are used to monitor the quantity, movement and other characteristics of that compound by "tracing" the isotope in the body.

Additional noninvasive techniques include plain x-rays and noncontrast high-resolution computed tomography (CT scan). These methods have several advantages over CTC, in that they are generally cheaper, painless and carry no risk of infection (Creamer, et al., 1992).

[a] Dural Grafts

Once the dural defect is located, a dura mater graft is constructed to close it. This procedure has been performed since the nineteenth century, with a wide variety of materials. In more recent times, these materials have included (Thammavaram, et al., 1990):

- metallic foils made from gold, silver, platinum and tantalum (a rare, malleable, noncorrosive metallic element often used to make plates that replace cranial defects);

- nonviable membranes, including amniotic membrane (the membrane containing the fetus and amniotic fluid);

- autologous grafts (grafts made from tissue taken from another part of the same body) using pericranial tissue (connective tissue covering the outer surface of the skull), temporalis fascia (a sheet of strong, fibrous tissue covering the temporal muscle, which is responsible for closing the jaw) or fascia lata (a sheet of fibrous tissue covering the outer surface of the thigh muscles);

- homologous grafts (grafts made from tissue taken from another individual) using freeze-dried or lyophilized dura (dura mater tissue that has undergone lyophilization, a process of rapid freezing and dehydration under a strong vacuum in order to stabilize the tissue); and

- other materials, including polyethylene film, fibrin film (a thin coating made from fibrin, an essential component of blood clots), Silastic-coated Dacron® (a synthetic polymer coated with a silicone substance that has the consistency of rubber) and Gelfoam® film (a thin coating made from an absorbable gelatin sponge).

The best results are obtained when graft material is inert, nontoxic, strong, elastic, suturable and easily prepared. The preferred choice is tissue that lies adjacent to the dural defect, such as pericranial tissue or temporalis fascia. Fascia lata has also been used successfully as a dural graft, even though it requires a second incision in a distant area of the body (Thammavaram, et al., 1990).

Two types of graft materials have been increasingly employed in recent years: lyophilized dura and Silastic-coated Dacron®. Lyophilized dura is expensive and difficult to obtain. Most important, it has been associated with transmission of Creutzfeld-Jakob disease, a frequently fatal degenerative nerve disorder characterized by progressive dementia and, in some cases, muscle wasting, tremor and spastic dysarthria (loss of control of muscles involved in speech articulation). Silastic-coated Dacron® has been associated with spontaneous formation of intracranial hematomas and myelopathy (nonspecific pathologic disturbances in the spinal cord). Because of the complications associated with these and other processed and synthetic materials, autologous grafts are preferred (Thammavaram, et al., 1990).

[b] Methods of Repair

The approach and method of repair vary with the type of fracture. Fractures in the ethmoid-cribriform plate (a thin, horizontal layer of the ethmoid bone that forms the roof of the nasal cavity and is perforated for the passage of olfactory nerves) and frontal sinus areas may be approached extracranially (from outside the skull). Ethmoid–cribriform plate fractures may be approached initially by external ethmoidectomy (removal of a portion of the ethmoid bone) and fixed with mucoperiosteal flaps (wound covers created from connective tissue lining the bones of the skull) created by tissue taken from a variety of donor sites. Frontal sinus leaks are usually repaired with an osteoplastic (related to bone-producing cells) flap or a fascial graft (a graft made from fascia, fibrous tissue surrounding muscle), with the defect filled in with abdominal fat (Daly, et al., 1992).

[3] Complications of Surgery

A craniotomy may be accompanied by hydrocephalus (accumulation of fluid in the ventricles of the brain), in which case the fistula may never close. Hydrocephalus may be overlooked in these patients because the ventricles do not increase in size; in fact, they sometimes become smaller.[6]

Craniotomies made in the base of the skull, including those performed for patients with trans-sphenoid fractures, place the patient in danger of injury to several key structures within that region, including the optic nerves, optic chiasm (segment of the optic tract in which some of the optic nerves cross from one side of the brain to the other), hypothalamus (region of the brain that regulates the activity of the pituitary gland), carotid arteries (which carry blood from the heart to the brain) and cranial nerves (Rowland, et al., 1991). Potential complications include:

Visual impairment. In patients with trans-sphenoid fractures, visual impairment is more likely to result from damage to local blood vessels than from direct damage to the optic nerve. A perforated blood vessel can result in optic nerve ischemia (lack of blood supply) or a hematoma that presses against the nerve (Greenfield, 1990).

Infection. More than 5 percent of patients undergoing a clean craniotomy develop an infection after surgery. The longer the procedure and the more frequently it is performed in the same patient, the

---

[6] *See* 5.60 *infra* for further discussion of hydrocephalus.

greater the risk of infection. Prolonged use of steroids (from 2.5 to 3 weeks) also appears to increase the risk of postsurgical infection. The most common types of infection include meningitis, ventriculitis (inflammation of the lining of the ventricles of the brain), subdural empyema (accumulation of pus within the subdural space), cerebritis (inflammation of brain tissue) and brain abscess (Greenfield, 1990).

Hemorrhage. Hemorrhage is a rare but potentially fatal complication of craniotomies involving the base of the skull. Injuries are more likely to result from perforations made in the unexpected twists and turns of an abnormal vasculature than from poor surgical technique, though the latter cannot automatically be ruled out. The risk of such injuries can be reduced by means of preoperative angiography (x-ray examination of the blood vessels) (Greenfield, 1990).

Endocrine disorders. Damage to the pituitary gland or anterior hypothalamus (area at the base of the brain that controls the amount and types of hormones secreted by the pituitary gland) can result in such endocrinologic disorders as diabetes insipidus (a condition characterized by inadequate levels of the antidiuretic hormone ADH, which inhibits excessive loss of fluids through the kidneys). Signs of diabetes insipidus include the production of copious amounts of dilute urine and an abnormally low concentration of sodium in the urine (Greenfield, 1990).

A craniotomy may also result in the collection of CSF, blood and other fluids within the subgaleal space (the region below the area of the scalp that attaches to the occipitofrontalis muscle extending from the eyebrows to the back of the head). This is essentially dead space, and consequently the need to drain it is controversial. Some experts (Greenfield, 1990) prefer to limit drainage to cases in which the pressure exerted by accumulated fluid threatens to disturb local sutures; causes swelling around the orbits, thereby hampering any attempts to evaluate pupillary light reflexes; or becomes contaminated with bacteria. A few drainage attempts should eliminate the problem.

If fluid continues to reaccumulate after several attempts, hydrocephalus should be suspected. Hydrocephalus can force the subarachnoid space to press against the subgaleal space, causing the intrasubgaleal pressure to rise. In this case, treatment efforts should focus on eliminating hydrocephalus rather than draining the subgaleal space. Continued drainage attempts can increase the risk of creating new CSF fistulas (Greenfield, 1990).

5.22 Otorrhea

A CSF leak from the auditory canal (otorrhea) suggests the possibility of a fracture in a bone at the base of the skull. The temporal bone is most often involved (Brandrick, 1989).

Otorrhea may also result from an injury or a surgical procedure performed in the inner ear. Inner ear surgery is performed primarily to remove tumors. A favored surgical approach to these tumors—the retrosigmoid approach—is also useful in treating patients with other neurologic disorders. A meticulous drill curettage (use of a small drill to remove tissue) is performed in the posterior wall of the inner ear canal to adequately expose the tumor or nerve lesion. Unfortunately, traditional approaches to this region block the view of much of the bone, preventing the surgeon from seeing all the exposed air cells (small air pockets). Unsealed or inadequately sealed air cells carry a risk for CSF leakage through the middle ear space and the eustachian tube (a membrane-lined channel extending from the tympanic cavity to the back of the throat).

Because the procedures that can lead to CSF otorrhea involve a bone that extends into the basal part of the skull, the risks associated with surgical correction procedures are similar to those discussed for CSF rhinorrhea.[7] The potential for pituitary damage is greater because of the location of the temporal bone. Thus postoperative monitoring for endocrinologic disorders may be more critical for patients with CSF otorrhea than for those with CSF rhinorrhea.

5.30 TRAUMATIC MENINGITIS

Individuals who experience a penetrating head injury or undergo invasive neurologic procedures are at risk for traumatic meningitis (an infection of the arachnoid and pia meninges surrounding the entire brain and spinal cord) (Luby, 1992; Rhee, et al., 1993). Meningitis may also arise in the absence of trauma. The infection is spread by the cerebrospinal fluid flowing between these two layers to the ventricles of the brain. The pus-filled exudate of this infection usually remains confined within the subarachnoid layer, concentrating primarily over the basal cisterns and cerebellum, and occasionally reaching the cerebrum. The fact that it is carried by CSF places individuals

---

[7] *See* 5.21[3] *supra.*

with meningeal or ventricular tears at particular risk for infection of adjacent brain tissue and subsequent abscess formation, a condition that is usually prevented by an intact pia layer.

A CSF leak in the cerebellar region is especially dangerous because of the potential for compromise of life-sustaining functions, including respiration. Even in the absence of a tear, the infection can block the flow of CSF and blood to brain tissue, causing brain edema (swelling),[8] brain tissue infarction (death of a discrete area of brain tissue, due to the blockage of the local blood supply), nerve damage, especially to the third and sixth cranial nerves (respectively, the oculomotor and abducens nerves, both of which help control eye movements) and subdural effusions (Swartz, 1992).

The pyogenic (pus-producing) form of meningitis, which affects at least 20,000 Americans annually, is an acute condition that is usually caused by bacteria (Treseler and Sugar, 1990). In most cases, a single aerobic (the type that needs oxygen to survive) microorganism is responsible for the infection. Simultaneous mixed infections and anaerobic infections (infections caused by organisms that thrive in the absence of oxygen) are so rare that their presence strongly suggests an anatomic breach, such as might occur through neurosurgery, a penetrating head injury, erosion of cranial bones by a tumor or rupture of an intraventricular abscess (Swartz, 1992).

5.31   Etiology

Specific organisms have become associated with meningitis that develops in individuals with certain types of head trauma (Swartz, 1992; Luby, 1992). They include:

- Gram-negative bacilli such as *Escherichia coli* (Swartz, 1992), as well as *Acinetobacter calcoaceticus, Klebsiella pneumoniae* (Schonwald, et al., 1989) and *Pseudomonas aeruginosa* (Winkelman and Galloway, 1992; Schonwald, et al., 1989);

- *Streptococcus pneumoniae* (previously called pneumococcus), which is often seen in individuals who have had a serious head injury in the past. It is often accompanied by CSF rhinorrhea,[9] usually as a result of a fracture or defect

---

[8] *See* 5.80 *infra.*

[9] *See* 5.21 *supra.*

in the cribriform plate (thin shelf of bone in the ethmoid bone
that forms the roof of the nasal cavity);

- *Staphylococcus epidermidis,* which is seen in patients who
  have had extensive neurosurgical procedures, especially in
  large urban hospitals; and

- *Haemophilus influenzae* type B, a highly age related organism. It is so uncommon in adults that its presence strongly
  suggests an anatomic defect, as may occur through trauma.

The risk for meningitis is even greater for trauma victims who are
already immunocompromised, since poor immune function increases
the risk of meningitis by *Listeria monocytogenes* and *Streptococcus
pneumoniae* (Swartz, 1992). Patients who are immune compromised
secondary to human immunodeficiency virus (HIV) infection are also
at high risk, especially for pyogenic (pus-producing) pneumococcal
meningitis. Alcoholism also complicates the prognosis for pyogenic
meningitis, because it is often associated with a compromised immune
state (Swartz, 1992).

Immunosuppression increases the risk of meningitis from organisms
that are normally rarely associated with it, such as *Staphylococcus
aureus.* In neonates and neurosurgical patients, *S. aureus* meningitis
has been associated with high mortality (Kim, et al., 1989).

5.32 Signs and Symptoms

Symptoms of meningitis include stiff neck, drowsiness and decreased mental activity. Meningitis is also highly suspected in the
presence of positive Kernig's and Brudzinski's signs. Kernig's sign
is positive when the patient cannot extend his or her leg completely
while in a seated position or while lying down with the thigh flexed
against the abdomen. Brudzinski's sign is positive when flexion of
the neck is accompanied by flexion of the hip or knee, or the passive
flexion of one of the lower limbs is accompanied by a similar
movement in the other limb. These signs are readily overlooked in
certain individuals, especially infants, obtunded individuals (persons
with dulled senses) or elderly persons with pneumonia (Swartz, 1992).
If meningitis is suspected even in the absence of typical meningeal
signs, the CSF should be examined.

Most patients with pyogenic meningitis complain of a sudden onset
of fever as well as headache, vomiting and stiff neck. Backache and

general weakness are also common. These initial symptoms, which may last several days or as long as a week, may be followed by the rapid development of confusion, obtundation and loss of consciousness (Swartz, 1992).

Other signs of meningitis are discussed in the following sections.

[1]   Cranial Nerve Abnormalities

Approximately 15 percent of patients with meningitis exhibit abnormal activity in the third (oculomotor), fourth (trochlear) and sixth (abducens) cranial nerves, which innervate muscles involved in eye movements, as well as in the seventh cranial nerve (facial), which innervates the teeth as well as the muscles, joints and skin of the face and mouth. The effect is often temporary, though children may experience persistent sensorineural hearing loss (hearing loss caused by damage to sensory fibers in the auditory nerve) (Swartz, 1992). *(See Figure 5-6.)*

[2]   Seizures

Generalized or focal seizures develop in approximately 25 percent of patients with meningitis, as a result of damage caused by cortical vein phlebitis (blood clots in the veins of the cerebral cortex) developing approximately one week after the onset of meningitis (Swartz, 1992).

[3]   Brain Edema and Cerebral Hypertension

These conditions may develop as the blood-brain barrier, which is designed to control the concentration of substances across the vascular border, breaks down in response to infection. These two conditions may accompany seizures, abnormal functioning of the oculomotor nerve, coma, systemic hypertension and bradycardia (abnormally slow heart rate) (Swartz, 1992).

[4]   Focal Cerebral Signs

Herniation (outpocketing) and brain edema cause brain tissue to press against adjacent brain structures, damaging these structures and compromising their normal functions. Common signs of abnormal pressure include visual field defects (inability to see images appearing within discrete regions visible to both eyes), hemiparesis (muscle weakness on one side of the body) and dysphagia (inability to swallow) (Swartz, 1992).

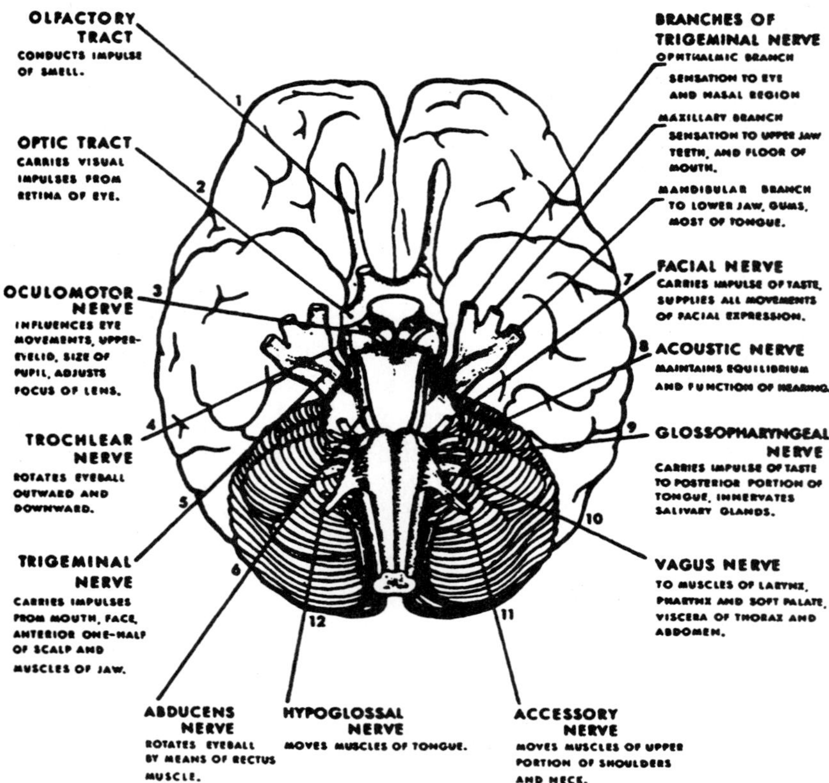

Fig. 5-6. View of the underside of the brain, showing the location of the 12 pairs of cranial nerves.

5.33　Diagnosis

Making a presumptive diagnosis of meningitis is relatively easy in a patient with a fever and meningeal signs, especially if these symptoms develop in high-risk settings. In all cases, an accurate diagnosis requires laboratory analysis of CSF and blood. Radiologic studies may be used to monitor any focal lesions associated with meningitis after antimicrobial therapy has begun. However, x-rays should not be obtained if the procedure will cause a delay in the CSF exam, which can identify the causative pathogen and allow early institution of an effective therapeutic regimen (Swartz, 1992).

The CSF is examined for the presence of a specific pathogen, the presence of pathogen-fighting immune cells, glucose concentration, protein concentration (which is often elevated in cases of pneumococcal meningitis) and other abnormalities. The search for the causative organism begins with a Gram-stained smear. A specimen prepared for viewing under a microscope is stained with crystal violet, then counterstained with another dye in order to identify any microorganisms in the sample as either Gram-negative (retaining only the counterstain) or Gram-positive (retaining the violet color of the first dye) (Lim, 1989). This technique identifies the organism in approximately 75 percent of cases (Swartz, 1992). When the organism is not found by Gram staining, the CSF is tested for the presence of specific bacterial antigens (proteins that are identified by the host as foreign and attacked by antibodies). The CSF should always be cultured, and if the culture is positive, the bacteria are tested for antibiotic sensitivity.

Blood tests are used mainly to find evidence of complications of meningitis. Abnormal creatinine and electrolyte levels are important indicators of abnormal antidiuretic hormone levels and the abnormal kidney functions associated with them (Swartz, 1992).

Certain pre-existing conditions that could result in meningitis may have to be ruled out before concluding that an infection is a result of trauma. These include:

- parameningeal infections (chronic infections of the ear or nasal sinuses, as well as lung abscess), all of which can predispose the patient to developing a brain or spinal abscess, subdural empyema (accumulation of pus within the subdural space) or pyogenic venous sinus phlebitis (inflammation of the venous structures, accompanied by the production of pus) (Swartz, 1992);

- bacterial endocarditis (a pyogenic bacterial infection of the inner layer of the heart, which can spread to the brain and cause an infarct, or death of tissue), capable of causing meningeal signs; and

- "chemical meningitis" (the development of meningeal signs as a result of exposure to contaminants in medical equipment or an anesthetic).

5.34 Non-neurologic Complications

Complications of meningitis that do not involve the nervous system include shock, coagulation disorders, septic complications and prolonged fever.

[1] Shock

Shock is a significant reduction in the circulating volume of blood accompanying pyogenic (pus-producing) meningitis when bacteremia (bacteria in the blood) is present. Immunocompromised individuals are at significant risk for going into shock.

The patient will require the same type of treatment that is provided to patients with septic shock (sudden circulatory failure associated with massive infection) (Swartz, 1992). This includes administration of fluids, respiratory support, parenteral (intravenous) antibiotics, vasoactive drugs (medications that cause blood vessels to dilate or constrict, in an attempt to normalize the rate of blood flow and blood pressure) and, when necessary, surgery in order to drain or remove abscesses (Berkow and Fletcher, 1992).

[2] Coagulation Disorders

These disorders may develop as a result of bacteremia (presence of bacteria in the blood), which can lead to thrombocytopenia (a drop in the number of blood platelets, which play an important role in blood coagulation) or disseminated intravascular coagulation (DIC). DIC, which is characterized by the production of a protein known as tissue factor activity (TFA) in the blood, occurs in persons with head injuries that involve a breach in the blood-brain barrier. It is most likely to accompany a Gram-negative infection, since Gram-negative organisms secrete an endotoxin capable of generating TFA in monocytes (a type of immune cell) that releases it into the blood (Swartz, 1992).

[3] Septic Complications

Septic complications of meningitis include endocarditis and pyogenic arthritis. Endocarditis is an inflammation of the innermost muscle layer of the heart. Pyogenic arthritis is an inflammation of a joint that is accompanied by the production of pus. It has been seen in individuals who develop meningitis from *S. pneumoniae*, *H. influenzae* and other organisms (Swartz, 1992).

A fever that accompanies meningitis should subside within two to five days in patients who are treated quickly and effectively. A prolonged fever may be a sign of neurologic complications, such as cortical venous thrombophlebitis (inflammation of veins in the area of the cerebral cortex), ventriculitis (inflammation of the lining of the ventricles of the brain) and subdural fluid collections, as well as inadequate or inappropriate antimicrobial therapy. The patient's CSF should be re-evaluated to identify the causative organisms accurately, as well as any other abnormal conditions. The patient should also be evaluated for the possibility of the spread of an infection from another part of the body (Swartz, 1992).

5.35   Recurrent Meningitis

Repeated episodes of meningitis usually indicate an anatomic defect or an immunocompromised host. It is most likely to develop in individuals who are infected with *S. pneumoniae, H. influenzae* or *N. meningitidis* in community settings. Nosocomial (arising in a hospital setting) cases are more likely to be caused by Gram-negative bacilli and *S. aureus* (Swartz, 1992).

Recurrence is most likely to occur in individuals with a history of head trauma, especially if there is a defect in the cribriform plate, a basilar skull fracture, erosion of the mastoid bone (posterior portion of the temporal bone), congenital craniospinal defect, penetrating trauma or the patient had invasive neurosurgery. CSF rhinorrhea or, less commonly, otorrhea, may create an anatomic defect that serves as a route for bacterial invasion of the meninges. Meningitis may recur months or years after the initial injury (Swartz, 1992).

Patients with recurrent bacterial meningitis should be examined for evidence of congenital or post-traumatic anatomic defects as well as for CSF fistulas, especially those running through the cribriform plate, pericranial air sinuses or temporal bone. Evidence of such fistulas includes a salty taste in the throat, cribriform plate leak, hearing loss or "full" feeling in the ear, as well as CSF rhinorrhea occurring only when the patient is in a side-lying or prone position (Swartz, 1992).

Recurrent pneumococcal meningitis can be evaluated by polytomography (radiograph of tissue along several predetermined planes) of the frontal and mastoid (rear portion of the temporal bone) regions of the skull, as well as by radioisotope techniques (addition of radioactive isotopes to compounds in order to quantitate or monitor their activity), such as radioiodine-labeled albumin injected intrathecally (within the subdural space) or radioisotopic cisternography (the use of isotopes to monitor the activities and flow of CSF within the basal cisterns). Intrathecally injected fluorescein (injection into the subdural space of an orange-red dye, also known as resorcinolphthalein sodium) can be used as a visual tracer, under ultraviolet light, to find CSF leaks (Swartz, 1992). When found, the fistula should be surgically closed immediately to prevent further recurrence of infection.

5.36 Treatment

Antimicrobial therapy should begin as soon as possible. The initial drug selection should be based on clues to the most likely organism responsible for infection, using such evidence as the patient's age, history of head trauma or neurologic procedures, or the presence of CSF rhinorrhea. Once the causative organism has been identified, specific therapy should be adjusted as necessary (Swartz, 1992).

The blood-brain barrier presents several important issues regarding the administration of antibiotics. Although this barrier usually prevents the penetration of brain tissue by medications in the blood or CSF, it becomes more permeable in the presence of inflammation. As a result, most antimicrobial agents can be effective when they are administered intravenously, and this route of administration is recommended throughout the treatment period. Because of this barrier, however, drug levels in the CSF are lower than optimal. First-and second-generation cephalosporins and clindamycin should be avoided, because they do not reach effective levels in the CSF. Because of the difficulty in achieving adequate drug levels in the CSF, dosages of drugs should not be reduced in patients showing signs of improvement (Swartz, 1992).

The recommended treatment regimens for meningitis of known cause are summarized in *Table 5–2*.

During treatment, the CSF analysis should be repeated in 24 to 48 hours if the patient shows no signs of satisfactory improvement. Routine follow-up lumbar punctures are not necessary for individuals who recover satisfactorily, especially those who have recovered from community-acquired (in a nonclinical setting) meningitis. Exceptions to this include patients being treated for Gram-negative bacillary meningitis or pneumococcal meningitis, both of which may develop following head trauma or penetrating neurosurgical procedures. The treatment for these patients is prolonged—10 to 14 days for pneumococcal meningitis and at least three weeks for Gram-negative bacillary meningitis. CSF examinations are recommended during and after the treatment program, to determine whether the causative organisms have been eradicated (Swartz, 1992).

TABLE 5-2
Microbe-Specific Treatment of Meningitis in Adults

Organism	Antimicrobial Agent	Dosage
Pneumococcus or Meningococcus	penicillin	24 million units/day in divided doses, every 2-3 hours
	ampicillin	12 gm/day in divided doses, every 2-3 hours
Pneumococcus in penicillin-allergic patients	chloramphenicol*	4-6 gm IV daily
Penincillin-resistant pneumococcal infection	chloramphenicol cefotaxime ceftiaxone	
H. influenzae, ampicillin-resistant	cefotaxime	12 gm daily
	chloramphenicol + ampicillin	4 gm IV daily + 12 gm IV
S. aureus	nafcillin	10-12 gm IV daily
	nafcillin + rifampin	600 mg daily, oral or IV
S. aureus in penicillin-resistant patients	vancomycin	2 gm IV in divided doses every 6 hours

TABLE 5-2
Continued. . .

Organism	**Antimicrobial Agent**	**Dosage**
	+ intrathecal vancomycin	slow administration of 5-20 mg vancomycin in 10 mL of 5% dextrose-0.85% sodium chloride
Enterococcus	penicillin + gentamicin	24 million units daily 3-5 mg/kg IV daily in divided doses, every 8 hours
	ampicillin + gentamicin	12 grams daily 3-5 mg/kg IV daily in divided doses, every 8 hours
Gram-negative bacilli: *E.coli, Klebsiella, Proteus,* etc. (not suitable for *Acinebacter* or *P. aeruginosa*	cefotaxime +	12 gm daily IV in divided doses, every 4 hours
	gentamicin	5 mg/kg daily IV, in divided doses, every 8 hours

Intrathecal gentamicin may also be indicated if there is no response to systemic treatment.

P. aeruginosa	ceftazidime + an aminoglycoside	2 gm IV every 6-8 hours
	piperacillin or azlocillin + an aminoglycoside	3-4 gm IV every 4-6 hours

* Chloramphenicol-resistant pneumococcal organisms have been reported.

During the treatment of meningitis, certain complications may arise that require immediate care. These include:

- Severe brain swelling, with CSF pressure exceeding 450 mm H_2O (normal is 100 to 150 mm H_2O). Untreated, it can cause herniation of brain tissue into the temporal lobe or cerebellum.

- Seizures.

- Pyogenic foci (localized masses of pus-producing material), which may require surgery for their removal.

5.37   Prognosis

Because of the routine practice of administering antimicrobials to patients with meningitis in a timely manner, mortality and morbidity for this condition tend to be low (Swartz, 1992), even among individuals with fractures at the base of the skull (Ash, et al., 1992). The highest mortality rates are seen in individuals with pneumococcal meningitis (25 percent), followed by adults with Gram-negative bacillary disease (20 to 30 percent). Although the rate for recurrent community acquired meningitis is only 5 percent (Swartz, 1992), it is considered particularly life threatening in children. Those who survive this condition are often left with inner ear abnormalities or unilateral deafness, which can be quite challenging to diagnose (Quiney, et al., 1989). The prognosis is worst for individuals with advanced age, other foci of infection, underlying diseases (especially those that compromise the immune system, including leukemia and alcoholism), coma and delayed treatment (Swartz, 1992).

5.40   PNEUMOCEPHALUS

Trauma that results in the formation of an abnormal communication between the meningeal layers and the surface of the body introduces the risk of pneumocephalus (intracranial accumulation of air). This uncommon complication arises most often after fracture in the base of the skull that is accompanied by a tear in the subarachnoid space. As CSF leaks out, air enters from the exterior, usually through the paranasal sinuses. In fact, the presence of air is often used as a clue for the finding of a CSF leak (Orebaugh and Margolis, 1990; Greenfield, 1990).

Pneumocephalus may result from trauma or surgery, especially surgical procedures in which the trans-sphenoid region or any of the paranasal sinuses is disturbed. It may also develop during the use of a lumbar subarachnoid drain to remove CSF from the area of a basal fracture during surgery.

In most cases, this is a benign condition. However, if a significant increase in air pressure develops, pneumocephalus can have the same effect as a mass lesion, causing postoperative deterioration of the patient's neurologic status (Greenfield, 1990).

The diagnosis of pneumocephalus is based on clinical signs and radiologic evidence. It should be suspected in patients with recent trauma to the head, nose or orbit of the eye, accompanied by headache, CSF rhinorrhea or a characteristic splashing sound heard when the patient moves his or her head (Orebaugh and Margolis, 1990). A single lateral (from the side) x-ray view is usually adequate; a brow-up lateral radiograph taken soon after any type of surgery or trauma that could result in a CSF fistula or pneumocephalus can prevent a delay in diagnosis and treatment while reducing the risk of serious complications, such as meningitis (Greenfield, 1990).

When treatment is required, a twist-needle drill or burr hole can be used to remove air from intracranial spaces and achieve decompression. A single aspiration is usually enough to relieve pressure and prevent the lesion from recurring (Greenfield, 1990).

5.50 ARACHNOID CYSTS

An arachnoid cyst is a cavity lined with arachnoid (the second meningeal layer, located between the dura mater and pia mater) tissue and filled with a fluid resembling cerebrospinal fluid. This space-occupying lesion alters normal intracranial function by causing the displacement of adjacent structures and increasing intracranial fluid pressure. Arachnoid cysts are generally categorized as primary, secondary or arachnoid diverticuli.

Primary arachnoid cysts are congenital in origin. These CSF-filled structures lie completely within the arachnoid membrane and are lined with arachnoid cells and collagen.

Secondary cysts arise as complications of trauma, infection and other insults. The walls of a secondary cyst may contain nonarachnoidal tissue, such as inflammatory cells and hemosiderin (the form in which iron is stored in the cell).

Arachnoid diverticuli are abnormal, pouchlike structures that, unlike primary and secondary arachnoid cysts, permit the CSF contained within to communicate with the CSF in the subarachnoid space (James, 1989).

Arachnoid cysts tend to affect males more than females, and they usually develop within the first two decades of life (James, 1989).

5.51 Diagnosis

The diagnosis of arachnoid cysts is based on patient history and neurologic findings. Patient complaints, though they tend to be somewhat general in terms of neurologic conditions, may offer important clues.

[1] Signs and Symptoms

Typical symptoms of arachnoid cysts are nonspecific and include headache, seizures and, in children, mental retardation. Additional signs vary with the location of the lesion. For example, intracranial hypertension and hydrocephalus are common in individuals with cysts in the posterior fossa (an indentation in the base of the skull beneath the pons, medulla and cerebellum), the most common site for cyst formation. Other common sites for arachnoidal cysts to develop include the cerebral convexity, the posterior region of the third ventricle and the middle fossa (a depression in the base of the skull beneath the temporal lobe of the brain) (James, 1989). A cyst in the suprasellar region of the brain (the area overlying a depression in the sphenoid bone that surrounds the pituitary gland) may cause visual problems as it presses against the optic nerve.

These anomalies must be differentiated from other conditions. For example, a cyst within the posterior fossa may be mistaken for a Dandy-Walker malformation (absence of an opening in the foramen of Magendie, causing an obstruction in the flow of CSF), which may require surgery to correct, or a rather large cisterna magna (cisterna cerebellomedullaris; an enlargement in the subarachnoid space lying between the cerebellum and the medulla oblongata), which usually requires no treatment (James, 1989).

Sudden changes in the status of the cyst can cause neurologic deterioration. A rapidly growing cyst may press against surrounding structures, causing them to shift their position so dramatically that they seriously impede the flow of CSF, causing obstructive hydrocephalus. Rupture of the cyst can cause the sudden pooling of CSF outside the subarachnoid space, which, in turn, can also displace brain structures. Deterioration of the patient's status may also indicate that blood has entered the cyst, causing an increase in the size of the lesion. This may occur spontaneously or as a result of trauma (James, 1989). Any neurologic signs that accompany arachnoid cysts should raise suspicion of a subdural hematoma or hygroma,[10] with which the cyst can communicate. A communication of this type can be detected by technetium–99 brain scintigraphy (a means of visualizing brain tissue using the radioisotope technetium–99) (Yokoyama, et al., 1989).

[2] Radiography

Cysts may be detected by plain radiographs of the skull, which reveal signs of intracranial hypertension and erosion of the cranium, as well as abnormally shaped or misplaced structures, especially in young children. CT scans will identify the cyst as well as distortions in structures surrounding the cyst. An arachnoidal cyst will appear as a large, round, clearly demarcated structure, varying in shape according to the region of the brain in which it is found. For example, cysts that develop within the sylvian fissure (sulcus lateralis cerebri; a deep cleft that stretches laterally between the frontal and temporal lobes of the brain and posteriorly between the temporal and parietal lobes) are often trapezoidal or triangular in shape.

Cysts may extend to neighboring structures, causing complications. In children, for example, cysts within the area of the temporal lobe, which contains nerves associated with hearing, may extend into the orbit through the optic canal. Suprasellar cysts (cysts that develop above the sella, a depression in the sphenoid bone that surrounds the pituitary gland) may extend in any and all directions. Magnetic resonance imaging (MRI) is highly effective in differentiating between cysts and tumors in the brain (James, 1989).

5.52 Treatment

Treatment is usually reserved for arachnoid cysts that cause significant symptoms. These can be drained through shunts, one of the simplest being a low-pressure, arachnoid cyst–peritoneal shunt that

---

[10] *See* 5.10 *supra* for further discussion of subdural hygroma and hematoma.

is employed to drain fluid from the cyst into the peritoneal cavity. In many cases, this will reduce the size of the cyst and allow surrounding brain tissue to expand to its normal dimensions.

Surgery, consisting of craniotomy and excision (removal) of the cell wall, has also been used to treat these patients. Surgical results can be less than favorable, however, because cyst recurrence and postoperative scar formation prevent complete or permanent drainage (James, 1989). Surgery may be warranted, however, for arachnoid cysts that develop in the middle cranial fossa (a depression in the base of the skull beneath the temporal lobe, optic chiasm and pituitary gland). These cysts are particularly vulnerable to trauma, which may cause bleeding into the cyst and, possibly, the subdural space as well. The result is a mass lesion that displaces midline structures and raises intracranial pressure significantly. The surgical procedure involves a craniotomy and resection (removal of part or all of a body structure) of the cyst as deep as the tentorial notch (an opening at the upper part of the cerebellum), with an opening made in the basal cisterns (von Wild, 1992).

After surgery, the patient should be followed carefully for signs of clinical deterioration. This may occur, even after a successful drainage procedure, because of unresolved hydrocephalus accompanying the lesion (James, 1989).

5.60 HYDROCEPHALUS

Hydrocephalus is a condition characterized by swelling of the cerebral ventricles and accumulation of cerebrospinal fluid within the skull. It is differentiated from brain edema, an accumulation of fluid within brain tissue,[11] by the fact that the accumulated fluid is usually contained within the CSF pathway. A breach in this pathway, however, may allow fluid to seep into brain tissue.

Hydrocephalus occurs as a result of blockage of the CSF pathway due to local hemorrhaging, crush injuries or congenital defects. It may also develop if CSF drainage from the subarachnoid space into the local venous system is blocked, for example, by scars on subarachnoid surfaces left by infection or hemorrhage.

The accumulated fluid may or may not cause the intracranial pressure to rise. Signs and symptoms of hydrocephalus include brain

---

[11] *See* 5.80 *infra.*

tissue atrophy, mental deterioration and convulsions; in children whose skull bones are still pliable, the forehead is often enlarged.

The onset of hydrocephalus may be sudden or gradual. In approximately 5 to 15 percent of severe traumatic cases, it is delayed. Therefore, it should be suspected in patients who deteriorate or reach a plateau after showing signs of improvement over a period of time.

Hydrocephalus is often characterized as *communicating* or *noncommunicating*. Although this division is useful in understanding the underlying pathology of the disease, it is an artificial classification system. For example, a single cerebellar hemorrhage can act as a blockade (noncommunicating hydrocephalus) and also create enough force to rupture a meningeal compartment and allow CSF to flow from one ventricle to another (communicating hydrocephalus).

5.61 Communicating Hydrocephalus

With communicating hydrocephalus, there is a free flow of CSF between the ventricles and down into the subarachnoid space of the spinal cord. Communicating hydrocephalus is an indication that the flow of CSF from the fourth ventricle into the venous system has been blocked, possibly as a result of damage to the subarachnoid villi (through which CSF reaches local venous structures) or the fourth ventricle. The blockage may be caused by residual scars from infection or a hemorrhage into the subarachnoid space, the latter being most common in postoperative cases (Greenfield, 1990). *(See Figure 5–7.)*

[1] Signs and Symptoms

The onset of symptoms of hydrocephalus is insidious and progressive. An unusual persistence of post-traumatic symptoms or a gradual deterioration after a partial recovery not associated with intracranial hypertension (elevated blood pressure within the brain) points to the possibility of the development of hydrocephalus.

Mental symptoms begin as apathy and inertia. Irritability and lack of communication follow until the patient loses complete contact with the world and fails to react to painful stimuli.

In addition to mental changes, other characteristic symptoms include urinary and fecal incontinence, which appear early; dementia; headaches; cranial nerve palsies and gait disturbances.

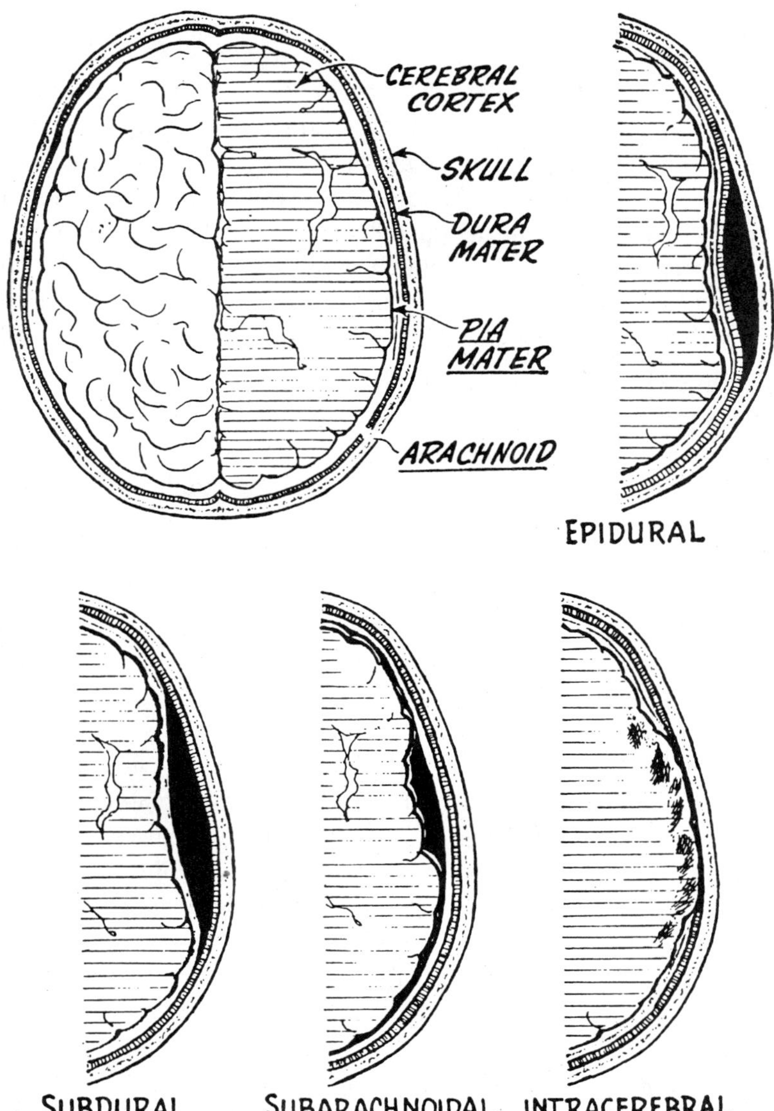

Fig. 5-7. The meninges (top left) and common types of intracranial hemorrhage.

[2]   Diagnosis

Diagnostic procedures include computed tomography (CT) scans, ventriculography (x-ray of the ventricles of the brain, taken after CSF has been removed from the ventricles and replaced with air or a contrast medium), angiography (x-ray of the blood vessels in the brain after a contrast medium has been introduced) or pneumoencephalography (x-ray of the skull and its contents after CSF has been removed and replaced with air), all of which are used to identify enlarged ventricles. A lumbar puncture may be performed to determine intracranial pressure and take a CSF sample for analysis (Greenfield, 1990).

Intracranial pressure is not the most reliable evidence of hydrocephalus, because it is not always elevated (Greenfield, 1990). Signs and symptoms of normal-pressure hydrocephalus include gait changes, cognitive deterioration and incontinence. These conditions are also commonly accompanied by other neurologic conditions, including post-traumatic amnesia. Normal-pressure hydrocephalus may also be characterized by signs of raised intracranial pressure, including nausea, headache and visual disturbances of unknown etiology, but no change in CSF pressure. As a result, early recognition of normal-pressure hydrocephalus is difficult (Mysiw and Jackson, 1990).

[3]   Treatment

Mild cases of hydrocephalus may subside without treatment. If the cause is known (e.g., meningitis or subarachnoid hemorrhage), the hydrocephalus may subside when the underlying condition is treated; this is limited mainly to milder cases. A ventriculostomy (surgical creation of an opening between the third ventricle and the area below it), lumbar puncture or placement of a temporary lumbar subarachnoid drain may be required for moderately severe cases in which the cause of hydrocephalus is known and can be corrected within a reasonable amount of time.

Permanent shunting may be required for more serious cases. Shunts are often made to drain excess fluid from the ventricles into the atria (upper chambers of the heart) or the peritoneum. Complications associated with these ventriculoperitoneal shunts in children with hydrocephalus resulting from trauma, meningitis, congenital defects and tumors include infection and blockage; rare complications include displacement of the shunt, CSF ascites (accumulation of CSF within the abdominal cavity) and abdominal cysts (Okoro and Ohaegbulam,

1992). Adjustable transcutaneous pressure valves (e.g., Sophy SU 8®) have been used with these shunts to control the rate of CSF flow from the ventricles and, thus, regulate the intracranial pressure (Sindou, et al., 1993). Valve adjustments allow the physician to prevent intracranial hypotension (abnormally low fluid pressure) from an excessive CSF flow, or subdural hygroma (accumulation of fluid in the subdural space) from an inadequate CSF flow; the valve system is most beneficial for patients with normal-pressure hydrocephalus.

Shunts have also been devised to drain excess CSF from the lumbar region of the spinal canal into the peritoneum. This type of shunt may reduce the risk of intracranial complications by redirecting some of the excess fluid. A retrospective study of 207 patients treated over an 11-year period revealed a lower rate of malfunction and infection with this lumboperitoneal shunt than that seen in patients treated with a ventriculoperitoneal shunt. The researchers concluded that the lumboperitoneal shunt would be most beneficial to patients with communicating hydrocephalus resulting from a subarachnoid hemorrhage due to a ruptured aneurysm (Aoki, 1990).

5.62   Noncommunicating Hydrocephalus

In noncommunicating hydrocephalus, CSF cannot exit from the fourth ventricle. The passageway may be blocked by a tumor, edema or hemorrhage. A CT scan may demonstrate the blockage, along with enlarged lateral and third ventricles. In some cases, the fourth ventricle looks abnormally small in comparison to the lateral and third ventricles; in others, all three sets of ventricles are enlarged, making an accurate diagnosis more difficult to achieve (Greenfield, 1990).

[1]   Signs and Symptoms

When increased intracranial pressure is suspected, all possible causes associated with CSF blockage must be ruled out, including the Arnold-Chiari anomaly (malformation of the cerebellum, causing compression of the fourth ventricle) and the Dandy-Walker malformation (absence of an opening in the foramen of Magendie). In infants, the signs and symptoms of hydrocephalus are modified because of open sutures and enlarged fontanelles, which tend to compensate for the increased pressure by causing an increase in head size. Vomiting, irritability, lethargy and failure to thrive may be encountered in rapidly developing hydrocephalus. The following signs may also develop in infants:

- bulging of the fontanelles;

- dilation and pronounced engorgement of the scalp veins, especially when the infant cries;

- separation of the cranial sutures;

- depression of the eye axis;

- impairment of visual acuity;

- nystagmus (rapid back and forth motion of the eyeballs);

- strabismus (squint); and

- hyperactive reflexes.

In older children and adults, the major manifestations include headache, nausea, vomiting, diplopia (double vision) caused by sixth nerve palsy, visual blurring, papilledema (swelling of the optic disc) with eventual optic atrophy, gait changes and pathologic alteration of reflexes.

[2] Diagnosis

Noncommunicating hydrocephalus is most often diagnosed by computed tomography (CT) scans, which reveal a mass causing blockage, hematoma (pooling of blood outside the blood vessels) or edema (swelling) blocking the ventricular passageway. The third and lateral ventricles appear enlarged, and the fourth ventricle may seem small by comparison. The diagnosis is more difficult when all the ventricles are enlarged, since this comparison cannot be made (Greenfield, 1990).

[3] Treatment

Treatment often consists of a temporary ventriculostomy (surgical creation of an opening between the floor of the third ventricle and the subarachnoid space below); in some cases, a permanent shunt is required. In contrast with patients with communicating hydrocephalus, patients with noncommunicating hydrocephalus should never undergo a lumbar puncture because of the risk of a tonsilar herniation (an outpocketing of the tonsilla cerebellum, a round mass on the base of the cerebellum), which may result in rapid deterioration of the patient, respiratory arrest and death (Greenfield, 1990).

5.70 PORENCEPHALY

Porencephaly is characterized by the presence of cavities or cysts within a cerebral hemisphere. The cavity may be completely enclosed by brain tissue, or it may communicate with an adjacent ventricle or arachnoid mater through a pore. It may develop before or after birth, either through malformation of brain structures or a destructive lesion created, for example, by inflammation, hemorrhage or damage to brain tissue lying close to a ventricle (Greenfield, 1990). Lesions that develop close to the ventricles pose a special risk in individuals who develop hydrocephalus, because hydrocephalus often causes the ventricles to expand, thereby weakening the integrity of brain tissue around porencephalic lesions, causing even more damage to brain tissue (Greenfield, 1990).

5.71 Diagnosis

Porencephaly is characterized by abnormal neurologic signs. The diagnosis is confirmed by CT scans or ultrasonography (use of sound waves to visualize internal body structures) (Berkow and Fletcher, 1992).

5.72 Treatment and Prognosis

For persons with porencephaly who also have hydrocephalus,[12] it is important to drain excess CSF from dilated ventricles, usually by means of a shunt. The prognosis varies with the severity of each case. Individuals with minor neurologic signs often demonstrate normal intelligence after treatment (Berkow and Fletcher, 1992).

5.80 BRAIN EDEMA

Injury to the meninges or the ventricles can cause a breach in the blood-brain barrier, which allows fluid to leak into adjacent brain tissue and contributes to brain edema (increase in brain volume due to an increase in the fluid content of brain tissue). Such injuries include trauma, excessive retraction (the use of a mechanical device to separate the edges of a wound) during surgery, hemorrhage, infection or the cytotoxic (cell-damaging) effects of drugs and toxic substances.

---

[12] *See* 5.60 *supra.*

Brain edema may be generalized or localized. The latter is likely to cause herniation (outpocketing) of brain tissue into nearby openings, thereby increasing the risk of mechanical injury and CSF blockage (Greenfield, 1990).

In patients with head trauma, brain edema has been known to contribute to a significant rise in intracranial hypertension (elevated pressure within the skull). In severe cases, the rise in pressure makes it difficult to close the dura mater during surgery and contributes to continued neurologic deterioration after surgery. The use of devices to monitor intracranial pressure in these patients introduces the additional risk of infection, which occurs in approximately 5 percent of patients requiring such monitoring (Greenfield, 1990).

5.81   Types of Brain Edema

Destruction of the blood-brain barrier may result in either vasogenic, cytotoxic or interstitial edema.

[1]   Vasogenic Edema

Vasogenic edema is probably the most common type of brain edema (Nelson, 1990). Characterized by an increase in the volume of extracellular fluid surrounding brain cells, it occurs as a result of the blood-brain barrier becoming increasingly permeable to proteins and other large molecules. Such leaks involve damaged or necrotic (dead) cells, or neovascularization (growth of new blood vessels around damaged ones).

This type of brain edema is seen most often in individuals with head injuries, abscesses, tumors and hemorrhages (Nelson, 1990), as well as lead encephalopathy (brain tissue degeneration from exposure to lead), meningitis (Rowland, et al., 1991) and ischemia (diminished oxygen supply) following infarction (tissue death due to the blockade of local blood vessels). Its effects include focal neurologic (associated with injury to specific nerves) abnormalities, intracranial hypertension (abnormally high pressure within the cavities of the skull) and impaired consciousness (Rowland, et al., 1991).

[2]   Cytotoxic Edema

In cytotoxic edema, excess CSF enters brain cells. It is associated with intracellular swelling of neurons, glial cells (supporting nerve cells in the brain that do not conduct impulses but perform accessory functions) and endothelial capillary cells, causing a reduction in the amount of space surrounding brain cells.

Cytotoxic edema may accompany other types of edema that develop in patients with meningitis or encephalitis. Meningitis-associated cytotoxic edema must be distinguished from the type that develops as a result of water intoxication, i.e., in patients who have ingested too much fluid or who have conditions that cause hyponatremia (abnormally low levels of sodium in the blood), such as diabetes insipidus.

[3]   Interstitial Edema

Interstitial edema is the accumulation of excessive amounts of fluid and sodium in white matter (tissue composed of axons, the long extensions of nerve cells through which signals are transmitted from one cell to the next) surrounding the ventricles of the brain. This condition, often seen in patients with obstructive hydrocephalus,[13] is associated with excessive reabsorption of CSF across membranes lining the ventricles of the brain.

Another form of brain edema, known as *pseudotumor cerebri* or *benign intracranial hypertension,* is characterized by a simultaneous rise in CSF production and development of interstitial edema. Unlike other forms of brain edema, this type is usually not accompanied by a reduction in mental functioning. It is often accompanied instead by headaches and papilledema (swelling of the optic disc). The condition may persist for months or years but is often self-limited.

5.82   Diagnosis

Brain edema can be detected by CT scans. Postoperative edema may appear only as a slight shift in brain position and reduced tissue density in the affected region. Since this condition often accompanies other complications of surgery and trauma and adds to the amount of space taken up by existing lesions, patients with tumors, intracerebral hemorrhage (bleeding within brain tissue) and contusions (bruises on brain tissue) should be evaluated for edema, as its reduction may reduce the mass effect of the accompanying lesion. When brain edema accompanies cerebral infarction, a severe stroke should be suspected.

---

[13] *See* 5.60 *supra.*

In some patients, the involved area can herniate (expand, thereby pressing against adjacent brain structures), and the condition can become fatal (Greenfield, 1990).

5.83   Treatment

The primary goal of treatment is to reduce intracranial pressure. The treatment of choice depends, in part, on the cause of the lesion. Steroids, such as dexamethasone, are used somewhat routinely in patients with brain edema associated with tumors and inflammatory lesions. The standard dosage is 4 to 20 mg administered every 4 to 6 hours.

The use of steroids in patients with brain edema associated with trauma, infarction or anoxia (lack of oxygen) is not so readily accepted. Methylprednisolone and dexamethasone have been used, but their effectiveness in terms of reducing patient morbidity or mortality has not been well established (Greenfield, 1990).

The preferred agent for reducing intracranial pressure in these patients is mannitol (a form of alcohol, chemically, that is generally regarded as a sugar). In emergency conditions, it is given as a rapid intravenous infusion of 1.0 to 1.5 g/kg of body weight for a period of 20 to 30 minutes (Greenfield, 1990). Other methods of reducing intracranial pressure include hyperventilation and barbiturate coma (LeRoux, et al., 1991).

Patients must be carefully monitored for signs of hypotension (abnormally low blood pressure), hypovolemia (abnormally low blood volume) and electrolyte imbalances during therapy (Greenfield, 1990). They should also be monitored for signs of a secondary rise in intracranial pressure, especially if the head injury responsible for the rise in pressure was severe.

5.90   AMA EVALUATION OF IMPAIRMENT

The American Medical Association (AMA) considers an impairment to be a condition that disrupts the individual's ability to perform the activities of daily living, such as those required for personal hygiene, eating, communicating, caring for one's home and personal finances, and maintaining one's posture, as well as recreational, social and work-related activities. The nature of the impairment and its consequences are based on clinical protocols as well as an evaluation of current and previous patient medical records. This information, in turn, is used to estimate the degree to which the individual's ability to carry out daily activities has been diminished by the impairment. This estimate, which is specific for each condition, is expressed as an impairment percentage, or "percentage impairment of the whole person."

The AMA's *Guides to the Evaluation of Permanent Impairment* (1993) includes sets of criteria for evaluating permanent impairment in specific regions of the central nervous system (brain and spinal cord) and peripheral nervous system (nerves outside the brain and spinal cord). Individuals with meningeal or ventricular tears are likely to experience some degree of impairment in one or more segments of either or both systems.

The AMA *Guides* identifies nine specific categories of cerebral impairment:

1. abnormal mental status and integrative functioning;
2. communication disorders;
3. disturbances of awareness and consciousness;
4. episodic neurologic disorders;
5. emotional or behavioral disturbances;
6. specific types of preoccupation or obsession;
7. major abnormalities in motor or sensory function;
8. movement disorders, including changes in station and gait; and
9. sleep disorders.

Individuals with impairments stemming from ventricular or meningeal tears may experience a certain degree of difficulty in more than one of these categories. Multiple impairment is best represented by the most severe of the first five categories; any degree of impairment in the last four categories may be combined with the worst of the first five to estimate total cerebral impairment. A special formula for calculating the final estimate—referred to as the combined value—is provided.

The categories that are most likely to be seen in individuals with meningeal or ventricular tears include all the foregoing except communications disturbances and preoccupation or obsessive disorders. Motor and sensory abnormalities also arise and, in some cases, are serious enough to cause severe impairment. However, it is not always immediately clear whether they are due to damage within the cerebrum, the spinal cord or the peripheral nerves. An accurate diagnosis is essential to predict the permanence and extent of impairment.

5.91 Disturbances in Mental Status and Integrative Functioning

Diminished mental activity is seen in some patients who develop hygroma or meningitis; mental retardation is also seen in children who develop arachnoid cysts. The criteria for mental status impairment range from impairment with continued ability to perform most activities of daily living satisfactorily (1 to 14 percent) to inability to care for oneself and remain safe without supervision (50 to 70 percent).

5.92 Behavioral or Emotional Disturbances

Some individuals who experience hygroma exhibit personality changes. Criteria for impairment range from mild limitations in daily social and interpersonal skills (0 to 14 percent) to severe limitations that result in total dependence on another person to carry out daily social and interpersonal activities (50 to 70 percent).

5.93 Disturbances in Level of Consciousness and Awareness

Individuals who develop traumatic meningitis or vasogenic brain edema are at risk for experiencing impaired levels of consciousness. Criteria for impairment range from brief repetitive or persistent alterations in consciousness during which the patient's ability to carry out daily activities is limited (0 to 14 percent), to a persistent vegetative state or irreversible coma for which total medical support is required (50 to 90 percent).

5.94 Episodic Neurologic Disorders

Episodic neurologic disorders include convulsive disorders, such as seizures, which are experienced by some individuals with arachnoid cysts or meningitis. Sleep disorders, such as the drowsiness experienced by some individuals with meningitis, are included in this category.

These impairments may involve other body systems, especially the cardiovascular and respiratory systems and the autonomic nervous system. Criteria have been established for impaired convulsive disorders and sleep/arousal disorders. The least amount of impairment for convulsive disorders is characterized by predictable signs and unpredictable occurrences, which do not disrupt the patient's usual activities but pose a risk to the patient or limit daily activities (0 to 14 percent); the greatest amount of impairment is associated with uncontrolled, severe and constant seizure activity and completely limits daily activities (50 to 70 percent). Criteria for sleep and arousal disorders range from reduced daytime alertness and altered sleep patterns that do not prevent the individual from carrying out most daily activities (1 to 9 percent), to impairments that severely reduce daytime alertness, to the point that the individual cannot care for himself or herself under any circumstances or in any manner (40 to 60 percent).[14]

5.95   The Brain Stem: Cranial Nerves

Cranial nerves III, IV, VI and VII may be affected in patients who experience traumatic meningitis. Cranial nerves III and IV (oculomotor and trochlear) are located within the midbrain. In cooperation with cranial nerve VI (abducens), they innervate the muscles responsible for moving the eyeball and controlling the size of the pupil. Permanent impairment of any of these three muscles may result in the patient's inability to see a single image with both eyes. Calculation of whole-person impairment—which can be severe—should incorporate impairment criteria established for the visual system.

Cranial nerves VI and VII (abducens and facial) lie within the pons and cerebellum. The primary role of the abducens nerve is to move the eyeball laterally. This nerve lies close to the facial nerve and other cranial nerves in this segment of the brain, including the sensory nuclei ("control centers") of the trigeminal nerve—which innervates structures of the face, mouth and teeth—and the auditory nerve, a branch of cranial nerve VIII (vestibulocochlear) that is involved in hearing and balance.

Criteria for facial nerve impairment range from complete loss of taste bud function (1 to 4 percent) to severe bilateral facial paralysis involving at least 75 percent of facial structures (20 to 45 percent).

---

[14] *See also* ch. 11 for a discussion of epilepsy.

Criteria for auditory nerve impairment range from minimal impairment of equilibrium that limits only daily living activities that are carried out in dangerous surroundings (1 to 9 percent), to severe impairment that limits the individual so much that assistance is necessary for personal hygiene and ambulation, and confinement may be necessary (50 to 70 percent).

5.96 Gait

The spinal cord plays a significant role in helping the individual sense joint position and triggering the contraction of all muscles involved in maintaining desired positions or changing them in order to achieve a particular type of gait. The change in gait seen in some patients with hydrocephalus may result from damage to cerebral nerves. It may also result from the effect of cerebral nerve damage on motor nerve fibers extending from the brain to the spinal cord. Gait impairment criteria range from mild impairments, which allow the patient to rise to a standing position and walk but make it difficult for the patient to handle stairs, deep chairs or long walks (1 to 9 percent), to severe impairment, which results in the patient not being able to stand without assistance, mechanical support or a prosthesis.

5.97 Peripheral Nervous System Deficits

Both motor and sensory function may be impaired in individuals with positive Kernig's and Brudzinski's signs, which include some individuals with traumatic meningitis. Such extremity impairments are not easily converted to whole-person impairment, since they must be evaluated in terms of loss of motion, vascular disorders and neurologic deficits, as well.

Sensory impairment criteria generally range from no loss of sensation and no pain (0 percent), to reduced sensation and severe pain or causalgia that prevents activity (81 to 95 percent). Criteria for impairment due to a loss of motor function and muscle power due to peripheral nerve disorders range from active movement against gravity with full resistance (0 percent), to no muscle contraction (100 percent).

5.100 BIBLIOGRAPHY

Text References

American Medical Association: Guides to the Evaluation of Permanent Impairment. Chicago: American Medical Association, 1993.

Aoki, N.: Lumboperitoneal Shunt: Clinical Applications, Complications, and Comparison with Ventriculoperitoneal Shunt. Neurosurgery 26(6):998–1003, June 90.

Ash, G. J., et al.: Antimicrobial Prophylaxis for Fractured Base of Skull in Children. Brain Inj. 6(6):521–527, Nov.-Dec. 1992.

Bahr, W. and Stoll, P.: Nasal Intubation in the Presence of Frontobasal Fractures: A Retrospective Study. J. Oral Maxillofac. Surg. 50(5):445–447, May 1992.

Bannister, C. M., et al.: Nasal Endotracheal Intubation in a Premature Infant with a Nasal Encephalocele. Arch. Dis. Child. 69(1Spec. No.):81–82, July 1993.

Berkow, R. and Fletcher, A. J. (Eds.): The Merck Manual of Diagnosis and Therapy, 16th ed. Rahway, N.J.: Merck Research Laboratories, 1992.

Brandrick, J. T.: Traumatic CSF Fistula Presenting Late as a Middle Ear Effusion. J. Laryngol. Otol. 103(1):97–98, Jan. 1989.

Creamer, M. J., et al.: Coronal Computerized Tomography and Cerebrospinal Fluid Rhinorrhea. Arch. Phys. Med. Rehabil. 73(6):599–602, June 1992.

Daly, D. T., et al.: Extracranial Approaches to the Repair of Cerebrospinal Fluid Rhinorrhea. Ear Nose Throat J. 71(7):311–313, July 1992.

deGroot, J. and Chusid, J. G.: Correlative Neuroanatomy, 20th ed. East Norwalk, Conn.: Appleton & Lange, 1988.

Fransen, P., et al.: Highly Sensitive Detection of beta 2 Transferrin in Rhinorrhea and Otorrhea as a Marker for Cerebrospinal Fluid (CSF) Leakage. Acta Neurochir. Wien 109(3–4): 98–10, 1991.

Greenfield, L. J. (Ed.): Complications in Surgery and Trauma, 2nd ed. Philadelphia: Lippincott, 1990.

Hasegawa, M., et al.: Traumatic Subdural Hygroma: Pathology and Meningeal Enhancement on Magnetic Resonance Imaging. Neurosurgery 31(3):580–585, Sept. 1992.

James, H. E.: Encephalocele, Dermoid Sinus and Arachnoid Cyst. In: McLaurin, R., et al. (Eds.): Pediatric Neurosurgery, 2nd ed. Philadelphia: Saunders, 1989.

Kim, J.H., et al.: Staphylococcus aureus Meningitis: Review of 28 Cases. Rev. Infect. Dis. 11(5): 698–706, Sept.-Oct. 1989.

Kupfermann, I.: Hypothalamus and Limbic System: Peptidergic Neurons, Homeostasis and Emotional Behavior. In: Kandel, E. R., et al. (Eds.): Principles of Neural Science, 3rd ed. Norwalk, Conn: Appleton and Lange, 1991.

Le Roux, P. D., et al.: Pediatric Intracranial Pressure Monitoring in Hypoxic and Nonhypoxic Brain Injury. Childs. Nerv. Syst. 7(1):34–39, Feb. 1991.

Lim, D.V.: Microbiology. St. Paul: West Publishing, 1989.

Luby, J. P.: Infections of the Central Nervous System. Am. J. Med. Sci. 304(6):379–391, Dec. 1992.

Lusins, J. O. and Levy, E. R.: MRI Documentation of Hemorrhage into Post-Traumatic Subdural Hygroma. Mt. Sinai J. Med. 60(2):161–162, Mar. 1993.

McLaurin, R. L. and Towbin, R.: Post Traumatic Hematomas. In: McLaurin, R. L., et al. (Eds.): Pediatric Neurosurgery, 2nd ed. Philadelphia: Saunders, 1989.

Milhorat, T. H.: Treatment of Hydrocephalus. In: Dudley, H., et al. (Eds.): Rob and Smith's Operative Surgery: Neurosurgery, 4th ed. London: Butterworth, 1989.

Miner, M. E. and Wagner, K. A. (Eds.): Neurotrauma: Treatment, Rehabilitation and Related Issues. No. 3. Boston: Butterworth, 1989.

Mysiw, W. J. and Jackson, R. D.: Relationship of New Onset Systemic Hypertension and Normal Pressure Hydrocephalus. Brain Inj. 4(3):233–238, July-Sept. 1990.

Nelson, J. S.: Pathology of the Nervous System. In: Kissane, J. M. (Ed.): Anderson's Pathology, 9th ed. St. Louis: Mosby, 1990.

Okoro, B. A. and Ohaegbulam, S. C.: Ventriculo-Peritoneal Shunts in Children. A Ten-Year Experience at the University of Nigeria Teaching Hospital, Enugu, Nigeria. West Afr. J. Med. 11(4):284–291, Oct.-Dec. 1992.

Orebaugh, S. L. and Margolis, J. H.: Post-Traumatic Intracerebral Pneumatocele: Case Report. J. Trauma 30(12):1577–1580, Dec. 1990.

Quiney, R. E., et al.: Recurrent Meningitis in Children due to Inner Ear Abnormalities. J. Laryngol. Otol. 103(5):473–480, May 1989.

Rhee, K. J., et al.: Does Nasotracheal Intubation Increase Complications in Patients with Skull Base Fractures? Ann. Emerg. Med. 22(7):1145–1147, July 1993.

Ropper, A. H.: Trauma of the Head and Spinal Cord. In: Wilson, J. D., et al. (Eds.): Harrison's Principles of Internal Medicine, 12th ed. New York: McGraw-Hill, 1991.

Rowland, L. P., et al.: Cerebrospinal Fluid—Blood Brain Barrier, Brain Edema and Hydrocephalus. In: Kandel, E. R., et al. (Eds.): Principles of Neural Science, 3rd ed. Norwalk, Conn.: Appleton and Lange, 1991.

Schonwald, S., et al.: Ciprofloxacin in the Treatment of Gram Negative Bacillary Meningitis. Am. J. Med. 87(5A):248S–249S, Nov. 30, 1989.

Shapiro, S. A. and Scully, T.: Closed Continuous Drainage of Cerebrospinal Fluid via a Lumbar Subarachnoid Catheter for Treatment or Prevention of Cranial/Spinal Cerebrospinal Fluid Fistula. Neurosurgery 30(2): 241–245, Feb. 1992.

Sindou, M., et al.: Transcutaneous Pressure Adjustable Valve for the Treatment of Hydrocephalus and Arachnoid Cysts in Adults. Experiences with 75 Cases. Acta Neurochir. Wien 121(3–4):135–139, 1993.

Swartz, M. N.: Bacterial Meningitis. In: Wyngaarden, J. B., et al.: Cecil Textbook of Medicine, 19th ed. Philadelphia: Saunders, 1992.

Teasdale, G. M. and Galbraith, S.: Head Injuries. In: Dudley, H., et al. (Eds.): Rob and Smith's Operative Surgery: Neurosurgery, 4th ed. London: Butterworth, 1989.

Thammavaram, K. V., et al.: Fascia Lata Graft as a Dural Substitute in Neurosurgery. South. Med. J. 83(6):634–636, June 1990.

Treseler, C. B. and Sugar, A. M.: Fungal Meningitis. Infect. Dis. Clin. North Am. 4(4):789–808, Dec. 1990.

von Wild, K.: Arachnoid Cysts of the Middle Cranial Fossa. Neurochirurgia Stuttg. 35(6):177–182, Nov. 1992.

Vrankovic, D. and Glavina, K.: Cranioplasty of the Anterior Fossa Traumatic Bone Defect using Autologous Cancellous Bone. Neurochirurgia Stuttg. 32(4):110–115, July 1989.

Winkelman, M. D. and Galloway, P. G.: Central Nervous System Complications of Thermal Burns. A Postmortem Study of 139 Patients. Medicine (Baltimore) 71(5):271–283, Sept. 1992.

Yokoyama, K., et al.: Scintigraphic Demonstration of Intracranial Communication between Arachnoid Cyst and Associated Subdural Hematoma. Clin. Nucl. Med. 14(5):350–353, May 1989.

Additional References

Baker, A. J., et al.: Excitatory Amino Acids in Cerebrospinal Fluid following Traumatic Brain Injury in Humans. J. Neurosurg. 79(3):369–372, Sept. 1993.

Leonetti, J. P., et al.: Posterior Internal Auditory Canal Closure following the Retrosigmoid Approach to the Cerebellopontine Angle. Am. J. Otol. 14(1):31–33, Jan. 1993.

Reider-Groswasser, I., et al.: Late CT Findings in Brain Trauma: Relationship to Cognitive and Behavioral Sequelae and to Vocational Outcome. Am. J. Roentgenol. 160(1):147–152, Jan. 1993.

Ronty, H., et al.: Cerebral Trauma and Alcohol Abuse. Eur. J. Clin. Invest. 23(3):182–187, Mar. 1993.

Unterberg, A., et al.: LongTerm Observations of Intracranial Pressure after Severe Head Injury. The Phenomenon of Secondary Rise of Intracranial Pressure. Neurosurgery 32(1):17–23; Discussion 23–24, Jan. 1993.

Vrankovic, D. and Glavina, K.: Classification of Frontal Fossa Fractures Associated with Cerebrospinal Fluid Rhinorrhea, Pneumocephalus or Meningitis. Indications and Time for Surgical Treatment. Neurochirurgia Stuttg. 36(2): 44–50, Mar. 1993.

CHAPTER 6

Skull Fractures

SCOPE

Fractures of the skull result from many types of trauma and are especially related to motor vehicle accidents, including those involving motorcycles. Skull fractures are likely to result when the head strikes, or is struck by, a blunt object. The two basic fracture categories are simple and compound. Fractures of the skull vault may occur alone, but they often extend to the base. Basilar fractures are usually extensions of vault lesions, but a few occur by themselves. The presence of a fracture does not always mean that the underlying tissue is damaged, but a depressed fracture is very likely to be accompanied by a contusion of the brain or an intracranial hemorrhage. Other complications of fractures include cranial nerve injuries, post-traumatic epilepsy, meningitis, hemorrhage and leakage of cerebrospinal fluid. Myriad potential complications of fractures make imperative such radiographic studies as routine skull x-rays and CT scanning in the evaluation of a head trauma victim.

SYNOPSIS

6.00 IN GENERAL

Skull fractures involve a break in the bony skeleton of the head that encases and protects the brain. Skull fractures arise as a consequence of head trauma. They are not a common result of such trauma, however, occurring in less than 20 percent of patients who are x-rayed for head trauma (McClean, et al., 1984).

Most skull fractures are not significant injuries, cause no internal complications and require little management or long-term care. However, they are an indication that head trauma has occurred, and as such, they raise the possibility of serious intracranial vascular or neurologic injury. Although such intracranial injury can occur in the absence of skull fracture, it is more common when a skull fracture is present. This probably reflects the violence and severity of force required to fracture the skull, as is evident by the motor vehicle accidents, falls from heights and assaults (in which gunshots are a principal agent of fracture) that are the most frequent causes of skull fracture.[1]

6.10 CLASSIFICATIONS

Skull fractures can be classified in a number of ways—by the type of fracture into linear, depressed or comminuted; into simple (or closed) or compound (open) fractures by the respective absence or presence of a break in the overlying skin and tissue; and by the location of the fracture, depending on whether it occurs in a bone of the base of the skull or in a bone of the calvaria (or skull vault, the upper, domelike portion of the skull).

6.11 Type of Fracture

Skull fractures may occur as linear fractures, in which horizontal, straight-line cracks occur in cranial bone; depressed fractures, in which vertical cracking and separation of bone occurs and a fragment of the inner surface, or table, of the skull is driven inward into the cranial cavity; or comminuted fractures, in which the bone breaks into multiple fragments.

[1] Linear Fractures

Linear skull fractures occur when the bone at the point of impact is forced inward, and a reflexive outward force is exerted on surrounding bone. The bone cracks along the line of these diverging forces. (*See Figure 6–1.*) Typically linear fractures are straight, single-line

---

[1] *See* 6.20 *infra.*

fractures, although a stellate (starlike) pattern of cracks radiating outward from the point of impact may also occur. In the case of straight-line fractures, the fracture usually runs from the point of impact toward the base of the skull. Simple linear fractures that do not cross meningeal vessels (arteries or veins in the three membranes, or meninges, that cover the brain and spinal cord) or involve bones of the skull base do not usually pose a serious clinical situation.

Linear fractures are the most common form of skull fracture. A study of 1,100 individuals with a history of skull fractures occurring over a 40-year period in Olmsted County, Minnesota, found that slightly more than half had simple linear fractures (Nelson, et al., 1984). Other estimates of the frequency of linear fractures range as high as 70 to 80 percent (Moses, 1984).

[2] Depressed Fractures

Depressed skull fractures are characterized by inward displacement of bone from the inner table of the calvaria. Simple depressed fractures can occur if a small, hard object traveling at high speed, such as a golf ball, hits the head. Although it does not penetrate the skin, such an object strikes the head with such force that the area of impact bends inward until its inner surface fractures, with the bone fragments propelled inward. In such a case, it is possible for the inner table of the skull to fracture without a fracture of its external surface (Bagchi, 1980).

A compound depressed fracture results if an object, such as a bullet, penetrates or perforates the skull. These fractures are often comminuted as well, involving multiple bone fragments (Zimmerman and Bilaniuk, 1983).

In the Minnesota series, about 15 percent of reported skull fractures were depressed fractures. About two thirds of these were simple fractures (Nelson, et al., 1984). In a number of other series, however, compound fractures have accounted for 75 to 90 percent of depressed fractures (van den Heever and van der Merwe, 1989). Over 50 percent of depressed fractures occur in the frontal area (Becker, et al., 1982), and in one report of 300 depressed fractures, over 90 percent occurred in the frontal or parietal bones (Braakman and Jennett, 1975). (*See Figure 6–2.*) Depressed fractures seem to occur most often in older children, adolescents and young adults.

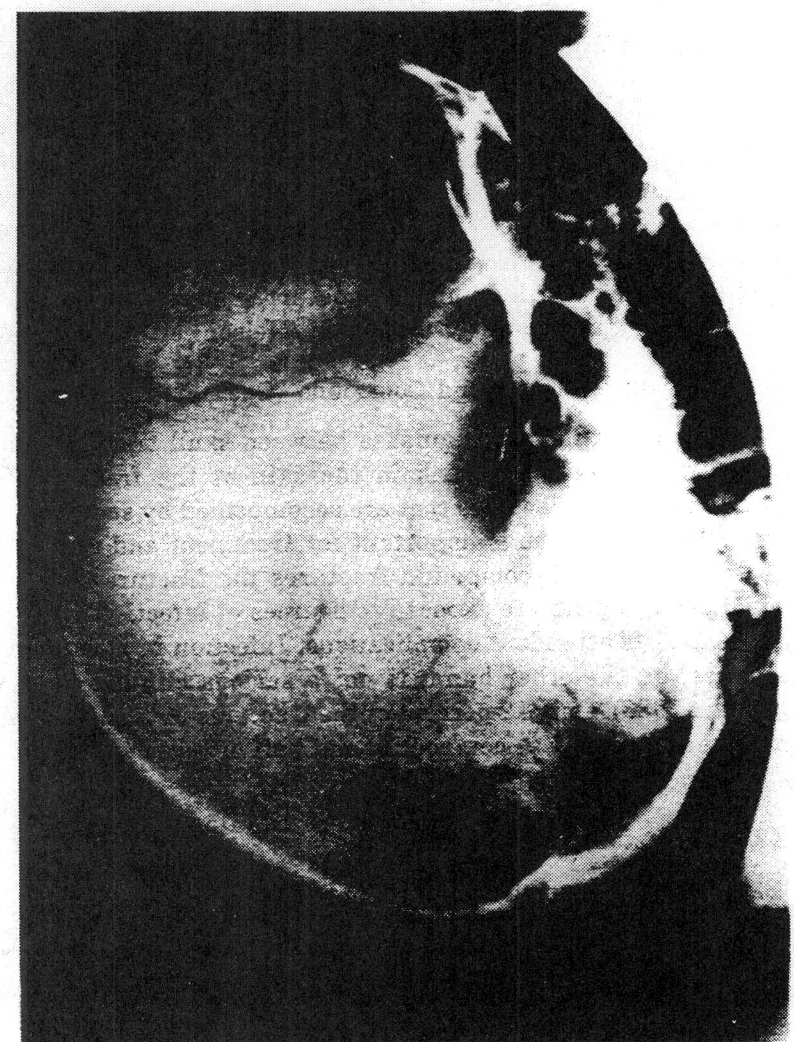

Fig. 6-1. X-ray of a linear skull fracture.

[3] Comminuted Fractures

Comminuted fractures, in which the bone fractures into multiple fragments, are rare, particularly in the absence of an associated linear or depressed fracture. In the Minnesota series, less than 2 percent were isolated comminuted fractures. In another 5 percent, however, comminution occurred along with linear or depressed fractures, mostly the latter (Nelson, et al., 1984).

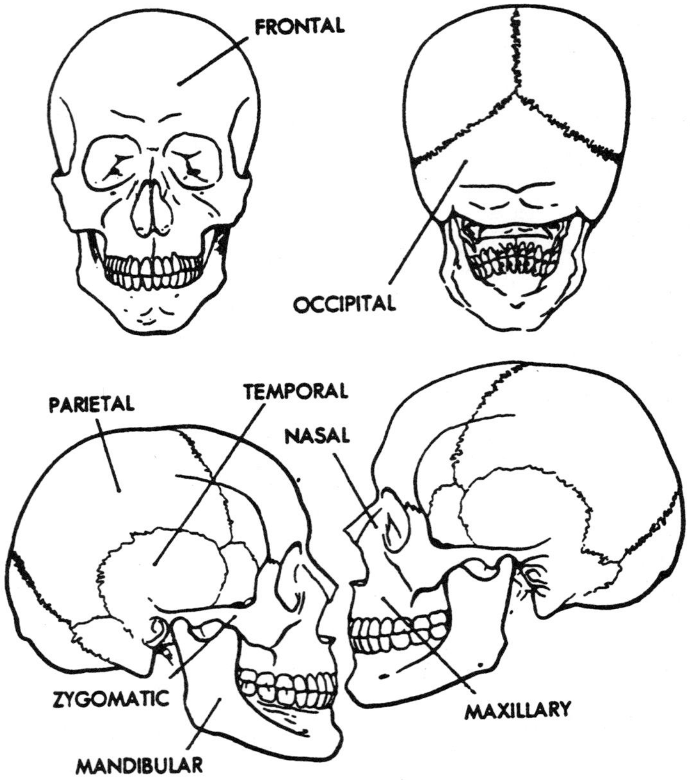

Fig. 6-2. The bones of the skull (external view).

6.12　Simple (Closed) and Compound (Open) Fractures

This classification distinguishes between skull fractures that are associated with no break in the skin at the fracture site (closed) and those fractures that are accompanied by such a break (open). The distinction is important for treatment and control of infection, since with compound fractures, the fracture area and cranial cavity within are exposed to sources of infection from the outside and the attendant complications of infection. In most simple fractures, on the other hand, infection is not a serious clinical concern (Lehman, 1988). Only 12 percent of the fractures in the Minnesota study were reported as compound, and half of these were caused by penetrating force (Nelson, et al., 1984).

6.13　Fracture Location

Skull fractures can also be classified according to their location. The structure of the skull is such that a number of bones constitute its base and several others constitute the calvaria, or skull vault. Because basilar skull fractures have a number of particular characteristics, they are usually distinguished as such, while fractures in the vault of the skull are usually classified as linear, depressed or comminuted, and as simple or compound.[2]

[1]　The Skull Base

The basilar skull consists of the ethmoid bone surrounding the eye and nose cavities; the petrous bone (the pyramidal portion of temporal bone wedged between the sphenoid and occipital bones); the lower part of the occipital bone; and the sphenoid, the bone at the front of the skull base that articulates (forms a joint) with every other cranial bone. (*See Figure 6–3.*) Fractures in these areas, which are always linear (Bagchi, 1980), occurred in nearly 20 percent of the patients studied in the Minnesota series, making basilar fracture the second most common type of skull fracture (after linear fracture) (Nelson, et al., 1984).

By virtue of its location, the skull base is not as exposed to direct outside forces as is the vault of the skull. Basilar fractures, therefore, usually occur as a result of indirect force being transmitted from the point of extreme external trauma. Motor vehicle accidents are a common source of basilar fractures, accounting for more than 60 percent of this type of injury (Nelson, et al., 1984).

External force is usually transmitted to the skull base through the bones of the calvaria but may also be transmitted by frontal attachments to the head, such as facial protection devices attached to motorcycle and football helmets. A study of fatal motorcycle accidents in Sweden, for example, found that 11 of 38 motorcyclists wearing full-face helmets suffered basilar skull fractures, compared with only 6 of 64 who wore open-face helmets (Krantz, 1985). Although they protect the energy-absorbing facial bones, therefore, such devices may sometimes also provide a pathway for the force to bypass these bones and follow a course to the basilar skull (Cooter, et al., 1988).

---

[2] *See* 6.10 *supra.*

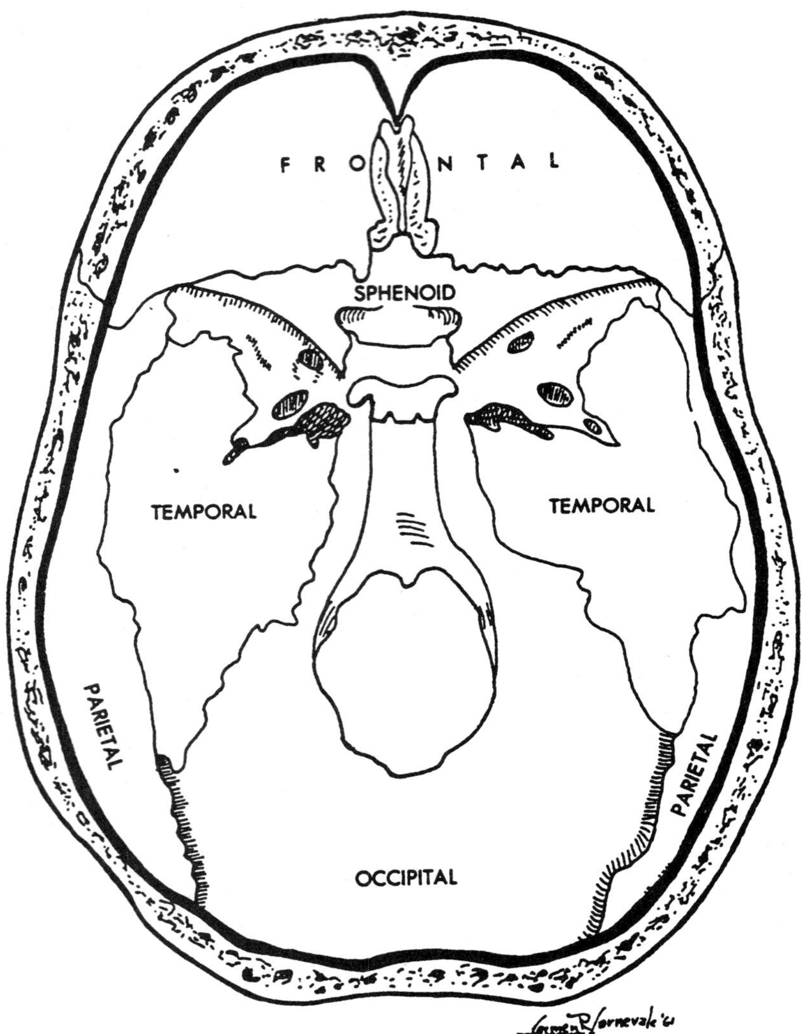

Fig. 6-3. A cross section of the base of the skull. The ethmoid bone and its cribriform plate are located between the right and left frontal bones. The cribriform plate directly overlies the uppermost portion of the nasal passages.

The sphenoid bone may be particularly susceptible to indirect force because of its articulation with other cranial and facial bones. In one study, 65 percent of 78 patients with fractures of the sphenoid also had a facial fracture, and 22 percent had a fracture in the cranial vault. Only 13 percent of fractures affected the sphenoid alone.

The sphenoid is subject to fracturing at multiple sites, as evidenced by the 178 sphenoid fractures in the 78 patients (Unger, et al., 1990). In addition to the sphenoid, the petrous portion of the temporal bone is a common site of basilar skull fracture, especially those that extend from the temporal or occipital bones to the central area of the cranial fossa, the inner hollow of the skull base that encase the lower structures of the brain.

Basilar skull fractures are characterized clinically by a particular set of symptoms, including leakage of cerebrospinal fluid (CSF) from the ear (otorrhea) and nasal passages (rhinorrhea), bleeding in the middle ear accompanied by surface discoloration ("Battle's sign") and bruising about the eyes ("raccoon face") caused by periorbital hemorrhage.

[2]   The Calvaria

The bones of the calvaria include the frontal bone of the forehead, the parietal bones forming the sides and roof of the skull, the squamous portions of the temporal bones at the side of the skull and the squamous portions of the occipital bone at the skull's lower rear.

The frontal and parietal bones are highly resistant to trauma. Their respective capacities for resistance have been measured at 1,100 and 550 pounds per square inch, compared with the resistance of the zygoma (cheekbone), which is afforded greater protection by overlying soft tissue, of 225 pounds per square inch. Nonetheless, since the lateral areas of the frontal and parietal bones form the largest surface area of the skull, lack significant soft tissue protection and are the parts of the skull most exposed to trauma, they are the most common site of fracture in the calvaria. In children, the occipital bone is a frequent site of linear fracture (Bagchi, 1980).

Fractures in the skull vault may be the origin of basilar fractures. For example, in one series of 134 occipital skull fractures, the fracture line in 52 patients extended from the occipital bone to a bone of the skull base. The most common extended occipital fractures were transverse (crosswise) fractures of the petrous pyramid. This is in contrast to fractures of the temporal and parietal bones, which are more likely to produce longitudinal (lengthwise) fractures of the petrous pyramid (Young and Schmidek, 1982).

Fractures in the bones of the calvaria are usually classified as linear or depressed and simple or compound.

6.20   MECHANISMS

Two major mechanical factors are at work in fractures of the skull: (1) the surface area of the skull striking or being struck by the impacting force, and (2) the speed at which the skull is struck. In addition, directional factors, such as linear or rotational forces exerted upon the head and neck, may also be involved and have particular implications for intracranial injury.

6.21   Surface Factors

Fractures of the skull can occur under circumstances in which the skull is struck by a broad, blunt surface or a limited focal surface. Examples of the former might include a wall, an automobile windshield or a dashboard. In the latter instance, the skull might strike a car bumper or steering wheel, the corner of a wall or edge of a step, a fist or hand implement such as a tool or baseball bat, or a small projectile.

[1]   Blunt Injuries

Upon blunt impact, the exterior bone of the skull is compressed, resulting in an in-bending of the interior surface of bone. This in-bending produces a tensile, or stretching, pressure on the inner table of the skull. If the impact is of sufficient force and the skull sufficiently thin at the point of impact, a linear fracture begins in the area of tensile pressure on the inner table of the skull. If, on the other hand, the impact occurs at a thick portion of the skull, such as the midfrontal, midoccipital or petrous portion of the temporal bone, the in-bending of the inner table is insignificant. Instead, the inner table is compressed, and tensile forces are exerted outward to areas of the skull surrounding the area of impact. If this periphery is a thin area of the skull, a linear fracture may occur here, or, if the impact is of sufficient magnitude to disperse tensile forces some distance, the linear fracture will occur at a thin area of the skull farther away (Gennarelli, 1982).

Fractures are generally propagated along the cranial paths of least resistance. Trauma on the lower forehead may propagate fractures up the vault along the frontal bone or down along the base of the skull into the anterior cranial fossa. In the latter case, the fracture line usually carries on along the lines of the cribriform structures of the basilar skull, separating bone much as postage stamps are separated along their perforated edges (Bagchi, 1980). Fractures from higher frontal forces are usually confined to the vault of the skull.

Frontolateral trauma sends fracture lines through the thin temporal bone of the lower side of the skull rather than over the thick frontal bone. Such trauma may result in fractures of the squamous portion of the temporal bone or of the orbital roof above the eye. High lateral forces can transmit energy through the lower portion of the temporal bone, causing fractures that originate some distance away in the floor of the middle cranial fossa and extending back toward the original site of impact. Posterior trauma at the occipital or posterior parietal regions sends fracture lines downward through the occipital bone toward the foramen magnum, the opening in the skull where the spinal cord attaches to the medulla oblongata of the brain. (*See Figure 6–4.*)

Crushing injuries can cause a particular form of skull fracture. Such injuries occur when the skull is crushed between two surfaces. This may occur when a heavy object falls on the side, front or back of the head of a person in a prone position with her or his head at rest on the ground or another surface. It might also result from a headfirst fall from a height, in which the skull is interposed between the ground or floor and the body above it. Under these circumstances, the skull is squeezed and its diameter is shortened along the axis of the direction of the force exerted between the opposing surfaces. The perpendicular axis, in response, is lengthened, and the skull fractures at its opposite ends, which may be 90 degrees away from the site of impact.

[2] Focal Injuries

A focal injury may be sustained when the head is struck by an object with a small surface area and the area of impact bends inward until the inner table of the skull fractures, with the bone fragment or fragments pushed inward. In noncomminuted simple fractures, the injured area may rebound to a configuration close to its original contour, leaving only an indentation in the outer skull and no significant interior displacement. However, the depressed fragment may also

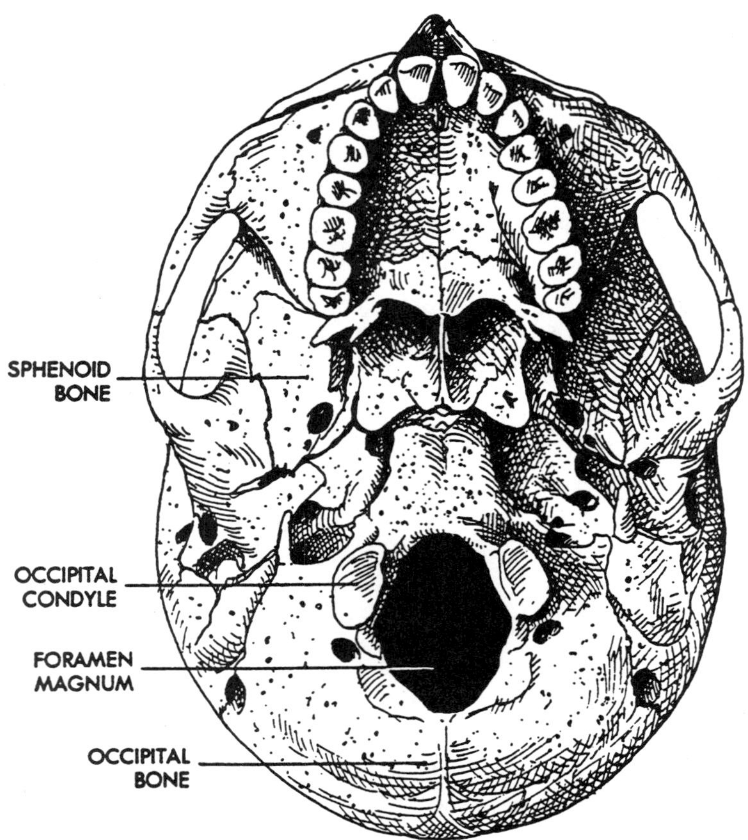

Fig. 6-4. The base of the skull, as seen from below. Special anatomic features of this aspect of the skull include the sphenoid bone; the occipital bone; the occipital condyle, which articulates with the atlas (first cervical vertebra); and the foramen magnum, the skull opening through which the brain stem exits before joining the spinal cord and the occipital bone.

slip and its outer surface become wedged beneath the edge of the adjacent intact bone. In this case, the fragment remains depressed. This situation fits the operational definition of depressed fractures that is sometimes adopted in the medical literature.

Focal injuries tend to cause fractures at the point of impact, and the smaller the offending object, the greater the likelihood of the fracture being localized in a small area of the skull surface. However, focal injuries are highly associated with depressed fractures, which carry a threat of intracranial damage caused by the inward extension or propulsion of skull fragments that penetrate the dura (the outermost of the three fibrous, protective membranes encompassing the brain and spinal cord) and the brain itself.

6.22 Speed Factors

The pattern of skull fracture also depends on the speed at which the impact on the skull occurs. In general, low-velocity forces will cause linear fractures, while high-velocity forces are more likely to cause depressed fractures.

[1] Low-Velocity Injuries

Objects that produce low-velocity injuries will be blunt, broad, immovable and large; the impact thus results in linear fracture. The force required to cause such fractures has been estimated at 900 to 1,700 pounds delivered to the skull in one millisecond or less (Thomas, 1985).

A fall from a standing position with the head striking a wall, floor, pavement, ice or rocky or hard ground is an example of such a low-velocity injury. In one study of skull fractures, over half of the simple linear fractures resulted from falls (Nelson, et al., 1984). Such falls are unlikely to result in severe complications or disability (Adams, et al., 1984). A low-speed automobile accident in which the forehead is propelled against a dashboard surface (as opposed to its edge) but with a minimum of trauma (described by a patient perhaps as bumping the forehead) is another example of this type of low-velocity injury.

Low-velocity focal injuries may occur, as well. Injury that is inflicted in a personal assault with a fist, hammer, wrench, baseball bat or similar implement might be typical of low-velocity injury. Assaults were the second major cause of depressed fractures in the Minnesota series (after motor vehicle accidents) (Nelson, et al., 1984). Occupational injuries on construction sites in which the head is struck by a heavy, slowly swinging suspended object are other examples of low-velocity focal injuries. The only evidence of a fracture in these instances is often an indentation in the skull at the point of impact, although, depending on the site and force of the blow, a more severely depressed fracture may occur.

[2] High-Velocity Injuries

High-velocity injuries are likely to result in depressed fractures. Depending on its size and shape as well as speed, the offending object may penetrate the skin and skull, resulting in compound and comminuted depressed fractures.

Objects that are propelled at moderately high velocity must have sufficient size and weight to cause skull fracture. Objects that typically cause simple depressed skull fractures include golf balls and baseballs. Because of their size and shape, such objects do not penetrate the skull and do not necessarily incur skin wounds at the point of impact.

High-velocity skull fractures that are likely to be compound (open) include head injuries incurred in high-speed automobile or motorcycle accidents, in which the skull itself is propelled at high velocity by inertial forces after a collision. High-velocity penetrating injuries caused by gunshots or explosive fragments such as shrapnel or debris from explosions are necessarily compound and often comminuted. They have the greatest potential for intracranial damage with severe neurologic consequences, as the penetrating object disrupts the dural covering of the brain and structures of the brain in its path. Such damage is not usually caused by the fracture of the skull itself but by the penetrating object that caused the skull fracture. It is possible, however, for fragments of bone to cause similar damage as they are driven some depth inward.

6.23 Directional Factors

A sufficiently forceful tangential blow to the head may fracture the skull while setting the head in rotational motion. Under these circumstances, linear skull fractures that have a tendency to come apart or fractures in which the fractured portions tend to be displaced underneath one another are common.

The head itself may already be in linear or rotational motion at the time of impact. The latter might typically occur in motor vehicle accidents in which accelerating forces set the head turning as a victim is thrown sideways from the vehicle. Rotational acceleration has been suspected as a factor in particularly severe basilar skull fractures known as ring fractures. These fractures usually occur during high-speed motor vehicle accidents and probably result from the torsion of the skull vault upon its base. They are characterized by a transverse fracture that encircles the bone surrounding the foramen magnum.

Severe accelerating and decelerating forces, whether they are linear or rotational, can cause internal brain injury without fracturing the skull. Such injuries are known as brain contusions and occur when the brain is dislodged from its normal position and forced against the interior of the skull.[3]

6.30 CLINICAL PICTURE

Most skull fractures present few clinical signs of external or internal damage. Since most are simple fractures, external signs are often absent. In most patients, internal signs are likewise absent, because only a small proportion of skull fractures result in intracranial injury. Under these circumstances, it is not surprising that a great many skull fractures are diagnosed radiologically and then receive little further treatment other than short-term observation. Indeed, if not for the widespread use of x-ray or other diagnostic technologies, it is likely that a great many skull fractures would go undiagnosed—with few adverse consequences to the patient (Clarke and Adams, 1990).

The clinical picture of the patient with a skull fracture has become controversial in recent decades, precisely because of the widespread use of x-rays, with their disadvantages of cost and radiation exposure. Nearly all studies of head trauma and x-ray findings report that skull fracture occurs in a small minority of cases—usually less than 20 percent (McClean, et al., 1984), and in many of these patients with positive findings, no further treatment is required. Thus the utility of "scattershot" x-raying for skull fractures after minor or mild head trauma has been questioned.

As an alternative to routine skull x-rays, there has been an effort to identify clinical signs that raise the suspicion of skull fracture and enable the physician to classify patients into so-called low-risk, moderate-risk and high-risk categories. Implementation of such guidelines in one British hospital was found to reduce the number of skull x-rays taken by 27 percent over a one-year period, at considerable cost savings (Clarke and Adams, 1990).

6.31 History and Examination

The details of the accident—including the nature of the offending object and the speed and location of its impact on the skull—should be obtained from the patient, witnesses or attendants at the site of the

---

[3] *See also* ch. 3 for a discussion of contusions of the brain.

trauma. These details are helpful in determining whether a linear, depressed or basilar skull fracture has occurred and where potential fracture sites exist according to typical fracture patterns.

Visual and palpable examination of the skull will reveal lacerations or entry and exit wounds, indicating sites of potential compound fractures. Nonpenetrating small missiles that nick the scalp may result in depressed fractures accompanied by small wounds that are easily overlooked, yet detecting the wound provides the most clear indication of a possible fracture in the underlying skull. Gentle palpation of the skull can reveal indentations characteristic of depressed fractures, displacement and motion along linear fractures, and contusions at potential fracture sites.

A baseline neurologic examination will assess the patient's level of consciousness, pupillary response, ocular movements, motor function and vital signs for indications of neurologic damage. Level of consciousness should be observed in terms of both cognition and wakefulness. Pupils should be checked for size and bilateral equality. Ocular movements should be checked for parallel tracking and disconjugate gaze (disconnected movements between both eyes). Motor functions can be tested by checking for movement and strength in the extremities and for decerebrate and decorticate posturing (characteristic reaction of the extremities to stimuli in the presence of specific, serious brain injury). The symmetry of deep tendon reflexes should also be checked, and temperature, respiration, pulse and blood pressure should be measured.

6.32 Findings and Likelihood of Skull Fracture

Findings in patients with potential skull fractures may range from the asymptomatic in "low-risk" patients to obvious neurologic symptoms of intracranial damage in "high-risk" patients. However, one major study of 7,000 patients admitted to hospital emergency rooms found that even patients with intracranial damage have only about a 50 percent chance of actually having a skull fracture (Masters, et al., 1987).

[1] Low-Risk Patients

Patients at low risk of having incurred a skull fracture may present with headache, dizziness, scalp hematomas (collections of blood under the skin), lacerations, contusions (bruises) or abrasions. Others may be asymptomatic. One study of low-risk patients found that skull fractures existed in 3 percent and intracranial injury in less than 1 percent of asymptomatic patients. The respective incidences of skull fracture and intracranial injury were 4 percent and 2 percent in patients with headache; 5 percent and 0 percent in patients with dizziness; 7 percent and 1 percent in patients with scalp hematomas; and 4 percent and 2 percent in patients with scalp lacerations (Thornbury, et al., 1984). In a series of 7,000 patients admitted to hospital emergency rooms with head trauma, only 0.4 percent of patients characterized as low risk were found to have skull fractures (Masters, et al., 1987).

Lacking more serious symptoms, it is unlikely that a skull fracture exists. If a fracture is present, it is most likely a simple linear fracture that probably warrants little diagnostic attention or management beyond short-term observation of the patient at home (Masters, et al., 1987).

[2]   Moderate-Risk Patients

Patients with a history of altered consciousness at or subsequent to the time of injury, progressive headache, post-traumatic seizures,[4] vomiting, post-traumatic amnesia, multiple trauma and serious facial injury are at a moderate risk of having a skull fracture. In one study (Masters, et al., 1987), 4.2 percent of patients with these symptoms had skull fractures, most of them simple linear fractures, although depressed, basilar and complex fractures (involving two or more breaks) were also observed.

Headache, nausea and vomiting have been reported in patients with occipital fractures who exhibit mild neurologic impairment, suggested by drowsiness, lethargy and lapsing into sleep (Young and Schmidek, 1982). These findings are also seen in children with skull fractures accompanied by intracranial complications (Rosenthal and Bergman, 1989). These patients have not only a moderate risk of skull fracture but a higher risk for intracranial complications than do those in the low-risk category.

Patients who present with leakage of cerebrospinal fluid (CSF) from the ear and nasal passages (otorrhea and rhinorrhea, respectively) and raccoonlike ecchymoses (black and blue marks) about the eyes also have a moderate possibility of having incurred a skull fracture, in

---

[4] *See also* ch. 11 for a discussion of post-traumatic epilepsy.

particular, a basilar type. These signs may also suggest the possibility of a linear fracture in the calvaria (vault), since these are often the origin of basilar skull fractures (Zimmerman and Bilaniuk, 1983).

When the patient history indicates trauma characteristic of depressed skull fracture—that is, the history includes a possible penetrating wound or a blow with an object—the patient should also be considered at moderate risk of skull fracture. Such patients are candidates for further observation and investigation, and they may evidence a palpably depressed fracture (Masters, et al., 1987).

[3] High-Risk Patients

Patients who are most likely to have a skull fracture are those with depressed or decreasing level of consciousness not clearly due to alcohol, drugs or other causes; focal neurologic deficiencies; and an obvious penetrating wound. In one large study, 21.5 percent of patients with any of these clinical signs had skull fractures, usually simple linear fractures or depressed fractures (Masters, et al., 1987).

Unconsciousness lasting for more than 30 minutes, a combination of head wound and hematoma, and amnesia are also signs that should raise suspicions of a skull fracture. In a series of 281 patients, 30 percent of those who were unconscious for 30 minutes or more had a skull fracture. Combined wound and hematoma signified a fracture in 23 percent of patients, and amnesia correlated with fracture in 15 percent. The study also found that 18 percent of patients with a reduced level of consciousness had skull fracture. Patients with any of these signs had an overall 14 percent chance of having a skull fracture, compared with a 3 percent chance in patients who exhibited none of the signs (Tunturi, et al., 1982).

6.40 DIAGNOSIS

When clinical signs suggest moderate or high suspicion of skull fracture, the diagnosis may be confirmed through radiography or computed tomography (CT). Plain film x-rays are adequate in most cases of linear fractures in the skull vault. However, these are probably the least important skull fractures to identify, since many require no treatment (Cooper and Ho, 1983). Plain film radiography continues to be used to diagnose depressed fractures, although computed tomography may demonstrate these, as well as basilar fractures, more clearly (Macpherson and Teasdale, 1989).

6.41 Radiography

The utility of skull radiographs in cases of minor and mild head trauma has come into question in recent decades. The use of skull x-rays is strongly advised when the trauma is accompanied by any of the following (Clarke and Adams, 1990):

- unconsciousness;
- impaired level of consciousness;
- abnormal neurologic signs or symptoms;
- discharge of cerebrospinal fluid, blood or both from nose or ears;
- blood in the middle ear or bruising behind the ear;
- periorbital ecchymosis;
- suspected skull penetration or depressed fracture;
- scalp laceration in combination with hematoma; and
- amnesia.

The guidelines also recommend taking x-rays in injuries in which an unusually strong force has struck the skull. The guidelines suggest considering x-rays when co-existing conditions such as stroke, mental handicap, epilepsy, intoxication or psychological state are obstacles to obtaining an accurate history or clinical evaluation, and for patients who will not be under the observation of family or friends. In patients with minor head trauma, with no abnormal signs or symptoms or with minor scalp laceration without associated hematomas, x-rays are not usually necessary (Clarke and Adams, 1990).

Because of the spatial relationships and superimposition among the skull and facial bones, a complete radiographic picture of the skull can only be obtained through a series of x-rays. These require at least four views—anteroposterior (front-to-back) (*see Figure 6–5*), posteroanterior (back-to-front) (*see Figure 6–6*) and lateral views from both sides. These views, plus a view perpendicular to the foramen magnum, cover the complete skull.

Depending on the angle of the beam, anteroposterior views can afford images of the frontal, ethmoid and occipital bones and the petrous pyramids. The petrous ridge can be seen with the posteroanterior view, while lateral views provide images of the temporal and parietal bones and the ethmoid, sphenoid and frontal sinuses.

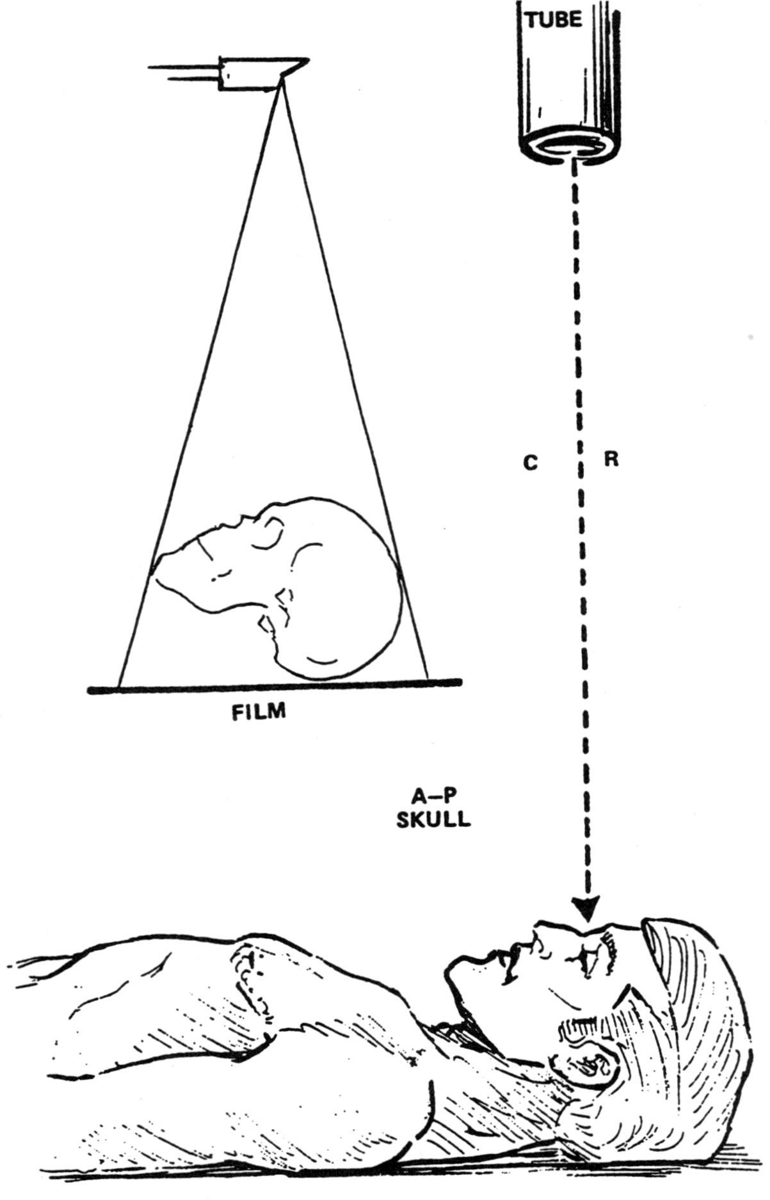

Fig. 6-5. A routine skull x-ray series includes an anteroposterior (A-P) view.

When specific areas of concern do not show well on the routine set of views, coned-down views, oblique-angle views and stereoscopic views may provide a better image (Pavlov, 1982).

[1] Linear Fractures

X-ray diagnosis of linear fractures remains widespread even as clinical guidelines for determining the need for such x-rays are increasingly espoused. The radiographic appearance of linear fractures is that of a long, straight lucency with sharp edges. Two contiguous or crisscrossing lines may appear when the fracture involves both the inner and outer tables of the skull. The fracture line rarely exceeds 3 millimeters at its maximum width and typically narrows at either end.

Fractures in the calvaria typically course toward the base, and basilar fractures take an opposite path toward the calvaria. Fracture lines tend to follow the cranial sutures (the channels of fibrous membrane adjoining the component bones of the calvaria). In young patients, extension of the fracture into the suture and separation of the suture is not uncommon, and this is suggested radiographically by widening of the sutures to 3 millimeters in the presence of contiguous fracture lines (Zimmerman and Bilaniuk, 1983).

Fractures in thin areas of the skull, such as the temporal bone, or in portions of the skull that in young people have not yet developed into their mature thickness, may be difficult to visualize. Lines in the normal structure of the skull, such as sutures, synchondroses (other areas where bones adjoin) and vascular grooves, may appear similar to fracture lines, but many of these may be distinguished from fractures by their symmetry and smooth edges. Lacerations of the scalp, dirt, foreign bodies and hair may also produce images that simulate fractures (Zimmerman and Bilaniuk, 1983).

[2] Depressed Fractures

In addition to routine x-ray views, stereoscopic and oblique projections and tangential views are often necessary for the best imaging of depressed fractures. Stereoscopic views are obtained by taking two exposures at slightly different angles while the patient remains stationary. Oblique views are taken with the skull slightly rotated, so that the fracture site is on a tangent to the x-ray beam. The latter are especially useful for evaluating the depth of the fragments in a depressed fracture (Pavlov, 1982).

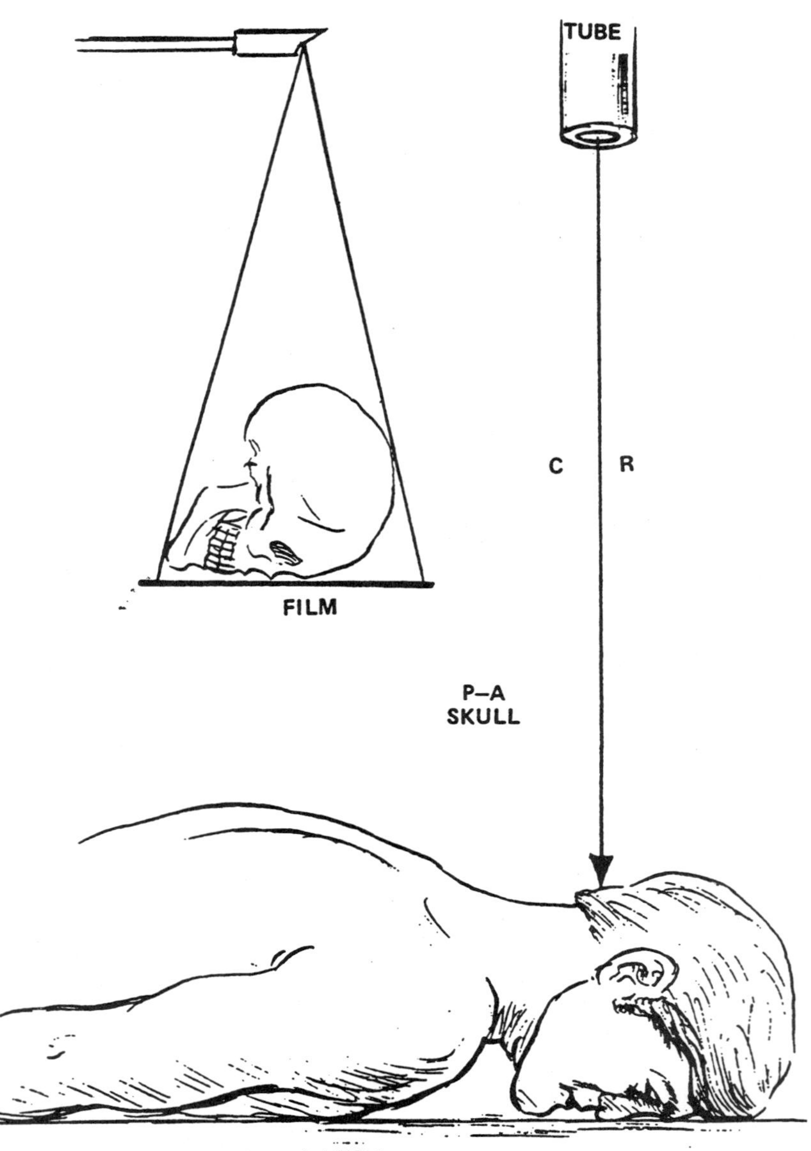

Fig. 6-6. A routine skull x-ray series also includes a posteroanterior (P-A) view.

Depressed fractures will show up as areas of increased density, representing bone overlying bone at the fracture site or the rotation of fragments to a position parallel to the x-ray beam (Zimmerman and Bilaniuk, 1983). Sometimes tangential views reveal depressed fractures that appear similar to the usual configuration of linear fractures (DeLuca and Rhea, 1983).

[3] Basilar Fractures

Basilar fractures are often difficult to detect radiographically, due to the superimposition of the paranasal sinuses and facial structures on the skull base. Stereoscopic views from the submento-vertex position (from beneath the chin toward the topmost point of the vault of the skull) may afford the best angles, but these are difficult to obtain and may be dangerous to attempt if spinal injury is present.

Other radiographic findings may suggest a basilar fracture. Identification of a fracture in the calvaria descending toward the skull base suggests a concomitant basilar fracture. The presence of an air mass (pneumocephalus) or fluid (characterized clinically by rhinorrhea or otorrhea) in the basilar sinuses, particularly the sphenoid sinus, is often a sign of a basilar fracture. These can be demonstrated by lateral skull radiographs exposed in a brow-up position with a horizontal x-ray beam (Zimmerman and Bilaniuk, 1983).

Fluid resulting from basilar fractures may also be detected through radionuclear medicine (using substances containing isotopes as tracers). The intrathecal (into the cerebrospinal fluid) isotope is injected, a cotton plug placed in the nose or ear, and the isotope collection is measured 6 to 24 hours later. The presence of the isotope on the cotton confirms the discharge of cerebrospinal fluid.

6.42 Computed Tomography (CT)

High-resolution, thin-section computed tomography can provide detailed three-dimensional images of very thin planar sections of the skull. It is especially useful in diagnosing basilar and depressed fractures, images of which may be difficult to obtain with plain-film radiography. Evaluation by computed tomography can also suggest optimal approaches in cases requiring surgery (Lehman, 1988).[5]

----

[5] *See also* ch. 8.

Computed tomography with bone windows of the skull base has been found more effective than plain film x-rays in diagnosing and describing fractures of the petrous bone arising from trauma to the temporal area (Fritz, et al., 1989) and fractures of the clivus (the body of the sphenoid bone where it articulates with the occipital bone). Fractures of the clivus are seldom detectable by x-ray and, although they remain rare, only began to appear with some frequency in the medical literature with the advent of computed tomographic diagnosis (Joslyn, et al., 1988).

Computed tomography may also confirm basilar fractures that occur as an extension of linear fractures in the calvaria when plain x-rays reveal only the vault fracture. They may not be as effective as plain x-rays in detecting linear fractures, however, particularly those that occur in the front or back of the skull (Macpherson and Teasdale, 1989). For depressed fractures, computed tomography is very useful for revealing the number and location of in-driven bone fragments in comminuted depressed fractures (Lehman, 1988).

Computed tomography can also evaluate potential intracranial complications and damage such as air masses, fluid leaks, hematomas, subarachnoid hemorrhage and cerebral swelling (Pavlov, 1982). It may be justified to detect such sequelae even in patients who appear neurologically stable at the time of presentation. It is particularly indicated when a linear fracture crosses the middle meningeal groove, in order to detect an epidural hematoma (collection of blood around the dura, the rigid, fibrous layer surrounding the brain), the most serious complication of this type of fracture (Lehman, 1988).

6.50   TREATMENT

Management of skull fractures depends largely on the type of fracture and extent of damage at the fracture site. Unless neurologic or vascular signs require surgical access to the interior, conservative treatment is suitable for most simple fractures. The bones of the skull do not heal in the same manner as other bones; neither are they as important in providing structural support to the anatomy. Thus fractured bones in the skull usually do not require reduction, stabilization and fixation as do other bone fractures, and there is no need to approach a fracture surgically if other findings do not warrant surgery. Simple depressed fractures that require reduction for cosmetic reasons are exceptions to this rule.

Compound fractures frequently require surgical management, which, at the minimum, cleans the wound area and debrides (removes nonviable tissue) bone fragments and foreign material. The neurosurgeon may also have to relieve intracranial pressure, vacate hematomas and attend to other vascular or neural damage.

Surgical procedures on the skull include *craniectomy* (removal of part of the skull), *craniotomy* (opening a bone flap in the skull to approach the underlying dura or brain) and *cranioplasty* (surgical repair of a defect in the skull with a bone graft or transplant). Surgical management may require the combined skills of a neurosurgeon and a reconstructive surgeon (Poole and Briggs, 1989).

6.51   Simple Fractures

Patients with simple linear and basilar fractures are usually kept under observation for 24 to 48 hours. This may be the extent of treatment in the absence of further adverse signs or developments. With most basilar fractures, otorrhea and rhinorrhea stop with time and when the patient is positioned in a posture to encourage complete drainage. After 48 hours of persistent drainage, antibiotic therapy may be warranted to prevent infection; after three weeks, surgical correction may be necessary (McLaurin and McLennan, 1982).

Surgical elevation of the depressed area of the skull may be required. This is done in some cases of simple depressed fractures, usually for cosmetic reasons but sometimes to repair a dural laceration caused by the depression of the bone at the time of the fracture or by continuing pressure from the depressed bone. In young children with simple depressed fractures, in whom dural laceration is uncommon, elevation may be accomplished by a small incision at the border of the fracture site that allows access to the inner side of the depression and leverage from below to position it back to its original location. Adults usually require a more complex approach, however, which may compromise the cosmetic benefits of surgical repair and the introduce risks that are inherent in any surgery (Becker, et al., 1982).

6.52   Compound Fractures

Compound fractures require attention to the wound site in addition to evaluation of the fracture itself. In compound linear fractures, local debridement of the wound followed by wound closure without drainage is usually sufficient. Because of the risk of infection, compound depressed fractures and fractures resulting from penetrating or perforating wounds usually must be surgically debrided, irrigated and elevated. Indications for surgical management include severe wound contamination, established wound infection, ragged scalp laceration, severely comminuted fracture, the presence of brain or cerebrospinal fluid in the wound, undue bleeding from the fracture, involvement of the frontal sinus, an intracranial lesion requiring surgery and the presence of cosmetically unacceptable depressions (van den Heever and van der Merwe, 1989).

Debriding of all foreign matter is essential in managing any compound fractures caused by penetrating or perforating objects. Gross contamination of the wound and fracture sites warrants antibiotic prophylaxis after debridement and irrigation (Lehman, 1988). Penicillin is often the antibiotic of choice.

Elevation of most depressed fractures, whether they are simple or compound, requires a surgical approach that allows satisfactory viewing and access. This necessitates leaving a wide margin (2 to 3 centimeters) between the incision and the depressed area. Loose fragments should be lifted out in such a way as to avoid further lacerations or pressure on adjacent or nearby fragments. Impacted fragments should not be removed until the surgeon has a clear view of dural damage and the operating team is ready to respond to hemorrhaging. Bone removal should continue until the surgeon is sure of the state of the dura (Becker, et al., 1982). Bone fragments that are not grossly contaminated may be soaked in antibiotic and reinserted as an alternate to later cosmetic cranioplasty (Lehman, 1988).

Whenever possible, a complete watertight closure of a lacerated dura should be carried out, in order to reduce the risk of infection and protect the underlying cortex against epileptogenic effects. This may not be possible if the depression is adjacent to major vascular structures, however. If closing a dural laceration is contraindicated, the insertion of an absorbable gelatin sponge may be an alternative course. Anticonvulsant therapy may be given in the event of a laceration of the dura and contusions in an area of cortical motor function (Lehman, 1988).[6]

---

[6] *See also* ch. 8 for a complete discussion of surgical treatment of head injuries.

Some compound depressed fractures with fresh, clear-cut, uninfected and relatively uncontaminated lacerations and with large fragments that are still attached to the pericranium may be treated more conservatively. In such cases, sufficient treatment may consist of shaving and antiseptic cleaning of the wound area, sterile removal of foreign objects and loose bone fragments, suturing, treating the area with antiseptic, and dry bandaging. The patient should follow a 10–day course of antibiotics and have the wound inspected regularly. If signs of infection appear, the patient should be scheduled for imminent surgical management (van den Heeven and van der Merwe, 1989).

6.60 SEQUELAE

The sequelae associated with skull fractures can be divided into short-term and long-term complications. The former occur at the time of trauma, either as a result of or in conjunction with the skull fracture. The latter may continue for a prolonged period after the fracture and its immediate complications have been treated. It should be noted that conditions in both categories may arise as a result of head trauma in which no fracture occurs, and in some instances, sequelae are more common in patients without fractures than those with. Although no causal link between a skull fracture and the presence of sequelae necessarily exists, their occurrence in conjunction with skull fracture (or certain types of skull fracture) is nonetheless frequent enough to associate them with skull fracture.

6.61 Short-term Complications

The principal short-term complications and associated injuries seen with skull fracture include infection, post-traumatic amnesia, intracranial hematomas and brain stem injury. In addition to these most common occurrences, subarachnoid hemorrhage, venous sinus thrombosis and ischemic brain damage may also occur in patients with skull fractures.

[1] Infection

An infection resulting in meningitis is a possible complication whenever compound linear and depressed fractures occur. In one large study, intracranial infections occurred in 14 percent of the patients with compound fractures who survived the trauma for one or more days, compared with about 5 percent of those with simple fractures (Wiederholt, et al., 1989). Infection can occur in simple basilar fractures by spread from the exterior through the roof of the frontal sinus, mastoid air cells and middle ear (Bagchi, 1980). The appearance of an infection may sometimes be delayed for as long as days or weeks if cerebrospinal fluid is trapped by swollen tissue or fragments of bone (McLaurin and McLennan, 1982).

[2] Post-traumatic Amnesia

Temporary amnesia in the aftermath of head trauma is common among patients with or without skull fracture. Well over half of all skull fracture patients endure some period of either retrograde (pertaining to events preceding the injury) or anterograde (pertaining to events after the injury) amnesia (Wiederholt, et al., 1989). The duration of memory loss apparently correlates with the severity of the injury and appears to be shorter in patients without skull fracture. In one study, amnesia lasted from between one day to more than one week in nearly half of patients with a skull fracture but less than one day in 85 percent of patients without skull fracture (Cartlidge and Shaw, 1981). As day-to-day memory returns to normal, memory of the "blanked out" period is gradually restored in most patients.

[3] Intracranial Hematomas

The brain is surrounded by three meningeal (membranous) layers. These, from the outside in, are the dura mater, arachnoid and pia mater. Intracranial hematomas—consisting of epidural (or extradural), subdural and intracerebral masses of extravasated blood—are among the common complications accompanying skull fracture and are a sign of potentially fatal trauma. They are most likely to occur in patients in whom a skull fracture is accompanied by impairment of consciousness or disorientation. About 25 percent of such patients develop a hematoma, compared with just 3 percent of skull fracture patients who do not lose consciousness or become disoriented (Mendelow, et al., 1983).

Epidural hematomas are closely associated with skull fractures—some 80 to 85 percent of patients with an epidural hematoma have a skull fracture (Rivas, et al., 1989). These hematomas result from the extravasation (leakage) of blood between the skull and the dura caused by tearing of blood vessels, typically a meningeal artery but sometimes a vein or a dural sinus. As the hematoma develops, it can strip the dura from the skull, forming an ovoid mass that progressively indents the brain, resulting in brain displacement and rising intracranial pressure.

Most epidural hematomas occur in the temporal, parietal and frontal regions (Jellinger, 1983). They also occur in the posterior fossa, particularly in cases of occipital fractures (Young and Schmidek, 1982). In a small number of patients, an epidural hematoma may not appear for some hours or days after the trauma (Rivas, et al., 1988).

A subdural hematoma is a hemorrhage in the space between the dura and the arachnoid covering of the brain. The source of the hemorrhage is usually a tear in the veins that bridge the cortex and venous sinuses. Such a tear can be caused by stretching of the vein during rapid rotation or movement of the brain (Jellinger, 1983). Subdural hematomas may also be caused by intracerebral hematomas erupting into the subdural space (Young and Schmidek, 1982). Bleeding from a subdural hematoma tends to be extensive and to displace and distort the brain and brain stem. Blood in the cerebrospinal fluid often signifies a subdural hematoma.

Subdural hematoma is associated with acceleration forces, such as a severe whiplash injury. In many types of head trauma, such as those occurring in motor vehicle accidents, acceleration and impact occur together, so about half of head trauma patients with a subdural hematoma have a concomitant skull fracture. Subdural hematoma leads to death in an estimated 50 to 60 percent of cases (Jellinger, 1983).

An intracerebral hematoma can occur when direct penetration of the brain by a foreign object causes extensive bleeding. Depressed skull fractures, some of which are caused by penetrating objects, are more closely associated with intracerebral hematomas than linear or basilar fractures. In one study of patients with depressed fractures who survived more than one day, 7.5 percent had intracerebral hematomas, compared with 0.8 and 2.3 percent, respectively, of patients with linear and basilar fractures (Wiederholt, et al., 1989). Like epidural hematomas, intracerebral hematomas may make a delayed appearance in some patients (Zimmerman and Bilaniuk, 1983).

[4] Brain Stem Injury

Brain stem injury is fairly common in fatal head trauma involving any kind of simple skull fracture. It occurs in about a quarter to a third of such cases. However, in one study, it was much more common in cases of basilar fractures than other fractures, occurring in 13.8 percent compared with 2.4 percent of linear fractures, 2.2 percent of depressed fractures and 7.1 percent of compound fractures (Wiederholt, et al., 1989). In another study of 42 accident fatalities involving pontomedullary tearing (separation of the pons from the medulla) and other brain stem injury, basilar fractures were the only type of fracture that occurred, appearing in 28 cases (Simpson, et al., 1989). Brain stem injury, when it is not fatal, may be associated with long-term disabilities such as motor impairment, defects in memory, and emotional and psychosocial sequelae (Thomsen, 1984.)

6.62 Long-term Complications

Complications that commonly occur in long-term survivors of head trauma involving skull fracture include headache, dizziness, seizures, cranial nerve damage and "growing" fracture.

[1] Headache

Headache is not a particularly meaningful symptom of skull fracture in the immediate aftermath of head trauma, as similar percentages (35 to 40 percent) of head trauma victims experience headaches whether a skull fracture is present or not. Patients with skull fracture are more likely to continue to have headaches over a prolonged period, however. In one study, three quarters of skull fracture patients with headaches in the immediate aftermath of the trauma continued to experience headache two years later, compared with about half the patients in a nonfracture group who had headaches for the same period (Cartlidge and Shaw, 1981).

[2] Dizziness

Dizziness is also cited as a long-term consequence of skull fracture. Although 15 to 20 percent of head trauma victims in one study experienced short-term dizziness irrespective of skull fracture, the percentage of those experiencing dizziness declined over time for those without skull fracture and increased slightly for those with (Cartlidge and Shaw, 1981). Dizziness or vertigo (sensation of whirling in space) is a symptom of possible damage in the nerves of the ear (Boles, 1982).

[3] Seizures (Post-traumatic Epilepsy)

Seizures, or post-traumatic epilepsy, are most associated with depressed fractures, probably because penetrating injuries are most likely to provoke them. Factors that increase the likelihood of developing post-traumatic epilepsy include penetration of the dura, injury in the parietal area as opposed to other areas and prolonged unconsciousness at the time of penetrating head trauma. Patients who do not experience seizures in the short-term postinjury period are unlikely to later, while close to half of those who do have seizures shortly after injury will remain at risk of having occasional seizures for years to come (Cartlidge and Shaw, 1981). According to a study of penetrating head injuries in veterans, this risk is associated with a shortened life span (Corkin, et al., 1984).

[4]   Cranial Nerve Damage

Cranial nerve damage is particularly associated with basilar fractures. The damage occurs where the nerves exit through the basilar foramina. Fractures of the cribriform plate (ethmoid bone) are likely to result in injury to the olfactory nerves, possibly resulting in anosmia (loss of the sense of smell). Fractures of the sphenoid bone may injure the cranial nerves passing through the cavernous sinus, namely nerves III, IV and VI affecting eye movement and trigeminal (V) nerve branches that give sensation to the face. Fractures of the temporal bone involving the petrous pyramid nearly always result in some hearing impairment, as do occipital fractures that extend to the petrous bone. In 10 percent of petrous bone fractures, dislocation of the ossicular chain produces a surgically correctable form of deafness. Deafness may also occur as a result of damage to cranial nerve VIII if the fracture extends through the internal auditory canal, cochlea and vestibular areas (inner ear structures that are essential for hearing) (Zimmerman and Bilaniuk, 1983). Nerve damage in the area of the ear may also cause tinnitus (ringing in the ears), dizziness and vertigo (Boles, 1982). As the facial nerve crosses the petrous bone, this may also be damaged by a fracture there, resulting in facial palsy.

[5]   Growing Fracture

Growing skull fracture (cephalohydrocele) refers to a condition in which a linear skull fracture progressively enlarges in width instead of healing. It is an uncommon delayed complication of skull fracture in infants and young children. In this group, the dura is more firmly attached to the skull than in adults and is more readily torn when the skull breaks.

The development of a growing fracture depends on the presence of a torn dura, local hemorrhage and interposition of tissue of the dura and arachnoid between the edges of the fracture. A cyst may eventually form that prevents the fracture from healing and allows it to enlarge (Jellinger, 1983). Growing fractures develop most frequently in the frontal and parietal regions. They may appear radiographically within eight weeks of the original fracture, but in some cases, months or years pass before they are evident (Zimmerman and Bilaniuk, 1983).

6.70 PROGNOSIS

The prognosis for patients with skull fracture is dependent on them surviving the immediate trauma and its aftermath and the extent of accompanying brain injury. In one large study, 91 percent of patients who survived the initial trauma for one day were alive 10 years later. Nearly 30 percent of patients with skull fracture died within one day of the trauma, however, compared with 2 percent of trauma victims without skull fracture (Wiederholt, et al., 1989). Thus skull fracture is an indicator of the existence of brain injury that is potentially severe enough to result in early death.

Patients whose fractures involve a subdural hematoma, intracerebral hematoma or brain stem injury—respectively associated with compound fractures, depressed or penetrating fractures and basilar fractures—generally have a less favorable outlook than those who incur an epidural hematoma. When the fracture is associated with epidural hematoma and after prompt surgical intervention, many patients can expect a good recovery, with only minor if any disability (Bergman, et al., 1987).

Patients with simple linear fractures have the best prognosis, as these are the least likely to be accompanied by life-threatening injuries. Although such injuries point to an impact of considerable force, many patients suffering this trauma show no evidence of brain damage and make an uneventful recovery.

6.100 BIBLIOGRAPHY

Text References

Adams, J. H., et al.: Diffuse Axonal Injury in Head Injuries Caused by a Fall. Lancet 8417(18):1420–1422, Dec. 22/29, 1984.

Bagchi A. K.: An Introduction to Head Injuries. Calcutta: Oxford University Press, 1980.

Becker, D. P., et al.: Diagnosis and Treatment of Head Injury in Adults. In: Youmans, J. R. (Ed.): Neurological Surgery, Vol. 4, 2nd ed. Philadelphia: Saunders, 1982.

Bergman, T. A., et al.: Outcome of Severe Closed Head Injury in the Midwest: A Review and Comparison With Other Major Head Trauma Studies. Minn. Med. 70:397–401, July 1987.

Boles, R.: Facial, Auditory, and Vestibular Nerve Injuries Associated With Basilar Skull Fractures. In: Youmans, J. R. (Ed.): Neurological Surgery, Vol. 4, 2nd ed. Philadelphia: Saunders, 1982.

Braakman, R. and Jennett, B.: Depressed Skull Fracture (Non-missile). In: Vinken, P. J. and Bruyn, G. W. (Eds.): Injuries of the Brain and Skull, Part I. Amsterdam: North-Holland Publishing Company, 1975.

Cartlidge, N. E. F. and Shaw, D. A.: Head Injury. London: Saunders, 1981.

Clarke, J. A. and Adams, J. E.: The Application of Clinical Guidelines for Skull Radiography in the Accident and Emergency Department: Theory and Practice. Clin. Radiol. 41:152–155, Mar. 1990.

Cooper, P. R. and Ho, V.: Role of Emergency Skull X-ray Films in the Evaluation of the Head-Injured Patient: A Retrospective Study. Neurosurgery 13:136–140, Aug. 1983.

Cooter, R. D., et al.: Helmet-Induced Skull Base Fracture in a Motorcyclist. Lancet 8577:84–85, Jan. 16, 1988.

Corkin, S., et al.: Prognostic Factors for Life Expectancy After Penetrating Head Injury. Arch. Neurol. 41:975–977, Sept. 1984.

DeLuca, S. A. and Rhea, J. T.: Skull Fractures. Am. Fam. Phys. 28:125–126, Sept. 1983.

Fritz, P., et al.: Radiological Evaluation of Temporal Bone Disease: High-Resolution Computed Tomography Versus Conventional X-Ray Diagnosis. Brit J. Radiol. 62:107–113, Feb. 1989.

Gennarelli, T. A.: Head Injury Mechanisms. In: Torg, J. S. (Ed.): Athletic Injuries to the Head, Neck, and Face. Philadelphia: Lea & Febiger, 1982.

Hayward, R. H.: Management of Acute Head Injuries. Oxford: Blackwell Scientific Publications, 1980.

Jellinger, K.: The Neuropathology of Pediatric Head Injuries. In: Shapiro, K. (Ed.): Pediatric Head Trauma. Mount Kisco, N.Y.: Futura Publishing Company, 1983.

Joslyn, J. N., et al.: Complex Fractures of the Clivus: Diagnosis With CT and Clinical Outcome in 11 Patients. Radiology 166:817–821, Mar. 1988.

Krantz, K. P. G.: Head and Neck Injuries to Motorcycle and Moped Riders—With Special Regard to the Effect of Protective Helmets. Injury 16:253–258, Jan. 1985.

Lehman, L. B.: Skull Fractures: Dispelling Some Misconceptions Affecting Management. Postgrad. Med. 83:53–63, Feb. 15, 1988.

Macpherson, P. and Teasdale, E.: Can Computed Tomography Be Relied Upon to Detect Skull Fractures? Clin. Radiol. 40:22–24, Jan. 1989.

Masters, S. J.: Evaluation of Head Trauma: Efficacy of Skull Films. A.J.R. Am. J. Roentgenol. 135:539–547, Sept. 1980.

Masters, S. J., et al.: Skull X-ray Examinations After Head Trauma: Recommendations by a Multidisciplinary Panel and Validation Study. N. Engl. J. Med. 316:84–91, Jan. 8, 1987.

McClean, P. M., et al.: Skull Film Radiography in the Management of Head Trauma. Ann. Emerg. Med. 13:607–611, Aug. 1984.

McLaurin, R. L. and McLennan, J. E.: Diagnosis and Treatment of Head Injury in Children. In: Youmans, J. R. (Ed.): Neurological Surgery, Vol. 4, 2nd ed. Philadelphia: Saunders, 1982.

Mendelow, A. D., et al.: Risks of Intracranial Haematoma in Head Injured Adults. Brit. Med. J. 287:1173–1176, Oct. 22, 1983.

Moses, H.: Trauma to the Head and Neck. In: Harvey, I. and McGhee, A. (Eds.): The Principles and Practice of Medicine. Norwalk, Conn.: Appleton-Century-Crofts, 1984.

Nelson, E. L., et al.: Incidence of Skull Fractures in Olmsted County, Minnesota. Neurosurg. 15:318–324, Sept. 1984.

Pavlov, H.: Radiographic Evaluation of the Head and Facial Bones. In: Torg, J. S. (Ed.): Athletic Injuries to the Head, Neck, and Face. Philadelphia: Lea & Febiger, 1982.

Poole, M. D. and Briggs, M.: Cranio-Orbital Trauma: A Team Approach to Management. Ann. Roy. Coll. Surg. 71:187–194, May 1989.

Rivas, J. J., et al.: Extradural Hematoma: Analysis of Factors Influencing Courses of 161 Patients. Neurosurg. 23:44–51, July 1988.

Rosenthal, B. W. and Bergman, I.: Intracranial Injury After Moderate Head Trauma in Children. J. Pediatr. 115:346–350, Sept. 1989.

Simpson, D. A., et al.: Pontomedullary Tears and Other Gross Brainstem Injuries After Vehicular Accidents. J. Trauma 29:1519–1525, Nov. 1989.

Thomas, L. M.: Skull Fractures. In: Wilkins, R. H. and Rengachary, S. S. (Eds.): Neurological Surgery. New York: McGraw-Hill, 1985.

Thomsen, I. V.: Late Outcome of Very Severe Blunt Head Trauma: A 10–15 Year Second Follow-Up. J. Neurolog. Neurosurg. Psychiatry 47:260–268, Mar. 1984.

Thornbury, J. R., et al.: Skull Fracture and the Low Risk of Intracranial Sequelae in Minor Head Trauma. A.J.R. Am. J. Roentgenol. 143:661–664, Sept. 1984.

Tunturi, T., et al.: Head Injuries and Skull Radiography: Clinical Factors Predicting a Fracture. Injury 13:478–483, May 1982.

Unger, J. M., et al.: Sphenoid Fractures: Prevalence, Sites, and Significance. Radiology 175:175–180, Apr. 1990.

van den Heever, C. M. and van der Merwe, D. J.: Management of Depressed Skull Fractures: Selective Conservative Management of Non-Missile Injuries. J. Neurosurg. 71:186–190, Aug. 1989.

Wiederholt, W. C., et al.: Short-Term Outcomes of Skull Fracture: A Population-Based Study of Survival and Neurologic Complications. Neurology 38: 96–102, Jan. 1989.

Young, H. A. and Schmidek, H. H.: Complications Accompanying Occipital Skull Fractures. J. Trauma 22:914–920, Nov. 1982.

Zimmerman, R. A. and Bilaniuk, L. T.: Radiology of Pediatric Craniocerebral Trauma. In: Shapiro, K. (Ed.): Pediatric Head Trauma. Mount Kisco, N. Y.: Futura Publishing, 1983.

CHAPTER 7

Brain Tumors (Malignant and Nonmalignant)

SCOPE

Brain tumors are among the most lethal and difficult-to-treat tumors. Because their growth within the confined space of the cranium leads to compression of brain structures and increased intracranial pressure, they can produce damage and clinical symptoms even when they are not malignant. Even when they are benign according to cellular type, they have a high morbidity and mortality unless they are treated. Because tumors can arise from any one of the varied specialized structures of the nervous system, identification and classification can be difficult. Diagnosis has been advanced by the development of highly sensitive imaging techniques, in particular, magnetic resonance imaging. These imaging techniques are also used in conjunction with stereotactic methods to permit more accurate biopsies, more precise radiotherapy and improved precision of surgical resection. Nevertheless, surgical excision continues to effect a cure in only a small proportion of cases. Even with apparently complete tumor removal followed by radiation therapy, the rate of recurrence is high. Current treatments also have a high incidence of severe adverse short-term and long-term effects.

SYNOPSIS

7.00　INTRODUCTION: EPIDEMIOLOGY AND DISTINCTIONS

Brain tumors are the second most common cause of death from intracranial (within the skull) disease, surpassed only by stroke (Greenberg and Polachini, 1995). In 1995, about 13,300 persons in the United States died from primary nervous system tumors, of which about 95 percent were in the brain (Preston-Martin, 1996). The prevalence in the United States population is about 1 to 2 percent (Harsh, 1994). Each year in the United States, about 35,000 new intracranial neoplasms (tumors) are diagnosed, for an incidence of about 16.5 per 100,000. Of these, slightly fewer than half are primary (originating within the brain), with the rest being metastases (secondary tumors arising from other sites).

Unlike tumors elsewhere in the body, a tumor in the brain can be considered life-threatening whether or not it consists of cancerous cells. A tumor composed of benign cells that occupy or impinge on a vital area is still a serious problem. A benign brain tumor has distinct boundaries, may be located in a vital or nonvital area and consists of benign, noncancerous cells. It may be curable by surgery alone. Because benign tumors as well as malignant ones tend to grow, most eventually reach a stage that they impinge on vital structures and cause neurologic symptoms.

Primary intracranial neoplasms may arise from the meninges (membranes covering the brain and spinal cord) or parenchyma (specific organ cells, supported by the connective tissue framework) of the brain. An intra-axial tumor is found mainly within the parenchyma or ventricular system (series of cavities that carry cerebrospinal fluid), and an extra-axial tumor is located in the meninges or subarachnoid space (between the outer arachnoid membrane covering the brain and spinal cord and the inner pia mater membrane).

7.01　Incidence, Prevalence and Distribution of Brain Tumors

The incidence of brain tumors increases with age from about 2 per 100,000 among individuals at age 10 to 20 per 100,000 among those at age 70 (Harsh, 1994). The incidence then decreases somewhat.

Tumors of the central nervous system (CNS; the brain and spinal cord) constitute 1 to 2 percent of all adult malignancies but 20 percent of childhood malignancies (Wisoff, 1994). Brain tumors are the second most common type of cancer in children, after leukemia, and the largest group of solid neoplasms in young people (Pollack, 1994; Wisoff, 1994). They are the third leading cause of death in children under the age of 16 years. About 1,500 to 2,000 children are diagnosed with brain tumors each year in the United States. The incidence of central nervous system tumors appears to be increasing, from about 2.4 new cases per 100,000 in 1973 to 3.3 per 100,000 in 1986 (Rorke, 1994; Wisoff, 1994).

The most common primary brain tumors in adults are gliomas (tumors composed of or derived from the less differentiated, more primitive supporting cells than the more specialized neurons)[1] and meningiomas (tumors that arise from the arachnoid cells on the inner surface of the dura mater, the outermost of the meninges surrounding the brain and spinal cord).[2] The incidence of gliomas, which comprise 45 to 60 percent of primary brain tumors, follows the pattern found for brain tumors as a group. Glioblastomas[3] show a sharp rise in incidence with increasing age. Other specific tumor types differ in age-based incidence (Harsh, 1994). Meningiomas, for example, comprise 15 to 20 percent of adult brain tumors but are rare in children.

Most tumors in adults arise in or near the cerebral hemispheres. In children over a year old, on the other hand, nearly 50 percent of tumors are infratentorial (below the membrane separating the cerebral hemispheres from the cerebellum and other structures) (Rorke, 1994). *(See Figure 7-1.)* Common tumors in children are medulloblastomas[4] (a type of glioma) and low-grade astrocytomas[5] (a type of glioma); the most common in children are astrocytomas. Cerebellar astrocytoma, optic glioma and brain stem glioma occur almost exclusively in children (Abbott, et al., 1994; O'Brien and Krisht, 1994). Tumors involving the optic nerve and optic chiasm comprise about 4 percent of pediatric brain tumors; even when these are treated successfully, vision deficits often result (Johnson and McCullough, 1994).

The incidence and mortality from primary brain tumors are higher for males than for females (Preston-Martin, 1996). They are also

---

[1] *See* 7.61 *infra.*

[2] *See* 7.62 *infra.*

[3] *See* 7.61[2] *infra.*

[4] *See* 7.61[6] *infra.*

[5] *See* 7.61[1] *infra.*

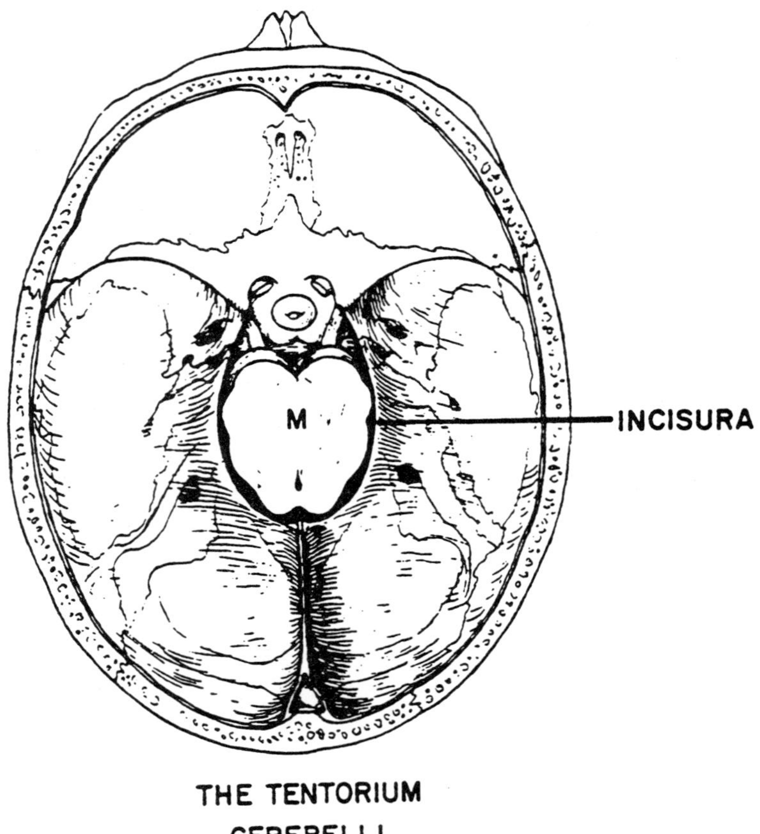

Figure. 7-1. The tentorium is a tough, fibrous membrane that separates the upper cerebral hemispheres from the structures in the posterior fossa below. It lies in a roughly horizontal plane, attached at its sides and behind to the bones of the base of the skull. M = midbrain (mesencephalon) in cross section.

higher for whites than for blacks. However, ratios vary for different types of tumor. Cerebellar medulloblastomas and glioblastoma multiforme are more common in males; meningiomas and schwannomas occur more frequently in females. Meningiomas and pituitary adenomas[6] are more common in blacks than in whites. The incidence of most types of primary brain tumors rises with increasing socioeconomic level, particularly among men. (Because the trend differs between men and women, this rising incidence is not thought to be due to better diagnosis.)

---

[6] *See* 7.70 *infra.*

7.02 Mortality

Brain tumors have a high mortality. Even with aggressive, multimodal treatment, only about half of patients diagnosed in the United States with primary brain tumor are alive one year after diagnosis (Preston-Martin, 1996). Survival time is dependent on the individual's age and functional state at diagnosis, as well as on the type and extent of the tumor (Harsh, 1994).

7.03 Etiology

Although they are matters of controversy, statistics gathered since the 1970s indicate a steadily increasing incidence of central nervous system (CNS) malignancies, particularly among the elderly (Preston-Martin, 1996). Thus age is a determinant for the development of brain tumors, with the incidence different tumors peaking at different ages.

The actual cause of brain tumors is not understood, however. Studies have identified some of the genetic alterations leading to tumor development, and three factors have been implicated as possible mutagens (agents that induce permanent changes in a cell's building blocks, known as deoxyribonucleic acid, or DNA). These are radiation, chemical agents and viruses (Harsh, 1994). Heredity is also considered to play a role.

[1] Radiation

Ionizing radiation, as found in diagnostic and therapeutic x-rays and particle irradiation, is an established risk factor for brain tumor development (Harsh, 1994). An increased incidence of nerve sheath tumors, meningiomas and malignant gliomas has been seen among persons who were treated with radiation for childhood tumors (Preston-Martin, 1996; Starshak, 1996).[7] The criteria for regarding a second tumor as radiation-induced are (Halperin and Anscher, 1994):

- occurrence in the irradiated region;

- different histologic type of the second tumor from the original tumor; and

- interval of four or more years since the completion of irradiation.

---

[7] *See* 7.54[6] *infra.*

Other forms of irradiation that have been implicated in tumorigenesis are scalp irradiation for tinea capitis (ringworm), which is no longer done, and dental x-rays. Prenatal exposure to pelvic radiation has also been implicated as a cause of primary pediatric brain tumors.

[2]　Chemical Mutagens

A variety of industrial organic chemicals have been implicated in the generation of brain tumors, but study results have been conflicting (Preston-Martin, 1996). Suspected chemicals include organic chlorides, which are used as pesticides; nitroso compounds, used in the rubber industry; and various petrochemicals.

[3]　Viruses

Although animal studies show that certain viruses can induce brain tumors, the role of viruses in human tumor etiology has not been substantiated in epidemiologic studies (Harsh, 1994).

[4]　Brain Injury

Anecdotal evidence and evidence from animal studies indicate that brain trauma, for example, contusions, gunshot wounds and incisions, can lead to tumor formation, but firmer epidemiologic evidence is needed (Harsh, 1994). Evidence for a possible association with head trauma is strongest for meningiomas (Preston-Martin, 1996). Some observations indicate an increased risk for development of acoustic neuroma, a nerve sheath tumor of the acoustic nerve, with exposure to extremely loud noise over several years. There also seems to be an association between brain tumor formation and multiple sclerosis.

[5]　Heredity

Patterns of hereditary predisposition to brain tumor development seem rare (Harsh, 1994). Usually an increased incidence within a family is due to one of the phakomatoses, a group of hereditary quasi-neoplastic diseases involving the skin, nervous system and sometimes other organs (Preston-Martin, 1996). These diseases include neurofibromatosis, tuberous sclerosis and von Hippel-Lindau disease.

7.10　ANATOMY OF THE BRAIN

All discussions of tumors of the brain refer to its structures, both macroscopic and cellular. The brain consists of several structures, each of which is connected and integrated with the others, both anatomically and functionally (Westmoreland, et al., 1994). These structures vary in their cellular composition and thus in the type of tumor that may occur in them.

7.11 Divisions of the Brain

The brain is divided by the tentorium cerebelli, one of the fibrous membranes called meninges, into the supratentorial and infratentorial levels (Westmoreland, et al., 1994). The supratentorial level, above the tentorium, consists of the cerebral hemispheres, basal ganglia, thalamus, hypothalamus and olfactory and optic nerves. The infratentorial, or posterior fossa, level consists of the brain stem and the cerebellum.

Each cerebral hemisphere is divided by fissures into four major lobes: frontal, parietal, temporal and occipital. *(See Figure 7-2.)* Specific areas of each lobe have been determined (mapped) to specific functions, such as speech, hearing, sight and memory. The two hemispheres are connected by the corpus callosum, a tract of nerve fibers that transfers information between them. Other important supratentorial structures are the thalamus, which acts as an integration center for sensory input and motor and cognitive output; the hypothalamus, which regulates endocrine function, body temperature, sleep, food intake and other visceral functions; the basal ganglia, which modulates motor activity; and the pineal and pituitary glands. *(See Figure 7-3.)*

The outer layer of the cerebral hemisphere is gray matter, composed of neuronal cell bodies and their dendritic processes (extensions of nerve cells that transmit impulses to them) and is called the cortex. White matter, lying beneath, is composed of nerve fibers, many of which are covered or sheathed with a white substance known as myelin. Subcortical structures include other white matter and the basal ganglia.

The cerebellum, the largest structure in the posterior fossa, is composed of two lobes or hemispheres, with a midline structure called the vermis. *(See Figure 7-4.)* It plays a primary role in the integration and modulation of motor activity, particularly posture, gait, equilibrium and voluntary movements.

The brain stem, in the posterior fossa level, consists of the pons, medulla oblongata and midbrain. It is continuous with the spinal cord

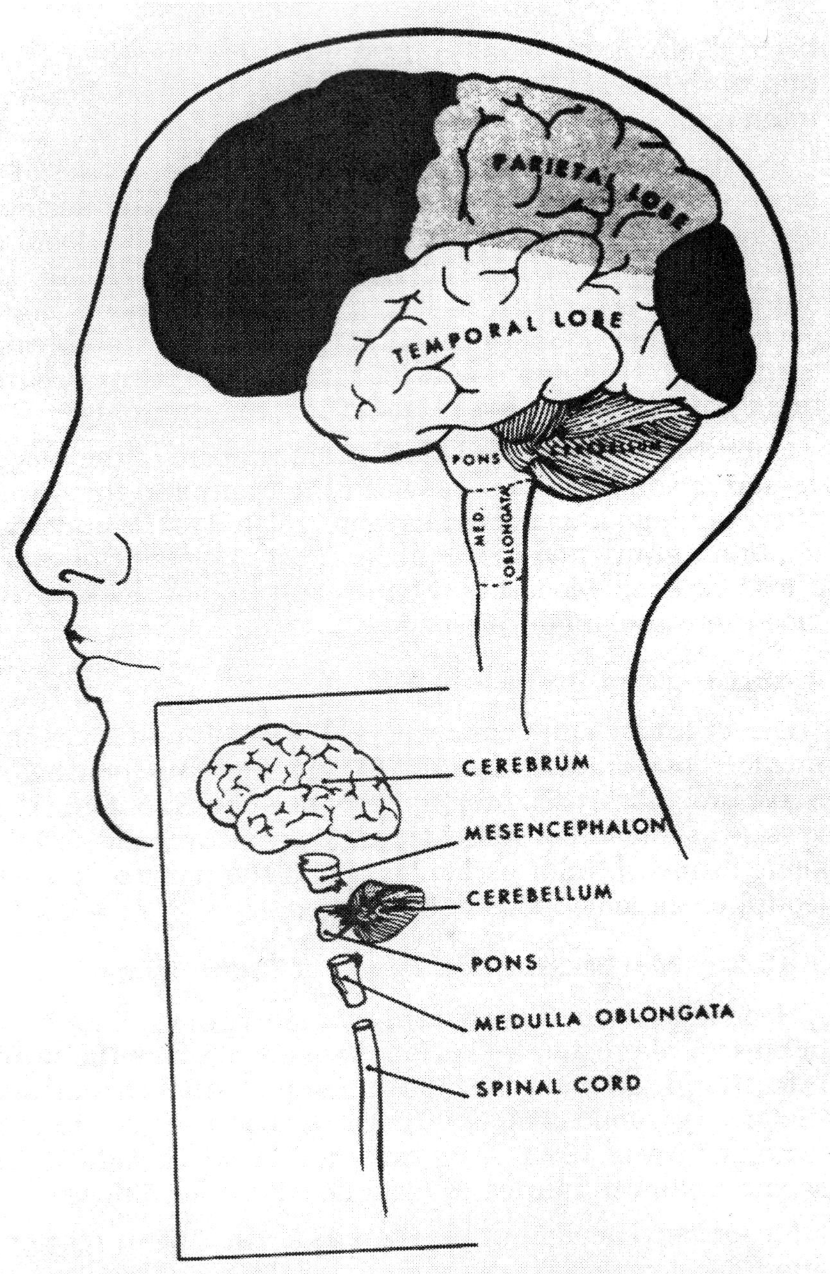

Figure 7-2. The brain and spinal cord. The front shaded portion is the frontal lobe, and the rear shaded portion is the occipital lobe. The pons and medulla oblongata are part of the brain stem. The mesencephalon is the midbrain.

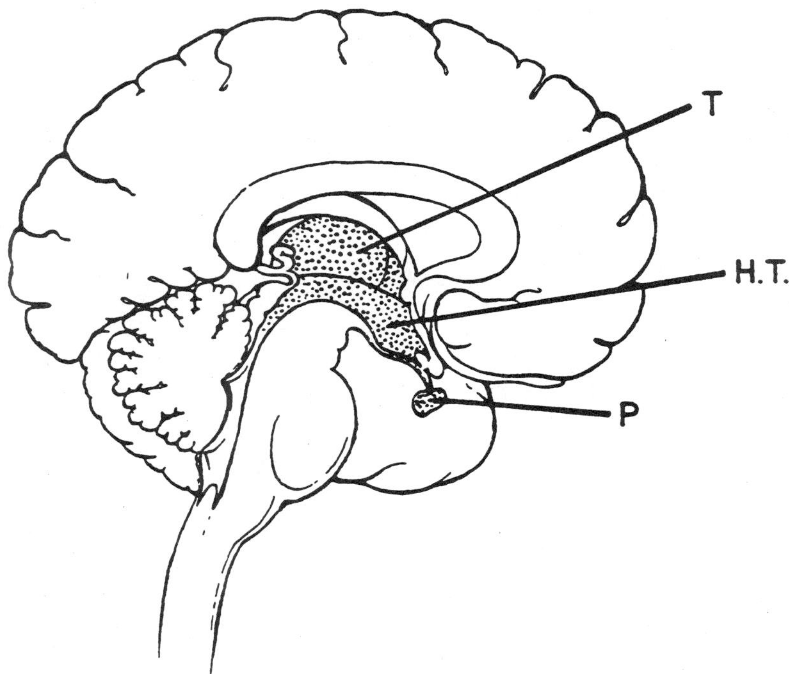

Figure 7-3. The position of the thalamus (T) in relation to other brain structures: the hypothalamus (HT) and pituitary gland (P).

at the foramen magnum (the opening of the skull through which the spinal cord enters to meet the brain). The brain stem structures are responsible for the integration and control of visceral functions. Serious damage to this area results in death. Cranial nerves III though XII exit from the brain stem.

The brain ventricles (several small cavities within the brain) contain choroid plexus, which secretes and absorbs the cerebrospinal fluid (CSF). *(See Figure 7-5.)* This fluid is circulated throughout the ventricles.

The entire central nervous system is covered by a system of membranes called meninges. *(See Figure 7-6.)* The outermost layer is the dura mater. Below it is the arachnoid, and the innermost layer is the pia mater.

7.12　Cranial Nerves

The twelve cranial nerves provide the pathways for central control of visceral functions. *(See Figure 7-7.)* In order from I to XII, their

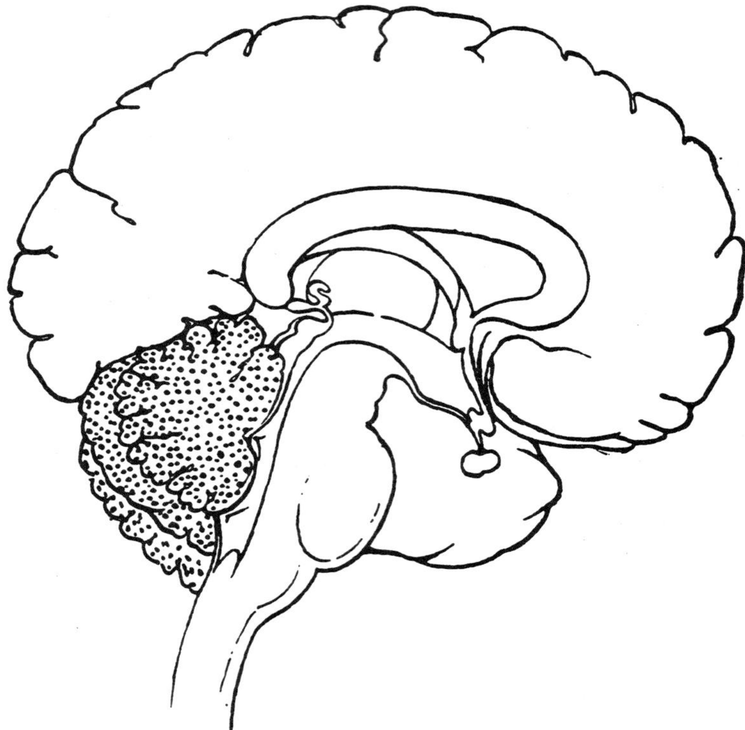

Figure 7-4. The cerebellum (shaded area) lies below the occipital lobe of the hemisphere and behind the midbrain and brain stem.

areas of control are as follows: olfactory (smell), optic (vision), oculomotor (eye movement), trochlear (eye movement), trigeminal (facial sensation), abducens (eye movement), facial (facial movement), cochlear-vestibular (hearing and balance), glossopharyngeal (throat movement), vagus (throat and larynx movement; control of visceral organs), spinal accessory (shoulder and neck movement), and hypo-glossal (tongue movement).

7.13   Cellular Architecture

The nervous system is composed of several kinds of highly special-ized cells with specific functions. Neurons, or nerve cells, are the basic functional unit of the nervous system. They receive, integrate and transmit electrical or chemical impulses. Most neurons have a single axon and one or more other processes, called dendrites. *(See Figure*

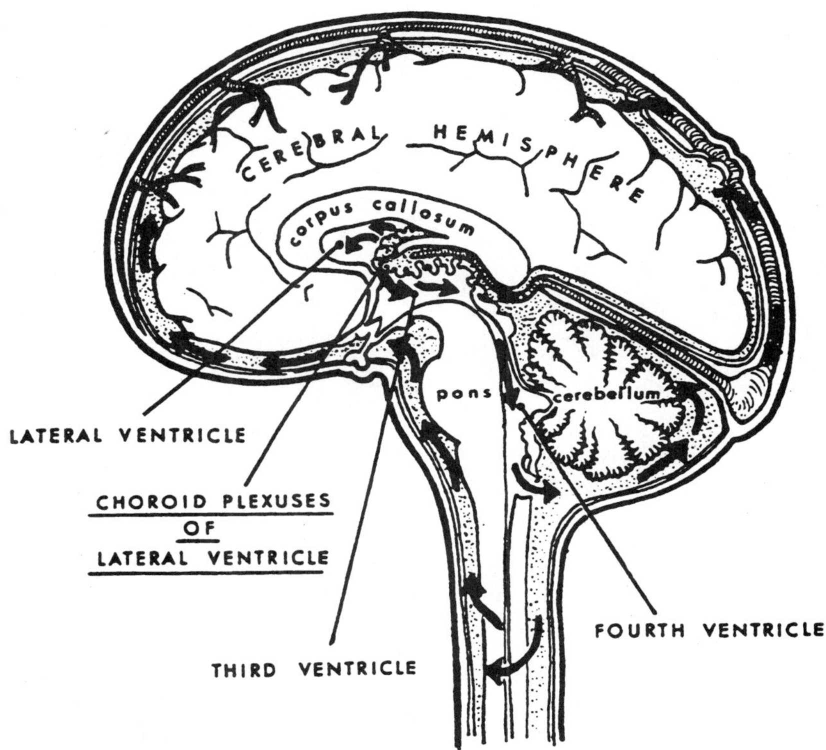

Figure 7-5. The ventricles of the brain contain choroid plexus, which, through its secretion and absorption of cerebrospinal fluid—a colorless liquid contained in the subarachnoid space that surrounds all the cavities in and about the brain and spinal cord—regulates intraventricular pressure. Arrows show the direction of circulation of CSF.

7-8.) Many axons are covered with a white insulating layer called myelin, which plays an important role in the conduction of electric impulses. Support cells include oligodendroglia, which form the myelin; astrocytes, which may function in the transport of molecules between the capillaries (small blood vessels) and the neurons; and ependymal cells, which line the ventricular system. These support cells and the neurons are derived embryologically from neuroepithelial cells. The connective tissue cells, such as those comprising the meninges, derive not from neuroepithelium but from embryonic mesoderm.

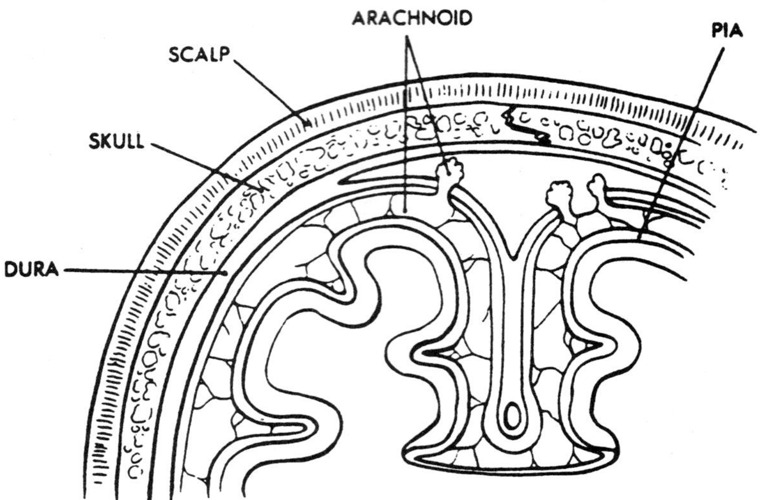

Figure 7-6. The coverings of the brain, from the outermost to the innermost: the scalp, skull, dura mater, arachnoid and pia mater.

7.20   BRAIN TUMOR CLASSIFICATION, GRADING AND PROGNOSIS

The classification, malignancy grade and biochemical/molecular characteristics of a brain tumor are important in determining therapy and prognosis (Harsh, 1994). Tumors are classified and graded at biopsy or removal, based on the cellular appearance under the light microscope. The correlation between appearance as seen in computed tomography (CT) or magnetic resonance imaging (MRI) and gross and microscopic pathology is helpful in making later diagnoses on the basis of the images.[8] Newer methods of grading look at molecular indices of malignancy, using biochemical, immunohistochemical or genetic markers.[9]

The prognosis varies greatly with tumor type. Some tumors, including meningiomas and pilocytic astrocytomas, are curable with surgical resection.[10] Others, such as glioblastoma multiforme, have a mean survival of a year or less, even with aggressive treatment.

---

[8] *See also* 7.43 *infra.*

[9] *See also* 7.22[2] *infra.*

[10] *See also* 7.51 *infra.*

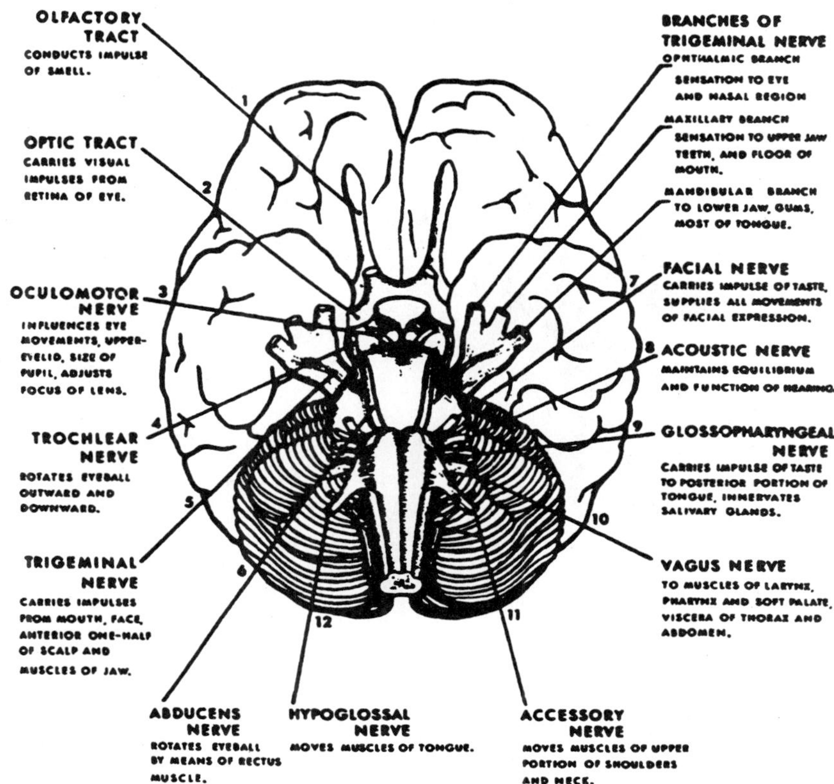

Figure 7-7. The cranial nerves are numbered I through XII.

Factors in a favorable prognosis include a patient of young age and good health and functional status at diagnosis, and near-total removal of the tumor (McDonald and Rosenblum, 1994). Survival-extending treatment adjuncts to surgery include targeted methods of radiation therapy, such as interstitial brachytherapy, and chemotherapy.[11]

7.21   Classification of Brain Tumors

Brain tumors may be classified on the basis of location, aggressiveness (tendency to spread malignantly) and cell type. The most commonly used approach—classification by cell morphology—is based on the premise that each tumor stems from a single cell type (Harsh, 1994). Such systems rely on histologic (referring to microscopic anatomy) patterns seen at the light microscope level and, more

---

[11] *See* 7.54[2] and 7.55 *infra,* respectively.

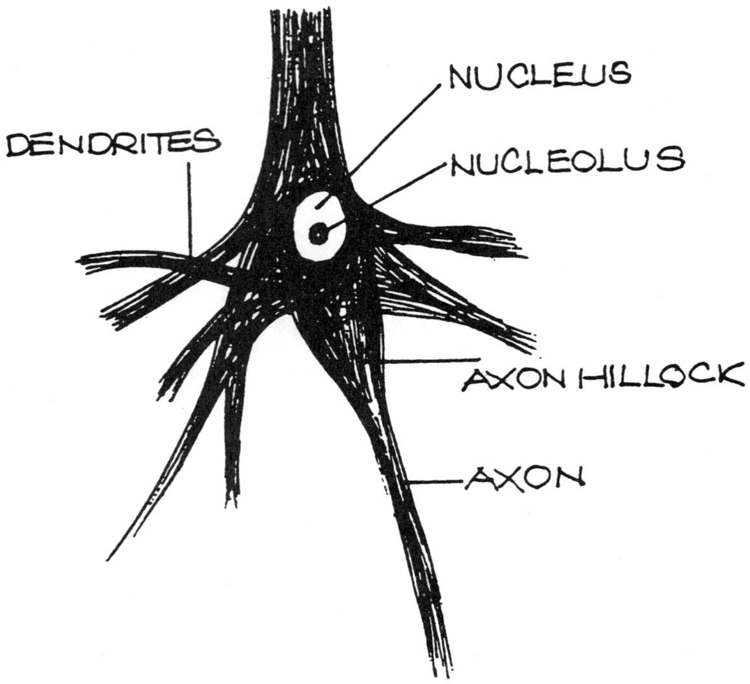

Figure 7-8. A neuron (nerve cell) has a single axon, which carries impulses away from the nerve to the brain, and a number of dendrites, which carry impulses to the nerve cell.

recently, on immunohistochemical analysis that uses antibody markers for specific cell types (Burger and Fuller, 1991). The microscopic approach works best with tumors composed of a high percentage of differentiated cells, which may be compared and correlated to the normal cells of the tissue from which they stemmed (Rorke, 1994).

Such systems do not allow, however, for mixed tumors composed of more than one cell type or for those with a major cell type that appears unrelated to normal adult cells. An additional problem is that classification systems for adult tumors are inadequate for pediatric tumors (Burger and Fuller, 1991).

[1] Tumor Classification by Tissue Type (Histologic)

Among several classification schemes for grouping brain tumors, the most widely used is the WHO (World Health Organization) system (Harsh, 1994). (*See Table 7-1.*) This system distinguishes tumors by principal cell type and by degree of anaplasia (loss of structural differentiation, as occurs in the development of malignant characteristics) within a cell type (McDonald and Rosenblum, 1994). It is based on tumor histogenesis (the type of tissue from which the tumor arises).

Table 7-1

WHO Histologic Classification of Tumors of the Nervous System

---

I.	Tumors of Neuroepithelial Tissue
	A. Astrocytic tumors (gliomas derived from astrocytes; includes astrocytomas of all malignancy grades)
	B. Oligodendroglial tumors
	C. Ependymal and choroid plexus tumors
	D. Pineal cell tumors
	E. Neuronal tumors (includes gangliocytomas and neuroblastomas)
	F. Poorly differentiated and embryonal tumors (includes glioblastomas and medulloblastomas)
II.	Tumors of Nerve Sheath Cells
III.	Tumors of the Meninges and Related Tissues (includes meningiomas)
IV.	Primary Malignant Lymphomas
V.	Tumors of Blood Vessel Origin
VI.	Germ Cell Tumors (includes germinomas, embryonal carcinomas, choriocarcinomas)
VII.	Other Malformative Tumors and Tumorlike Lesions (includes craniopharyngiomas)
VIII.	Vascular Malformations
IX.	Tumors of the Anterior Pituitary (includes pituitary adenomas)
X.	Local Extensions from Regional Tumors
XI.	Metastatic Tumors
XII.	Unclassified Tumors

---

[2] Tumor Classification by Site

Tumor subsites used in official diagnostic classifications of tumors of the central nervous system are the brain, cranial nerve, cerebral meninges, spinal cord and spinal meninges (Preston-Martin, 1996). Descriptions of tumors further specify anatomic sites by familiar names, such as cerebellar. Thus a tumor may be named as a cerebellar astrocytoma.

7.22   Tumor Grading

As with other types of cancer, brain tumors are graded according to the degree of tissue anaplasia (loss of structural differentiation), which generally corresponds with malignant behavior (Harsh, 1994). Cellular characteristics of rapidly growing malignant tumors of the central nervous system include an increased number of cells, many with features indicating uncontrolled multiplication and lack of differentiation. The tumors seldom metastasize (spread to another part of the body), but they do invade and destroy surrounding tissue.

Grading systems assign a low grade, such as grade I, to benign tumors with relatively well differentiated cells, and a high grade, such as grade IV, to rapidly growing malignant tumors with poorly differentiated cells (McDonald and Rosenblum, 1994). Benign tumors grow slowly and do not infiltrate nearby tissue. They tend to be well defined and to be surgically resectable (removable). Malignant tumors tend to infiltrate surrounding structures and to be difficult, if not impossible, to remove.

The value of grading schemes depends on the type of tumor (Harsh, 1994). For some types of tumors, such as astrocytomas, the cellular appearance has strong prognostic value, and grading is important in decision making. For others, such as ependymomas, the grading has little utility for prognosis.

[1]   Cytologic Grading

Cytologic grading looks at the cellular characteristics of a tumor, such as the number of mitotic figures (components that indicate cells are undergoing division), variability in cell size and shape, lack of cytoplasmic differentiation (presence of cell-type-specific characteristics in the area surrounding the nucleus) and nuclei with varying shapes. Other important variables are the extent of invasion into nearby tissue, growth of blood vessels and tissue necrosis (death).

[2]   Molecular Neuropathology

Other measurements of malignancy rely on objective molecular criteria. One of these is the index of proliferation (increase in number), found by injecting and measuring a biochemical that labels dividing cells. Such indices have been found to correlate well with tumor recurrence and clinical outcome (Harsh, 1994).

The index of proliferation is highest in tumors with the lowest differentiation and the highest invasiveness. Among brain tumors, the generally benign ependymoma has an index of less than 1, mixed glioma an index of 2.1, highly anaplastic astrocytoma an index of 2.7, glioblastoma multiforme an index of 7.3 and medulloblastoma one of 9.5.

Immunohistochemical markers rely on the reaction of specially prepared antibodies with tumor tissue. This method assists in assigning cell type as well as determining degree of differentiation. (The use of genetic markers, such as DNA content and chromosome appearance, is still at the research stage.)

7.30 SYMPTOMS AND SIGNS OF BRAIN TUMORS

Symptoms of intracranial neoplasms depend on the tumor location, its tendency to spread and the potential for increasing intracranial pressure (McDonald and Rosenblum, 1994). Many symptoms arise from increased intracranial pressure (IICP), which may result from mass effect as the tumor expands, from blockage of cerebrospinal fluid (CSF) circulation or from swelling (edema) of surrounding tissue. These symptoms include headache, which is typically worst upon awakening but diminishing during the day; vomiting, with or without nausea, also usually just after waking; mental changes, such as sluggishness or drowsiness; ataxia or other loss of coordination; and seizures.

Symptoms may develop gradually over time, particularly if the tumor is a benign, slowly growing one. Symptoms that occur suddenly may be due to a rapidly growing tumor or to acute obstruction of CSF circulation. A slowly growing tumor can also cause apparently sudden symptoms, such as seizures, when it impinges on a critical region of the brain. Tumors in an area of the cerebrum related to judgment may cause personality or intellectual changes that the patient may not notice.

Although headaches and alterations in neurologic function are the most common symptoms of brain tumors, disturbances of other, non-neurologic processes may occur. Focal (localized) lesions may lead to motor or sensory disturbances of areas controlled by the affected area of the brain, but pressure on nearby areas may result in diffuse dysfunction (Haerer, 1992). Also, depending on its intracranial location, a brain tumor can mimic a more benign disorder elsewhere in the body. Thus a thorough knowledge of neurologic structure and function correlates is essential for establishing the presence and location of an intracranial lesion.

7.31 Pain

Headaches are the initial symptom of brain tumors in about 40 percent of patients (Adelman, 1995). Each year up to 95 percent of the American population suffers one or more headaches, most of which are benign; however, a headache may signal a pathologic process.

The history and nature of a headache can be important for diagnosis. A neoplasm (tumor) should be suspected and sought in cases of slowly progressive, throbbing morning headaches that worsen with coughing or other exertion, or with postural change (Adelman, 1995). Other types of headaches that should lead to the performance of imaging studies include rapid-onset headache, which may be due to sudden obstruction of CSF flow by a midline tumor; headache with cognitive changes or other neurologic abnormalities; progressively worsening headache (over days or weeks) with rapid onset; or headache associated with fever and/or nausea and vomiting.[12]

7.32 Sensory Disturbances

Early neurologic symptoms of brain tumor may include mild to moderate visual or auditory alterations. Among these are progressive loss or blurring of vision (especially in only one area of the visual field) and unilateral (on one side of the body) hearing loss or tinnitus (ringing in the ear). Anosmia (loss of the sense of smell) may also occur. The diagnostician should be alert to such specific, localized symptoms that may point to the involvement of particular cranial nerves.[13] Numbness or sensory loss, particularly when it is localized to one side of the body or to one or more (adjacent) regions, may indicate the presence of an intracranial growth.

7.33 Motor Disturbances

Progressive paralysis is a symptom of possible intracranial neoplastic growth. Convulsions, either focal or diffuse, may point to a tumor.

---

[12] *See also* ch. 10 for further discussion of headache.

[13] *See* 7.12 *supra.*

Weakness or ataxia (failure of voluntary muscle coordination) may indicate a cerebellar growth. Swallowing difficulty and loss of the gag reflex are also symptoms referable to the brain stem or cranial nerves and may result from pressure exerted by a tumor on this area.

7.34   Other Symptoms

Emotional, mental or personality changes, such as confusion, dementia, listlessness, irritability and somnolence, are also possible symptoms of brain tumors. They may indicate the presence of growths in the cerebral areas or an increase in intracranial pressure.

The appearance of such endocrine abnormalities as lactation (milk production), acromegaly (progressive enlargement of such peripheral body parts as the head and face, hands or feet) or Cushing's syndrome (a disorder caused by increased cortisol secretion, characterized by round face, acne, trunk obesity, hypertension, decreased carbohydrate tolerance and other abnormalities) may indicate a pituitary tumor.

7.35   Symptoms in Children

In infants and young children, symptoms of an expanding tumor may include head enlargement and bulging fontanels (membranous intervals between the angles of the cranial bones; the "soft spots"). Listlessness, irritability and failure to thrive are common symptoms (Pollack, 1994). Macewen's sign, in which percussion (tapping) of the skull gives a cracked-pot sound, is another important sign of brain tumor in the infant. Vomiting may be a symptom in older children.

7.40   DIAGNOSIS OF BRAIN TUMORS

The brain is complex, and a lesion in one area may cause either focal or widespread lesions. The diagnosis of neurologic problems can be difficult and demands an integration of information from patient history, neurologic examination and other clinical findings. Advances in neuroimaging have enhanced the clinician's ability to visualize changes in the brain and spinal cord and to make accurate diagnoses. A neurologic evaluation may not be complete without computed tomography (CT) or magnetic resonance imaging (MRI).

7.41 History

A history of the onset and development of symptoms is essential to accurate diagnosis. Intracranial neoplasms usually lead to symptoms that are gradual in onset and worsen progressively (Haerer, 1992; McDonald and Rosenblum, 1994). The symptoms may occur suddenly, however, if the tumor blocks cerebrospinal fluid flow or impinges on a blood vessel. Acute symptoms may also indicate the presence of an aggressive tumor, such as a glioblastoma multiforme.[14]

Because the probability of occurrence of specific tumors is age related, the patient's age is important in arriving at a diagnosis.[15] Although most CNS tumors arise spontaneously, family history is helpful to ascertain or rule out the possibility of hereditary disease.[16]

7.42 Neurologic Examination

A thorough clinical examination is essential and should precede neuroimaging studies. The neurologic examination looks for alterations in mental status, cranial nerve deficits and weakness of the extremities. Early neurologic signs may include unequal reflexes and papilledema (swelling of the optic disk on the retina at the back of the eyeball). The syndrome of increased intracranial pressure, characterized by bifrontal or bioccipital headaches upon awakening, vomiting, mental lassitude, gait unsteadiness and papilledema, may result from mass effect (displacement and functional damage or destruction of brain tissue by any type of mass that compresses it) of a tumor or from obstructive hydrocephalus (accumulation of cerebrospinal fluid due to obstruction of its circulation or failure of its reabsorption in the brain). If this syndrome occurs suddenly, it is an acute situation that may signal a sudden blockage from tumor growth. Benign tumors with a particular tendency to cause increased cranial pressure include medulloblastomas, which may compress or obstruct the fourth ventricle, and ependymomas, which may block the ventricles.

---

[14] *See* 7.61[2] *infra.*

[15] *See* 7.60 *infra.*

[16] *See* 7.02[5] *supra.*

7.43 Imaging Studies

Appropriate imaging studies are essential—and usually sufficient—for diagnosis and localization of intracranial neoplasms (Greenberg and Polachini, 1995). If both computed tomography (CT) and magnetic resonance imaging (MRI) scans are normal, the existence of a tumor is unlikely.

CT and MRI have revolutionized the diagnosis of brain tumors. They provide information about structures within the skull that was previously available only during craniotomy (surgical opening of the skull). As the use of these sophisticated imaging devices increases, the use of skull x-rays and cerebral angiography is diminishing (Adelman, 1995; Haerer, 1992). Echoencephalography (use of ultrasound), pneumoencephalography (x-ray imaging after injection of air or other gas into the cerebral ventricles and subarachnoid spaces) and ventriculography (radiography of cerebral ventricles by injection of radiopaque contrast material or gas) are seldom used.

Although a CT scan can show bone involvement, calcifications or mass effect leading to anatomic displacement, MRI has greater sensitivity and frequently can demonstrate masses that may not be seen by CT. Thus MRI has become the method of choice for confirmation and visualization of suspected tumors (Greenberg and Polachini, 1995). However, MRI may not be widely available in medical facilities outside urban areas (Preston-Martin, 1996).

Once a structure has been detected, several important characteristics that are obtained by interpretation of the computerized images help diagnose the type of lesion. These include size, diffuseness, degree of impingement on normal tissue and whether the structure is extra-axial (extraparenchymal; outside the "body" or functional tissue of the brain) or intra-axial (intraparenchymal).

The existence, pattern and degree of accumulation of contrast material, also called contrast enhancement, differ among various types of lesions and thus have diagnostic value (Greenberg and Polachini, 1995). Intense contrast enhancement may indicate breakdown of the blood-brain barrier (the structures and physiologic mechanism that limits the passage of blood constituents to the cerebrospinal fluid and brain tissue) or tumor location outside this endothelial barrier. Malignant tumors tend to show more contrast enhancement than nonmalignant bodies.

Precise three-dimensional information about tumor location, extent and shape is essential to ensure removal of as much neoplastic tissue as possible with minimal damage to surrounding normal tissue. Much research has been aimed at improving the translation of images from CT and MRI into three-dimensional visualization during open surgery. The demarcation between normal and tumor tissue may be clear on films but ambiguous within the skull, and locating the tumor itself may be difficult. Volumetric stereotaxis is an important approach to this problem.[17]

[1]   Computed Tomography (CT)

In computed tomography, a series of scans is captured by multiple detectors as a fan beam of x-rays is rotated in a plane through 360 degrees. Three-dimensional computerized reconstruction results in images that show brain structures with great contrast and clarity. This method captures images of most neural structures with one set of scans.

In most imaging series, CT scans are made both before and after administration of a contrast medium, typically an iodine compound. CT scanning is now widely available, and a large body of data exists for image-tumor correlations. The use of CT and MRI frequently complement each other (Brody, 1991).

[2]   Magnetic Resonance Imaging (MRI)

Magnetic resonance imaging has greater sensitivity than CT and generally provides better definition of the tumor and associated structures, such as cysts, vessels and necrotic (nonviable) tissue (Edelman and Warach, 1993). Despite its greater cost, it has become the most frequently used method of brain tumor diagnosis, because of its ability to pinpoint tumors and their anatomic relationship to other structures (Greenberg and Polachini, 1995). MRI is preferred for extra-axial tumors such as meningiomas, acoustic neuromas and pituitary adenomas. Usually both T1-weighted images, in which tumors and other tissue with mobile water appear dark, and T2-weighted images, in which they appear bright, are used (Edelman and Warach, 1993).

New imaging techniques significantly shorten scan times, increasing the utility of MRI in tumor diagnosis, but a cooperative patient who limits movement is still necessary. MRI cannot be used in the presence of a pacemaker or a metallic implant that could affect the magnetic

---

[17] *See* 7.43[3] *infra.*

field (Westmoreland, et al., 1994). Children often must be sedated for the procedure.

Despite the excellent tissue contrast attained with MRI, optimum diagnosis requires the injection of a contrast material, gadolinium chelate (a magnetically active rare earth element with an excellent margin of safety), prior to scanning (Edelman and Warach). For some tumors, diagnostic accuracy can be increased by attention to timing of scanning after administration of the contrast material.

[3] Stereotactic Techniques

Volumetric stereotaxis is used to derive precise three-dimensional information in preparation for surgery[18] (Kelly, 1991). The patient's head is held in a rigid, calibrated frame during the scans, and the images are localized in relation to the frame calibrations. Use of the same frame during later biopsy and surgery enables precise localization of the intracranial lesion in the surgical field.

Volumetric stereotaxis is used by the surgeon during preoperative planning and computerized simulation, enabling selection of the surgical approach that will maximize the preservation of normal brain tissue and vascular structures. The procedure is mathematically complex and computer-intensive. It requires high-quality image acquisition and processing, ability to display the reconstructed brain image in real time and an interactive stereotactic surgical system.

A simpler stereotactic procedure is the point-in-space technique, which is used for biopsy (removal of a portion of tissue for analysis) or radiation therapy. Although such procedures can be performed without computer assistance, computerized planning improves accuracy, safety and efficiency.

[4] Angiography

Angiography of the brain is radiographic (x-ray) imaging of the blood vessels after injection of a radiopaque material. This technique has been supplanted by CT and MRI for many uses, but it remains useful to show vascular changes associated with the disease (Haerer, 1992). It also helps in planning of surgery on tumors that have developed extensive, possibly abnormal new vascularization (blood vessels supplying an area) and in planning the safest, least vascular approach (Al-Mefty and Origitano, 1994).

---

[18] *See* 7.46[1] *infra.*

[5]   Positron Emission Tomography (PET)

Positron emission tomography (PET) is sometimes used to identify aggressive astrocytomas or to differentiate recurrent tumor from radiation necrosis (tissue death), but its resolution is poor for most purposes (Greenberg and Polachini, 1995). Also, the technique is expensive and not widely available.

PET is sometimes used to evaluate the uptake and metabolism of chemotherapeutic agents (Rozental, 1991). It may also be used to differentiate tissue necrosis from tumor recurrence, an assessment that may spare a patient from reoperation.

7.44   Electroencephalography (EEG)

Electroencephalography (EEG), the measurement of electric impulses in the brain, recorded from the scalp, is of limited utility in tumor diagnosis, because many brain irritants such as tumors and abscesses lead to similar EEG patterns (Haerer, 1992). However, EEG can help in narrowing the possible causes of seizures, which are often an early symptom of brain tumor as well as other central nervous system disorders. Such specialized neurophysiologic tests as evoked response testing (stimulation of particular nerves to record the electric response in the brain), visual field testing (for a tumor near the optic chiasm, the region in the brain where the fibers of the right and left optic nerves converge) and audiography (for a cerebellopontine angle tumor) may be useful to assess functional deficit and prognosis in some cases. When a tumor has been localized to an important functional area, intraoperative direct cortical stimulation and computerized mapping, with the patient awake, can help guide the surgeon to minimize damage to normal tissue.

Noninvasive mapping methods include magnetoencephalography (MEG), PET scanning, transcranial magnetic field motor stimulation and functional MRI. MEG detects small magnetic fields associated with neuronal activity and may be used for localization of a tumor in relation to functional areas.

7.45   Lumbar Puncture

Lumbar puncture (spinal tap) with analysis of cerebrospinal fluid may be needed to rule out infection and look for metastases. It may aid in staging medulloblastoma. However, its use is generally postponed until imaging studies have indicated that it is essential (Haerer, 1992).

A lumbar puncture is usually contraindicated when intracranial pressure is elevated due to tumor growth or to obstructive hydrocephalus (accumulation of cerebrospinal fluid due to obstruction of its circulation or failure of its reabsorption).

7.46 Biopsy

Usually surgery, once it is begun, aims at resection (surgical removal) of as much of the tumor as possible. Although biopsy is a surgical procedure that leaves the lesion in place, in certain instances, a biopsy is preferred (McDonald and Rosenblum, 1994). Biopsy is useful for diagnosis, for example. One reason is that an abscess (localized focus of infection) can have an appearance similar to many types of tumors. A biopsy is therefore important in the differential diagnosis of brain tumor versus abscess (which is treatable by drainage plus antibiotics) (Pauker and Kopelman, 1993). Also, because tumors differ in their responsiveness to radiation or chemotherapy, biopsy is needed to confirm the diagnosis before institution of either as a stand-alone therapy (Friedman and Spiegelmann, 1992).

[1] Closed Stereotactic Biopsy

If imaging studies show that a patient has a small lesion and the individual is experiencing few symptoms, a biopsy may be indicated, particularly if the lesion site is deep (McDonald and Rosenblum, 1994). This use of biopsy avoids the potential morbidity of open resection and allows the use of local anesthesia in an older person or one with medical problems. If the problem is partially or wholly cystic, simple drainage may significantly improve neurologic functioning.

Closed stereotactic biopsy is a commonly performed, easy procedure with a mortality rate of less than 1 percent and a morbidity rate of less than 5 percent (Friedman and Spiegelmann, 1992). With the aid of a stereotactic frame, which was used previously during CT and/or MRI, the surgeon inserts a probe into the targeted tumor in order to obtain a specimen for pathologic diagnosis. The point-in-space stereotactic procedures used for biopsy are simpler than volumetric stereotactic surgery, which requires computerized reconstruction and guidance in the approach to the tumor.[19]

A possible diagnostic pitfall in biopsy is the choice of the correct target, based on CT or MRI (Friedman and Spiegelmann, 1992). Frequently a tumor has edematous (swollen) but otherwise normal brain tissue on the periphery, with necrotic tissue in the interior. The goal is to sample the specimen from the contrast enhancing ring, if one is present. Another pitfall is the variability of some brain tumor tissue and the possibility that the retrieved tissue may be from an adjacent area (Kepes, 1994).

Despite these possible problems, accuracy of tissue identification by stereotactic biopsy is over 90 percent (McDonald and Rosenblum, 1994).

[2] Open Biopsy

Craniotomy (surgery using an opening into the skull) is necessary for biopsy if the lesion is highly vascular (has many blood vessels) or if there is a risk of bleeding diathesis (constitutional tendency to bleed spontaneously or from trivial trauma due to a clotting or vessel defect) (McDonald and Rosenblum, 1994). The open procedure is also essential if electrocorticography (mapping of cortical function) is needed to determine the functional effects of tumor resection.

7.47 Delayed Diagnosis

Because of the deleterious effects of pressure on the brain from a tumor, as well as the possibility of rapid tumor growth, early diagnosis is vital. In addition, a patient may have delayed seeking medical attention. However, in some cases, the patient's condition, whether it is due to systemic disease or increased cranial pressure from obstructive hydrocephalus, requires a delay in performing the biopsy. In such an instance, the patient may be treated with steroids to decrease the brain swelling. In a few cases, it may be advisable to install a shunt to drain excess CSF.

---

[19] *See* 7.52 *infra.*

7.50   TREATMENT OF BRAIN TUMORS

Treatment of both metastatic and primary brain tumors consists of surgery, radiation therapy and chemotherapy. Each of these treatment modalities is an area of active basic and clinical research, which aims at improving both survival time and quality of life for affected patients.

Both benign and malignant tumors should be resected (surgically removed) whenever this is possible. Types of benign tumors for which resection offers a cure include meningiomas, low-grade astrocytomas, craniopharyngiomas, pituitary adenomas and hemangioblastomas.[20] Although resection by itself does not cure a malignant tumor, removal of as much neoplastic tissue as possible is essential.

Surgery, either by craniotomy or stereotactically, is the most common approach to treating brain tumors. Resection of as much of the tumor as possible offers the best chance for improved survival time and neurologic function (McDonald and Rosenblum, 1994). The goal in surgery is to accomplish this while minimizing damage to normal tissue.

Evidence indicates that total resection of most tumors, along with adjacent tissue (which may have metastatic disease that is more malignant than the original tumor), is the best way to prevent recurrence (Berger and Ojemann, 1994). Most tumor recurrence seems to arise within 2 centimeters of the boundary seen in CT or MRI, and removal of this adjacent tissue may therefore be beneficial. Although resection of large lesions presents an increased risk of neurologic deficit, large size of the tumor does not significantly increase the risk of the surgery itself. However, the type, location, vascularity and grade of tumor play a significant role in the patient's postoperative functional status and thus dictate the specific surgical approach used.

As have surgeons in other fields, neurosurgeons have adopted microsurgical techniques in which fine instruments and microscopes are used to perform precise resections with minimal disturbance to surrounding tissue. In the central nervous system, however, diseased tissue may touch areas of normal tissue that must be spared to minimize postoperative functional deficit. Thus a method for precise guidance of surgical instruments has been developed. In stereotactic surgery, a geometric frame is affixed to the head, so that cross-matching of coordinates between the brain and its diagnostic MRI or

---

[20] *See* 7.60 *infra.*

CT images directs the surgeon precisely to the target area (Tasker and Bernstein, 1994). This methodology has not supplanted open surgery, however, and a surgical team chooses the approach that is best suited to the tumor and its location.

7.51   Open Surgery

Open surgery for brain tumors involves a craniotomy, in which the scalp is peeled back, and a plate of skull bone is removed to expose the dura mater, the outer membrane covering the brain. Cutting the dura exposes the surface of the brain. The surgeon proceeds with the operation to remove (or biopsy) the tumor according to preplanning, possibly with computerized simulation, based on the MR (or CT) images. When this is completed, the dura is sutured shut, and the plate of bone is replaced and wired into place.

Tumor location dictates patient positioning and surgical approach (McDonald and Rosenblum, 1994). Although access to the tumor must be optimized, each position carries specific risks (Turner, 1994).

7.52   Stereotactic Surgery

In stereotactic surgery, also called volumetric stereotaxis, the patient's head is held in the same rigid frame (called a stereotactic frame) that was used in the computerized imaging studies to localize the lesion (Kelly, 1991; Tasker and Bernstein, 1994). During surgery, the surgeon views a scaled real-time display of the tumor and its surrounding tissue. The computer-generated three-dimensional reconstruction of the tumor volume, based on CT and MRI scans, may be superimposed on the intraoperative view to assist in defining the tumor boundaries.

The precision of the three-dimensional calibrations enables the surgeon to direct probes into the brain through one or more small holes in the skull, thus using the safest and least invasive route to reach deep-seated or centrally located tumors. Open stereotactic surgery is used for deep tumors, such as tumors of the basal ganglia or thalamus (Kelly, 1991).

Advantages of the stereotactic approach include precise localization of the tumor, enabling maximal resection of tumor tissue with minimal injury to healthy tissue. Because of the complexity of neural connections in the integration of motor and sensory functions, any damage to normal tissue can lead to neurologic deficit, with consequent prolongation of rehabilitation, which should be avoidable. As with any neoplasm, complete tumor removal is essential to prevent or postpone recurrence.

In general, the stereotactic approach improves postoperative neurologic results, in comparison to conventional, nonstereotactic surgical techniques (Kelly, 1991). Because computed simulation is used during preoperative planning, surgery may be performed with improved efficiency, usually in less time than with conventional techniques. Some tumors that are deemed inoperable by conventional open surgery may be reached by volumetric stereotactic methodology.

7.53   Perioperative Risks and Their Management

The risks in neurosurgery include those related to the nervous system, systemic problems and general surgical risks (Turner, 1994). Potential neurologic problems include those related to the tumor itself, increased intracerebral pressure and seizures. In addition, pre-existing systemic disorders can dispose the patient to cardiovascular and respiratory distress during surgery.

The goals of treatment for brain tumors are to prolong survival time and improve quality of life (McDonald and Rosenblum, 1994). Thus the potential effects of surgery must be evaluated carefully. Partial resection of a large infiltrating tumor may improve the patient's neurologic and functional state, whereas an attempt at total extirpation may increase the neurologic deficit.

The location, composition, vascularity and invasiveness of the tumor are important considerations in planning the surgical approach. The patient's overall condition is an important factor, and sometimes postponement of surgery is advisable to allow time for improvement.

The mortality rate from craniotomy is 1 to 2 percent (McDonald and Rosenblum, 1994).

[1]   General Surgical Risks

The typical risks encountered in surgery are sometimes exacerbated in neurosurgery, due to the length of the procedures. Intraoperative risks include complications from anesthesia and bleeding. Possible delayed problems include embolism (vessel obstruction by a detached blood clot), phlebitis (vein inflammation), infection and wound healing. These risks are increased for the elderly, the medically ill and those with impaired neurologic function.

[2]　Neurologic Risks

Any tumor can cause increased intracranial pressure, through mass effect or by blocking CSF drainage. When pressure is caused by hydrocephalus (accumulation of CSF in the ventricles), drainage may be necessary to stabilize the patient and protect against pressure-caused damage. If surgery must be delayed, steroid administration may be used. Induction of general anesthesia may increase the pressure further, possibly causing secondary damage, and thus must be carefully controlled.

Prior therapy plays a prominent role in treatment decisions. Recent chemotherapy may have left the patient in a debilitated condition, resulting in an increased risk that must be weighed against the benefits of prompt surgery.

Neurologic surgery can worsen coexisting neurologic disorders, such as Parkinson's disease or multiple sclerosis. These conditions should be maximally stabilized prior to surgery.

Anticonvulsant medications may be administered preoperatively if the surgery carries a significant (greater than 5 to 10 percent) risk of causing seizures (Turner, 1994).

Postoperative swelling from the surgery is a frequent (11 percent) occurrence (McDonald and Rosenblum, 1994). Both this and intracranial hemorrhage can cause transient or permanent neurologic deficit.

Neurologic risks are increased in the elderly, in those with a profound neurologic deficit and in those with a deep-seated bilateral or midline tumor (McDonald and Rosenblum, 1994).

[3]　Functional Mapping to Minimize Neurologic Risk

Surgical outcome is improved for some procedures by intraoperative mapping of functional areas and by monitoring evoked potentials from areas that might be at risk (Berger and Ojemann, 1994; Levine, et al., 1994; Moller, 1995). In this method, electric potentials are evoked in the neural tissue in response to sensory stimulation. This permits mapping of functional areas so that they may be avoided during tumor resection (removal).

Some surgical teams are using this method during surgery in the cerebellar pontine angle, where surgery poses risks to the brain stem and to many of the cranial nerves, including the facial nerve. An alternative method for this region, based on the fact that cranial nerves V through XI have some motor function, is to stimulate the area near the nerve and observe whether there is a twitch of the appropriate muscle (Levine, et al., 1994). Mapping techniques seem more applicable for some functions than for others, and attempts to monitor visual evoked potentials to prevent damage to optic pathways during surgery for craniopharyngiomas or pituitary tumors has had equivocal results (Strauss, et al., 1994).

[4] Systemic Risks

Systemic conditions that increase intraoperative risk include diabetes, hypertension (high blood pressure), cardiac arrhythmias (irregular heartbeat patterns), coagulation (blood clotting) disorders, platelet abnormalities and renal (kidney) compromise. When it is possible to do so, these conditions should be maximally controlled prior to surgery.

Potential medical complications include pneumonia, deep vein thrombosis (clotting) and myocardial infarction (heart attack)[21] (McDonald and Rosenblum, 1994).

7.54 Radiation Therapy

A totally nonsurgical approach to treating a brain tumor is rarely indicated. Radiation and chemotherapy are used more often as adjuncts to surgery than as stand-alone therapies. Radiation therapy following surgery has been shown to improve survival time in patients with anaplastic astrocytomas, glioblastoma multiforme and ependymomas (McDonald and Rosenblum, 1994).[22]

Radiation therapy is the chief means of managing brain tumors nonoperatively. More frequently, radiation plays a major role in the postsurgical treatment of most tumors. Its use can increase the cure rate or survival time (McDonald and Rosenblum, 1994). It is commonly used in the treatment of recurrences.

[21] *See also* ch. 8 for discussion of surgical treatment of head injuries.

[22] *See* 7.61 *infra.*

The method and timing of radiation therapy are thought to play a critical role in its effectiveness. In the case of anaplastic astrocytomas, some advocate deferring postsurgical irradiation until the tumor resumes growth. Controversy also exists over the choice between high-dose and low-dose irradiation.

The method of delivering radiation ranges from an external beam delivered to the whole brain to implantation of radioactive seeds within the tumor or its remnants (McDonald and Rosenblum, 1994). Many variations have been tried, with the goal of delivering a high dose to a focal area while sparing surrounding tissue.[23]

[1] Conventional Radiation Therapy

External-beam radiotherapy, also called teletherapy, is the conventional method of delivering radiation to a tumor (Halperin and Anscher, 1994). A linear accelerator (LINAC) transfers high-energy x-rays, or a cobalt-60 machine administers gamma rays, with targeting assisted by use of a CT or MRI scan.

The radiation is typically delivered in multiple fractions. Protocols vary for different tumors and among institutions, but most patients receive a total of 60 to 65 Gy (grays, the measure of absorbed radiation dose, equivalent to one joule per kilogram of tissue; 1 Gy = 100 rad, where 1 rad is equivalent to 100 ergs of energy per gram of tissue) over a six-week period of time, with treatment delivered five days per week in doses (fractions) of 1.8 to 2.5 Gy (Freeman and Lehnert, 1991). When a stereotactic frame is used to improve the accuracy of radiation delivery, this is called stereotactic radiation therapy (Coffey, 1994).

[2] Interstitial Brachytherapy

In brachytherapy, also called stereotactic interstitial irradiation, radioactive seeds of the radioactive isotopes iridium-192, iodine-125 or palladium-103 are implanted into the tumor as delineated by CT and/or MRI scan ((Halperin and Anscher, 1994; Kun, 1991). The radiation emitted by these sources is calculated to deliver a lethal dose to the tumor, while the dose fall-off results in a much lower amount of radiation being transmitted to the nearby normal tissue (Friedman and Spiegelmann, 1992). The dose rate is considerably lower than in conventional external beam irradiation (40 to 50 centiGrays, with 1

---

[23] *See* 7.54[6] *infra.*

centiGray or cGy = 100 Grays or 1 rad, per hour, compared with 200 cGy per minute).

Interstitial irradiation often serves as an adjunct to external beam radiation therapy, in order to increase the dosage to the targeted area. The drawback of this method is the necessity for surgery both to place the radioactive seeds and to remove them after the total desired dosage has been reached; this may be followed later by further surgery to remove dead tissue. In addition to tissue necrosis (death of tissue), possible complications include bleeding, infection, tumor swelling and cerebrospinal fluid (CSF) leak.

This treatment is appropriate for tumors that are localized rather than diffuse. Usually the maximum diameter is 5 to 6 centimeters (Kun, 1991). Larger tumors require a higher dose, which increases the probability of necrosis. The tumor should be surgically accessible and should not be too close to vascular midline structures.

In general, patients with a low functional score are not good candidates for brachytherapy (Friedman and Spiegelmann, 1992). The technique has been used successfully to treat children.

[3] Radiosurgery

In stereotactic radiosurgery, multiple focused beams of irradiation are delivered to the tumor with precise targeting that uses stereotactic methodology, resulting in a single, high dose to a small area (Coffey, 1994; Kun, 1991; Larson and Coffey, 1993). An immobilization frame is used during both diagnostic imaging and radiotherapy. The goal is to maximize the dose delivered to the tumor, in the hope that the precise targeting will completely destroy abnormal tissue while minimizing damage to surrounding normal tissue. In a variation, the total desired dosage is delivered in several fractionated sessions.

Specific radiation delivery techniques include use of a gamma knife with multiple independent beams, linear acceleration focusing multiple arcs on a single point, dynamic rotation in which both the patient couch and the linear accelerator beam move, and use of a focused proton beam (Larson and Coffey, 1993). Another modality—charged particle-beam therapy, using accelerated protons or helium ions—has been used for treating pituitary adenomas (Coffey, 1994).

This method has low morbidity and is attractive because it is noninvasive. It shows promise for the treatment of brain tumors in children, in whom the potential damage to the growing brain with conventional radiotherapy may outweigh the therapeutic benefits (Lew and LaVally, 1995). At present, it is only useful for circumscribed tumors with little or no infiltration into surrounding tissue. Generally the tumors must be 4 centimeters or smaller in diameter, because as the target becomes larger, the risk of irradiating normal tissue increases (Friedman and Spiegelmann, 1992).

[4]   Use of Radiosensitizers

Various agents, for example, hyperthermia (elevated temperature), have been used to attempt to sensitize tumor cells selectively to radiation. This is still in the experimental stages.

[5]   Hyperfractionated Irradiation and Accelerated Fraction Radiation

In hyperfractionated radiotherapy, smaller doses of radiation are administered more frequently to achieve approximately the same or higher total dosage, in a similar time span as with conventional radiotherapy (Freeman and Lehnert, 1991). Typically low doses in the range of 100 to 120 cGy are administered twice daily (Pollack, 1994). The total dosage, in the range of 7,000 cGy, is higher than in conventional radiation therapy, but it is thought that the sublethal damage from lower single doses is more easily repaired by normal cells between doses.

The rationale for the frequent doses is the hypothesis that this increases the probability of irradiating tumor cells during a sensitive part of the cell cycle. It is thought, on the basis of the cell cycle, that the interval between doses should be at least 4 to 6 hours (Freeman and Lehnert, 1991). Studies to date do not show a significant increase in disease-free survival time with this approach, but survivors seem to have fewer adverse neurologic effects.

In accelerated fraction radiation, the overall treatment time is reduced by more frequent delivery of doses similar to those used in conventional radiotherapy (Freeman and Lehnert, 1991). The aim is improved tumor control by limiting the opportunity for tumor cell regeneration and repopulation. This regimen is best for patients with rapidly growing tumors. It results in more early complications but fewer late adverse effects. Survival rates have not been improved, however.

[6]   Adverse Effects of Radiation Therapy

Acute adverse effects of radiation therapy, occurring during or within hours after treatment, include tissue swelling, with resulting temporary neurologic deficits (McDonald and Rosenblum, 1994). This may be alleviated by steroid administration.

Nausea, vomiting, difficulty in swallowing and neurologic dysfunction can occur in the weeks or months following treatment (Al-Mefty, et al., 1990). Other short-term delayed effects include alopecia (hair loss), tinnitus (ringing in the ears) and skin changes.

Radiation therapy has serious delayed adverse effects, particularly for children. Occurring months to years later, radiation-induced brain necrosis can result in deficits in mental function. The effects of radiotherapy on the developing nervous system can be devastating, and irradiation is now seldom used to treat children under two or three years of age (Pollack, 1994). A child receiving standard whole-brain radiation at the age of four may experience a 40-point decrease in IQ over the next two years (Duffner and Cohen, 1991; Sutton and Packer, 1994).

Even in adults, radiation to the brain can lead to cerebral atrophy and necrosis, visual disturbances, seizures and endocrine problems (Al-Mefty, et al., 1990; Slavin and Ausman, 1994). The incidence of radiation necrosis is estimated at 5 percent. Symptoms range from mild confusion to organic mental syndrome with dementia. Paralysis, coma and death are also possible outcomes. The latency period ranges from 2 months to nearly 20 years. The larger the radiation dosage, the sooner the symptoms appear. Most reported cases of radiation necrosis have occurred subsequent to radiotherapy performed with accepted dosages and timing (total dosage of less than 5000 cGy, in fractions of less than 200 cGy) (Al-Mefty, et al., 1990).

Visual impairment can be severe and may be either sudden or progressive. Reported latency ranges from five months to seven years.

Hormonal derangement may occur after radiotherapy. Cranial irradiation can cause hypothyroidism (undersecretion of thyroid hormone), growth hormone deficiency and retarded growth (Duffner and Cohen, 1991). Hormonal disturbance is thought to result from hypothalamic or pituitary damage (Al-Mefty, et al., 1990). The pituitary is more sensitive to radiation damage than is the rest of the brain (Halperin and Anscher, 1994).

Among the late effects of radiation therapy is induction of new tumors (Duffner and Cohen, 1991; Halperin and Anscher, 1994; Preston-Martin, 1996). The excess risk for tumorigenesis has been calculated at 1.8 per 10,000 persons per year (Al-Mefty, et al., 1990). Latency has been reported to range from 4 to 30 years. Sarcomas, meningiomas and gliomas are the most frequently induced.[24] Children seem particularly susceptible.

These findings emphasize the need for careful patient selection and dosage calculation. Any improvement in precision of targeting, particularly if it permits a lower total dosage, should help preserve brain and endocrine system function.

A specific complication of radiation therapy combined with methotrexate chemotherapy is the development of leukoencephalopathy (multifocal destruction of the white matter around the ventricles) (Duffner and Cohen, 1991). Characterized clinically by dementia and ataxia (lack of muscular coordination), this condition may lead to death.

7.55 Chemotherapy of Brain Tumors

Chemotherapy is most commonly used an as adjunct to surgery and radiation therapy. It may prolong survival with some tumors, including anaplastic astrocytomas, medulloblastomas and some germ cell tumors (McDonald and Rosenblum, 1994).

Chemotherapy is used infrequently as the primary approach to brain tumors because of problems relating to the blood-brain barrier (the structures and physiologic mechanism that limits the passage of blood constituents to the cerebrospinal fluid and brain tissue) (Schold, 1994). There is at present no effective chemotherapy for benign brain tumors. Most metastatic tumors in the brain do not respond to the generalized chemotherapeutic approach to other body systems because of the blood-brain barrier.

A variety of agents are available for chemotherapy. BCNU (carmustine; 1,3-bis(2-chloroethyl)-1-nitrosourea) is the standard for treatment of gliomas (McDonald and Rosenblum, 1994; Schold, 1994). Two oral agents that are effective against brain tumors are procarbazine and CCNU (lomustine; 1-(2-chloroethyl)-3-cyclohexyl-1-nitrosourea).

---

[24] *See* 7.03[1] *supra.*

Frequently two or more drugs are administered. Vincristine and carboplatin may be effective therapy for low-grade astrocytomas in children under age five. A regimen of vincristine, procarbazine and CCNU (lomustine; 1-(2-chloroethyl)-3-cyclohexyl-1-nitrosourea) prolongs survival in patients with anaplastic astrocytomas. Some glioblastomas respond to procarbazine or BCNU.

Chemotherapy is used as the postsurgical therapy for young children to avoid use of radiation with its effects on the developing brain. It may also be used for young children as the primary treatment for nonresectable tumors. Chemotherapy is also used to treat medulloblastomas in children under the age of three.

Although most chemotherapy involves intravenous infusion, the use of other pathways for drug delivery is under investigation. These include intrathecal delivery (into the subarachnoid or subdural space) and intratumoral chemotherapy, with stereotactic implantation of a sustained-release drug into the tumor.

Other approaches attempt to modify the permeability of the blood-brain barrier to permit chemotherapeutic and radiation-sensitizing agents to enter the brain.

7.56 Immunotherapy

A variety of immunology-based therapies are being studied. Restorative immunotherapy attempts to enhance the patient's own immune system with such agents as tumor necrosis factor and other cytokines, interferons or interleukins (McDonald and Rosenblum, 1994). In adoptive immunotherapy, immune system cells such as lymphocytes are conditioned to attack specific or nonspecific brain tumor antigens and are then injected into the tumor. Passive immunotherapy, in which anti-tumor antibodies are injected, either alone or attached to radioactive or chemotherapeutic agents, shows more promise than active immunotherapy, in which tumor-specific antigens are injected in the hope of stimulating the patient's own immune system.

In a gene therapy approach, the brain is infected by a virus that has been genetically engineered to attack tumor cells while ignoring normal tissue.

7.57   Treatment of Recurrent Tumors

A recurrent tumor may be treated with surgery, radiation or chemotherapy; commonly a combination is used. Reoperation for recurrent anaplastic astrocytoma or glioblastoma multiforme increases patient survival time. The factors involved in the decision for initial surgery also apply to the choices for recurrent tumors (McDonald and Rosenblum, 1994).

7.60   PREVALENT PRIMARY BRAIN TUMORS

Primary brain tumors include gliomas, meningiomas, pituitary adenomas, vestibular schwannomas, lymphomas and a number of rarer tumors. Their names generally indicate the primary cell type from which they are derived.

The majority of intracranial neoplasms in adults occur above the tentorium cerebelli (the membrane separating the cerebral hemispheres, basal ganglia and thalamus, above, from the posterior fossa structures—cerebellum, midbrain, pons and medulla—below). Most of those in children occur below the tentorium.

7.61   Gliomas

About 50 percent of all intracranial neoplasms are gliomas (Haerer, 1992; McDonald and Rosenblum, 1994). Gliomas are primary tumors composed of or derived from the embryonic percursors to glial cells, the major supporting cells of the brain. They are usually classified by their histogenesis (type of tissue from which they arise), but several naming systems and much disagreement exist. Commonly included in the term *gliomas* are most of the tumors of neuroepithelial tissue in WHO Class I: astrocytic tumors, oligodendrogliomas, ependymomas and glioblastoma multiforme.[25] Tumors of mixed cell type also occur. The characteristics, biology, prognosis and treatment of these tumors vary greatly.

Mitotically active (undergoing cell division) cells of malignant gliomas are often motile, migrating along fiber tracts and cortical surfaces to invade neighboring areas (Harsh, 1994). The tumor cells secrete enzymes that destroy normal tissue.

---

[25] *See* 7.21[1] *supra.*

Most gliomas are treated by surgical resection, usually followed by radiation therapy and sometimes chemotherapy. For most glial tumors, such a multimodal approach gives the best possibility for long-term survival. Gliomas tend to recur, however, and the patient should be aware of the probability of long-term, repeated treatment. Even when the long-term outcome is poor, surgery or radiation therapy may improve the patient's quality of life and neurologic function, particularly if elevated intracranial pressure is relieved.

In a few cases, a small, nonenhancing and thus apparently nonmalignant tumor that does not cause symptoms may be followed radiographically (McDonald and Rosenblum, 1994). Large tumors in elderly, debilitated patients may be treated with palliative radiotherapy. Advances in stereotactic volumetric surgery[26] are decreasing the number of tumor sites that are regarded as inaccessible. However, except for resection of small tumors near the surface, the risks of permanent neurologic deficit resulting from the surgical procedure need to be weighed against the potential for increased survival time and quality of life. The use of electrophysiologic mapping during surgery can assist in avoiding eloquent (highly functional) areas.[27]

Many gliomas have a poor prognosis despite aggressive treatment combining surgery, radiation therapy and chemotherapy, usually with a nitrosourea (Schold, 1994). Factors contributing to a favorable outcome in adults include young patient age; normal or near-normal functional status presurgically; absence of metabolic, cardiovascular or pulmonary disease; small, well-defined, nonmalignant tumor without significant new vascularization; superficial tumor location or location not requiring resection of highly functional areas (McDonald and Rosenblum, 1994). Neurologic functional status is often quantitated by means of the Karnofsky Performance Scale, which assesses functioning on a scale from 100 (normal) to 10 (moribund, death imminent). Patients with a score of 70 (able to care for self but unable to carry on most normal activities) or better have a survival rate more than twice that of patients with lower scores.

[1]　Astrocytomas

About a third of gliomas are astrocytomas, which are the single most common primary intracerebral neoplasm (McDonald and Rosenblum,

---

[26] *See* 7.52 *supra.*

[27] *See* 7.44 *supra.*

1994). Astrocytomas are derived from astrocytes, cells with radiating processes that play a role in neuron migration during embryogenesis and in chemical and mechanical maintenance of neurons thereafter (Westmoreland, et al., 1994). Astrocytomas are most common in adults, in whom they are found mainly in the cerebral hemispheres. In children, they are most frequent in the cerebellum. In both children and adults, the prognosis depends on tumor site and resectability and on degree of anaplasia (loss of structural differentiation).

Several astrocytoma grading schemes attempt to provide pathologic and prognostic information. Included in these are pilocytic astrocytomas, which comprise about 2 percent of gliomas; low-grade astrocytomas, which represent 5 to 25 percent; anaplastic astrocytomas, with an incidence of 10 to 30 percent of gliomas; and glioblastoma multiforme, which constitute 45 to 50 percent (McDonald and Rosenblum, 1994). The least malignant tumors, termed grade I, low-grade or mildly anaplastic, grow slowly. Their main characteristic is an increase in cell number. They tend to occur in the third and fourth decades of life (Greenberg and Polachini, 1995).

Symptoms of grade I astrocytomas may include epileptic seizures from brain irritation and signs of increased pressure, such as headaches, paralysis or personality change. These tumors are often difficult to diagnose by CT scan but may be well defined by MRI (McDonald and Rosenblum, 1994). Lesions appear homogeneous and tend not to show contrast enhancement (Greenberg and Polachini, 1995), so that the tumor is diffuse.

Surgery may be required to relieve pressure, but the prognosis is generally good. A problem with tumor resection is that the tumor is often diffuse, with poorly demarcated borders, and intact brain tissue may be resected along with tumor (Greenberg and Polachini, 1995). Stereotactic methods often are helpful to map and plan as precise a resection as possible. Another problem is that isolated cells may infiltrate normal tissue. This leads to a dilemma about the amount of tissue to resect, because resection of functional tissue leads to neurologic deficit. In children, however, low-grade gliomas, particularly pilocytic astrocytomas, tend to be better defined.

Pilocytic astrocytomas, sometimes classified as grade I astrocytomas, are most common in young people, in whom 80 to 90 percent occur, and tend to occur in the cerebellum (61 percent) or the region of the optic chiasm and hypothalamus (28 percent) (McDonald and

Rosenblum, 1994; O'Brien and Krisht, 1994). Symptoms depend on tumor site: Cerebellar tumors cause cerebellar symptoms (problems with equilibrium or motor coordination) or such signs of increased intracranial pressure as headache, nausea and vomiting; visual loss or endocrine dysfunction results from tumors in the optic chiasm and hypothalamus; cerebral tumors may cause seizures, weakness or headache.

A tumor may be solid or cystic (composed of one or more abnormal fluid-containing sacs). After injection of contrast material, MRI images show variable enhancement and a macrocystic appearance; borders are usually well defined, normally enabling a clean resection (Greenberg and Polachini, 1995).

Most pilocytic astrocytomas follow a benign course and can be cured by complete resection (McDonald and Rosenblum, 1994). Complete removal results in a 25-year survival rate of 90 percent (O'Brien and Krisht, 1994). Even subtotal resection results in a 2-year survival rate of more than 50 percent. Rarely, a malignant variant occurs (Burger and Fuller, 1991).

Grade II, or low-grade, astrocytomas are moderately anaplastic, with hypercellularity and some enlarged nuclei with increased chromatin, but with a majority of clearly astrocytic cells. They are invasive but grow slowly, are not necrotic and have no vascular proliferation. They occur predominantly in the cerebral hemispheres, with about 40 percent in the frontal lobe and 25 percent each in the temporal and parietal lobes. Symptoms include seizures, headaches and other symptoms of increased intracranial pressure. They are usually well defined in imaging studies but rarely show contrast enhancement. The usual treatment is surgical resection, often followed by radiation therapy. Median survival time is about 3.5 years.

Grade III—anaplastic—astrocytomas, resulting from malignant transformation of low-grade astrocytomas, are invasive and aggressive (Greenberg and Polachini, 1995). They occur most frequently in the cerebral hemispheres. Moderate pleomorphism (varied cell forms) is found in both cells and their nuclei. Some necrosis may be present, and there may be some vascular proliferation. Symptoms include seizures and symptoms of intracranial pressure, sometimes accompanied by changes in mental status. Imaging studies typically show enhancement with contrast, mass effect and edema (seen as a hypodense area).

Treatment is surgery followed by radiation or chemotherapy with BCNU. Treatment at recurrence may be repeated surgery, radiosurgery, interstitial brachytherapy (implantation of radioactive seeds in the tumor)[28] or chemotherapy. Up to half of aggressively treated patients survive for two years.

[2] Glioblastomas

Sometimes classified as grade IV astrocytomas, glioblastoma multiforme comprise about half of cerebral gliomas (Greenberg and Polachini, 1995; McDonald and Rosenblum, 1994). Peak incidence is in the fifth and sixth decades. Occurring mainly in the cerebral hemispheres, this is one of the most malignant brain tumors, with primitive, anaplastic cells (Haerer, 1992). A glioma may arise independently or as a result of differentiation of an astrocytoma (Greenberg and Polachini, 1995; McDonald and Rosenblum, 1994).

Common symptoms are headache, nausea and vomiting, focal weakness and changes in mental status. This tumor tends to have an irregular shape, with areas of solid growth and necrotic regions (dead tissue) due to the tumor's outgrowing its blood supply. The appearance of abnormal blood vessels also helps diagnose this tumor type. Typically a hypodense (in CT) or hypointense (in MRI) area is surrounded by a contrast-enhancing somewhat hyperdense area, with edematous (swollen) tissue on the periphery. There may be hemorrhage.

Treatment for glioblastoma multiforme is surgical resection, followed by radiation and chemotherapy. Chemotherapy may prolong survival time, which is generally a year or less with aggressive therapy.

[3] Oligodendrogliomas

Oligodendrogliomas, arising from oligodendroglia (oligodendrocytes), which form central nervous system myelin by wrapping around the axons, comprise 4 to 15 percent of gliomas (Greenberg and Polachini, 1995; McDonald and Rosenblum, 1994). They most frequently occur in the fourth to fifth decade. They arise most often in the white matter of the cerebral hemispheres or in the brain stem in adults (Haerer, 1992). Although they are rare in children, when they occur, oligodendrogliomas tend to arise in the region of the optic nerve and chiasm. Symptoms include seizures, headache, visual changes and

---

[28] *See* 7.54[2] *supra.*

focal deficits. Imaging studies show irregular regions of calcification; contrast enhancement is usually seen only with anaplastic changes.

Treatment is surgical excision, followed by radiation therapy if excision is subtotal. Oligodendrogliomas appear to be more sensitive to chemotherapy than do astrocytomas; a combination of CCNU, procarbazine and vincristine is used (Schold, 1994). Median survival time is 35 to 60 months for well-differentiated tumors, less for anaplastic oligodendrogliomas. The presence of calcifications is a favorable prognostic sign.

[4] Ependymoma

Although they are rare in adults, ependymomas are the third most common intracranial tumor in children (McDonald and Rosenblum, 1994), occurring most frequently in individuals between the ages of 10 and 15 (Greenberg and Polachini, 1995). They arise from the cells of the ventricular system in the posterior fossa level (the region below the tentorium cerebelli and above the opening to the spinal canal; this area includes the midbrain, pons, medulla and cerebellum) or above the tentorium. Ependymoma symptoms include headache, nausea and vomiting. Imaging studies show a heterogeneous mass with calcified or cystic areas; it usually enhances with contrast.

Most ependymomas are benign; transformation to anaplastic tumors is rare. Treatment is by surgical resection, followed by radiation therapy. Radiation delivery and dosage appear to play a critical role in outcome. The five-year survival rate is 35 to 60 percent. In contrast to many other brain tumors, the prognosis is somewhat better for older patients.

The relatively rare choroid plexus tumors, arising from choroid plexus epithelial cells, are classed with ependymoma in the WHO system. Choroid plexus papillomas, which comprise 3 to 5 percent of pediatric intracranial tumors, are relatively benign (Greenberg and Polachini, 1995). They occur mainly in the lateral ventricles in children but in the fourth ventricle in adults. The initial symptom is usually obstructive hydrocephalus. Cure is possible by total resection.

Anaplastic choroid plexus papilloma is a malignant variant. It tends to invade nearby brain parenchyma.

[5] Gangliogliomas

Gangliogliomas, composed of neoplastic astrocytes and neoplastic neurons, comprise 3 percent of brain tumors in children (Greenberg and Polachini, 1995). The neurons have varied shapes and sizes, including binucleate and giant. They occur most frequently in the cerebral hemispheres, typically the temporal lobe. Imaging studies show a cystic solid that is hypodense in CT, hypointense in MRI. About 35 percent have calcifications.

Symptoms depend on location and often include seizures. This type of tumor grows slowly.

[6] Medulloblastomas

The highly malignant medulloblastomas are found almost exclusively in children and young adults (Sutton and Packer, 1994). Comprising about 15 percent of all gliomas, medulloblastomas represent slightly less than 30 percent of posterior fossa tumors in children, making them one of the most common of these (Greenberg and Polachini, 1995; Haerer, 1992). They are the most common malignant brain tumor in children, with peak incidence within the first decade of life. This tumor is thought to arise from immature germinal matrix stem cells of the cerebellum, which normally form the external layer of the cerebellum (Greenberg and Polachini, 1995; Westmoreland, et al., 1994). The cerebellum is the primary site affected. Hydrocephalus (collection of fluid in the brain) occurs in 80 to 90 percent of patients, and the symptoms are usually those of increased intracranial pressure. Both CT and MRI studies typically show a well-defined cerebellar mass with little or no edema.

Because of the hydrocephalus, a child is frequently acutely ill at diagnosis. Controversy exists about the relative value of using preoperative steroids, drainage or shunting (Sutton and Packer, 1994).

Surgical resection is followed by radiation therapy, but the possibility of brain damage usually precludes radiation for children under the age of three. Some centers add chemotherapy to a low dosage of radiation, using such standard drugs as vincristine and cisplatin. There is a high rate of recurrence with medulloblastomas, and, unlike most other brain tumors, a high rate of metastases to other parts of the body (Sure, et al., 1995). Despite more complete resections with improved surgical techniques and targeted radiation therapy, the long-term prognosis is unfavorable.

[7] Mixed Gliomas

Mixed gliomas contain elements of two or three different cell types, usually astrocytoma with oligodendroglioma and/or ependymoma. The prognosis is determined largely by the most malignant cells in the tumor.

[8] Brain Stem Gliomas

Until recently, any type of glioma occurring in the brain stem was considered to be inoperable and to have a poor prognosis (Walker and Petronio, 1994). Many brain stem tumors are low-grade astrocytomas in which malignancy and potential for surgical excision correlate with location.

Brain stem gliomas comprise 10 to 20 percent of pediatric brain tumors. These fall into four categories: diffuse, focal (solid or cystic), exophytic (extending into the fourth ventricle) and cervicomedullary (Abbott, et al., 1994). The majority are diffuse, with rapid motor degeneration; therapy is only palliative. Tumors in the other categories are treated by radical surgical resection, with care taken to minimize cranial nerve deficits.

The most common brain stem tumor in adults is a pontine glioma, which is found on biopsy to be an anaplastic astrocytoma or a glioblastoma. Treatment with hyperfractionated radiotherapy gives relief of symptoms, but maximum survival time is 12 to 15 months (Walker and Petronio, 1994).

7.62 Meningiomas

Meningiomas arise from the arachnoid cells on the inner surface of the dura mater, the outermost of the meninges (membranes) surrounding the brain and spinal cord (Al-Mefty and Origitano, 1994). They constitute the most common benign intracranial tumor type and comprise 13 to 19 percent of all brain tumors (Greenberg and Polachini, 1995). Peak incidence is at age 45, and they are rare in childhood. Meningiomas usually have receptors for the hormone progesterone and occur in women twice as frequently as in men. Multiple tumors occur in 5 to 15 percent of patients. They tend to occur, along with gliomas and acoustic neuromas, in neurofibromatosis (also known as von Recklinghausen's disease).

Most meningiomas occur adjacent to the skull. Ninety percent are supratentorial. Meningiomas are discrete, varying from a few millimeters to several centimeters in diameter (Al-Mefty and Origitano, 1994). They may be multilobulated or flat. About a third have bone involvement. They can be visualized in skull x-rays and by CT or MRI. CT shows a meningioma as a homogeneous tumor with well-defined borders and contrast enhancement.

Symptoms are related to the tumor's mass effect or to seizure-provoking irritation. Typically meningiomas press inward against the brain; over time, this can result in edema, which is out of proportion to tumor size, and eventual tissue atrophy (Greenberg and Polachini, 1995). Sometimes bone involvement results in hyperostosis (abnormal bone growth, which may progress to the point that it is visible through the skin). Bone destruction and extracranial growth may also occur (Greenberg and Polachini, 1995).

Some symptoms are specific to tumor location. These include weakness or numbness of the lower extremities (arising from a parasagittal tumor involving the dura channels at the top of the skull), visual disturbances (from a tumor at the base of the skull), hydrocephalus (resulting from posterior fossa involvement) and impaired sense of smell (from a tumor in the olfactory groove). A tumor originating from the tentorium can grow both upward and downward and involve one or more cranial nerves.

Frequently meningiomas can be cured by complete removal, but they tend to recur. A residue from partial removal will tend to regrow. Although the goal of surgical treatment is complete removal, some meningiomas adhere to vascular and neural structures or wrap around cranial nerves, making dissection difficult (Al-Mefty and Origitano, 1994). Radiation therapy should not be used for these benign tumors unless there is a nonresectable residue or recurrence. A small meningioma may be watched, rather than removed, if it is not causing symptoms. Follow-up is usually by CT.

Meningiomas can undergo transformation, increasing in mitotic activity, forming atypical cells and infiltrating other sites (Greenberg and Polachini, 1995). Malignant variants, defined by frequency of mitoses and invasiveness, are malignant meningioma, hemangiopericytoma, papillary meningioma and meningeal sarcoma. Atypical appearance on CT or MRI, such as poorly defined borders and multilobular appearance, indicate an increased tendency to malignant transformation. Malignant variants are treated aggressively, like other malignant brain tumors, with attempted surgical resection followed by radiation therapy.

7.63 Primary Central Nervous System (CNS) Lymphomas

Primary central nervous system lymphomas account for less than 2 percent of intracranial tumors (Greenberg and Polachini, 1995). Histologically they resemble systemic non-Hodgkins lymphomas, but they occur in the absence of this disease. Peak incidence is in the sixth decade for patients without predisposing factors. Risk factors are acquired immunodeficiency syndrome (AIDS), congenital immunodeficiency disorders and autoimmune diseases such as lupus or rheumatoid arthritis. The disease is more common in males than females, with a ratio of about 3 to 2.

Personality and behavioral changes are the most common symptoms.

The disease may appear as a single tumor, well-defined or diffuse, or as multifocal infiltrates (Greenberg and Polachini, 1995). Multiple lesions are common in AIDS patients. Lymphoma may affect the cerebral hemispheres, the cerebellum or the brain stem. Anaplastic lymphocytes tend to have a perivascular (around blood vessels) arrangement. Lymphoma is poorly defined in either CT or MRI without contrast but enhances with contrast with both modalities. In such studies, lymphoma is sometimes difficult to distinguish from malignant glioma. Definitive diagnosis is often by stereotactic biopsy.[29]

Surgery is seldom possible. Treatment is with radiation, to which lymphoma is highly sensitive (Schold, 1994). Nevertheless, the prognosis is poor, with a median survival time of less than a year in treated patients (Greenberg and Polachini, 1995). The use of drugs that may be effective for systemic lymphoma (cyclophosphamide, adriamycin, vincristine) is being studied (Schold, 1994).

7.64 Pineal Region Tumors

Tumors of the pineal region are rare in adults, comprising less than 1 percent of primary brain tumors, but they comprise 3 to 8 percent of pediatric intracranial tumors (Edwards and Baumgartner, 1994; Slavin and Ausman, 1994). They are a heterogenous group, placed together by region rather than histology (Greenberg and Polachini, 1995).

---

[29] *See* 7.46[1] *supra.*

The pineal gland is a photoreceptive organ in some vertebrates and in humans plays a role in regulating circadian rhythm by secretion of melatonin in response to light (Westmoreland, 1994). It lies in the posterior wall of the third ventricle, below the corpus callosum.

Pineal region tumors are classified by cell origin (Greenberg and Polachini, 1995). Tumors of germ cell origin, accounting for more than half of pineal region tumors, include germinoma, arising from primitive germ cells, embryonal carcinoma, teratoma and others (Slavin and Ausman, 1994). Those of pineal cell origin are less common and include the slow-growing pineocytoma and the more malignant, rapidly growing pineoblastoma. More common types of tumors, such as astrocytomas, can also occur in the pineal region.

Pineal germinoma is a malignant tumor that destroys the pineal gland and may metastasize via the cerebrospinal fluid (Greenberg and Polachini, 1995; Slavin and Ausman, 1994). Although most germ cell tumors arise in the pineal region, some also arise in the suprasellar (above the sella turcica, a bony cavity in the sphenoid bone at the base of the skull, which contains the pituitary gland) region (Allen, 1991).

Symptoms and imaging characteristics vary with the tumor type, size and location. Headache and papilledema (swelling of the optic disk) are common (Slavin and Ausman, 1994). Precocious puberty occurs in about 10 percent of male patients with a tumor in this region.

Controversy exists over the treatment of pineal region tumors (Allen, 1991; Slavin and Ausman, 1994). Historically most (70 to 85 percent) of these tumors have been treated by focal radiation, because of the difficulties in surgical resection (Allen, 1991). This has led to radiation for benign tumors, which can be treated by surgical resection alone. Optimal treatment requires tissue biopsy (Edwards and Baumgartner, 1994), for therapy decisions depend on whether the tumor is benign or malignant.

Germinomas respond well to radiation, but nongerminoma tumors tend to respond poorly to radiation but well to chemotherapy. A treatment algorithm that has improved long-term survival includes hydrocephalus control, total resection of benign tumors, and radiation and/or chemotherapy for nonresectable tumors, based on histology (Slavin and Ausman, 1994).

7.65 Craniopharyngiomas

Craniopharyngiomas, the most common nonglial brain tumor of children, comprise up to 9 percent of pediatric nervous system tumors but only 2.5 percent of adult brain tumors (Friedman and Spiegelmann, 1992; Hoffman and Kestle, 1994; Sanford and Muhlbauer, 1991). About half of all craniopharyngiomas occur in patients below age 18.

While they are usually benign, craniopharyngiomas may affect endocrine or visual function through their proximity to the pituitary and hypothalamus and to the optic nerve (Hoffman and Kestle, 1994). Imaging shows suprasellar calcification (Greenberg and Polachini, 1995).

About 60 percent of craniopharyngiomas can be removed completely, but sometimes adherence to vessels or the hypothalamus prevents resection (Hoffman and Kestle, 1994). Recurrence is decreased by postsurgical radiation therapy. Use of interstitial brachytherapy stereotactic implantation of radioactive seeds in the tumor)[30] for cystic craniopharyngioma has been successful when surgical resection was not possible (Friedman and Spiegelmann, 1992).

7.66 Acoustic Schwannomas

An acoustic schwannoma, often called an acoustic neuroma, arises from the sheath of the vestibular-acoustic nerve (Wilkins, 1994). It is a benign, slowly growing tumor that may not create symptoms until it has grown quite large. Symptoms are generally due to compression of the brain stem or cerebellum.

Possible symptoms are sensorineural hearing loss, tinnitus (ringing in the ears), vertigo, facial palsy or numbness and difficulty in swallowing. As the tumor develops over time, the patient may compensate for a gradual loss of vestibular function. Unless there are other symptoms, such as hearing problems, the patient may delay seeking medical attention. Sometimes the symptoms for which medical attention is sought are referable to hydrocephalus.

Acoustic neuromas occur in the internal auditory canal or cerebellopontine angle as smoothly circumscribed lesions. There are two types (Greenberg and Polachini, 1995):

---

[30] *See* 7.54[2] *supra.*

- Antoni A: small, densely packed tumors; and

- Antoni B: larger, porous tumors.

Type B tumors are more likely to have cystic degeneration.

Imaging by MRI shows the acoustic neuroma more clearly than does CT (Greenberg and Polachini, 1995). MRI with contrast is often necessary for diagnosis.

Microsurgical techniques have improved the prognosis for patients with this type of tumor. When the tumor is detected early, hearing and facial nerve function can be preserved. Radiosurgery may stop tumor growth, with a low risk of complications.

7.67   Relatively Uncommon Primary Tumors

A tumor can arise from any cell type, at nearly every site in the brain. Thus there are a wide variety of seldom-seen tumors. These can be the hardest to diagnose.

[1]   Primitive Neuroectodermal Tumor (PNET)

The primitive neuroectodermal tumor, traditionally known as cerebral neuroblastoma, is rare, with a peak incidence in children between ages one and five. The tumor tends to arise in the deep white matter of the frontoparietal regions (Greenberg and Polachini, 1995). Imaging studies show a large, well-defined mass with heterogeneous contrast enhancement, calcification and cystic changes. Symptoms are usually those of increased intracranial pressure.

The use of the term "primitive neuroectodermal tumor" is somewhat controversial, with some neuropathologists using it to refer to all tumors derived from neuroepithelial precursors, including medulloblastoma and pineoblastoma (Greenberg and Polachini, 1995).

[2]   Tumors of the Base of the Skull

Tumors arising at the base of the skull are rare. They include osteomas, fibromas, lipomas, teratomas and others. Most are benign.

[3]   Hemangioblastomas

Cerebellar hemangioblastomas are benign, circumscribed cystic tumors that account for 1 to 2.5 percent of intracranial tumors (Greenberg and Polachini, 1995). They tend to occur in the third to fifth decades. Symptoms are those of increased intracranial pressure. The prognosis is excellent with total surgical resection.

7.70 PITUITARY TUMORS

The pituitary gland is a small neuroendocrine structure located in a small cavity of the sphenoid bone called the sella turcica. It has three lobes—the anterior (adenohypophysis), the posterior (neurohypophysis) and the intermediate. *(See Figure 7-9.)* The adenohypophysis does not have a neural connection to the brain, but the neurohypophysis is continuous with the hypothalamus, the gland that controls pituitary function through blood vessels in the case of the anterior lobe and via neural input in the case of the posterior lobe. Pituitary adenomas are benign tumors of the adenohypophysis. They constitute about 5 percent of brain tumors (Harsh, 1994).

Because the pituitary gland produces a large number of hormones that are vital to regulation of glands throughout the body, any disorder affecting it will have wide-ranging effects (Laske and Oldfield, 1994). *(See Figure 7-10.)* The anterior lobe produces six hormones: prolactin, growth hormone, adrenocorticotrophic hormone (ACTH; adrenocorti-

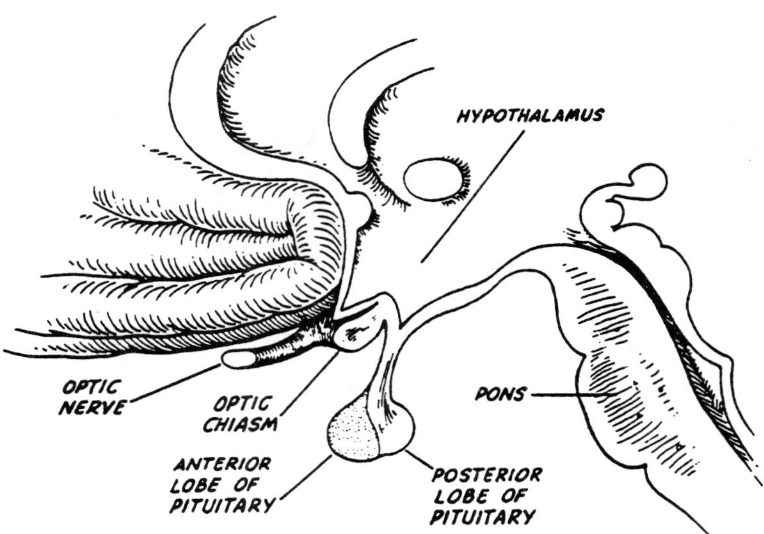

Figure 7-9. The relationship of the pituitary gland to surrounding structures.

cotrophin), thyroid-stimulating hormone (TSH, thyrotropin), luteiniz-
ing hormone (LH) and follicle-stimulating hormone (FH). The two
hormones secreted by the posterior lobe—vasopressin (antidiuretic
hormone; ADH) and oxytocin—regulate kidney resorption of water
and uterine contractions, respectively.

Symptoms of pituitary adenomas may be related to excessive
hormone secretion, deficient hormone production or mass effect on
nearby structures, such as the optic chiasm. Adenomas may be
functioning (producing hormone) or nonfunctioning.

7.71   Diagnosis and Treatment of Pituitary Adenomas

When symptoms suggest pituitary dysfunction, endocrine function
tests are typically the first step in diagnosis (Laske and Oldfield, 1994).

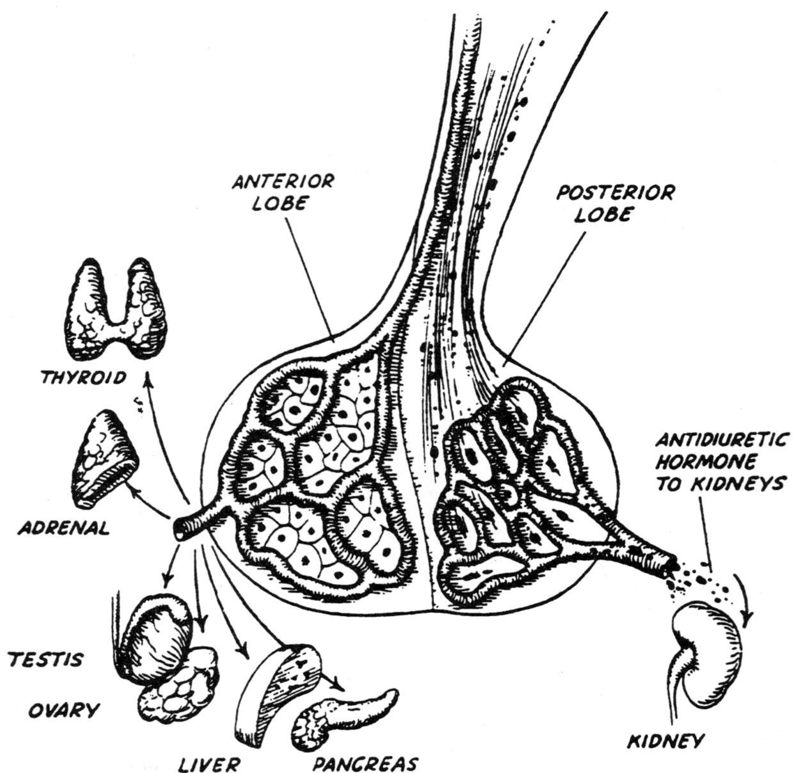

Figure 7-10. The distribution of hormones from the anterior lobe of the
pituitary gland to various structures affected by it.

These include assays of thyroid function, ACTH response and serum hormone levels (Eisenberg, et al., 1994). If these indicate the probability of a pituitary tumor, MRI studies are done.

MRI, both with and without contrast, is the imaging method of choice for suspected pituitary tumors, although CT is excellent for showing the sphenoid sinus anatomy (Greenberg and Polachini, 1995; Nelson, 1994). Timing of the studies in relation to contrast administration is more important for pituitary tumors than for most other types (Eisenberg, et al., 1994). Microadenomas may show contour abnormalities with stalk displacement.

Nonfunctioning pituitary adenomas are resected surgically (Nelson, 1994). Unless acute symptoms require prompt surgery, hormone replacement is instituted two to three weeks prior to surgery in order to optimize patient health. Medically unstable patients may be treated with radiation instead of surgery. Recurrence is about 20 percent after surgery alone and about 10 percent after surgery with radiation.

7.72 Functioning Pituitary Adenomas

Functioning tumors are usually microadenomas, 10 millimeters or less in diameter (Greenberg and Polachini, 1995; Laske and Oldfield, 1994). The clinical effects of these tumors result from excessive secretion of pituitary hormones. The most common secretions are prolactin, growth hormone and ACTH.

[1] Prolactinomas

The most common hypersecretory pituitary tumors are prolactinomas, which produce the hormone prolactin (Eisenberg, et al., 1994). They comprise about 40 percent of pituitary adenomas. More symptomatic in women than in men, they may produce deficiency of female gonad activity, with a decrease in estrogen secretion, osteoporosis, amenorrhea (cessation of menstruation) and galactorrhea (abnormal discharge of milk from the breasts) (Laske and Oldfield, 1994). Men experience loss of libido, impotence and infertility. Both may have visual impairment and headache.

Pharmacologic treatment with bromocriptine is useful for prolactinomas (Eisenberg, et al., 1994). This drug stimulates dopamine receptors on the prolactin-secreting cells and leads to tumor shrinkage. In most patients, the tumor re-expands when therapy is stopped. The usual side effects of this lifelong therapy are nausea and vomiting. In a few patients, however, the drug seems to have a permanent effect, and it is suggested that the drug be withdrawn every few years as a test.

Surgical resection is used to treat patients who cannot tolerate bromocriptine or who fail to respond to it. It is also used to treat women with tumors larger than 12 millimeters who wish to conceive. Surgery is followed by radiation therapy in patients with residual tumor who fail to respond to bromocriptine.

A few patients have asymptomatic microprolactinomas, in which the tumor size and secretion do not increase. These are often observed without treatment.

[2] Growth-Hormone-Secreting Adenomas

A pituitary adenoma may secrete excessive amounts of growth hormone, resulting in acromegaly in adults and gigantism in children. This is the most common cause of the syndrome (Eisenberg, et al., 1994). In acromegaly, facial features coarsen, hands and feet enlarge, sweating increases and organs enlarge. Headaches and osteoarthritis are common. Hypertension (high blood pressure) and atherosclerosis (deposits of fatty plaques in arteries) are increased. As the adenoma enlarges, it may compress the optic system and lead to visual deficits. Excessive growth hormone secretion is also associated with colon polyps.

Untreated acromegaly is eventually fatal. Trans-sphenoidal resection, usually through a sublabial (beneath the upper lip) or trans-septal (through the nasal septum) approach, is usually successful, with a low morbidity. Pituitary function is preserved in 95 percent of cases. In cases in which surgery is not possible, the somatostatin analog octreotide is effective in suppressing growth hormone production and shrinking the tumor. Unfortunately, it must be injected three times a day, and the incidence of the side effects of diarrhea and gallstones increases with continued use. The drug is sometimes used to shrink the tumor preoperatively. Radiation therapy has equivocal results.

[3] ACTH-Secreting Adenomas (Cushing's Disease)

A corticotrophin-producing pituitary adenoma secretes excessive ACTH, resulting in overproduction of cortisol by the adrenal gland. The result is Cushing's syndrome, for which a pituitary adenoma is only one possible cause (Laske and Oldfield, 1994). Symptoms include skin lesions, fatigue, lack of a feeling of well-being, muscle weakness, and pain and weight gain, with characteristic fat deposition in the face, shoulders and trunk. Patients may develop atherosclerosis, hypertension, diabetes and osteoporosis (Eisenberg, et al., 1994).

Distinguishing between an adenoma and other possible causes of Cushing's syndrome can be frustrating, for symptoms occur while the tumor is small and often not detectable in imaging studies. Studies include measurements of plasma baseline and stimulated cortisol and ACTH levels. In doubtful cases, ACTH is measured in a sample from the petrosal sinus.

Treatment is trans-sphenoidal microsurgical exploration with selective adenomectomy. Repeat surgery, sometimes with total resection, may be necessary to effect a cure. Eventual cure is attained in 90 percent of cases. The reported efficacy of radiation therapy ranges from 50 to 100 percent. The available drugs only treat the symptoms, and their side effects tend to be unpleasant. Ketoconazole, which blocks the enzymes involved in cortisol and testosterone production, may be used for interim treatment if surgery must be postponed.

[4] Glycoprotein-Secreting Adenomas (TSH, FSH, LH)

Adenomas secreting the gonadotropic hormones FSH or LH are rare. The tumors that do secrete these hormones do not produce a specific hypersecretory syndrome and are not discovered until they grow to a size that impinges on nearby structures, such as the optic chiasm (Eisenberg, et al., 1994). By the time of diagnosis, the possibility of surgical cure is usually low, because of sinus and suprasellar involvement.

Trans-sphenoidal resection is followed by radiation therapy if some tumor remains. This gives symptomatic relief. Twice-yearly follow-up is recommended.

Excessive TSH (thyroid-stimulating hormone) production is rarely the cause of hyperthyroidism. When such a tumor does arise, the symptoms are those of hyperthyroidism.

7.73 Nonfunctioning Pituitary Adenomas

About 30 percent of pituitary adenomas are nonfunctioning tumors that arise from nonsecreting pituitary cells (Nelson, 1994). These tumors are usually macroadenomas measuring more than 10 millimeters in diameter. They may be either cystic or solid but are usually solid.

Nonfunctioning pituitary adenomas are most common in the fourth and fifth decades. Because they do not lead to hormone overproduction, which would create symptoms, they are often not diagnosed until they are quite large (Nelson, 1994). Then they cause symptoms due to mass effect, by compression of the optic chiasm or cranial nerves III to VI. Headache or progressive visual field loss are common symptoms. Adenoma growth can also lead to enlargement of the sella. Impingement on the hypothalamus may cause temperature, hunger or sleep disturbances.

As the adenoma grows, pituitary function gradually diminishes. The usual order of loss of hormone secretion is: gonadotropin, growth hormone, thyroid-stimulating hormone, ACTH.

7.80   METASTATIC BRAIN TUMORS

Nearly 25 percent of cancer patients develop metastases to the brain; such metastases constitute about half to two thirds of all tumors in the brain (Young and Patchell, 1994). Cancers that commonly metastasize to the brain are lung (with a 30 percent incidence of brain metastases), breast (30 percent incidence), gastrointestinal and renal-cell cancer, and melanoma (22 percent incidence) (Greenberg and Polachini, 1995). About 15 percent of metastases involve the cerebral meninges; these frequently originate with leukemias, 11 to 70 percent of which metastasize to the meninges; lymphomas; small cell bronchial carcinoma or a primary CNS tumor. Disability or death in patients with brain metastases results from the brain involvement more often than from systemic disease (Young and Patchell, 1994). In a few cases, metastasis to the brain is the first sign of cancer elsewhere.

Metastases to the brain may be solitary or multiple. Most multiple brain tumors are due to metastases. Typical characteristics of metastatic brain tumors include prominent edema, cystic changes, necrosis and hemorrhage (Greenberg and Polachini, 1995). Most metastases show contrast enhancement in both CT and MRI. Because a single metastasis and an abscess can appear very similar in CT or MRI, a biopsy[31] is often necessary for definitive diagnosis (Pauker and

---

[31] *See* 7.46 *supra* for discussion of biopsy.

Kopelman, 1993; Young and Patchell, 1994). Biopsies have shown that about 10 percent of suspected solitary brain metastases in patients with systemic cancer were due to other causes.

A single discrete metastatic lesion in a patient with controlled systemic disease is usually treated by combined surgery and irradiation (Young and Patchell, 1994). However, in about half of patients with a single metastasis, surgery is not attempted because of a risk of neurologic deficit due to tumor location or because the systemic neoplastic disease is uncontrolled. Many cerebral metastases are in highly functional areas near the middle cerebral artery. Metastases often result in significant cerebral edema, which should be reduced by steroid administration prior to surgery, when this is possible.

Stereotactic microsurgical techniques are best for removal of a metastasis (Kelly, 1991). This enhances precise localization of the tumor, minimizes damage to nearby tissues and improves control of bleeding. When possible, incision is through a sulcus (groove) rather than a gyrus (ridge). Surgery followed by radiation prolongs survival, versus radiation alone (Greenberg and Polachini, 1995). Because of the high probability of multiple metastases, some experts advise searching for multiple lesions in MRI by use of a higher-than-normal dose of gadolinium prior to surgery (Greenberg and Polachini, 1995).

Disseminated brain metastases are treated by radiation alone (Young and Patchell, 1994). Chemotherapy may also be used. Sometimes multiple lesions may be removed by stereotactic radiosurgery.

7.90 PROGNOSIS

The prognosis of a brain tumor depends on its location, pathologic characteristics, stage at diagnosis, extent of involvement of intracranial structures, accessibility for surgery and responsiveness to radiation and chemotherapy (Haerer, 1992). Although survival time has increased somewhat as a result of better surgical and radiotherapeutic techniques, the outlook remains grim for most patients with malignant tumors. Even benign tumors tend to recur, and repeat surgery is often required.

Controversy exists about the type and frequency of surveillance that is most effective in detecting a recurrence in time for effective treatment. In children, the performance of follow-up imaging studies is generally recommended every three months for the first year and every six months for up to five years (Pollack, 1994). Some groups contend that outcome is better if any recurrence is detected at a presymptomatic stage, but others claim that the prognosis for recurrent disease is dismal whether it is detected before or after symptoms are evident.

7.100 BIBLIOGRAPHY

Text References

Abbott, R., et al.: Brainstem Tumors: Surgical Indications. In: Cheek, W. R. (Ed.): Pediatric Neurosurgery, 3rd ed. Philadelphia: Saunders., 1994.

Adelman, J. U.: Headache and Other Craniofacial Pains. In: Greenberg, J. O.: Neuroimaging. New York: McGraw-Hill, Inc., 1995.

Allen, J. C.: Controversies in the Management of Intracranial Germ Cell Tumors. Neurol. Clin. 9:441-452, 1991.

Al-Mefty, O. and Origitano, T. C.: Meningiomas. In: Rengachary, S. S. and Wilkins, R. H. (Eds.): Principles of Neurosurgery. London: Mosby-Wolfe, 1994.

Al-Mefty, O., et al.: The Long-Term Side Effects of Radiation Therapy for Benign Brain Tumors in Adults. J. Neurosurg. 73:502-512, 1990.

Berger, M. S. and Ojemann, G. A.: Techniques of Functional Localization During Removal of Tumors Involving the Cerebral Hemispheres. In: Loftus, C. M. and Traynelis, V. C.: Intraoperative Monitoring Techniques in the Nervous System. New York: McGraw-Hill, 1994.

Brody, A. S.: New Perspectives in CT and MR Imaging. Neurol. Clin. 9:273-286, 1991.

Burger, P. C. and Fuller, G. N.: Pathology—Trends and Pitfalls in Histologic Diagnosis, Immunopathology, and Applications of Oncogene Research. Neurol. Clin. 9:249-271, 1991.

Coffey, R. J.: Stereotactic Radiosurgery and Focused Beam Irradiation. In: Rengachary, S. S. and Wilkins, R. H. (Eds.): Principles of Neurosurgery. London: Mosby-Wolfe, 1994.

Duffner, P. K. and Cohen, M. E.: The Long-Term Effects of Central Nervous System Therapy on Children with Brain Tumors. Neurol. Clin. 9:479-495, 1991. Edelman, R. R. and Warach, S.: Medical

Progress: Magnetic Resonance Imaging. N. Engl. J. Med. 328:708-716, 1993.

Edwards, M. S. B. and Baumgartner, I.: Pineal Region Tumors. In: Cheek, W. R. (Ed.): Pediatric Neurosurgery, 3rd ed. Philadelphia: Saunders, 1994.

Eisenberg, M. B., et al.: Functioning Pituitary Adenomas. In: Rengachary, S. S. and Wilkins, R. H. (Eds.): Principles of Neurosurgery. London: Mosby-Wolfe, 1994.

Freeman, C. R. and Lehnert, S.: Radiotherapy Dose-Fractionation Schedules. Neurol Clin. 9:351-362, 1991.

Friedman, W. A. and Spiegelmann, R.: Stereotactic Surgery and Radiosurgery. In: Little, J. R. and Awad, I. A. (Eds.): Reoperative Neurosurgery. Baltimore: Williams & Wilkins, 1992.

Greenberg, J. O. and Polachini, I.: Intracranial Neoplasms. In: Greenberg, J. O.: Neuroimaging. New York: McGraw-Hill, Inc., 1995.

Haerer, A. F.: Differential Diagnosis of Intracranial Disease. In: Haerer, A. F.: DeJong's The Neurologic Examination, 5th ed. Philadelphia: Lippincott, 1992.

Halperin, E. C. and Anscher, M. S.: Radiation Therapy for Central Nervous System Tumors. In: Rengachary, S. S. and Wilkins, R. H. (Eds.): Principles of Neurosurgery. London: Mosby-Wolfe, 1994.

Harsh, G. R., IV: Neuro-Oncology: Overview. In: Rengachary, S. S. and Wilkins, R. H. (Eds.): Principles of Neurosurgery. London: Mosby-Wolfe, 1994.

Hoffman, H. J. and Kestle, J. R. W.: Craniopharyngiomas. In: Cheek, W. R. (Ed.): Pediatric Neurosurgery, 3rd ed. Philadelphia: Saunders, 1994.

Johnson, D. L. and McCullough, D. C.: Optic Nerve Gliomas and Other Tumors Involving the Optic Nerve and Chiasm. In: Cheek, W. R. (Ed.): Pediatric Neurosurgery, 3rd ed. Philadelphia: Saunders, 1994.

Kelly, P. J.: Tumor Stereotaxis. Philadelphia: Saunders, 1991. Kepes, J. J.: Pitfalls and Problems in the Histopathologic Evaluation of Stereotactic Needle Biopsy Specimens. Neurosurg. Clin. N. Am. 5:19-33, 1994.

Kun, L. E. Radiation Therapy: Trends in Treatment. Neurol Clin. 9:337-350, 1991.

Larson, D. A. and Coffey, R. J.: Radiosurgery: Devices, Principles, and Rationale. Clin. Neurosurg. 40:429-445, 1993.

Laske, D. W. and Oldfield, E. H.: Assessment of Pituitary Function. In: Rengachary, S. S. and Wilkins, R. H. (Eds.): Principles of Neurosurgery. London: Mosby-Wolfe, 1994.

Levine, R. A., et al.: Auditory Evoked Potentials and Other Neurophysiologic Monitoring Techniques During Surgery in The Cerebellopontine Angle. In: Loftus, C. M. and Traynelis, V. C.: Intraoperative Monitoring Techniques in the Nervous System. New York: McGraw-Hill, 1994.

Lew, C. M. and LaVally, B.: The Role of Stereotactic Radiation Therapy in the Management of Children with Brain Tumors. J. Pediatr. Oncol. Nurs. 12:212-222, 1995.

McDonald, J. D. and Rosenblum, M. L.: Gliomas. In: Rengachary, S. S. and Wilkins, R. H. (Eds.): Principles of Neurosurgery. London: Mosby-Wolfe, 1994.

Moller, A. R.: Intra-Operative Neurophysiologic Monitoring in Neurosurgery: Benefits, Efficacy, and Cost Effectiveness. Clin. Neurosurg. 42:171-179, 1995.

Nelson, P. B.: Nonfunctioning Pituitary Adenomas. In: Rengachary, S. S. and Wilkins, R. H. (Eds.): Principles of Neurosurgery. London: Mosby-Wolfe, 1994.

O'Brien, M. S. and Krisht, A.: Cerebellar Astrocytoma. In: Cheek, W. R. (Ed.): Pediatric Neurosurgery, 3rd ed. Philadelphia: Saunders, 1994.

Pauker, S. G. and Kopelman, R. I.: Clinical Problem-Solving: A Rewarding Pursuit of Certainty. N. Engl. J. Med. 329:644-656, 1993.

Pollack, I. F.: Brain Tumors in Children. N. Engl. J. Med. 331:1500-1507, 1994.

Preston-Martin, S.: Epidemiology of Primary CNS Tumors. Neurol. Clin. 14:273-290, 1996.

Rorke, L. B.: Introductory Survey of Brain Tumors. In: Cheek, W. R. (Ed.): Pediatric Neurosurgery, 3rd ed. Philadelphia: Saunders, 1994.

Rozental, J. M.: Positron Emission Tomography (PET) and Single-Photon Emission Computed Tomography (SPECT) of Brain Tumors. Neurol. Clin. 9:287-305, 1991. Sanford, R. A. and Muhlbauer, M. S.: Craniopharyngioma in Children. Clin. Neurol 9:453-465, 1991.

Schold, S. C., Jr.: Chemotherapy of Central Nervous System Tumors. In: Rengachary, S. S. and Wilkins, R. H. (Eds.): Principles of Neurosurgery. London: Mosby-Wolfe, 1994.

Slavin, K. V. and Ausman, J. I.: Tumors of the Pineal Region. In: Rengachary, S. S. and Wilkins, R. H. (Eds.): Principles of Neurosurgery. London: Mosby-Wolfe, 1994. Starshak, R. J.: Radiation-Induced Meningioma in Children: Report of Two Cases and Review of the Literature. Pediatr. Radiol. 26:537-541, 1996.

Strauss, C., et al.: Monitoring of Visual Evoked Potentials During Para-and Suprasellar Procedures. In: Loftus, C. M. and Traynelis, V. C.: Intraoperative Monitoring Techniques in the Nervous System. New York: McGraw-Hill, 1994.

Sure, U., et al.: Secondary Manifestation of Medulloblastoma: Metastases and Local Recurrences in 66 Patients. Acta Neurochir. 136:117-126, 1995.

Sutton, L. N. and Packer, R. J.: Medulloblastomas. In: Cheek, W. R. (Ed.): Pediatric Neurosurgery, 3rd ed. Philadelphia: Saunders, 1994.

Tasker, R. R. and Bernstein, M.: Stereotactic Surgery. In: Rengachary, S. S. and Wilkins, R. H. (Eds.): Principles of Neurosurgery. London: Mosby-Wolfe, 1994.

Turner, D. A.: Perioperative Care of the Neurosurgical Patient. In: Rengachary, S. S. and Wilkins, R. H. (Eds.): Principles of Neurosurgery. London: Mosby-Wolfe, 1994.

Walker, M. L. and Petronio, J.: Posterior Fossa Tumors. In: Rengachary, S. S. and Wilkins, R. H. (Eds.): Principles of Neurosurgery. London: Mosby-Wolfe, 1994.

Westmoreland, B. F., et al.: Medical Neurosciences, 3rd ed. Boston: Little, Brown, 1994.

Wilkins, R. H.: Cerebellopontine Angle Tumors. In: Rengachary, S. S. and Wilkins, R. H. (Eds.): Principles of Neurosurgery. London: Mosby-Wolfe, 1994.

Wisoff, J. H.: Tumors of the Cerebral Hemisphere. In: Cheek, W. R. (Ed.): Pediatric Neurosurgery, 3rd ed. Philadelphia: Saunders, 1994.

Young, B. and Patchell, R. A.: Metastatic Tumors. In: Rengachary, S. S. and Wilkins, R. H. (Eds.): Principles of Neurosurgery. London: Mosby-Wolfe, 1994.Additional References

Brain Tumor Foundation of Canada. URL: http://www.btfc.org/ Gilles, F. H., et al.: Childhood Brain Tumor Consortium. Histologic Feature Reliability in Childhood Neural Tumors. J. Neuropathol. Exp. Neurol. 53:559-571, 1994.

Kelly, P. J.: Stereotactic Surgical Procedures for Brain. URL: http://mcns10.med.nyu.edu/index.html

Maciunas, R. J., et al.: A Technique for Interactive Image-Guided Neurosurgical Intervention in Primary Brain Tumors. Neurosurg. Clin. N. Amer. 7:245-266, 1996. Pang, D.: Craniopharyngiomas. In: Rengachary, S. S. and Wilkins, R. H. (Eds.): Principles of Neurosurgery. London: Mosby-Wolfe, 1994.

Schiff, D. and Wen, P. Y.: Uncommon Brain Tumors. Neurol. Clin. 13:953-974, 1995.

Tatter, S.: A Primer of Brain Tumors. Des Plaines, Ill.: American Brain Tumor Association. URL: http://neurosurgery.mgh.harvard.edu/ abta/

CHAPTER 8

Surgical Treatment of Head Injuries

SCOPE

Head injuries are divided roughly into the categories of closed head injury, depressed fracture of the skull and compound fracture of the skull. In compound fracture, there is the likelihood that the pericranial tissues have been torn and that the brain is exposed or severely damaged. Blunt head injuries, even when they are relatively minor, present the potential for serious consequences such as hemorrhage or slow bleeding, with attendant complications involving, for example, the potentially life-threatening development of increased intracranial pressure. Management of intracranial bleeding and evacuation of clots and hematomas are major lifesaving aspects of the neurosurgical care of patients with head injury. Surgery is almost always indicated in open head injuries. The outcome of patients with head injuries is directly related to the nature of the injury, the severity of brain damage and the quality and speed of initial treatment and management. In general, a patient who survives critical brain injury has a good chance for recovery with minimal disability.

SYNOPSIS

8.00 OVERVIEW

The care and management of patients with significant head injuries is complex and requires the services of a variety of specialists. Although patients with head injury may be housed primarily in the facilities of departments of neurology, general surgery or other specialty groups, their care virtually always requires consultation and possibly treatment by neurosurgical specialists. In most major centers that have specialized neurosurgical services, patients with head injury are assigned to neurosurgery, and a neurosurgeon will have the primary responsibility for their care.

The initial treatment of patients with head injury takes place at the site of the traumatic event and in the emergency department of the facility. The role of the emergency department is to guarantee that patients are cared for according to the severity of their injuries (triaged) and that proper diagnosis and initial management are carried out expeditiously. The ultimate outcome of these patients depends largely on how vigorously the emergency personnel fulfill this role (Gennarelli and Kotapka, 1992).

The task of caring for the patient with head injury requires the integration of surgical and nonsurgical treatment, and often the boundaries between surgical and nonsurgical fields overlap. The following text will review the various measures used in treating patients with head injury that require invasive procedures of a primarily surgical nature.

8.01 Treatment Goals

The surgical and nonsurgical methods of management are limited by the extent of brain damage that is incurred at the moment of injury. Once the cells of the brain die, they do not regenerate; therefore, the major surgical goals must be to:

- preserve life during the initial acute period when shock, impaired respiration, hemorrhage and other problems may be life threatening;
- minimize the possibility of further damage to the brain from bony fragments of the skull, and from bleeding and brain swelling;
- minimize the possibility of intracranial infection in open and penetrating head injuries by removing devitalized tissue, cleansing the wound and repairing openings in the dura (outer membrane covering the brain) and skull that can allow microorganisms to enter the intracranial space;
- restore free flow of cerebrospinal fluid;

- repair and treat cranial nerve injuries;

- repair skull and scalp injuries; and

- combat infections and treat abscesses with methods that require intracranial surgery.

These goals cannot include restoration of function to nerve cells within the brain that are already hopelessly damaged. However, neurosurgical intervention may be lifesaving and sometimes can result in dramatic improvements in a patient's clinical state by removing conditions (intracranial blood clots, for example) that are impairing the function of neurons without actually causing the nerve cells to die.

8.02   Treatment Limitations

Much of the living brain is a soft, almost gel-like substance that is extremely fragile and readily injured. The neurosurgeon is limited by the extent of surgical manipulation that is possible without adding to the brain injury; minimal damage to overlying brain tissues and structures is unavoidable when the surgeon must reach deeper-lying brain structures. Other restraints stem from the fact that most neurosurgical procedures are lengthy and require general anesthesia, with its attendant risks. In addition, because they are usually severely injured and may have cardiovascular, respiratory and hormonal disturbances that add to these risks, patients with head injury are often relatively poor candidates for extensive surgery and general anesthesia.

When the patient has no chance for survival without surgical intervention, extensive "heroic" procedures may be attempted even though the chance of saving the patient is relatively small. The decision to undertake surgical treatment when the prognosis is unfavorable depends on many factors. If the decision is made to undertake surgical treatment even in unfavorable cases, the neurosurgeon is often dealing with a patient who has almost no chance of survival without surgery.

For many patients with head injury, care is largely limited to general supportive measures and careful attention to maintaining nondamaging levels of intracranial pressure (ICP). Monitoring a patient's intracranial pressure is most often accomplished through a ventriculostomy catheter; however, neurosurgeons also use fiberoptic ICP catheters, cerebral blood flow measurement probes, microdialysis catheters, jugular venous oxygen saturation catheters and brain oxygen content measurement electrodes.

8.10 EMERGENCY AND EARLY SURGICAL MANAGEMENT

The initial care of a patient with head injury requires an assessment of the severity of the injury and protection of the brain from further damage until a definitive diagnosis and treatment can be achieved. Care of the surgical patient with head injury requires coordinated teamwork by perioperative nurses, neurosurgeons, anesthesia care providers and emergency department staff members (Pieper, et al., 1996).

Most head injuries fall into two categories: focal and diffuse. *Focal* injury refers to brain injuries with a lesion large enough to be seen by the naked eye. *Diffuse* injuries are those associated with more widespread disruption of neurologic function and are not usually macroscopically visible. The outcome from head injury depends largely on which type of injury is present, the severity of the injury and how aggressively the injury has been managed (Gennarelli and Kotapka, 1992).

By evaluating three basic items, the severity of brain injury can be assessed in less than one minute:

1. level of consciousness;

2. pupillary function; and

3. lateralized weakness of the extremities.

Abnormality of all three is highly indicative of a focal mass lesion requiring surgery; level of consciousness may be the only abnormality in diffuse brain injury (Gennarelli and Kotapka, 1992).

Emergency management may include adequate oxygenation, rapid correction of hypotension (low blood pressure) and treatment of increased intracranial pressure (ICP). The ultimate goal is to prevent secondary brain damage in a patient with a recently injured and vulnerable brain. Transfer from the scene of injury to the emergency room and the intensive care unit increases the likelihood of secondary insult from hypoxia (inadequate oxygenation), hypotension or surges of increased intracranial pressure. In most cases, the neurologist and neurosurgeon become closely involved in patient care at this point (Wijdicks, 1995).

Patients who appear not to be seriously injured must be thoroughly evaluated in the emergency facility. Patients without open injuries and who are not in coma may nevertheless be neurologically abnormal. Patients with major trauma should be transported to hospitals with neurointensive care or neurosurgical facilities.

8.11 "On Site" Care and Transport

When a severe head injury occurs, a few minutes can make the difference between life and death. The first responders to an incident are typically law enforcement personnel and firefighters, who are trained in first aid and cardiopulmonary resuscitation (CPR), basic procedures to protect the cervical (neck) spine and control of any obvious hemorrhage. Emergency medical technicians (EMTs) and paramedics provide advanced life support, administer medications and fluids, and provide electrocardiogram (EKG) monitoring (Eckstein, 1995).

Patients with acute head injury may move about with their eyes open. However, although they are apparently awake and may be talking, they may not be fully conscious. Individuals in this state of confusion and panic have severely impaired judgment and may attempt to flee the scene or resist treatment, insisting that they are unhurt. Patients may also be in an obvious confused state, with grossly incoherent or absent speech. These individuals should be gently but firmly brought under control for appropriate treatment.

8.12 Initial Emergency Care in a Medical Facility

When the patient with head injury arrives at the hospital emergency department, several resuscitative and stabilizing measures have already been instituted by emergency personnel. It is essential for the surgeon providing definitive care to have a complete and thorough understanding of both the capabilities and the limitations of these initial interventions (Eckstein, 1995).

The initial triage in the emergency department is the same as in the field, focusing on the provision of an adequate airway and the control of major bleeding. A verbal report from the paramedics is important, not only for the physician to know what was done in the field but also to determine whether the patient's neurologic status is improving or worsening.

Convulsions can occur even after mild head injury, and they are a serious concern to the emergency physician. Seizures may indicate the development of an intracranial hemorrhage, or the seizure may be a manifestation of direct cerebral injury. The seizure itself can change the intracranial dynamics, causing further damage, bleeding or brain herniation. Some neurosurgeons feel that all traumatized unconscious patients should receive intravenous drug treatment to prevent seizures (Schwartz, et al., 1992). Phenytoin is the anticonvulsant medication that is most frequently used, since it can safely be given intravenously. When the drug is loaded (an initial bolus of a higher dose), seizure protection occurs within hours.

A simple neurologic examination is performed to assess the patient's level of consciousness. Associated injuries or medical conditions may require immediate treatment. Additional diagnostic procedures, such as baseline blood tests, simple x-rays, computed tomography (CT) scans or electroencephalogram (EEG), may be ordered. For example, a blood test may indicate that the unconscious patient is diabetic and that abnormally high or low blood sugar level rather than head injury is the medical cause of unconsciousness (Schwartz, et al., 1992).

8.13   Early Care in Neurologic Intensive Care Units

Most patients with severe head injuries are cared for in intensive care units, which allows for the constant monitoring of blood pressure, heart rate and respiration. Specialized neurologic intensive care units are available in some facilities. Continuous monitoring of intracranial pressure by insertion of a sensing device into some region within the cranium may also be available. Further neurologic evaluation may require performing CT scans, MRI, angiography or lumbar puncture.

The single most important component of neurologic examination following head injury is the determination of the level of consciousness of the patient. In unconscious patients or in those with a disturbed level of consciousness, the scope of the examination may be severely limited because of its dependence on patient cooperation. The unconscious patient's respiratory funciton, motor response to pain, pupillary reaction to light and corneal reflexes are noted. The presence of unilateral pupillary dilatation and unreactivity implies the existence of a mass lesion, requiring urgent diagnosis and surgical evacuation of the mass (Moulton, 1992).

The Glasgow Coma Scale[1] and the Rancho Los Amigos Scale are commonly used to evaluate level of consciousness. A person who is

---

[1] *See* 8.23[4] *infra.*

not comatose may nevertheless harbor a serious intracranial injury. Patients who have either pupillary or extremity abnormalities most likely have a focal lesion of insufficient size at the moment to compress the brain stem enough to produce coma. All such patients should be admitted for further testing.

8.20   INTRACRANIAL HEMORRHAGE AND HEMATOMA

Bleeding is inevitable in penetrating head wounds, since the scalp, skull, meninges (membranes enveloping the brain) and brain substances are richly supplied with blood. In many instances, bleeding is relatively minor unless major vessels are involved, and it can be easily controlled at the time of the initial treatment of the wound.

Blunt head injuries, even when they are relatively minor, present the potential for serious hemorrhage or slow bleeding. The blood clot becomes an expanding mass inside the tightly closed intracranial space, exerting pressure on brain tissues. The management of intracranial bleeding and evacuation of the well-formed clots and the organized form (hematoma) these clots rapidly assume is a major lifesaving aspect of the neurosurgical care of patients with head injury.

Bleeding within the skull is usually described in terms of the anatomic location relative to the membranous coverings (the meninges) of the brain and spinal cord. The outer meningeal layer (dura mater) is thick and fibrous; the inner layer (pia mater) is delicately thin and attached to the surface of the brain; the intermediate layer (arachnoid) is a loosely constructed tissue of honeycomb structure and not always well defined. Traumatic intracranial hemorrhage may be epidural (between dura mater and skull), subdural (between dura mater and arachnoid), subarachnoid (between arachnoid and pia mater) or intracerebral (within the substance of the brain proper). *(See Figure 8-1.)*

8.21   Subarachnoid Hemorrhage

Subarachnoid bleeding is the most common type of hemorrhage following trauma. Abrasions, contusions and lacerations of the cortical surface cause bleeding into the subarachnoid space, leading to meningeal irritation and headache, nuchal (pertaining to the back of the neck) rigidity and photophobia (sensitivity to light) (D'Angelo, 1994).

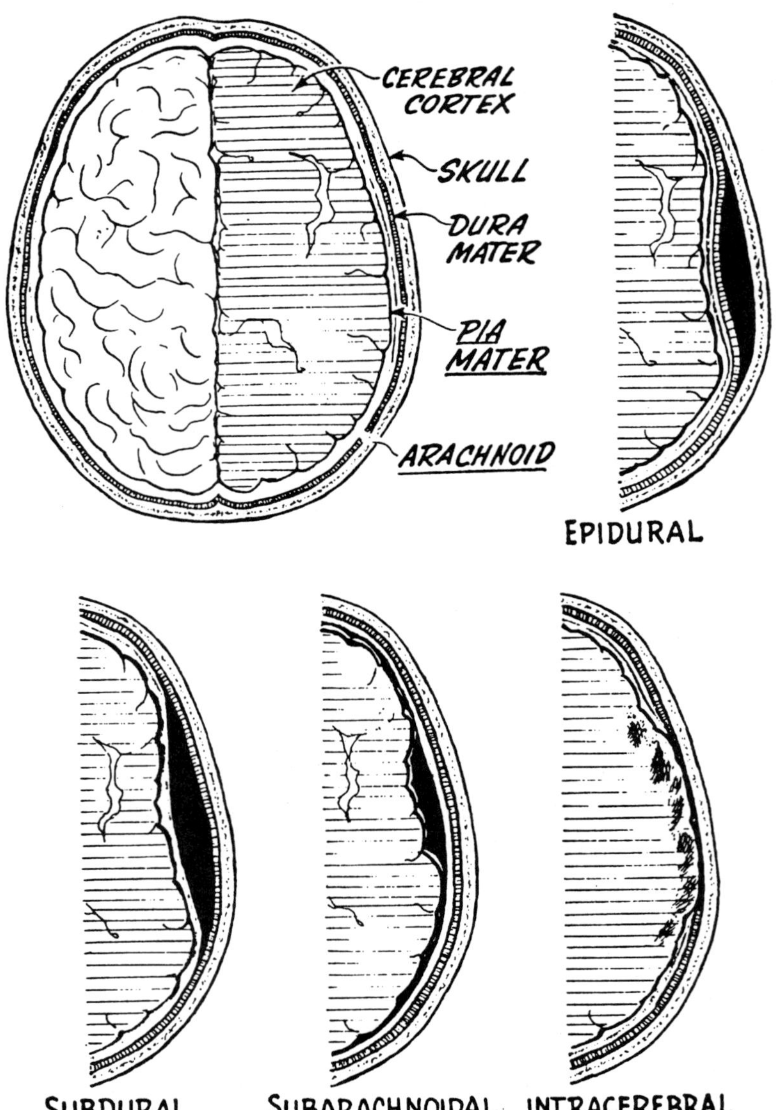

Fig. 8-1. The meninges surrounding the brain and spinal cord (top left) and common types of intracranial hemorrhage.

In most cases, serious clinical sequelae to subarachnoid hemorrhage are not observed, and subarachnoid hemorrhage is of little concern except to warn the physician that serious damage to the brain or its coverings may have occurred. No specific treatment is required; however, repeated CT scans are recommended to exclude the possibility of additional intracranial loculated (with small cavities) blood (Rowland, 1995).

8.22   Epidural Hemorrhage and Hematoma

Epidural hematoma (EDH) is caused by bleeding into the potential space between the inner surface of the skull and the dura mater, usually as a result of arterial bleeding from a rupture or tear in the middle meningeal artery or its branches. A dilated and fixed pupil is symptomatic of this injury; it is always on the same side as the clot and is caused by compression of the third cranial nerve.[2] In about 15 percent of patients, bleeding may occur from blood vessels of one of the dural sinuses (large channels in the dura mater that convey venous blood from the cerebrum into the veins of the neck). The hematoma is usually located over the convexity of the hemisphere in the middle fossa (the middle of three depressions in the floor of the skull, it supports the temporal lobe of the brain and the pituitary gland), but occasionally the hemorrhage may be confined to the anterior fossa (the convexity that supports the frontal lobes of the brain) (Rowland, 1995).

Since the body has no mechanism for the absorption of an epidural hematoma, the clotted blood must be removed surgically. Hemorrhage into the epidural space, if it is left untreated, causes death within a few days due to the pressure effects on the brain (Rowland, 1995).

[1]   Signs, Symptoms and Progression

The classic description of the progression of acute epidural hematoma is as follows: a blow to the head resulting in linear fracture crossing the middle meningeal groove of the temporal bone; brief loss of consciousness; a regaining of consciousness (lucid interval); arterial bleeding with an expanding epidural mass; increasing intracranial pressure with obtundation (the person is dazed); tentorial herniation[3]

---

[2] *See also* ch. 4 for a full discussion of the description and diagnosis of intracranial hematomas.

[3] *See* 8.51[2] *infra.*

with contralateral hemiparesis (paralysis of the opposite side of the body) and ipsilateral (pertaining to the same side) pupillary dilatation; decerebrate rigidity; respiratory irregularity and death (D'Angelo, 1994).

Surgical treatment of epidural hematoma can result in complete recovery if it is accomplished early. Delay can lead to ischemia (lack of blood supply) and other damaging effects of pressure.

[2] Management of Asymptomatic Hematoma

An important controversial issue concerns the management of patients with a small epidural hematoma that does not produce appreciable clinical signs. One study has shown that such patients, managed conservatively, had a 55 percent chance of delayed expansion requiring surgical intervention when associated skull fractures traversed the meninges or major dural vessels, such as the transverse sinus. Approximately 60 percent of these patients did not show signs of clinical deterioration in the course of conservative management (Wijdicks, 1995). Another study showed that conservative management of asymptomatic epidural hematomas may be appropriate, except when CT scan indicates a volume of more than 30 mL, thickness of more than 15 mm and a midline shift beyond 5 mm (Wijdicks, 1995).

[3] Surgical Pathophysiology

Bleeding in cases of epidural hematoma usually stems from the middle meningeal or posterior meningeal artery, both of which pass through the space between the skull and dura. The principal trunk of the middle meningeal artery is in the temporal region; other major branches are in the frontal and posterior parietal regions. *(See Figure 8-2.)* Epidural hemorrhage in the occipital region is less common.

Arterial bleeding physically strips the dura from the skull, forming a clot at the site of arterial damage. Commonly this occurs at the site of a skull fracture where the fracture line crosses the meningeal artery (in adults, this artery is partly embedded in grooves on the inner surface of the skull).

EDH may also result from blood oozing from torn veins. Venous blood is under lower pressure than blood in the arteries; therefore, venous bleeding occurs more slowly.

Depressed and linear skull fractures raise the possibility of underlying epidural hematoma. In these instances, the source of bleeding is

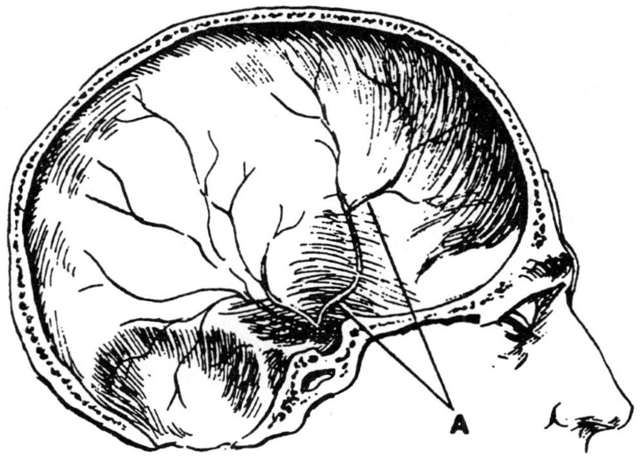

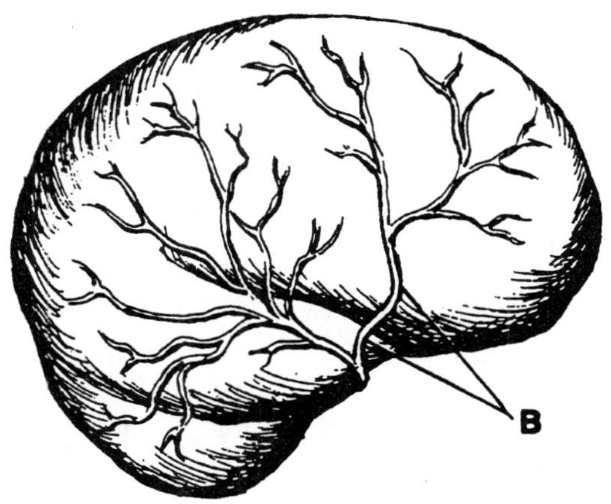

Fig. 8-2. The course of the middle meningeal artery. (A) Grooves of the middle meningeal artery. (B) Middle meningeal artery on the surface of the dura.

the diploic veins within the skull itself. Such bleeding is under relatively low pressure and usually is not life threatening.

Because the dura and skull are tightly bound together, there is significant resistance to expansion and separation of the dura from the skull, effectively slowing the early hemorrhage process. As the mass of the EDH expands, however, it forms a clot and continues to tear other vessels as the dura is stripped from the skull. If the region of clot and fresh bleeding is extensive or strategically placed, it can increase intracranial pressure rapidly and force brain tissue downward into the tentorial notch (a circular opening in the dura at the base of the cerebrum, through which the brain stem passes), compressing the vital centers in the brain stem that control heartbeat and respiration as well as the blood vessels that serve them, resulting in rapid death.

A clot that develops more slowly may change in structure from a loosely organized blood clot with fresh bleeding into an organized, solid mass. Part of this process includes the migration of cells from the dura into the clot, forming a more solid tissue mass. This occurs about a week after injury. Later, blood vessels invade the hematoma. In the early stages, draining a largely liquid mass and achieving control of bleeding is the principal surgical challenge. In chronic EDH, removal of a solid or semi-solid mass may also involve a developed blood supply that potentially can serve as a fresh source of bleeding.

[4] Diagnostic Procedures

Diagnosis of epidural hematoma is made by computed tomography (CT) scan rather than MRI scan, which is not as sensitive for blood. Lumbar puncture is no longer used, and CT supersedes the use of x-rays. The electroencephalogram (EEG) has also been superseded by CT scan as a diagnostic test for EDH. Patterns in the EEG are not consistent, and the EEG record might even be normal. EEG may be important, however, if there are seizures (Rowland, 1995).

[5] Surgical Treatment

Surgical removal of the clot is the treatment for epidural hematoma (EDH). In a patient with rapid neurologic deterioration, the initial procedure is the placement of one or two burr holes just anterior to (in front of) the upper ear, allowing immediate access to the hematoma. The burr holes may be in the temporal, frontal or other regions of the skull, based on information about the site of impact, site of fracture and known patterns of the locations of the major meningeal arteries. If the burr hole is situated well, the underlying hematoma may spontaneously evacuate if the intracranial contents are under extreme pressure. If this occurs, the patient's blood pressure and other hemodynamic parameters may change rapidly.

The hematoma is floated out with copious amounts of warm irrigation fluid. The clot may also be removed by suction or mechanically; however, an extremely adherent EDH is best left behind, because the force necessary to remove it may cause significant damage. The neurosurgeon must identify the source of bleeding, and every effort must be made to cauterize the bleeding vessels (Pieper, et al., 1996).

If the neurosurgeon suspects the presence of a concomitant subdural hematoma (bleeding into the space just below the dura), he or she creates a small dural opening to assess the subdural space. If evidence of subdural hematoma (SDH) is found, the neurosurgeon opens the dura and removes the SDH. The neurosurgeon may place extra dural tack-up sutures to anchor the dura to the inner table of the skull and may also place small, self-regulating suction drainage devices to minimize the likelihood of recurrent postoperative EDH (Pieper, et al., 1996). *(See Figure 8-3.)*

Postoperative treatment includes methods to combat shock and treatment of cerebral edema (swelling).

[6]   Results of Surgical Treatment

Epidural hemorrhage is the most commonly fatal complication of head injury, with a mortality rate of nearly 100 percent in untreated patients and more than 30 percent in treated patients. However, the relatively high mortality in treated patients is usually a result of delayed diagnosis and/or extreme severity of brain damage (Rowland, 1995).

To a great extent, the results of surgical treatment of epidural hematoma depend upon the degree of associated brain damage. If brain damage is slight, recovery is generally good. The prognosis is good for patients with EDH who undergo surgical evacuation before the onset of neurologic decompensation. Approximately 80 percent of these patients have a rapid recovery, with little neurologic deficit. Mortality rates of 16 to 32 percent are reported when surgery is performed early (Jastremski, 1996).

[7]   Epidural Hemorrhage and Hematoma in Infants and Children

In adults, epidural hematoma is almost always due to laceration of the middle meningeal artery or one of its branches. In children, however, EDH can result from even mild injury that has produced a tear in the dural veins, in the meningeal artery or its branches, in the accompanying middle meningeal veins or in the smaller emissary veins of the dural sinuses (Menkes and Till, 1995).

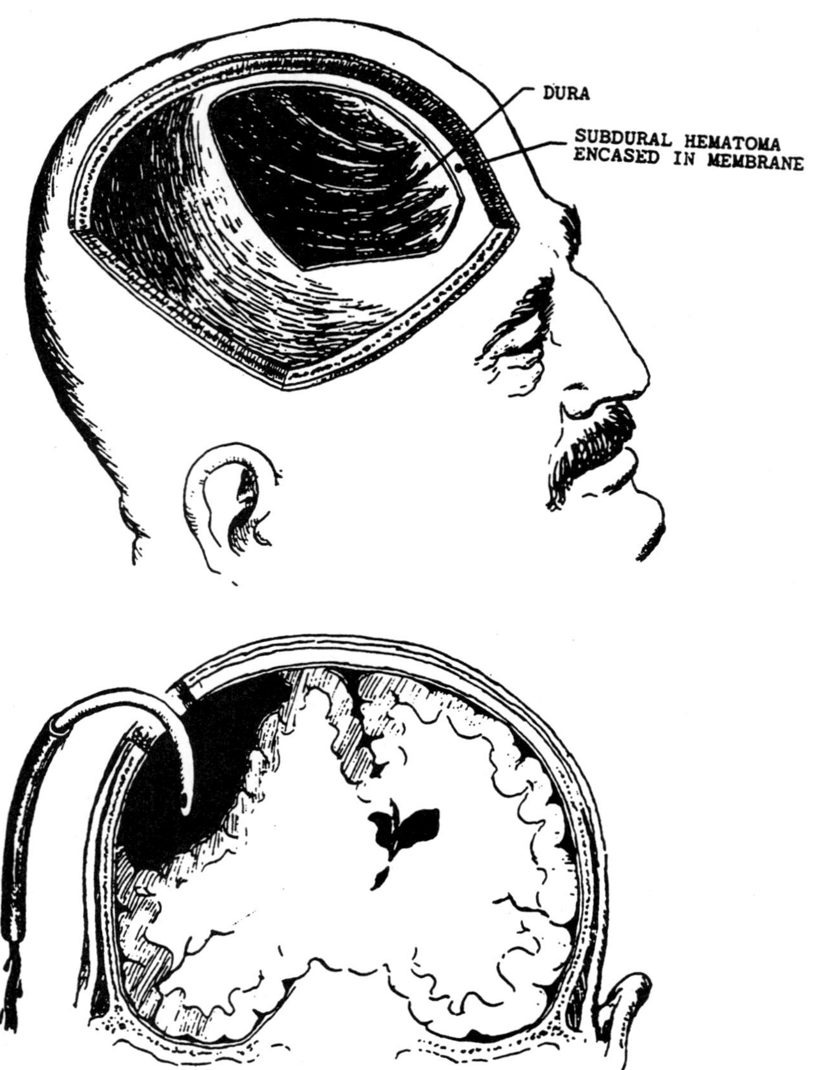

Fig. 8-3. Suction drainage devices to minimize the likelihood of recurrent postoperative EDH. Upper drawing shows the dura pulled back to expose a hematoma encased in a fibrous membrane. Lower drawing shows drainage of blood from the hematoma, which has compressed and distorted the brain.

Epidural hematoma is uncommon in children, although it is extremely important to consider in children with head injuries. Diagnosis of hematoma is difficult in young children. The following clinical symptoms are suggestive of EDH in newborn infants:

- difficulty breathing, altered breathing patterns;
- pale, bluish skin color;
- bulging of the anterior portion of the top of the head (fontanelle; the "soft spot");
- possible skull fracture, surface evidence of bruising of the skull, use of deep forceps or depressions in the skull; and
- convulsions.

In older children, symptoms are similar to those seen in adults; however, in many cases, the surgical treatment must be done so quickly that there is no time for imaging studies. In any event, 20 to 40 percent of children with EDH, a skull fracture is not detectable by radiographic examination or even at operation, so time should not be spent searching for fracture. EDH in children must be differentiated from acute subdural hematoma, intracerebral hematoma and severe brain swelling with or without contusion.

Operative removal of the clot is accomplished through burr holes or may require more complete procedures, similar to those used to treat adults. Although some patients show dramatic improvement, the general prognosis for young children with EDH remains grave (Menkes and Till, 1995).

8.23   Subdural Hematoma

Bleeding into the space just below the dura is known as subdural hemorrhage or hematoma (SDH). This is the most frequently occurring type of intracranial hematoma in patients with closed head injuries.[4] Subdural hematomas occur in as many as 20 percent to 40 percent of patients with severe head injury and arise from rupture of small veins bridging the space between the cortex and dura, although the source of bleeding may be a lacerated cortical artery. The SDH may expand within the potential space between the arachnoid membrane

---

[4] *See also* ch. 4 for full discussion of etiology, diagnosis, treatment and complications of subdural hematoma.

and the overlying dura. Acute SDHs require immediate surgical intervention (Pieper, et al., 1996).

[1] Surgical Pathophysiology

In contrast to epidural hematomas, which develop rapidly and are usually a result of arterial bleeding under the relatively high hydrodynamic pressure in the arteries, subdural hematomas usually develop more slowly and become symptomatic, since they are largely due to bleeding from veins that are under much lower hydrodynamic pressure than arteries.

When the rate of bleeding is sufficiently rapid to result in symptoms within hours of injury, the hematoma is termed *acute;* when signs of damaging effects do not appear for weeks or months, the hematoma is termed *chronic.* In chronic SDH, actual bleeding may have ceased shortly after injury, leaving a blood clot that typically becomes encapsulated with membranous tissue surrounding the boundaries of the clot. Fluids may be absorbed into the clot by osmotic pressure, due to differences in the chemical makeup of the fluids within the clot and those of the fluids that surround the membrane. Intracranial pressure rises as the clot enlarges. The expanding mass, located within a confined chamber that is almost full of nearly uncompressible contents, results in distortion and pressure on blood vessels and brain tissue. As intracranial pressure rises, the softer brain tissues are forced downward into the tentorial notch, compressing the vital centers in the brain stem that control heartbeat and respiration and the blood vessels that serve them, resulting, without treatment, in rapid death.

[2] Diagnostic Procedures

All patients with head injury should undergo computed tomography (CT) scan, especially those with skull fracture, those who score below 15 on the Glasgow Coma scale for 24 hours or more and all patients with seizures or a focal neurologic deficit (Miller, 1993). CT scanning clearly identifies space-occupying lesions, contusions and hemorrhagic or edematous areas in the brain. An accurate diagnosis can be made within minutes, allowing rapid initiation of treatment. CT scans have efficiently reduced mortality and morbidity from epidural hematoma (EDH), subdural hematoma (SDH) and intracranial hematoma (ICH) (Jastremski, 1996).

When CT scan reveals an intracranial hematoma, the decision must be made whether or not surgical evacuation is required. When a subdural hematoma is considered too small for surgical evaluation, CT scanning should be repeated after a few days to determine if the hematoma is expanding (Miller, 1993), if there has been no clinical deterioration of the patient.

[3]   Surgical Treatment of Acute Subdural Hematoma

Acute subdural hematoma requires surgical removal; however, the urgency with which surgical evacuation of an intracranial hematoma must proceed depends on the size of the hematoma, the presence of increased intracranial pressure (ICP) and the severity of the patient's neurologic deficits. An intracranial hematoma is considered significant if it measures at least 5 mm in size. Smaller hematomas may require immediate evacuation, however, if they are within the posterior fossa or if they are associated with increased ICP (Pieper, et al., 1996).

For acute hematomas, burr holes are usually insufficient, and most neurosurgeons prefer sufficient exposure to permit visualization from the midline to the base of the patient's skull, both because a subdural hematoma can cover most of the cerebral hemisphere and because the neurosurgeon may discover unexpected findings during the craniotomy procedure (Pieper, et al., 1996).

When rapid decompression is desired, the incision begins just anterior to the ear and extends upward from the zygomatic (cheekbone) arch for several centimeters. The neurosurgeon places burr holes and removes a small amount of additional bone. The dura is then incised, and as much as possible of the underlying clot is aspirated. Additional burr holes are placed, and the neurosurgeon performs the remainder of the dural opening, then evacuates the hematoma by floating it out with copious amounts of warm irrigation fluid; gentle traction with cup forceps may be required to remove any adherent hematoma. Extremely adherent hematoma is left behind, as its removal may cause significant damage to the underlying cortex.

The neurosurgeon must identify and control all sources of bleeding, usually by cauterizing the bleeding vessels. The use of hemostatic material is minimized to leave space into which the brain may expand when postinjury brain swelling occurs (Pieper, et al., 1996).

[4]   Results of Surgical Treatment of Acute Subdural Hematoma

The original state of the patient is greatly associated with the outcome of acute subdural hematoma. For patients with a Glasgow

Coma Scale score of 3 to 5, the mortality rate is 76 percent; with scores of 12 to 15, death is exceptional, and more than 90 percent of patients in this group have a good functional recovery. Adverse prognosticators include pupillary abnormalities, decerebrate posturing, age over 40 and high ICP but not necessarily concomitant intracerebral hematoma (Rowland, 1995).

[5]   Surgical Treatment of Chronic Subdural Hematoma

Symptomatic subacute or chronic SDHs are a common occurrence, and their treatment ranges from a conservative, nonoperative approach to a variety of surgical approaches. Surgical procedures include wide craniotomy (surgical opening of the skull) or craniectomy (surgical procedure in which a portion of the skull is removed), with or without neomembrane stripping, burr hole evacuation with subdural drainage, twist drill craniostomy (surgical opening into the skull) and ventricular expansion via a lumbar or ventricular catheter. Studies have shown that minimally invasive surgical techniques (notably a single burr hole placed over the hematoma) achieve effective drainage of the subdural space without need for large, extensive craniectomies or prolonged bed rest (Benzel, et al., 1994). Chronic subdural hematomas of significant size can be removed through burr holes, in procedures similar to those used in the removal of acute SDH.[5]

[6]   Results of Surgical Treatment of Chronic Subdural Hematoma

For surgical treatment of chronic subdural hematoma, the mortality rate is estimated to be 6 percent, the morbidity rate to be 14 percent and complete recovery to be 71 percent (Rowland, 1995). As with acute SDH, the outcome is largely dependent on the patient's general medical and neurologic state. Many patients with chronic SDH are elderly and may have arteriosclerosis, degenerative diseases of the nervous system, cerebral atrophy and/or multiple strokes as well as the traumatically induced hematoma.

[7]   Subdural Hematoma in Infants and Children

Subdural hematoma is a relatively common complication of head trauma in children and represents one of the two major neurosurgical problems of infancy. In 80 to 85 percent of cases, the hematoma is

---

[5] *See* 8.23[3] *supra.*

bilateral and is located in the frontoparietal region. In a large percentage of postnatal trauma hematomas, parental abuse can be suspected from evidence of soft-tissue bruising and from radiographic evidence of multiple episodes of skeletal trauma (Menkes and Till, 1995).

Clinical manifestations in children depend largely on the age of the child. In older children, as in adults, the hematoma can be acute or chronic, with symptoms of increased intracranial pressure predominating. Brain injury, usually in the form of acute subdural hematoma, is seen in a significant proportion of battered babies; SDH is the most common cause of death or physical disability in infants and must therefore be sought in all victims of child abuse (Menkes and Till, 1995).

In children over two years old, chronic subdural hematoma is a rare occurrence. Chronic SDH is much more common in infants, usually between the ages of two and six months. In about 60 percent of infants with chronic SDH, child abuse is the source of the trauma (Menkes and Till, 1995).

Evacuation of the hematoma is usually achieved by repeated subdural taps monitored by computed tomography (CT). If more than 10 taps are required, surgical intervention is necessary. The former practice of removing subdural membranes is no longer deemed necessary. Normal development is seen in 75 percent of these children, but 25 percent have some psychomotor retardation (Rowland, 1995). Unlike subdural hematomas in older children and adults, SDH occurring in infants tends to recollect repeatedly, even after total evacuation (Menkes and Till, 1995).

The prognosis for an infant with SDH is related to the extent of injury to the brain rather than the size of the hematoma. If brain injury is extensive, the brain will not expand, and the hematoma can calcify or ossify. Removal of a calcified or an ossified hematoma is of no advantage. The prognosis is particularly poor for children who are victims of nonaccidental trauma (Menkes and Till, 1995).

8.24 Intracerebral Hemorrhage and Hematoma

An intracerebral hematoma (ICH) is a well-defined blood clot within the brain tissue. The most frequent sites are the frontal and temporal lobes. Intracerebral hematomas result from tears in the brain parenchyma (functional tissue) at the points of greatest impact or injury.[6]

---

[6] *See also* ch. 4 for a full discussion of nonsurgical aspects of this condition.

Brain tissue in the frontal and anterior temporal lobes is often damaged from the rough surfaces of the underlying skull during the sudden deceleration that accompanies closed head injuries. *(See Figure 8-4.)* CT scan will show these areas of parenchymal bruising as small petechial (pinpoint) hemorrhages. When these are unaccompanied by significant mass effect, close observation without surgical intervention is the preferred treatment. However, the contused areas can coalesce into a large intraparenchymal hematoma, producing elevated intracranial pressure (ICP) and concomitant neurologic deterioration, usually during the first few hours or days following trauma. If this occurs, the patient must immediately undergo surgical evacuation (Pieper, et al., 1996).

Minutes or more than a week may pass between injury and clinical evidence of hemorrhage; 66 percent of operations are performed within the first 48 hours. Delayed hemorrhage, which is relatively uncommon, is diagnosed when the first CT scan shows no bleeding but a later one does. CT is mandatory for any patient showing clinical evidence of neurologic deterioration (Rowland, 1995).

Signs and symptoms of intracranial hematoma (ICH) are similar to those of contusions,[7] and the outcome depends on the size and location of the hematoma. Progressive focal edema and mass effect are complications of ICH. Delayed hemorrhage after ICH is known as delayed traumatic intracerebral hemorrhage (DTICH) and occurs in areas that were injured at the time of initial impact but appeared normal on CT scan. Clot formation and deterioration occur within a few days of the original trauma. DTICH is associated with a poor outcome and a high incidence of intracranial hypertension (Jastremski, 1996).

8.30 PENETRATING BRAIN INJURIES

Several terms are used in the description of craniocerebral missile injuries (CMI) in the literature, and they vary somewhat according to author. To some, the term *penetrating* refers specifically to gunshot or shrapnel injuries, whereas *perforating* is used to describe puncture and stab wounds. More commonly, CMI are classified as *superficial, tangential, penetrating* and *perforating.* Superficial injuries are those that occur when missiles are trapped within the scalp or skull at impact (e.g., spent bullets) without penetrating the cranial vault; tangential

---

[7] *See also* ch. 3.

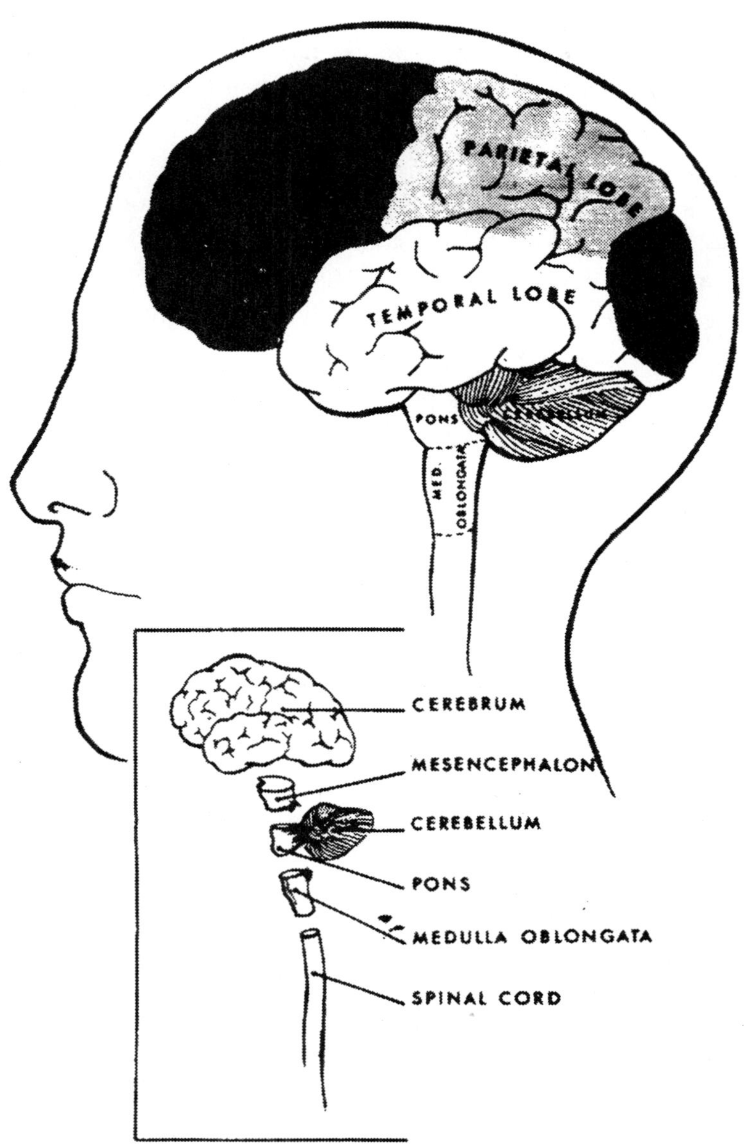

Fig. 8-4. The lobes of the brain. The dark area in front is the frontal lobe.

injuries are produced by a missile that grazes the head, sometimes producing extensive intracranial damage without passing through the cranial vault; penetrating lesions are those in which the bullet penetrates and lodges within the head; and perforating injuries are through-and-through lesions, with both entrance and exit wounds. This last term is misleading, however, in that most bullets that enter the cranial vault enter and exit the brain itself but are then trapped within the skull (Kim and Zee, 1995).

Similarly, many tangential injuries may also be considered penetrating injuries, because of the high frequency of deeply in-driven bone fragments, which in themselves are intracranial missiles. Overall, more than 80 percent of gunshot wounds penetrate the head (Kim and Zee, 1995).

8.31   Surgical Pathophysiology

In general, certain features of the brain result in greater damage when a bullet strikes the brain than in other regions of the body. These include the soft consistency of brain tissue, the containment of the brain in the rigid skull with no room for expansion at the moment of impact, the high vulnerability of nerve tissue to stretching damage and the importance of specific pathways within the brain.

The degree and extent of brain injury are dependent upon many factors, including the size and velocity of the penetrating object, the entrance location, the path it takes within the cranium, its exit location, the amount of ricocheting effect within the skull and whether the missile is relatively sterile.

[1]   Projectile Wounds

Projectile wounds may be roughly classified into high-velocity or low-velocity injuries. Low-velocity injuries are those resulting from BB guns or small-caliber guns, and they cause much less damage than high-velocity missiles, since much of their energy dissipates in penetrating superficial tissues and the skull. These projectiles may even fail to penetrate the skull or dura, due to loss of energy or deflection of their pathway.

The bullets discharged from many small-caliber rifles and pistols lose their velocity relatively rapidly as they travel from gun to target. The velocity of the bullet as it enters the head is critically important in determining the extent of brain damage incurred; small-caliber guns fired at a distance may result in damage restricted to the track of the bullet as it passes through the head and brain. Shotgun pellets have an even lower velocity, and the individual pellets spread out as they travel from gun to target. However, when they are fired at close range, the pellets remain tightly grouped, and the energy transmitted into the head represents the sum of that of all the pellets, making one large entrance wound and resulting in massive damage. Higher-velocity bullets are usually of higher caliber, lose less velocity in moving from gun to target and therefore carry tremendous energy on impact. These bullets maintain a relatively straight pathway, and as they encounter the resistant tissues, they dispel a portion of their energy, resulting in virtually a small explosion within the head and brain.

The alterations created by missiles may be described in three categories, depending on the velocity of the missile: (1) direct laceration, (2) shock wave transmission and (3) cavitation. Low-impact velocities result in minimal tissue damage, primarily by laceration, and include all stabbing injuries and many handgun injuries, particularly if the gun was fired from a distance. As velocity increases, shock wave and cavitation increase and become the predominant mechanisms for tissue damage. Shock waves are violent pulsations of high-pressure waves that travel at the speed of sound and emanate from the front of the advancing missile. Shock waves may reflect off the skull and summate, increasing the amount of damage (Kim and Zee, 1995).

Cavitation is the predominant mechanism of high-velocity missiles. The advancing missile pushes away tissues in a violent centrifugal motion, creating a temporary conical cavity that pulsates several times before collapsing. A negative pressure gradient is created, suctioning debris into the wound. With the highest velocities, the cavitational motion may be so centrifugally explosive that it literally bursts the skull (Kim and Zee, 1995).

Other clues to identifying entrance and exit sites are related to the anatomy of the skull. As a result of certain structural features, the skull is optimized for strength but lightweight. It consists of an outer table of compact bone; a central, less compact, lighter-weight layer and a more compact inner table. At entrance sites, beveling occurs on the inner table, which is always more comminuted (broken into fragments) than the outer table, although the reverse is true in perforating injuries at the exit site, where greater outer table fracturing and beveling is seen. Entrance wounds may also be identified by the presence of adjacent in-driven bone fragments (Kim and Zee, 1995).

At the point of impact, focal in-bending of the skull occurs, with concomitant out-bending of the skull occurring circumferentially at a distance from the point of impact, with inner and outer table stresses reversed. High-velocity missiles can impart an explosive movement of brain tissue against calvarial (upper portion of the skull) bone, sometimes causing extensive skull fracturing at a distance from the impact site (Kim and Zee, 1995).

The characteristic features of these and other bullet wounds assist in guiding the surgical treatment. Determining the track and extent of the wound is of obvious importance. Exit wounds are characteristically larger than entrance wounds, because the bullet is distorted or fragmented at exit and may exit at any angle. Depending on a variety of factors, however, the bullet may lose its original orientation and strike the tissue at a variety of angles, even sideways. Many bullets fail to exit and are retained; also the bullet and its fragments may ricochet off the interior of the skull, causing additional wound tracks. Higher-velocity bullets may ricochet in this manner and still exit the skull.

When a person has been shot at close range, powder burns or smoke stains may be visible at the entrance site. Shrapnel or other high velocity fragment wounds are relatively uncommon in civilian life but do occur occasionally during assault and in industrial explosions. Their pathophysiologic features are roughly similar to those caused by high-velocity bullets; however, in many instances, multiple projectiles are involved. Multiple injuries to other parts of the body are also common in these instances. The frequently large size and irregular shape of these penetrating objects make them particularly damaging. In addition, shrapnel from bombs or high-energy fragments from explosions are more likely to carry bone fragments, hair, dirt and other sources of infection into the wound. Bullets, by contrast, are heated to high temperatures when they are fired and may essentially be sterilized.

[2] Low Velocity Wounds

Penetrating wounds from broken glass and other sharp objects are uncommon but do occur, especially as a result of motor vehicle accidents. Intentional assaults with knives, ice picks and the like occur with greater frequency.

Penetrating head injuries from low-velocity missiles occur more frequently in children and infants than in adults, because the bones of the skull are relatively soft and more easily penetrated by sharp objects. In adults, the skull is not readily penetrated even by small, sharp objects, except at certain sites where the bone is thin. The bone behind the eyes is especially thin; as is the portion of the skull of the temporal region, just above the ears.

Low-velocity wounds fall into two categories of treatment: cases in which the penetrating object is retained in place at the time of examination, and those in which no such object is present at the time. When the object is retained, the major surgical goal is to remove it without causing additional brain trauma—a situation that often presents difficult challenges due to hemorrhage or damage to brain tissue or blood vessels. The risk of intracranial infection is also significantly greater than that associated with bullets or other high velocity injuries, both because low-velocity objects are frequently large in size and because of the absence of any partial sterilization, as occurs by the heat generated in firing a bullet.

8.32 Diagnostic Evaluation

The purpose of obtaining radiographic information is to determine the site of penetration, the extent of skull and neural injury, and the presence or absence of intracranial hematoma. CT scan is used to accomplish these goals. Although x-rays of the skull can provide a more easily understood indication of the actual entrance point, path and final location of the projectile, skull films cannot detect the presence or absence of a mass lesion or indicate the extent of brain injury.

When CT scan is obtained, the use of plain films becomes a diagnostic decision of the physician, and in many cases, plain films are considered unnecessary (Ward, et al., 1994). Plain x-ray films are useful if there are many fragments, which can degrade CT scans, and they are also used in the emergency department to diagnose skull fractures. Angiography (x-ray of blood vessels after injection of a contrast medium) may be done if there is a high probability of vascular lesions, particularly traumatic aneurysms (ballooning out of the wall of a blood vessel) (Kaufman, 1995).

Magnetic resonance imaging (MRI) is superior to CT scan in imaging extracerebral fluid collections (except subarachnoid hemorrhage), edema, nonhemorrhagic contusions and shear injuries, early or small cerebral infarctions (areas with lack of blood supply) and most lesions in the posterior fossa or brain stem; however, it is of little use in the acute setting. In addition, the presence of a metallic foreign body (such as a bullet) must be considered a relative contraindication to MRI, and a judgment must be made in individual cases, as bullets containing ferromagnetic materials carry the risk of rotation and movement during MRI (Kim and Zee, 1995).

Continuous cerebral blood flow studies, involving continuous monitoring of cerebral circulation, represent new technology in the care of patients with head injury. Cerebral blood flow studies have been used in the past to define no-flow states in brain death. Radiologically tagged xenon is delivered by a computerized ventilator that monitors xenon uptake as a reflection of cerebral blood flow. Although it is in limited use, this technology promises to be helpful in determining the effects of brain injury on blood flow and monitoring the effects of treatment to improve blood flow in ischemic areas (Jastremski, 1996).

8.33   Treatment

The initial treatment of penetrating injuries to the brain is similar to that for closed head injuries.[8] It should be noted that the more neurologically intact the patient is, the more extensive the neurologic examination should be in order to determine the true degree of impact (Ward, et al., 1994). The prognosis for patients with significant neurologic impairment from gunshot wounds is generally poor, and it may be that surgery is not indicated (Ward, et al., 1994).

[1]   General Surgical Considerations

The three major goals of surgery are to remove necrotic brain tissue, metal and bone fragments and prevent infections; to remove necrotic brain tissue to prevent further swelling and development of hematomas; and to remove masses, particularly hematomas (Kaufman, 1995). The decision to operate on a patient with a high-velocity penetrating head injury is based on many different factors. Surgery is generally performed in the following situations:

---

[8] *See* 8.10 *supra.*

1. The patient's condition could improve so that significant neurologic sequelae would be averted.

2. The patient is sufficiently stabilized and can tolerate surgery.

3. The neurologic condition is such that the patient could benefit from surgery.

4. The area of penetration is reasonably accessible to surgical intervention.

Once the patient is in surgery, every attempt is made to remove mass lesions, provide adequate debridement (removal of dead or nonviable tissue) of the missile track, remove bone fragments and provide adequate closure of dural openings. The neurosurgeon debrides and irrigates the injured brain tissue to minimize the potential for infection. If a limited debridement is planned, the neurosurgeon may incorporate the entrance and exit wounds into two separate "lazy S" incisions. The bone around the entry and exit sites may then be removed. A larger incision and bone flap may be required when there is intracranial hematoma.

Once devitalized tissue has been debrided and any underlying hematomas, bone fragments, contused brain tissue or foreign bodies have been evacuated, the surgeon repairs the dura in a watertight seal (Pieper, et al., 1996). The purpose of the watertight seal is to prevent leakage of cerebrospinal fluid and to prevent formation of a pathway for bacteria to get into the brain, which would result in either meningitis or brain abscess[9] (Ward, et al., 1994). The watertight dural repair also prevents the scalp from sticking to the brain if there is a bone defect (Kaufman, 1995).

The operative team may use several modalities to monitor the patient's cerebral metabolism during surgery. Ventriculostomy catheters provide both monitoring and treatment of elevated intracranial pressure; these may be placed before or during surgery if the patient develops acute brain swelling.[10]

Fiberoptic monitoring systems are used when the placement of ventriculostomy catheters is difficult. Cerebral blood flow probes may be used to monitor cerebrospinal fluid during a craniotomy procedure. Microdialysis catheters may be placed into the patient's cortex during

---

[9] *See* 8.90 *infra.*

[10] *See* 8.52[1] *infra.*

the craniotomy procedure, to monitor traumatically induced changes in the patient's extracellular metabolite concentrations. Jugular venous oxygen saturation catheters may be placed during surgery to monitor the patient's cerebral metabolism, help in determining the optimal timing of neurosurgical interventions and provide general information about the patient's prognosis (Pieper, et al., 1996).

In addition, intraoperatively and postoperatively, the patient is medicated with anticonvulsants. It has been shown that patients with penetrating injury to the brain have a 25 percent or higher chance of having post-traumatic seizures if they are not treated adequately with anticonvulsants (Ward, et al., 1994).

[2]　High Velocity Missile Injuries

In many cases, all the missile fragments are not removed during surgery. If fragments are in deep-seated locations, it may not be possible to retrieve them without causing severe damage to brain tissues. Even relatively large missile fragments embedded in the brain that are readily seen on imaging are often extremely difficult to locate at surgery. In addition, although bullets, particularly jacketed ones, may contain metals that cause electrolysis (decomposition by the passing through of an electric current) of bacteria, no systematic study of their biocompatibility has been done. Some authors have suggested that such bullets predispose patients to seizures and later fibroglial (pertaining to fine fibers in cells of the fibrous tissues of the body) scarring and epilepsy, while most others feel that metallic fragments pose no real threat if they are left in place (Kaufman, 1995).

Bone fragments, especially those that have carried bits of scalp and hair with them, can lead to infection; clusters of bone fragments indicate a potentially contaminated area. Complete removal of all bone fragments may not be needed in all cases (Kaufman, 1995).

[3]　Prognosis After Surgery for High Velocity Missile Wounds

Despite major advances and new technology, severe head injury remains a devastating condition. In gunshot wounds, 71 to 76 percent of all victims sustain injuries so severe that death occurs at the scene of the shooting (Ward, et al., 1994). However, if these patients do survive, few remain vegetative or severely disabled. Most are considered to have moderate disability or to have made a good recovery (Pieper, et al., 1996).

Other factors affect survival and outcome in the patient with penetrating wounds to the brain. Most often, it is the combination of the immediate effects of the penetrating missile and the secondary insults that follow that is responsible for high mortality rates. One of the most important factors is the path the bullet takes as it travels through the brain; injuries limited to a single hemisphere are associated with better outcome than those in which the bullet crosses the midline and causes bihemisphere injuries. Bullets that pass through the ventricles (hollow spaces within the brain) are associated with mortality rates as high as 90 percent. Bullets that cross both midsagittal and midcoronal planes or that come to rest in the posterior fossa are lethal in 100 percent of cases. The presence of intracerebral hematoma[11] or intraventricular blood has also been associated with poor outcome (Ward, et al., 1994).

In addition, the caliber and velocity of the bullet are factors: Large-caliber high-velocity bullets carry a greater wounding potential than smaller ones. However, the circumstances of the shooting correspond to the injuries and outcome. A small-caliber low-velocity bullet discharged inches from the head will result in a more devastating injury than a larger caliber high-velocity bullet discharged from a distance. Victims of assault stand a better chance of survival than victims of attempted suicide.

Patients who survive penetrating head injury generally experience relatively good functional outcomes. Only 3 to 6 percent survive in a vegetative state or with severe disability. Most studies indicate that a quarter to two thirds of all survivors achieve an independent life-style and even employment. The major factor is survival; if survival is achieved, a self-sufficient life-style most often follows (Ward, et al., 1994).

[4] Low Velocity Penetrating Injuries

Penetration by low-velocity objects, such as a knife, glass fragment, etc., may not result in dramatic symptoms. In some cases, particularly if the victim is intoxicated, a penetrating wound of this nature may leave only a minor entrance wound that is considered inconsequential or forgotten entirely by the victim.

The removal of large objects embedded in the skull requires careful evaluation of the situation, and removal is delayed, therefore, until

---

[11] *See* 8.24 *supra.*

the patient is in the operating room. Removal of the object may release tamponade (restraint of hemorrhage by a plug lodged in a cavity) of an injured intracranial vessel, resulting in rapid intracranial bleeding. If it becomes clear that the object is not near large vascular structures and is of relatively small diameter, it may reasonably be simply pulled out, although not without risk. It is therefore recommended that the patient be stabilized and the object removed in the operating room.

As with all penetrating injuries to the brain, infection is a major concern, especially when the injury is due to low-velocity penetrating objects.[12]

8.40   TRAUMATIC HYDROCEPHALUS

Hydrocephalus is characterized by an increased amount of cerebrospinal fluid (CSF) in the brain and dilation of the cerebral ventricles. The condition can take several forms; normal pressure hydrocephalus (NPH) is most commonly associated with head injury, often following subarachnoid hemorrhage.[13] In some patients, the obstruction of CSF is transient: Intracranial pressure increases, and hydrocephalus appears but then disappears spontaneously. Other patients exhibit progressive hydrocephalus requiring surgical intervention (Prockop, 1995).

In most cases, hydrocephalus develops insidiously over a period of time. Acute hydrocephalus can develop in a few hours in the patient with head injuries, however, and contribute significantly to increased intracranial pressure.

8.41   Surgical Pathophysiology

Inside the brain and spinal cord is a system of hollow spaces: the four ventricles of the brain, their connecting channels and the central canal of the spinal cord. It is thought that most of the cerebrospinal fluid is formed in the ventricles by the choroid plexuses, small pouches of specialized tissue in anatomic continuity with the pia mater. *(See Figure 8-5.)* The CSF is secreted by the plexuses continuously, normally at the rate of about a pint a day. Smaller amounts of CSF are produced by other regions, including the central canal of the spinal cord.

---

[12] *See* 8.90 *infra.*

[13] *See* 8.21 *supra.*

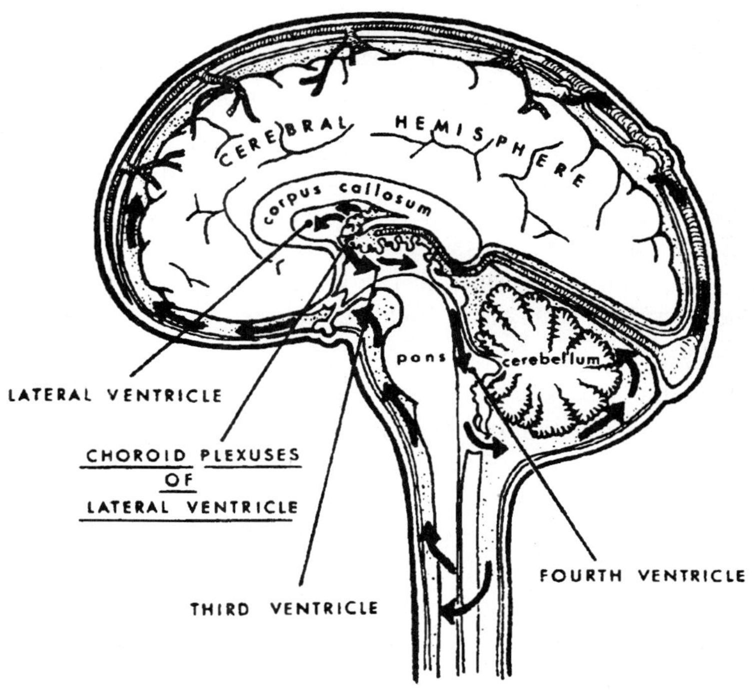

Fig. 8-5. Most of the cerebrospinal fluid is formed in the ventricles by the choroid plexuses. The CSF is secreted by the plexuses continuously; smaller amounts of CSF are produced by other regions, including the central canal of the spinal cord.

The body must maintain CSF pressure at or near equilibrium with the outside atmospheric pressure, and the fluid must be reabsorbed at about the same rate that it is formed. This is accomplished through the pacchionian granulations (hairlike projections of the arachnoid into the intracranial venous sinuses). The pressure of the CSF is maintained at levels slightly higher than the pressure of the blood in the sinuses, causing the CSF to flow into the venous channels.

[1]   Obstruction of Cerebrospinal Fluid Flow

Hydrocephalus occurs when the flow of cerebrospinal fluid is interrupted or obstructed, when there is an excessive formation of CSF or when the absorption of CSF is compromised.

The rate of CSF absorption is directly related to intracranial pressure. Normal pressure hydrocephalus (NPH) is thought to be a problem of CSF absorption, not of formation, primarily in the flow of fluid from the basal cisterns (spaces containing CSF) over the convexities to the sagittal and other sinuses and into the cranial nerve root pathways. Many aspects of CSF physiology, as well as normal NPH pathophysiology, are not entirely understood (Gleason, et al., 1993).

In traumatic hydrocephalus, head injury results in bleeding into the subarachnoid space between the arachnoid and pia mater at one or more critical sites. The presence of blood in this region begins an irritative reaction that results in fibrous scarring between the two meningeal layers. The scarring effectively blocks the flow of cerebrospinal fluid.

Another traumatic source is scarring of the lining of the walls of the ventricles. Herniation of brain substance through the tentorial gap at the base of the dura can cause acute hydrocephalus and is a life-threatening consequence of elevated intracranial pressure. In this instance, the symptoms of hydrocephalus are inconspicuous compared to the more dramatic symptoms of tentorial herniation.[14]

To result in hydrocephalus, obstructive scarring must block the flow from the source of the CSF fluid to its normal exit sites. The fourth ventricle, for example, is a small, tubular channel easily blocked by scarring. Another vulnerable region is the ventricular cisterns, where a relatively small opening permits CSF to flow out of the cerebral ventricles around the cerebellum, down into the spinal cord and then to the subarachnoid space over the surface of the brain. If the fourth ventricle or the exit from the cisterns is blocked by scarring, the fluid cannot escape through the cisternal system to its exit points over the brain surface, where the fluid is absorbed into the venous circulation. Intracranial pressure builds, and the increased pressure within the blocked ventricular region causes compression of the surrounding brain tissue.

[2] Symptoms of Hydrocephalus

The symptoms of hydrocephalus, whether it is due to bleeding into the subarachnoid space or scarring after traumatic meningitis, usually develop gradually for weeks after head trauma or hemorrhage. A clinical sign of this condition is regression of a critically injured patient to a lower level of consciousness following a period of gradual

---

[14] *See* 8.51[2] *infra.*

improvement. In addition, there is evidence of increased cerebrospinal fluid pressure.

Acute hydrocephalus presents with rapidly developing increased intracranial pressure and, if it is not promptly treated, results in deep coma and death. Normal pressure hydrocephalus develops more slowly; symptoms include declining memory; unsteady, broad-based gait with a history of falling; inattentiveness; indifference to self and urinary incontinence.

8.42   Diagnosis

Computed tomography (CT) scan and magnetic resonance imaging (MRI) are the best diagnostic tests for all forms of hydrocephalus. Lumbar puncture is sometimes indicated to measure CSF pressure (Prockop, 1995).

Isotope cisternography has been used to indicate CSF flow with cases of shunt-responsive normal pressure hydrocephalus; however, cisternography adds little to the accuracy of the combination of MRI scan and clinical criteria.

8.43   Neurosurgical Treatment

Numerous neurosurgical methods are used to treat traumatic obstructive hydrocephalus, all with the same goal of establishing an adequate drainage system or a shunt that bypasses the obstruction in the CSF flow pattern and diverts it to some other bodily site, from which it will be harmlessly excreted. Ventriculoperitoneal shunts have been the standard therapy, although this form of shunting is far from risk free. One end of a tube is placed in a lateral ventricle of the brain and fed beneath the skin to the upper peritoneal cavity of the abdomen. A burr hole must be drilled in the skull and the tubing passed through brain tissue into the lateral ventricle. The risks of shunt placement include shunt malfunction, infection, overdrainage resulting in subdural hematoma, epilepsy and, rarely, intracerebral hemorrhage (Gleason, et al., 1993).

Although many problems are associated with shunting, the procedure is almost always successful in arresting the brain-damaging effects of increased intracranial pressure within the ventricles. Traumatic hydrocephalus usually occurs only in severely or moderately brain injured patients whose symptoms represent a combination of the effects of other brain injury with the superimposed complication of obstructive hydrocephalus; the degree of improvement that can result from shunting can be major and make an important difference in the quality of life for the patient.

8.50   INCREASED INTRACRANIAL PRESSURE

Increased intracranial pressure (ICP) is a major complication of head injury and is the most frequent cause of death among patients with head injury (Jastremski, 1996).

Normal ICP refers to the intracranial volume within the rigid skull: 80 percent brain tissue, 10 percent cerebrospinal fluid and 10 percent blood within blood vessels. Increased ICP results from an increase in the volume of one of these three constituents without a compensatory decrease in one of the other two. Increased absorption of CSF, displacement of CSF into the subarachnoid space and decreased production of CSF are the major compensatory mechanisms. Vasoconstriction with reduced blood volume or shifts of brain tissue may also occur, but these are of time-limited assistance (Jastremski, 1996).

Understanding the concept of *compliance* also contributes to an understanding of ICP. Compliance refers to the relationship between volume and pressure within the skull. When compensatory mechanisms fail, compliance is minimal, and a small increase in volume causes a large increase in ICP (Jastremski, 1996).

Brain swelling (edema) and intracranial hemorrhage are the major causes of increased ICP. Although there are no operative procedures for reducing brain swelling, intracranial pressure may be reduced by opening the skull. When hematomas or hemorrhage are the cause of increased ICP, surgical management is necessary. In uncontrolled ICP, the terminal event is usually an increase of the ICP to a level at or slightly above the mean arterial blood pressure (Moulton, 1992).

In the infant or child with severe head injury, control of increased ICP is the most important problem of medical management. Children tend to have a lower incidence of surgically treatable mass lesions than adults but a higher incidence of ICP. Continuous ICP monitoring is advisable and is usually achieved from the ventricles or from the subarachnoid, subdural and epidural spaces, using fiberoptic monitors (Menkes and Till, 1995).

8.51 Surgical Pathophysiology

In closed head injury, cerebral edema may be localized or diffuse. Diffuse cerebral edema of one or both hemispheres is common in traumatic brain injury. Cerebral edema exaggerates the amount and severity of any neurologic deficit; the severity and extent of edema are related to the severity of the head injury. As the brain's compensatory mechanisms to accommodate additional brain mass fail, increases in ICP begin (Jastremski, 1996).

The skull is a closed, rigid, bony case that encloses three compartments: the brain tissue, the cerebrospinal fluid and the blood vessels. If the brain tissue swells, intracranial pressure rises and blood vessels are compressed. When the ICP is sufficiently elevated, the systemic blood pressure level is inadequate to ensure blood supply into the skull against a pressure gradient that is unfavorable due to swelling within the skull.

[1] Symptoms

The elevation of ICP within the fixed boundaries of the skull results in a common group of symptoms. The early stages are marked by headache and vomiting, elevation of blood pressure with a slow pulse, and slowed, stertorous (sonorous, similar to snoring) breathing. As the pressure increases, the blood pressure falls, pulse rate increases and body temperature rises. The pupils enlarge, and the eyelids droop. The eyes may be deviated outward, particularly if the elevated ICP is due to a localized hematoma. Consciousness becomes impaired, progressing from confusion to stupor to coma and, if the ICP is not brought under control, death. Frank hemorrhage can be seen in the retina when the ICP has been elevated for several days.

[2] Tentorial Herniation

The tough, fibrous dura that covers the cerebrum has a roughly circular opening in the center of its base through which the brain stem passes. This opening is called the tentorial notch.

As intracranial pressure rises, the softer brain tissues are forced downward into the tentorial notch (herniation), compressing the vital centers in the brain stem that control heartbeat and respiration and the blood vessels that serve them, resulting in death. Tentorial herniation is a particularly urgent emergency, since death occurs rapidly.

Clinical symptoms of elevated ICP include decerebrate posture (rigid body, with the arms turned inward at the wrist, elbow and shoulder, and the legs extended). This posture may come and go. Respiration and heart rate slow, blood pressure falls, and the patient becomes comatose. The pupils are fixed and dilated. Occasional recovery from advanced tentorial herniation may occur following treatment but is uncommon. In most advanced cases, death follows rapidly.

8.52 Diagnosis and Management of Increased Intracranial Pressure

Continuous ICP monitoring may be achieved through the use of various modalities. However, the issue of whether to monitor ICP is somewhat controversial, because current techniques are invasive and carry a risk of morbidity from intracranial infection, intracranial hemorrhage or epilepsy. However, when it is understood that the cerebral perfusion pressure is important and that levels of arterial pressure are meaningless unless ICP is known, then logic dictates that ICP should be monitored (Miller, 1993).

ICP monitoring allows for aggressive management of patients with potential or actual increased ICP. Monitoring also provides a means of evaluating the treatments being used to prevent or control the condition.

[1] Ventriculostomy Catheters

Ventriculostomy catheters provide both monitoring and treatment of elevated ICP. These are placed either before surgery or intraoperatively. After cannulating (inserting a tube or catheter into a body cavity) a ventricle, the neurosurgeon tunnels the ventriculostomy catheter away from the incision, bringing it out through a separate stab wound and securing it with sutures. The patient's cerebrospinal fluid can be drained through the catheter, and the monitors can be recalibrated after placement (Pieper, et al., 1996).

The probe of the fiberoptic ICP monitoring system is placed directly into the white matter of the brain. The effectiveness of this particular system has been validated; infectious complications and intracerebral hematoma at the site of the placement are extremely rare (Wijdicks, 1995).

Studies have shown that raised ICP is found in 80 percent or more of comatose patients with head injuries. Loss of image of the third ventricle and perimesencephalic cisterns on CT scans is indicative that ICP is or will become elevated; however, the absence of these findings is not a guarantee of normal ICP (Miller, 1993).

ICP monitoring is recommended for the following patients (Moulton, 1992):

- all comatose patients;

- patients who have had mass lesions evacuated and who are not sufficiently conscious to follow commands;

- patients in whom nonoperative treatments have been elected; and

- patients with head injuries and a disturbed level of consciousness, in whom pharmacologic paralysis is necessary for respiratory management.

[2]   Treatment Procedures

Increased ICP is medically managed by the drainage of cerebrospinal fluid, institution of chemical paralysis and sedation, hypothermia, administration of the osmotic agent mannitol and the anesthetic etomidate, and possibly hyperventilation and barbiturate therapy (Ward, et al., 1994).

Osmotically active agents have long been used to manage cerebral edema. Hypertonic solutions remove cerebral tissue fluid via the vascular osmotic pressure gradient, reducing brain volume and lowering ICP. The agent must remain in the intravascular compartment to be effective; if the blood-brain barrier has been compromised, the therapy becomes more harmful than beneficial. There is a potential for the hypertonic solution to move into the already edematous brain, increasing the edema in a rebound phenomenon (Jastremski, 1996).

Treatment with the osmotic agent mannitol is the cornerstone of ICP reduction. If the patient does not respond well to mannitol and there are no new CT scan findings other than diffuse abnormalities or cerebral edema, a more aggressive (but potentially harmful) treatment may be attempted with the use of furosemide with albumin. This treatment carries a high risk of complications and is only at times successful. Barbiturates can be considered, but there has been no clinical documentation showing that the use of barbiturates in head injury improves patient outcome (Wijdicks, 1995).

8.53 Surgical Treatment

The surgical options for controlling elevated ICP include frontal or temporal decompressive craniectomy, removal of an existing bone flap and internal decompression by removing a swollen or damaged frontal or temporal lobe (Moulton, 1992). Ideally therapy for increased intracranial pressure (ICP) is aimed at the cause of the increase in pressure.

Decompression involves opening the skull surgically in order to relieve increased intracranial pressure. The procedure is reserved for grave situations when other methods have failed and tentorial herniation[15] is imminent. Improvements in reducing elevated ICP through nonoperative means have largely made decompression outmoded; most patients benefit from nonsurgical treatment or more conservative surgical treatment.

In a comatose patient with extracerebral hematoma, it is important that the brain be decompressed as soon as possible. A standard procedure is to administer a bolus (concentrated) dose of mannitol rapidly while the patient is in the CT imaging suite and then transfer the patient to an operating room, where the skull can be opened and the hematoma evacuated from the epidural or subdural space. Epidural and subdural hematomas require more access than can be gained through burr hole techniques (Miller, 1993).

8.60 CRANIAL NERVE INJURIES

Damage to the peripheral and cranial nerves is a common occurrence in patients with moderate or severe head injuries. Operative treatment is not possible for most instances of traumatic cranial nerve dysfunction; however, a significant number of patients recover cranial nerve function spontaneously.

---

[15] *See* 8.51[2] *supra.*

8.61 Pathophysiology

Each of the 12 pairs of cranial nerves has a name that corresponds either to its function or its anatomic location. *(See Figure 8-6.)* Some of these nerves are more frequently or more severely traumatized than others, largely because of their location. A cranial nerve is most vulnerable and most frequently damaged at the point in its course where it enters or leaves the skull. Skull fractures may directly injure the nerve, and swelling of tissues around a fracture or hemorrhage can compress the nerve and impair function.

After nerve damage, the pathologic changes depend on the nature of the injury, which can also affect the regenerative process. Mechanical nerve injuries may be classified as:

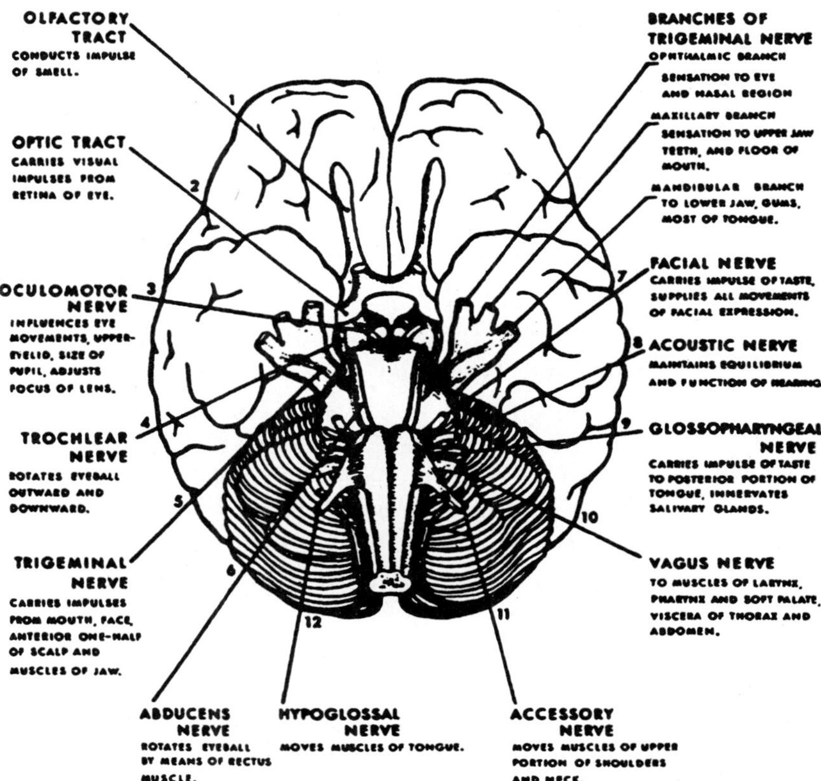

Fig. 8-6. The locations of the cranial nerves and their functions, as seen from the underside of the brain.

- *neurotmesis,* or complete severing of the nerve;

- *axonotmesis,* in which axons are interrupted by distal (below the site of injury) degeneration but the endoneurium (delicate membrane of connective tissue surrounding the nerve) is intact; or

- *neurapraxia,* involving a blockage of conduction due to compression at the site of the lesion, with normal distal conduction and no degeneration of distal fibers.

Damage may occur to cranial nerves in their course outside the skull, usually as a result of trauma to the face. The extent and permanence of dysfunction are directly related to the degree of injury to the nerve. If the nerve is severed completely and the distance between proximal (above the site of injury) and distal ends is great, regeneration is not possible unless the ends are apposed (brought together) at operation (Lange, et al., 1995).

In conditions in which intracranial pressure increases, cranial nerves may be compressed along their course within the skull. The nerve cell bodies forming the origins of the nerves within the brain stem may also be affected. When trauma is sufficient to traumatize the brain stem, ominous and frequently fatal disturbances of functions can occur. In these cases, altered cranial nerve function may coexist with deep coma.

8.62   Symptoms and Treatment

The 12 pairs of cranial nerves are divided so that in each pair, one supplies a particular side of the body. The symptoms and signs of cranial nerve injury depend on which nerve or branch of a nerve is affected; if the nerve is a motor nerve, then the result is flaccid paralysis with wasting of the muscles that are innervated (supplied) by the nerve. If the nerve is sensory, the result is loss of sensation in an area that is usually smaller than the anatomic distribution of the nerve. Stabbing pain, pins-and-needles sensations or burning pain may accompany partial injury or incomplete division of a nerve. Changes in skin, mucous membranes and bones (trophic changes) may occur following complete or incomplete interruption of a nerve (Lange, et al., 1995). The diagnosis of injury to cranial nerves is usually made clinically by the distribution of the motor and sensory abnormalities.

Damage to the peripheral and cranial nerves is a common sequel of blunt head trauma; the most commonly affected nerves are the olfactory (I), facial (VII) and acoustic (VIII), followed by the optic (II) and oculomotor (III) nerves. The prognosis for recovery is good for the facial nerve, intermediate for the oculomotor nerve and poor for the olfactory, optic and acoustic nerves. Treatment is usually symptomatic, although surgical decompression of the optic and facial nerves can lead to dramatic results in selected patients. Steroids are also effective in some instances (Keane and Baloh, 1992).

Other instances in which surgical intervention is appropriate are discussed in the following sections.

[1]   The Oculomotor Nerve

The oculomotor nerve (cranial nerve III) affects eye movements. Damage to this nerve results in loss of the ability to open the eye. The eyeball is deviated outward and slightly downward; the pupil is dilated, does not react to light and loses the power of accommodation. This nerve usually recovers spontaneously over a period of a few months; however, if the condition persists for longer than five to six months, additional symptoms may develop and the condition is probably permanent. Surgical repair of the eyes-outward position is possible, and restoration of normal eye movements can be expected.

[2]   The Trochlear Nerve

Damage to the fourth (trochlear) nerve is associated with basilar skull fractures affecting the wings of the sphenoid bone, which results in the inability to turn the eye downward and inward. Hemorrhage or physical damage to the pulley system of the muscle served by the nerve is the pathophysiologic mechanism of impairment. Recovery is usually spontaneous, and surgical repair is usually not indicated.

[3]   The Trigeminal Nerve

The trigeminal or fifth cranial nerve supplies sensation to much of the surface of the face. Injury to this nerve causes paralysis of the muscles of mastication, with deviation of the jaw toward the side of the lesion; loss of ability to appreciate soft tactile, thermal or painful sensations in the face; and loss of the corneal and sneezing reflexes (Lange, et al., 1995).

Spontaneous recovery is common. As sensation returns, severe, stabbing pain may develop, in some instances requiring repeated local anesthetic injection or surgical division of the nerve pathways.

[4] The Abducens Nerve

The sixth cranial (abducens) nerve has a long course from its point of emergence from the brain stem to the lateral rectus muscle in the orbit. When intracranial pressure increases, this nerve is peculiarly subject to injury by compression against the floor of the skull. Unilateral or bilateral paralysis of the lateral rectus muscle may develop in patients with elevated ICP (Lange, et al., 1995).

When this nerve is damaged, the eye turns inward, and outer-directed movements are impaired or lost. If improvement does not occur spontaneously, which may require up to a year, the persistent turned-in position of the eyeball may be corrected surgically.

[5] The Facial Nerve

The facial (seventh cranial) nerve has two divisions as it leaves the brain stem: the motor root and the nervus intermedius. Damage to the facial nerve causes paralysis of the facial muscles, with or without loss of taste on the anterior two thirds of the tongue. Secretion of the lacrimal and salivary glands may be altered, depending on the portion of the nerve involved.

Whether the seventh nerve has any somatic sensory function is a matter of controversy. Sensory loss is only rarely detected in patients with lesions of the seventh nerve (Lange, et al., 1995).

The branches of the seventh nerve are peripheral and are subject to injury by stab and gunshot wounds, cuts and birth trauma. Damage is often associated with fracture of the temporal bone and is usually evident immediately after injury or may go undetected for several days after the accident. The mechanism of the delayed paralysis is unclear. When nerve damage is associated with head trauma, the prognosis for improvement is usually good, although recovery may not be complete (Lange, et al., 1995).

When damage is severe, facial paralysis is obvious, even when the face is at rest. Surgical procedures may be required if spontaneous recovery does not occur. Neurolysis or end-to-end suture may be indicated in extracranial lesions of the nerve or its branches. End-to-end suture is not possible when the nerve is damaged proximal to the stylomastoid foramen, and innervation of the facial muscle can only be achieved by suturing the distal portion of the seventh nerve with the central portion of one of the other cranial nerves, usually the eleventh or twelfth (Lange, et al., 1995).

[6]   Cranial Nerves IX, X, XI and XII

Injury to these cranial nerves occurs primarily through trauma to the base of the skull. In some instances, isolated symptoms of dysfunction may be observed. In other instances, injuries to the base of the skull are so severe that the patient cannot survive.

The ninth cranial (glossopharyngeal) nerve contains both motor and sensory fibers. Damage results in loss of taste and the gag reflex. Damage to the tenth (vagus) nerve causes difficulty in swallowing and speaking. Damage to the eleventh (accessory) nerve results in impairment of rotary movements of the neck and shrugging movements of the shoulder. Damage to the twelfth (hypoglossal) nerve results in atrophy and paralysis of the tongue. Damage to these nerves warrants rehabilitation therapy, although most patients will be able to compensate for isolated loss of function.

8.70   SCALP INJURIES

Scalp injuries are among the most common head injuries; most can be managed by general surgeons, trauma specialists or emergency care physicians. Major scalp injuries often require the services of a plastic surgeon.

The scalp is highly efficient in protecting the skull from infection. Complete closure of the scalp is therefore an important factor in the surgical management of head injuries. Because of the extensive vascular system in the scalp and the poor contractility of these vessels, scalp wounds can result in significant blood loss and, occasionally, hypovolemia (low volume of circulating blood) (Jastremski, 1996).

8.71   Anatomy and Pathophysiology

The highly specialized, multilayered structure of the scalp protects the skull and brain from various minor injuries. *(See Figure 8-7.)* From the outside in, the five layers are skin, subcutaneous tissue, galea aponeurotica, loose areolar tissue and periosteum (membrane covering the bone of the skull). Laceration of all five layers obviously occurs when there is penetrating injury and in all but the most superficial tangential injuries.

The aponeurotica (a layer of dense fibrous tissue beneath the overlying skin) enables the scalp to absorb much of the energy from a blow to the head, partly because the aponeurotica can move readily

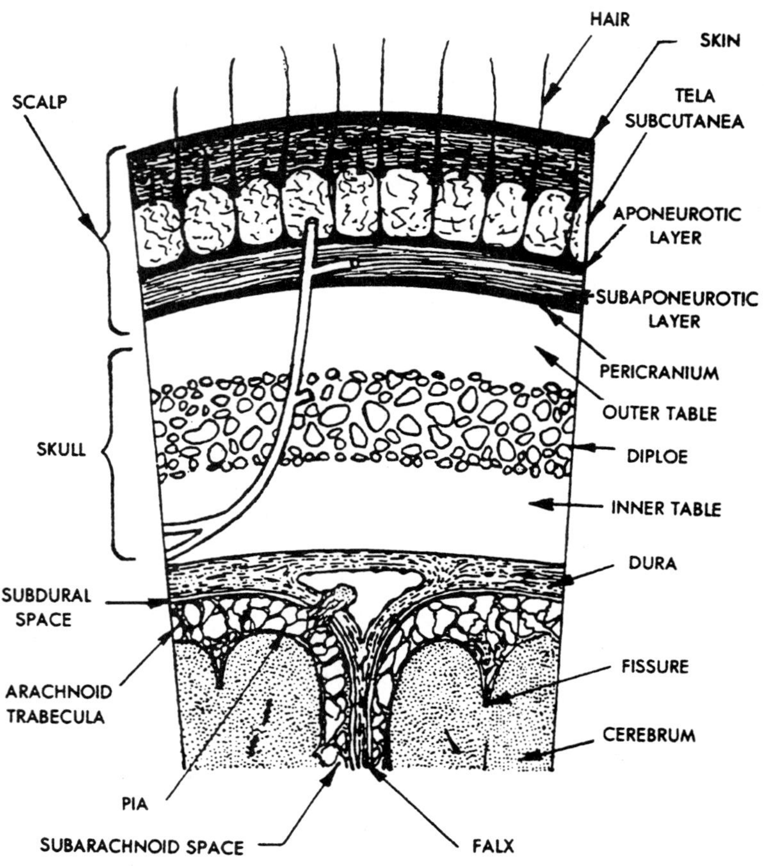

Fig. 8-7. Cross section of the scalp, skull and meninges. The five layers of the scalp are the skin, subcutaneous tissue, galea aponeurotica, loose areolar tissue and periosteum (membrane covering the skull bone). The layers of the skull consist of the pericranium, outer table, diploe and inner table. The brain (cerebrum) is protected by the three meningeal layers: dura mater, arachnoid and pia mater.

within the limits of its attached muscle supply (the frontalis and occipitalis muscles). This protective absorption of energy is particularly effective in ameliorating glancing, tangential blows. The hair, skin and fatty layers are also protective.

The subaponeurotic tissue beneath the galea aponeurotica is a layer of loose fibrous tissue that permits the relatively great mobility of the scalp on the skull. The subaponeurotic space, under normal conditions, is merely a potential space that readily yields to an accumulation of pus, blood or other fluid and is available to the surgeon or in occurrences of trauma as a cleavage plane. Infection in this location may lead to thrombosis (clot formation) in small emissary veins that communicate between the scalp and the cranial cavity. Such thrombosis can in turn lead to extension of infection. Therefore, it is of great importance that all traumatic deep scalp wounds be treated and adequately sutured.

Scalp injury is sometimes followed by persistent tenderness and pain (particularly in the occipital portion). Treatment includes drug therapy and, occasionally, resection (surgical removal) of the scar.

[1] Blood Supply

The scalp has a rich supply of blood vessels. Five pairs of arteries bring blood to the scalp, passing along the subcutaneous layer. This blood supply arises from the external carotid artery through several of its branches (the superficial temporal artery, ophthalmic artery and auricular and occipital branches of the external carotid artery). There are no blood vessels in the scalp from the bones of the skull, and few large arteries cross from the right to the left sides of the scalp. The vascular pattern is important in designing surgical procedures to gain access to the intracranial contents and in repairing scalp injuries.

The veins run roughly parallel in pattern with the arteries, but they communicate with the nervous return from the skull and the intracranial regions. Two surgically important consequences result from this arrangement:

1 Scalp injuries that tear these venous pathways can lead to serious hemorrhage.

2. These venous pathways create a potential route for infection to spread from the face and scalp inward to the brain, resulting in serious meningitis and other disorders. Even small wounds are potentially dangerous.

[2] Traumatic Hemorrhage

Traumatic hemorrhage in the scalp can occur in three anatomic levels, depending to some extent on the patient's age. Subcutaneous and subperiosteal hematomas are more common in children and are most frequently associated with minor birth trauma. Subgaleal hematomas are the most common type seen in adults with penetrating head injury.

CT scan shows high-attenuation collections overlying the temporalis muscle, which is below the galea in the subgaleal space. Hemorrhage in this location tends to spread diffusely over the skull because of lack of impedance within the subgaleal space. A subgaleal *hygroma* is a collection of CSF within the subgaleal space and may be distinguished on CT scan by its low attenuation. Its presence is ipso facto evidence of underlying skull fracture and dural laceration (Kim and Zee, 1995).

8.72 Cuts, Tears and Lacerations

Scalp lacerations should be treated promptly (after considering other injuries that might take precedence). The major considerations of repair are thorough cleansing and removal of damaged tissue, and adequate closure.

At the emergency room, the scalp is inspected carefully to identify regions where the skull is depressed, indicating skull fracture, and to search for bone fragments. When the scalp is torn over a depressed skull fracture, the possibility of infection makes it desirable to elevate the skull fracture back to its normal position and suture the overlying scalp laceration during the acute period.

Lacerations cannot be evaluated properly unless bleeding, which may be profuse, is controlled. Hemostats can be clamped to the galea and reflected (turned back) over the scalp to compress the vessels. Digital pressure may be applied to stop bleeding when the skull is intact. Self-retaining retractors can be used to spread the wound taut, providing a better view of the underlying pericranium and bone. If it is not possible to adequately view the wound, the examiner should palpate the bone (examine it manually). Linear fractures and depressed fractures are easily palpated but may not be apparent on skull films or CT/MRI scans.

Small scalp lacerations can be sutured following debridement. When the galea is also lacerated and the wound gapes, this layer too should be closed with nonabsorbable sutures. If the injury has produced a flap, the surgeon must make sure the edges of the flap bleed. If they do not, the edges may become necrotic. There is no urgency in suturing these lacerations in the emergency department; some neurosurgeons prefer not to close the wound when depressed fragments are present or suspected until they have elevated the wound (Schwartz, et al., 1992).

Injuries that lacerate the galea can result in excessive bleeding. Improper closure of the wound that does not tightly approximate the galea can lead to excessive bleeding into the loose areolar layer. This can result in a subgaleal hematoma that may extend throughout the areolar space, an area confined by the superior eyelids, zygomatic arch (the prominence of the cheekbone) and superior nuchal line (ridge at the back of the neck). If the areolar layer is contaminated during injury or wound closure, a subgaleal infection may result. Injuries that lacerate the periosteum result in subperiosteal bleeding, which further separates the periosteum from the underlying calvarium (a subperiosteal hematoma). This mass usually recedes without treatment (D'Angelo, 1994).

Skull radiographs, CT scans, MRI and other diagnostic procedures may be ordered to rule out concurrent injury.

8.73 Burns

The scalp has exceptional ability to heal following burn injuries; in the portions covered with hair, even deep burns heal well.

[1] Thermal Burns

When thermal burns injure the scalp, a generally conservative approach is advised, involving minimal trimming of tissue and avoiding removal of the eschar (hardened tissue) that forms. If reconstructive surgery is indicated, it is planned and executed after stable recovery of the patient.

[2] Chemical Burns

Industrial accidents are probably the most common source of chemical burns. They may also result from assaults, accidents and self-inflicted wounds.

Strong acids usually inflict maximal injury immediately. The reaction can be stopped by thorough washing. In contrast, alkali burns continue to damage tissue even after thorough washing, thus increasing the depth of injury.

[3] Electric Burns

The scalp is a relatively unusual site for serious burn injuries in patients who survive electric shock. Electric burns of the scalp usually require contact with high voltage sources, and the amount of heat generated depends on the resistance of tissue. When they do occur, electric burns to the scalp are likely to be more severe than they first appear. The surgical repair of electric burns of the scalp is usually conservative until the lesion is stable. Grafts may be a necessary part of surgical repair.

8.74 Avulsion

Avulsion—the frank tearing away of the scalp from the cranium (scalping)—occurs most often in industrial and farm machinery accidents, when long hair is caught in machinery. Dog bites, motor vehicle accidents and other types of trauma can also result in partial or total avulsion. Scalp avulsion is a rare occurrence, however; a review of literature up to 1988 documents only 16 cases (Buncke, 1996).

[1] Pathophysiology

The usual pathophysiologic mechanism is forceful traction (pulling) of the hair in a slightly off-center direction. Well-aligned vertical pulling simply tears the hair from the scalp. Separation of the scalp occurs at the subaponeurotic layer.

Although the immediate pain is often mild, it becomes severe shortly after the initial injury. Bleeding is profuse from widespread venous tearing and arterial damage and, in fact, could become life threatening (Cheng, et al., 1996).

[2] Surgical Repair

Surgical replantation of full scalp avulsion is a challenging and rare procedure. Since most or all of the avulsed scalp can usually be retrieved, replantation is attempted as soon as possible, either in part or using the whole scalp. Surgeons have been successful in replanting avulsed scalps that were amputated and then hemisectioned by machinery (Cheng, et al., 1996).

Since avulsion produces wide areas of vascular trauma that require multiple interpositional vein grafts, many surgeons recommend the use of anticoagulants, vasodilators and any other methods that may protect the traumatized repairs (Cheng, et al., 1996).

Surgical repair of an avulsed scalp must be accomplished relatively quickly following the injury, as the time to ischemia for an avulsed scalp is shorter than for other body parts. The scalp should be put on ice until it can be delivered with the patient to the operating room, as cooling prolongs the tolerance of ischemia in all tissues (Rivera and Gross, 1995).

The most recent surgical technology for scalp replantation involves the use of a microscope to assist surgeons in reconnecting the arteries and veins to re-establish adequate circulation. Several teams of surgeons may work on the patient at the same time; one team prepares the avulsed scalp, one team prepares the patient and another is ready for skin- and vein-grafting procedures. The avulsed scalp must be shaved of hair and cleansed, the small arteries and veins identified and the scalp assessed for damage and repair potential.

Leech therapy has been used to resolve venous insufficiency following scalp replantation. Leeches emit a heparinlike chemical that helps keep vessels from clotting, and they enhance circulation through the vasodilation that results from their feeding (Rivera and Gross, 1996).

[3] Prognosis

The outcome of scalp replantation varies with the extent of the injury, the adequacy of tissue repair, the degree of inflammatory response and scarring, and the absence of complications such as arterial or venous occlusion and infection (Rivera and Gross, 1995).

8.80 SKULL FRACTURES

The skull provides the framework, container and sheltering bony case for the brain, the cranial nerves, the organs of the special senses (eyes, ears, vestibular apparatus, nose and tongue), the face, the mouth and the upper respiratory cavities and passages. Its principal function is to protect the brain from outside forces; however, when it is exposed to trauma, the skull itself can become a source of injury to the brain. Movement of the skull with respect to the brain, its attachments and blood vessels, or their movement within the skull are factors of great importance in the production of brain injury in craniocerebral trauma.[16]

8.81   Surgical Treatment of Linear Fractures

Skull fractures are classified as linear, basilar or depressed, but they are also described as simple, comminuted (in which the bone is broken into fragments) and compound (in which the break causes a communication to the outside of the body).

Linear fractures are usually not displaced and do not require treatment unless the fracture extends into the orbit or paranasal sinuses, or crosses a major vascular channel. Surgery may be required to correct these secondary injuries (Jastremski, 1996). The scalp should be carefully examined for bruises, lacerations and evidence of blood collecting beneath it; x-rays and CT scans are helpful diagnostic procedures that will rule out such complications. *(See Figure 8-8.)* When the scalp is torn, it must be thoroughly cleansed and sutured to prevent potential infection.[17]

8.82   Surgical Treatment of Basilar Fractures

The base of the skull is weakened by numerous openings (foramina) through which the various nerves and blood vessels enter and leave the brain; basilar fractures, which occur at the base of the skull and include the anterior, middle or posterior fossa (depressions in the base of the skull that contain various brain structures), are considerably more common than fractures of the temporal bones.

When basilar fracture is present, CSF may leak through the nose or ear. Such leakage often stops spontaneously, and surgical repair is seldom necessary. CSF leakage through the nose (rhinorrhea) is more persistent and can result in a CSF fistula (a defect in the dura or arachnoid membranes that allows CSF to escape from the subarachnoid space) and delayed meningitis. Surgical repair may be indicated.

---

[16] *See also* ch. 6 for a complete discussion of skull fractures, including pathophysiology and diagnosis.

[17] *See* 8.72 *supra.*

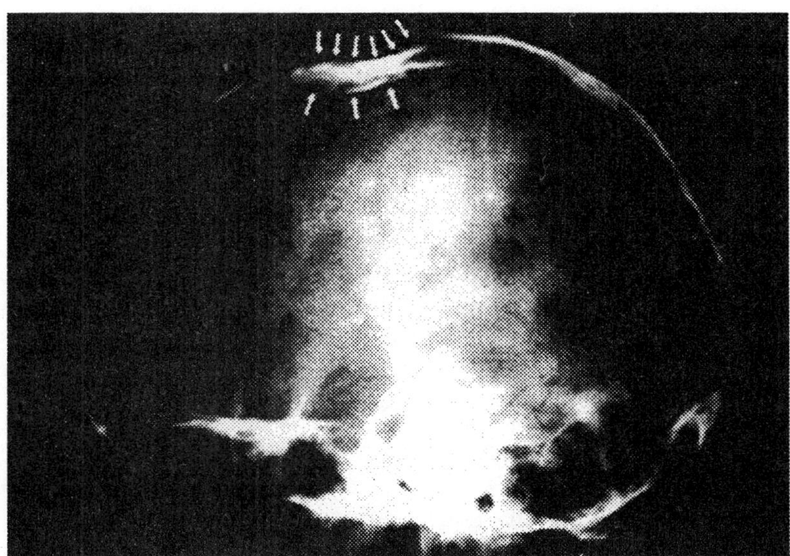

Fig. 8-8. Depressed skull fracture (arrows) indicated by an area of increased density of the x-ray film.

8.83 Surgical Treatment of Depressed Skull Fractures

Depressed skull fractures may be compound, or open, in the presence of a communicating scalp laceration. When a depressed skull fracture is open, there is an increased risk of infection. Surgical asepsis (operation performed with sterilized instruments and hands, etc., in a region made free of pathogenic microorganisms) is used to care for the scalp laceration, and surgery to elevate the depressed bone is usually performed within 24 hours. Fracture fragments must be removed from grossly contaminated wounds. When skull fragments have been driven into important vascular structures, removal of the fragment may result in rapid bleeding that can be difficult to control. When these fragments cannot be replaced, an acrylic or a metal plate may be needed to close the skull (cranioplasty). This procedure may be delayed to prevent local infection (Jastremski, 1996).

Depressed and compound fractures usually require surgical repair to restore the integrity of the dura and overlying tissues and to prevent infection. High mortality rates are seen in patients with depressed fractures in which treatment has been delayed and infection has been established.

8.84 Skull Fractures in Infants and Children

The skull of an infant differs from that of an adult or older child in several significant respects. It is remarkably flexible and moldable in order to permit passage through the narrow birth canal. The vault of the newborn skull is relatively pliable, since the bones have not yet formed secure junctures with one another. The "soft spots" of the fontanelles of the skull have sizable gaps where the membrane has not yet filled in with bone. The surgical relevance of these features of the infant skull includes its greater flexibility, leading to a tendency to indent rather than fracture, and the ease of access to the intracranial space through the fontanelles. These features are often important in the treatment of subdural hematoma, since burr holes and other openings in the skull are usually unnecessary.

Although the vault of the skull of the newborn can be distorted significantly, it will resume its normal configuration spontaneously. Because of this elasticity and ability to withstand a great degree of distortion, the skull of an infant absorbs the energy of physical impact and protects the brain better than the skull of an adult.

In younger children, most skull fractures are linear and asymptomatic, and in the older child, they are readily diagnosed by radiography or by CT using bone windows. Fractures may be irregular in infants and can sometimes be confused with a suture or wormian bone (one of a number of small bones situated in the sutures, where the bones of the cranium join). Closed linear fractures usually heal without surgical management in three to four months (Menkes and Till, 1995).

Depressed fractures are common in perinatal injury, often as a result of difficult forceps delivery; small indentations called Ping-Pong-ball fractures can occur, which are not true fractures and often resolve spontaneously. Most skull fractures in the infant can be treated nonoperatively, although there are instances when surgical management is indicated.

Depressed skull fracture can also occur with any localized skull trauma later in childhood. In the past, elevation and examination of the underlying dura was the recommended course of management. More recently a conservative approach has been suggested that reserves surgical intervention for infants with compound depressed fractures or those with focal neurologic signs; the outcome following surgical or conservative measures seems to be the same (Menkes and Till, 1995).

A complication of a closed head injury with linear fracture in an infant is the "growing fracture," which is associated most commonly with victims of child abuse. Dural tears occur in the parietal area and are unrecognized because the scalp is intact. A CSF-filled cyst develops between the cortex and overlying bone. At the same time, the bone edges along the fracture do not unite, apparently due to the fluid preventing direct contact. The bone is resorbed, so that radiographs taken after an interval of several months show an irregular bone defect with scalloped edges. Surgical separation of the bone from underlying arachnoid, dural repair or replacement, and closure of the bone defect with rib grafts is required. In some cases, normal pressure hydrocephalus[18] develops, which requires shunting (Menkes and Till, 1995).

Basal skull fractures are uncommon in children but should be suspected when the child has signs of bleeding from the nasopharynx or the middle ear. Fractures at the base of the anterior fossa can lead to hemorrhage into the orbit (Menkes and Till, 1995).

Compound fractures occur in about 20 percent of children with traumatic head injury. Management involves limited cleansing of the scalp, institution of antibiotic treatment and tetanus prophylaxis. Anticonvulsant therapy is used routinely when the bony fragments have penetrated beyond the dura (Menkes and Till, 1995).

8.90 CRANIAL AND INTRACRANIAL INFECTIONS

Although antibiotics and modern neurosurgical techniques have greatly reduced the occurrence of infection, it continues to be a major problem and is seen in approximately 5 to 7 percent of head injuries. Infectious complications may be delayed for years in the presence of an intracranial foreign body. Risk factors include external wound infection, cerebrospinal fluid fistula, paranasal sinus injury and retained organic material such as hair or clothing, but not retained bullets (the heat generated as a bullet is discharged effectively sterilizes it). Retained bone fragments may be a source of infection but have been shown to be less of a significant risk than was previously thought (Kim and Zee, 1995).

---

[18] *See* 8.40 *supra.*

8.91 Osteomyelitis

Skull infections may develop after compound fracture of the skull and may result in bony defects that require cranioplasty (plastic surgery to correct a defect in the bones of the cranium, i.e., those bones of the skull that form the sphere containing the brain) to restore normal appearance. Usually the responsible microbe is from one of the staphylococcus groups. The region may become tender, or the infection may be identified by CT scan or by the presence of obvious abscess. Osteomyelitis (bone infection) of the skull may be visualized with plain films as well as CT and is seen as irregular areas of lytic bony destruction (Kim and Zee, 1995).

Surgical treatment consists of removal of the devitalized layer and local treatment of abscesses, local irrigation with antibiotics and provision for drainage.

8.92 Meningitis

Meningitis is the infectious inflammation of the membranes surrounding the brain (the meninges). Any of the pathogenic organisms may be the cause of meningitis, which may follow compound fractures, penetrating missiles or linear fractures that extend into the nasal sinuses or middle ear. The incidence of meningitis following open depressed skull fracture is about 10 percent. Although it is not a common occurrence, the risk is greater when injuries are associated with cerebrospinal fluid fistula. CSF fistulae often manifest as CSF leakage from the nose or ears. Meningitis also occurs in approximately 3 to 50 percent of patients who have traumatic dural fistulae (abnormal connection from the dura, or outermost membrane surrounding the brain, to the outside of the body) (D'Angelo, 1994).

Meningitis commonly develops two to eight days after injury but may be delayed several months, particularly in patients with fractures through the nasal sinuses or mastoid, and may recur, with as many as seven or eight attacks. The presence of CSF fistulae with rhinorrhea or otorrhea favors recurrence. Treatment in such instances must include closure of the fistula (Rowland, 1995).

Meningitis is best diagnosed through cerebrospinal fluid analysis, but contrast-enhanced CT may show leptomeningeal (pertaining to the arachnoid and pia mater) enhancement within sulci (grooves in the brain tissue) or the basal cisterns (fluid-filled cavities) (Kim and Zee, 1995). Meningitis due to CSF fistulae should be aggressively treated with antibiotics.

8.93   Empyema

Abscesses and local collections of pus can accumulate on either side of the dura following penetrating injuries. A local collection of debris from reactions to infection in the space between the dura and the inner surface of the skull is known as epidural empyema. It can enlarge enough to cause elevated intracranial pressure and result in specific neurologic symptoms. On CT scan, epidural and subdural empyemas are similar in configuration to hemorrhagic collections in these locations, except they are usually of low attenuation and exhibit prominent enhancement of the adjacent meninges or dura (Kim and Zee, 1995).

Treatment is basically surgical. Multiple burr holes are drilled in the region, and the pus is removed by saline irrigation. Open craniotomy may be indicated if granulation (scar) tissue needs to be removed.

Subdural empyema is a similar infection located below the dura; it is associated with penetrating injuries that extend through the dura. Diagnosis may be difficult, especially in severely injured patients with impaired consciousness. Treatment usually requires craniotomy, exploration and evacuation of the abscess, irrigation with antibiotics and establishment of subdural drainage.

8.94   Abscess of the Brain

Intracerebral abscess may follow compound skull fractures and the entrance of penetrating missiles. Abscess of the brain is a rare complication of head injury, usually associated with infection of the scalp wound.[19] Symptoms commonly develop in the first few weeks after injury but may be delayed (Rowland, 1995).

The abscess grows and acts as any space-occupying lesion, raising intracranial pressure.[20] Headache, seizures and a variety of symptoms associated with increased ICP may be present. However, sometimes

---

[19] *See* 8.71 *supra.*

[20] *See* 8.50 *supra.*

even large abscesses are not symptomatic. CT scan usually identifies and localizes brain abscess.

The specific methods of treatment of cerebral abscess following head injury are the same as those of abscess from other sources— namely, drainage of the infection and administration of antibiotics— unless foreign material has accompanied the track infection and requires operative intervention (Rowland, 1995).

8.100   BIBLIOGRAPHY

Text References

Benzel, E. C., et al.: The Single Burr Hole Technique for the Evacuation of Non-Acute Subdural Hematomas. J. Trauma 36:190-194, 1994.

Buncke, H. J.: Microsurgical Replantation of the Avulsed Scalp: Report of 20 Cases: Discussion. Reconstr. Surg. 97:1107-1108, 1996.

Cheng, K., et al.: Microsurgical Replantation of the Avulsed Scalp: Report of 20 Cases. Plast. Reconstr Surg. 97:1099-1106, 1996.

D'Angelo, C. M.: Sequelae of Minor Closed Head Injuries. In: Weiner. W. and Goetz, C.: Neurology for the Non-Neurologist. Philadelphia: Lippincott, 1994.

Eckstein, M.: The Prehospital and Emergency Department Management of Penetrating Head Injuries. In: Mayberg, et al. (Eds.): Neurosurg. Clin. N. Am. Philadelphia: Saunders, 1995.

Gennarelli, T. A. and Kotapka, M. J.: Trauma to the Head. General Considerations. In: Schwartz, G. R., et al. (Eds.): Principles and Practice of Emergency Medicine. Philadelphia: Lea & Febiger, 1992.

Gleason, P. L., et al.: The Neurobiology of Normal Pressure Hydrocephalus. Neurosurg. Clin. 4:667-674, 1993.

Jastremski, C. W.: Patients with Head Injury and Brain Dysfunction. In: Clochesy, J., et al. (Eds.): Critical Care Nursing. Philadelphia: Saunders, 1996.

Kaufman, H. H.: Care and Variations in the Care of Patients with Gunshot Wounds to the Brain. In: Mayberg, et al. (Eds.): Neurosurg. Clin. N. Am. Philadelphia: Saunders, 1995.

Keane, J. R. and Baloh, R. W.: Posttraumatic Cranial Neuropathies. Neurol. Clin. 10:849-867, 1992.

Kim, P. E. and Zee, C. S.: The Radiologic Evaluation of Craniocerebral Missile Injuries. In: Mayberg, et al. (Eds.): Neurosurg. Clinics of North America. Philadelphia: Saunders, 1995.

Lange, D. J., et al.: Peripheral and Cranial Nerve Lesions. In: Rowland, L. P. (Ed.): Merritt's Textbook of Neurology. Baltimore: Williams and Wilkins, 1995.

Menkes, J. and Till, K.: Postnatal Trauma and Injuries by Physical Agents. In: Menkes, J. H. (Ed.): Textbook of Child Neurology. Baltimore: Williams & Wilkins, 1995.

Miller, D. J.: Head Injury. J. Neurol. Neurosurg. Psychiatry 56:440-447, 1993.

Moulton, R.J.: Closed and Open Head Injury. In: Hall, J. B., et al. (Eds.): Principles of Critical Care. New York: McGraw-Hill, 1992.

Pieper, D., et al.: Surgical Management of Patients with Severe Head Injuries. AORN J. 63:854-864, 1996.

Prockop, L. D.: Disorders of Cerebrospinal and Brain Fluids. In: Rowland, L. P. (Ed.): Merritt's Textbook of Neurology. Baltimore: Williams and Wilkins, 1995.

Rivera, M. and Gross, J.: Scalp Replantation After Traumatic Injury. AORN J. 62:175-184, 1995.

Rowland, L. P.: Trauma. In: Rowland, L. P. (Ed.): Merritt's Textbook of Neurology. Baltimore: Williams and Wilkins, 1995.

Schwartz, G. R., et al.: Management of Head Injuries. In: Schwartz, G. R., et al. (Eds.): Principles and Practice of Emergency Medicine. Philadelphia: Lea & Febiger, 1992.

Ward, J. D., et al.: Penetrating Head Injury. Crit. Care Nurs. Q. 17:79-89, 1994.

Wijdicks, E. F.: Neurology of Critical Illness. Philadelphia: Davis, 1995.

Additional References

Greene, K. A., et al.: Impact of Traumatic Subarachnoid Hemorrhage on Outcome in Nonpenetrating Head Injury. J. Neurosurg. 84:445-452, 1995.

Snoey, E. and Levitt, M. A.: Delayed Diagnosis of Subdural Hematoma Following Normal Computed Tomography Scan. Ann. Emerg. Med. 23:1127-1130, 1994.

Sullivan, T. E., et al.: Closed Head Injury Assessment and Research Methodology. J. Neurosci. Nurs. 26:24-29, 1994.

CHAPTER 9

Cerebrovascular Injuries (Stroke)

SCOPE

Cerebrovascular injuries may result from trauma to the head or as a result of cerebrovascular disease. Intracranial vascular injury can be caused by penetrating or closed head trauma, resulting in compressive hematomas (accumulations of blood) within the brain or its enveloping meningeal tissues. The manifestations of cerebrovascular disease are commonly referred to as stroke or cerebrovascular accident (CVA). Cerebrovascular disease can lead to intracranial hemorrhage, most commonly from a ruptured aneurysm. More often, cerebrovascular disease results in brain ischemia and infarction from thrombosis or occlusion of an artery by an embolus. Cerebrovascular injury can have a devastating effect on all body systems and ultimately be fatal. Many systemic diseases cause problems in the cerebral vasculature similar to those of stroke. CT scan, MRI and arteriography are the mainstays of diagnosis. Treatment includes the administration of antihypertensive, anticoagulant and thrombolytic medications, and surgical procedures, such as carotid endarterectomy, to correct problems in the arteries. Treatment is determined by the nature of the lesion, its size and site.

SYNOPSIS

9.50   REHABILITATION AFTER CEREBROVASCULAR INJURY
9.100   BIBLIOGRAPHY

9.00   THE CEREBROVASCULAR SYSTEM

The vascular system is composed of arteries, veins and capillaries. Arteries transport blood away from the heart to peripheral organs. Veins return blood to the heart. Thin-walled capillaries interposed between arteries and veins connect arterioles (small arteries) and venules (small veins continuous with capillaries) in organs and allow for the exchange of substances between tissues and the bloodstream. (*See Figure 9-1.*)

This network of vessels is referred to as the *peripheral vasculature.* Arteries transport oxygen and metabolic substrates (substances that are affected by enzymes) in the blood to peripheral organs, and veins return blood saturated with waste products to be eliminated.

Blood is circulated throughout the body as arterial pressure is generated by contraction of the heart, facilitated by contraction and relaxation of muscle fibers in arterial walls. Tension in these muscle fibers is controlled by an intricate system of nerves called the vasomotor nerves. The vasomotor system is part of the autonomic

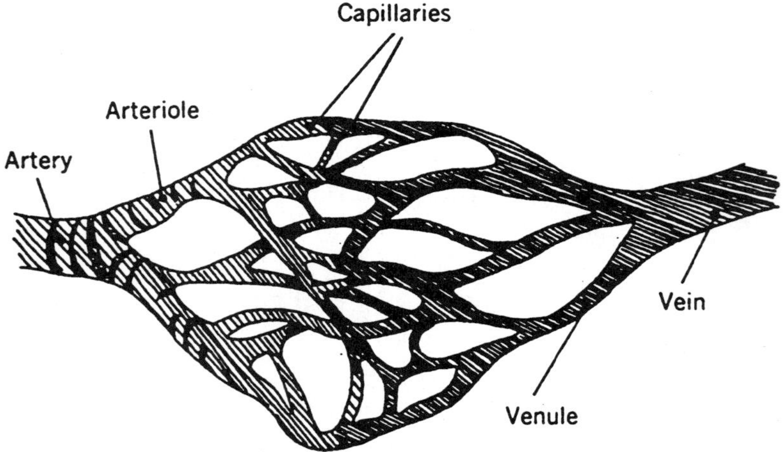

Fig. 9-1. The peripheral vascular system is composed of arteries, veins and capillaries. Capillaries connect arterioles and venules in organs and allow for the exchange of substances between tissues and the bloodstream.

(involuntary) nervous system and regulates the supply of varying amounts of blood to different organs, according to their metabolic requirements. The autoregulation of the intracranial arteries (the arteries that supply the brain) is very intricate, allowing for maintenance of critical amounts of blood flow and blood pressure in various parts of the brain.

9.01   Structure of Blood Vessel Walls

Each blood vessel is a hollow tube with walls composed of three tissue layers: the intima, the media and the adventitia. (*See Figure 9-2.*) The intima is a smooth inner lining of endothelial cells, which are important for metabolism and for maintaining a barrier to the cellular components of blood. The media, or middle layer, consists of connective tissue and smooth muscle and is important for regulating tissue tension in the vessel wall. Muscle fibers of the media form oblique concentric bands that can regulate vessel diameter and thus blood flow and perfusion pressure. Muscle contraction increases perfusion pressure but decreases blood flow. Muscular relaxation results in dilation (expansion), which decreases perfusion pressure and increases blood flow. Autoregulation of muscle tension in the media of cerebral arterioles is particularly well developed and allows for meticulous regulation of the distribution of regional blood flow in the brain. The adventitia—the outermost vessel wall layer—consists of elastic connective tissue that provides for vessel distension and structural maintenance.

Arterial walls must be relatively strong to withstand the force of blood being pumped under pressure, but this three-ply composition permits flexibility and resilience. Veins have a larger diameter than arteries, and thus venous blood is under lower pressure than arterial blood. Vein walls are thinner and more fibrous than artery walls, and they have less smooth muscle.

9.02   Brain Anatomy and Circulation

The brain and the spinal cord comprise the central nervous system. (*See Figure 9-3.*) The brain is divided into the cortical and subcortical cerebral lobes, the cerebellum and the various parts of the brain stem. (*See Figure 9-4.*) The brain and spinal cord are covered by three layers of meninges (connective tissue): the dura mater, arachnoid membrane

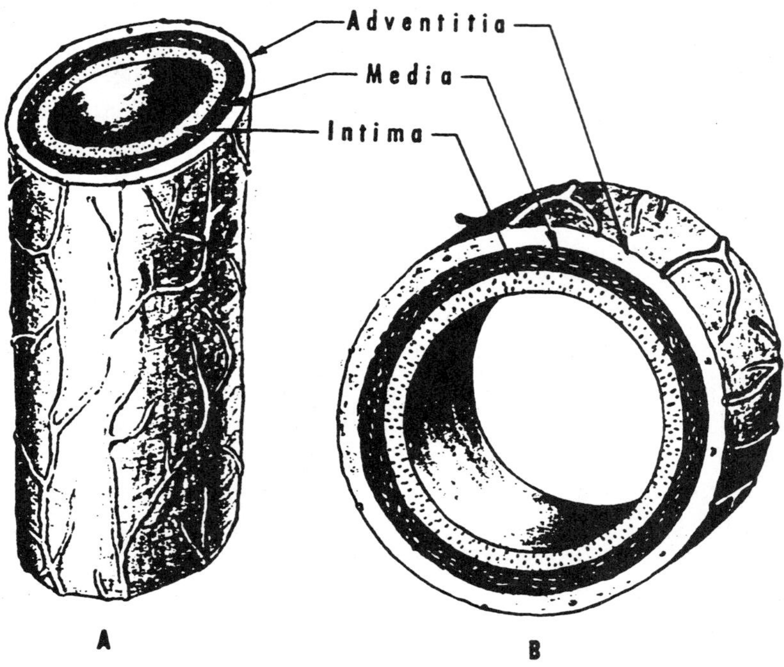

Fig. 9-2. The three layers of an artery wall.

and pia mater. Cerebrospinal fluid (CSF) circulates through the ventricles (cavities within the brain) and is also found in the subarachnoid space (the space separating the arachnoid from the pia mater). (*See Figure 9-5.*)

The brain is supplied with blood by the two internal carotid arteries and the two vertebral arteries. The two internal carotid arteries enter the skull anterior to (in front of) the foramen magnum at the skull base and branch to form the anterior and middle cerebral arteries. The two vertebral arteries enter the skull through the foramen magnum at the skull base and converge to form the basilar artery, which divides into the posterior cerebral arteries after supplying branches to the brain stem and cerebellum. (*See Figure 9-6.*) The internal carotid arteries and the posterior cerebral arteries are connected at the base of the brain by the posterior communicating arteries, forming the circle of Willis, an anastomotic (connected) vascular ring. (*See Figure 9-7.*) The basilar and cerebral arteries and their branches are positioned beneath the thin arachnoid membrane in the subarachnoid space.

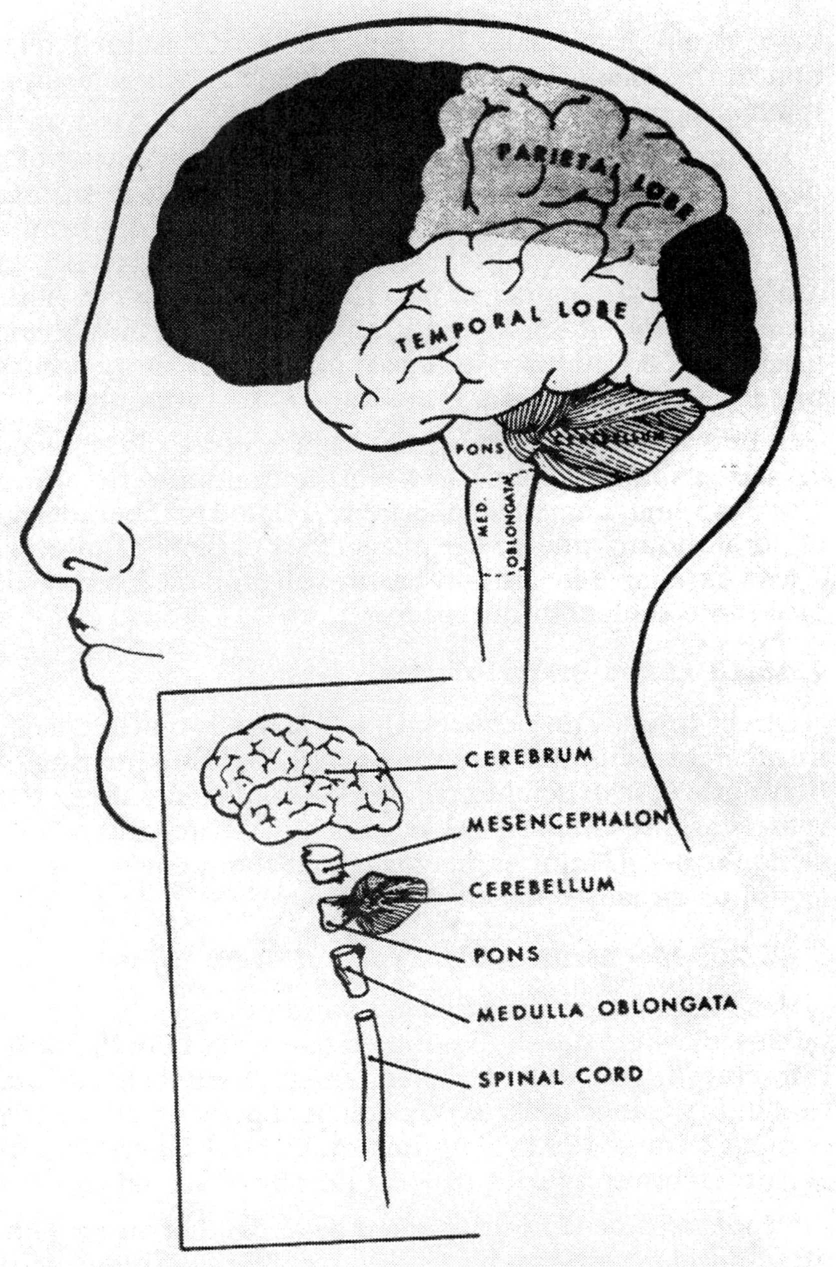

Fig. 9-3. The brain and spinal cord.

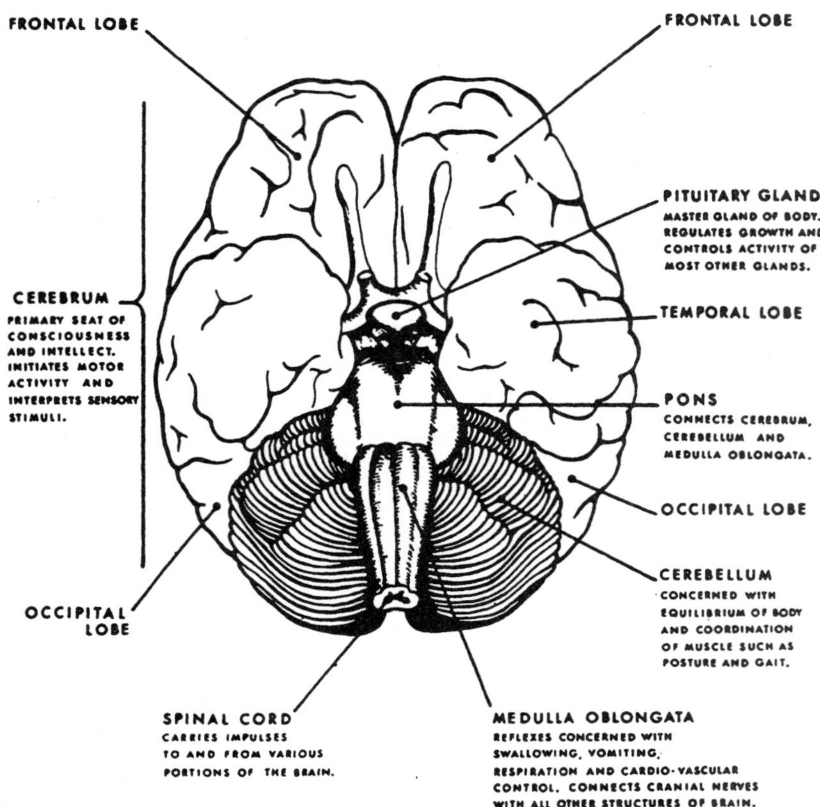

Fig. 9-4. View of the brain from beneath, showing the lobes, the cerebellum and various parts of the brain stem.

Blood is returned from brain tissue by a system of veins that tend to parallel the major arteries. These veins empty into venous sinuses (of no relation to the paranasal sinuses) that are formed between the two layers of the dura mater (the thickest of the brain meninges). The venous sinuses drain into the internal jugular veins, and thus blood is returned to the heart (Carpenter, 1991).

9.03   Diagnostic Techniques in Cerebrovascular Trauma and Disease

Neuroimaging and neurophysiologic diagnostic tests help locate the site of a central nervous system lesion and determine the cause and extent of injury. Computed tomography (CT), an x-ray procedure that

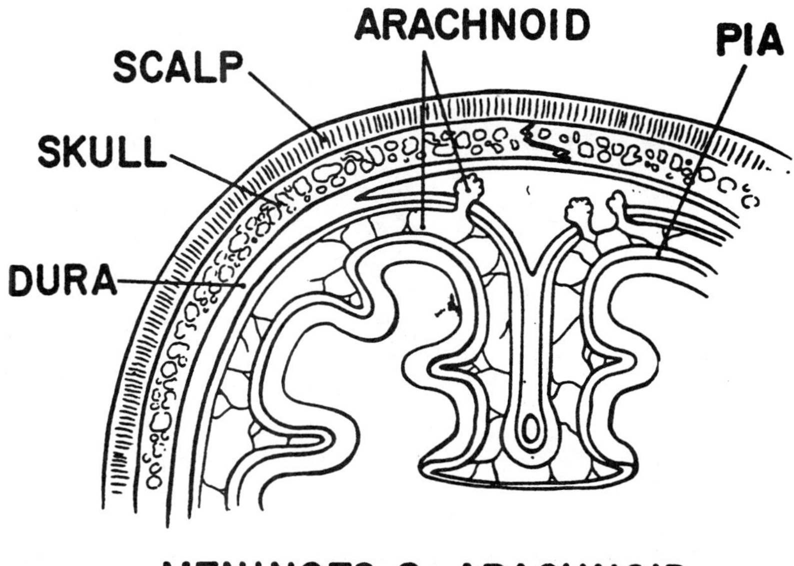

Fig. 9-5. The meningeal tissues and their relation to the brain.

generates cross-sectional "slice" views through the body, is noninvasive, rapidly provides good quality images of the brain and is widely available. Magnetic resonance imaging (MRI) utilizes radio waves and is completely noninvasive. CT is generally superior to MRI for the evaluation of acute trauma and acute hemorrhage, although MRI typically provides superior brain images in most other situations. Single photon emission computerized tomography (SPECT) is used to track a radioisotope that is administered intravenously and provides information about blood flow.

With the development of carotid duplex Doppler ultrasound and transcranial Doppler ultrasound, vascular imaging is becoming increasingly sophisticated. The resolution of magnetic resonance angiography (MRA) is also rapidly improving. Definitive vascular imaging still calls for arteriography (x-ray study of arteries that have been injected with a contrast medium), although this invasive procedure may become obsolete as the resolution of noninvasive neuroimaging techniques improves. Electroencephalography (EEG, which measures electrical activity in the brain) has a limited role in the evaluation of cerebrovascular injury, although it does provide functional information and is useful for identifying epileptiform (related to epilepsy) activity.[1]

---

[1] *See also* ch. 11 for a discussion of epilepsy.

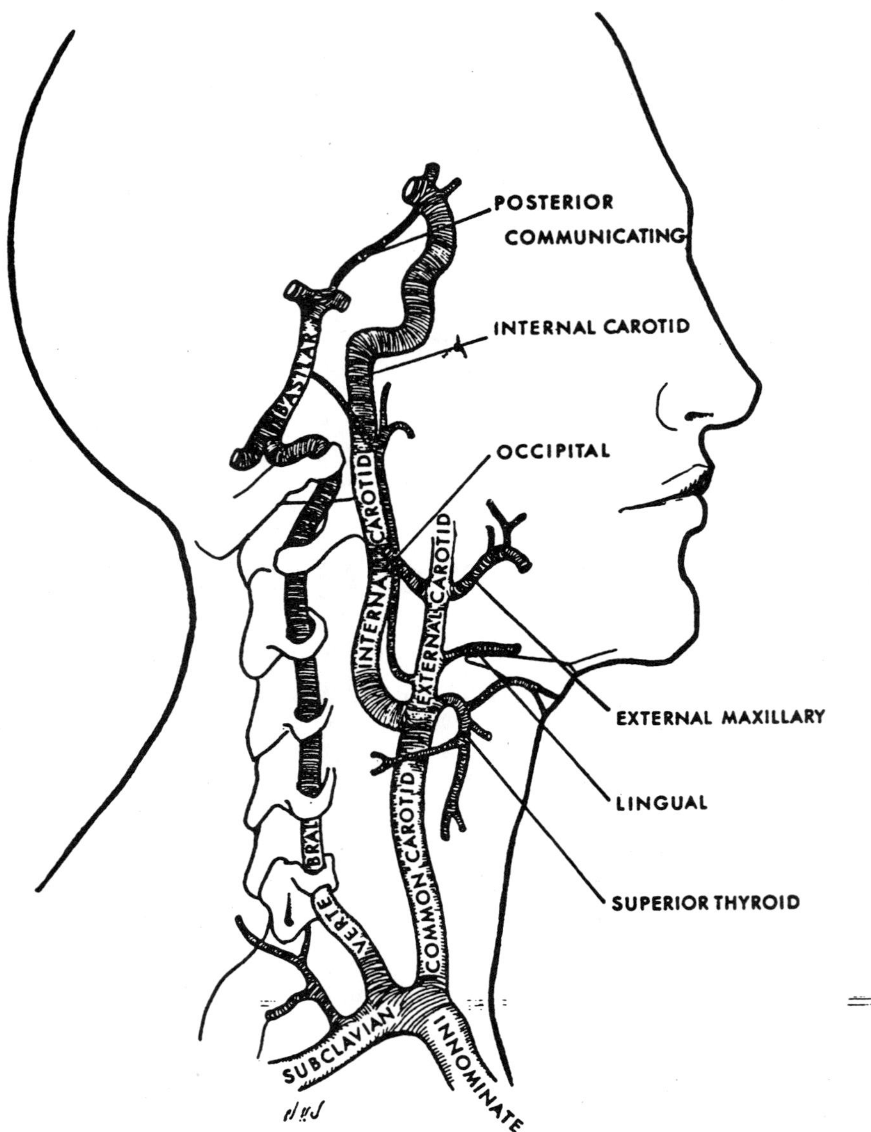

Fig. 9-6. The arteries that supply the head and neck. The carotid and vertebral arteries are the main blood source for the brain.

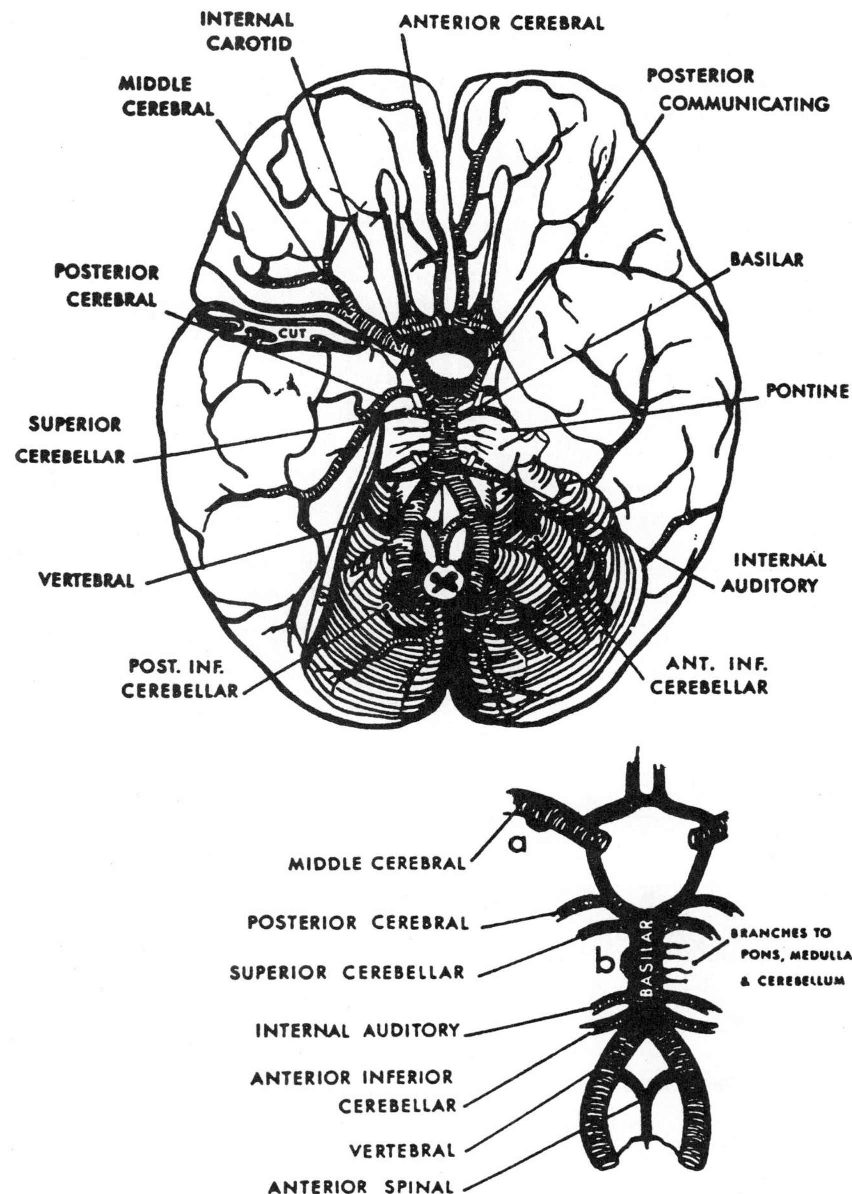

Fig. 9-7. The vascular system of the brain as seen from its underside. The centrally located Circle of Willis lies at the juncture of the cerebral and basilar arteries.

9.10 TRAUMATIC INTRACRANIAL VASCULAR INJURIES

Trauma to the intracranial vasculature most commonly produces symptoms that manifest acutely, within minutes or hours of the trauma. However, symptoms may develop in a more chronic manner and not become apparent for days or weeks. The two major causes of acute and chronic symptoms that represent abnormal function of various brain structures and pathways are *ischemia* and *mass effect*.

When trauma interrupts blood flow through an artery, tissues distal to (beyond) the injury may not be adequately perfused, and thus they will be deprived of oxygen and nutrients. *Ischemia* is the term used to describe the state of such tissue. The brain is particularly sensitive to ischemia. If ischemia persists, the ischemic brain tissue is irreversibly damaged, and infarction (permanent destruction) of the tissue occurs, accompanied by edema (swelling due to accumulation of fluid) of the infarcted tissue. Infarcted brain tissue cannot regenerate.

The brain is contained in a fixed and limited space by the skull. Normal brain tissue can be displaced (herniated) and functionally damaged or destroyed by any type of mass that compresses it. This mass effect can occur after intracranial vascular trauma by formation of a hematoma (accumulation of blood), edema, infarction or contusion (bruising) of tissue, or accumulation of an abnormal volume of CSF if the normal outflow route of the fluid is blocked (Poirier, 1990; Plum and Posner, 1980).

9.11 Mechanisms of Injury

A variety of traumatic mechanisms that affect blood flow to the brain or the integrity of the cerebral vasculature can contribute to cerebrovascular disorders.

[1] Ischemia

Ischemia, which refers to diminution or cessation of blood flow, can result from functional impedance or obstruction of arterial blood flow. When ischemia is sufficient, the supply of oxygen to tissue is inadequate, and the tissue is said to be hypoxic. This results in acidosis (intracellular accumulation of metabolic acids), edema (swelling of the cells due to fluid accumulation) and an influx of calcium ions into the neurons (nerve cells). If this process is prolonged, infarction (cellular death) of the ischemic tissue occurs.

The brain is the organ most vulnerable to ischemia, with permanent damage occurring within a few minutes. As the duration of ischemia continues, it becomes increasingly difficult to restore perfusion of blood to the tissue, and the likelihood of infarction rises.

Ischemic damage to the brain can be global (widespread) or regional (limited to a particular area). A common cause of global brain ischemia is hypoperfusion (low perfusion) resulting from a cardiac arrhythmia (irregular heartbeat) or myocardial infarction (heart attack), with inadequate cardiac output of blood to perfuse the brain. Another common cause is asphyxiation from strangling or choking. Regional ischemia can result from occlusion, laceration or spasm of an artery, or from compression of arteries by regional brain edema or hematoma (Poirier, 1990; Schochet, 1983; Adams, 1995; Yatsu, 1995a).

[2]   Arterial and Venous Laceration and Transection

Laceration (tearing) and transection of arteries occurs commonly, usually as a result of penetrating head injury. Traumatic intracranial arterial laceration can range in severity from a simple puncture to a ragged tear of the vessel wall or complete arterial transection. It is usually caused by a penetrating missile, such as a bullet, or a bone fragment after a skull fracture. Closed (nonpenetrating) head trauma can result in venous and, less commonly, arterial intracranial laceration.

Hemorrhage may be more severe after arterial laceration than after complete arterial transection. When a blood vessel is completely transected, the severed ends retract and constrict, facilitating thrombus (blood clot) formation. This does not occur after incomplete laceration, and the edges of the wound tend to gape and continue to bleed (Poirier, 1990; Schochet, 1983).

[3]   Arterial Contusion and Thrombosis

Contusion (bruising) of blood vessels usually results from blunt trauma that disrupts the intima of the vessel but does not lacerate the arterial wall.[2] The media and adventitia may also be contused. This can occur even after minor head trauma. Contusion tends to disrupt

---

[2] *See* 9.01 *supra* for further discussion of the structure of blood vessel walls.

the arterial intima, causing an effusion of blood and the formation of a hematoma (an accumulation of semi-clotted blood) within the adventitia of the vessel.[3] A large tear of the intima may result in a thrombus in the vessel wall that blocks blood flow through the artery. The thrombus may slowly enlarge and extend along the vessel wall. This is commonly referred to as arterial dissection.

Pieces of intravascular thrombi may break off and be carried in the blood vessel to distal sites (at which point the clots are called emboli), where they lodge in small blood vessels and promote further thrombus formation, tissue ischemia and infarction. This process is referred to as embolization (Poirier, 1990; Schochet, 1983; Adams and Victor, 1993).

[4]   Traumatic Vascular Spasm

Traumatic intracranial arterial spasm, or vasospasm, results from autoregulated contraction of the involuntary muscle of the media layer of the arterial wall. It may occur independently or in association with other vascular lesions, such as contusion or laceration. Spasm can result from blunt trauma and also from the force generated by the shock wave of a penetrating missile, such as a bullet. High-velocity missiles generate the greatest force. Severe spasm can completely obstruct distal blood supply, causing ischemia and infarction of brain tissue supplied by the artery in spasm (Poirier, 1990; Schochet, 1983; Mayberg, et al., 1994).

[5]   Traumatic Aneurysm

An aneurysm is an expansion in an artery caused by damage to the vessel wall. The pressure of blood within the artery creates a saclike enlargement at the weakened area.

Rupture, the most serious complication of an aneurysm, can occur if the weakened adventitia suddenly breaks down. This results in hemorrhage under arterial pressure into and around the brain, under the arachnoid membrane (subarachnoid hemorrhage).

Thrombi can form within aneurysms. Although this reduces the risk of rupture, thrombi can impede blood flow in the artery. Thrombi of this type also can embolize to distal arterial sites.

Aneurysms are usually caused by a congenital (present from birth) defect of the arterial wall. The role of arteriosclerosis (hardening of

---

[3] *See* 9.12 *infra* for further discussion of intracranial hematoma.

blood vessels, most commonly due to the deposition of fatty plaques in vessel walls) in aneurysm formation is uncertain. Infection of a blood vessel can also result in aneurysm formation. Venous aneurysms are rare (Poirier, 1990; Schochet, 1983; Mayberg, et al., 1994).

[6]   False Aneurysm

False aneurysm (pseudonaneurysm) usually occurs after laceration of all layers of an arterial wall from penetrating trauma, with the hemorrhage contained in the surrounding tissue. A fibrous membrane forms around the hematoma; the hematoma's interior liquefies, and the mass pulsates with arterial blood flow. (*See Figure 9-8.*) Arterial pressure progressively enlarges the false aneurysm, and rupture can occur. Although false aneurysms are common in the peripheral vasculature, they do not tend to occur intracranially. This is because brain tissue is too soft to contain a hematoma adjacent to an artery adequately for a false aneurysm to develop (Poirier, 1990; Schochet, 1983).

[7]   Traumatic Arteriovenous Fistula

An arteriovenous fistula is an abnormal direct communication between an artery and a vein. Arteriovenous fistulas may develop acutely following simultaneous perforation of an artery and an adjacent vein. In such cases, arterial blood is diverted from the injured artery into the adjacent vein immediately after the trauma. Sometimes a hematoma forms around the damaged artery and the fistula does not develop until the clot liquefies, days or weeks after the trauma.

The fistula diverts arterial blood flow directly into the venous system, because arterial pressure is greater than venous pressure. (*See*

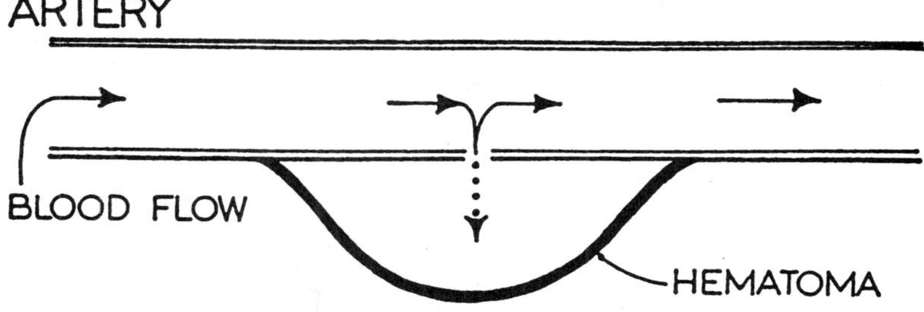

Fig. 9-8. A false aneurysm, in which hemorrhage through an artery wall is held in place by surrounding tissues.

Figure 9-9.) This diversion of blood flow into the venous system can result in a relative decrease in arterial blood flow to areas distal to (farther from the point of origin) the fistula that are normally supplied by the artery. The pathologic significance of the diverted blood depends on the size of the fistula, the sizes of the involved vessels and the duration of the fistula. With time, collateral blood vessels can develop around the fistula to enhance arterial circulation to tissue distal to the fistula.

Although extracranial arteriovenous fistulas develop commonly after penetrating trauma and procedures, traumatic intracranial arteriovenous fistulas are not common. Carotid artery to cavernous venous sinus fistulas are most often seen. The carotid artery passes directly through the cavernous venous sinus behind the orbit (eye socket). Penetrating or blunt trauma to the intracavernous portion of the carotid artery can produce a fistula. Patients with this type of fistula tend to develop exophthalmos (bulging of the eyeball) with ocular pulsation synchronous with the heartbeat. Congenital arteriovenous fistulas are usually referred to as arteriovenous malformations (Poirier, 1990; Schochet, 1983; Adams and Victor, 1993).

9.12   Traumatic Intracranial Hematoma

Traumatic intracranial hematomas may be epidural, subdural, subarachnoid or intraparenchymal in location.[4] (*See Figure 9-10.*)

[1]   Epidural Hematoma

Epidural (extradural; outside the dura mater) hemorrhage most commonly occurs acutely from head trauma resulting in a linear fracture of the temporal bone (on the side of the head), with subsequent laceration of the underlying middle meningeal artery. The hematoma accumulates in the space between the skull and the dura mater. (*See Figure 9-11.*)

It is common for patients with an extradural hematoma to experience a brief loss of consciousness at the time of injury, due to cerebral concussion, and then to regain consciousness. They often have a characteristic "lucid interval," followed in a few hours by increased intracranial pressure and compression of brain structures as the

---

[4] *See also* ch. 4 for further discussion of intracranial hematomas.

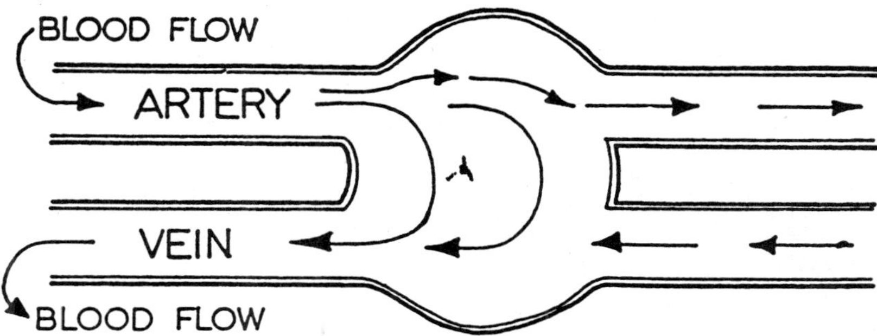

Fig. 9-9. An arteriovenous fistula diverts blood directly into the venous bed, owing to the higher pressure of arterial blood.

hematoma enlarges. Compression of the third cranial nerve by herniated brain tissue results in a dilated pupil that does not respond to bright light. There may be weakness of the contralateral (opposite) side of the body.

Epidural hematomas are often fatal if not rapidly diagnosed and surgically evacuated. Diagnosis is usually accomplished by computed tomography (Poirier, 1990; Schochet, 1983; Rowland, 1995a; Adams and Victor, 1993).

[2]   Subdural Hematoma

Subdural (between the dura mater and the arachnoid) hematomas result from arterial or venous bleeding in the subdural space, usually over the convexity of the cerebral hemisphere, and may be unilateral or bilateral (on one or both sides). (*See Figure 9-12.*) Symptoms result from painful stretching of the dura, increased intracranial pressure and displacement of brain structures as the hematoma enlarges.

Acute subdural hematoma typically follows acute trauma, as a result of arterial bleeding, and may combine with epidural hemorrhage, cerebral contusion and cerebral laceration. The clinical presentation is similar to that of epidural hematoma. CT is diagnostic, and prompt surgical evacuation is necessary if the hematoma causes mass effect.[5]

Chronic subdural hematoma results from venous bleeding and may not cause symptoms for weeks to months after head trauma. The trauma that precipitated the bleeding may have been so minor that

---

[5] *See* 9.10 *supra.*

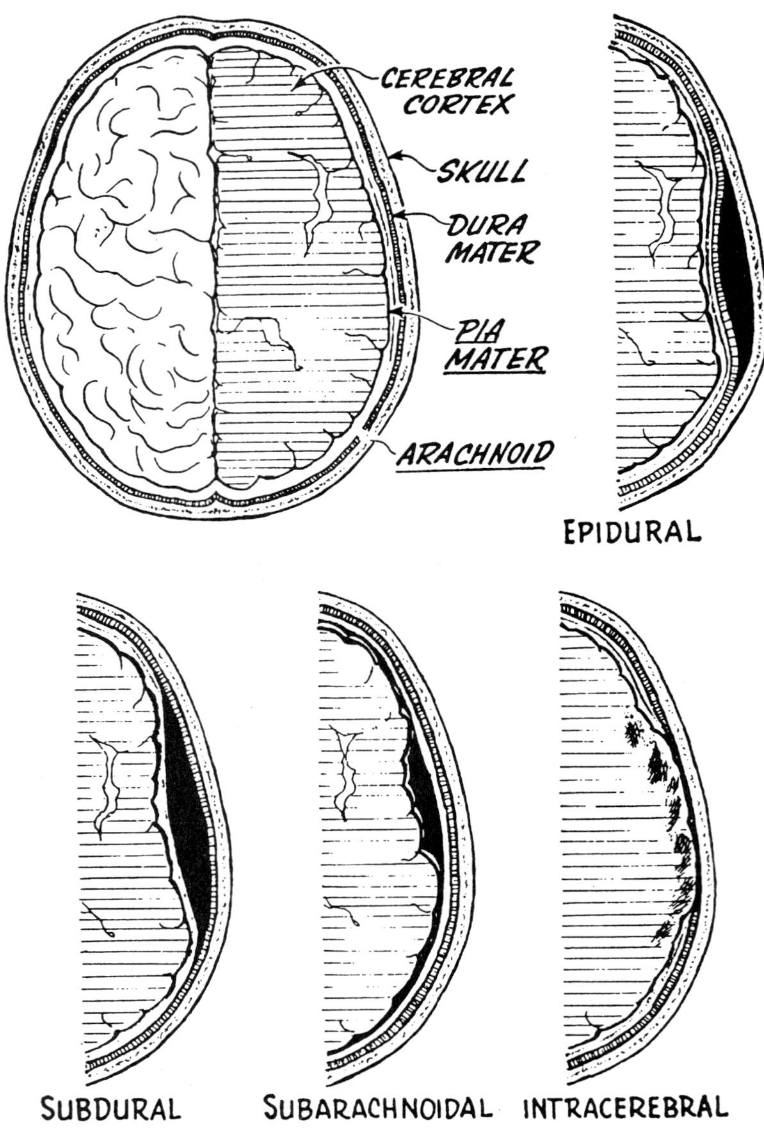

Fig. 9-10. The cerebral cortex (outer layer) and surrounding meninges, with different types of intracranial hematoma that may occur.

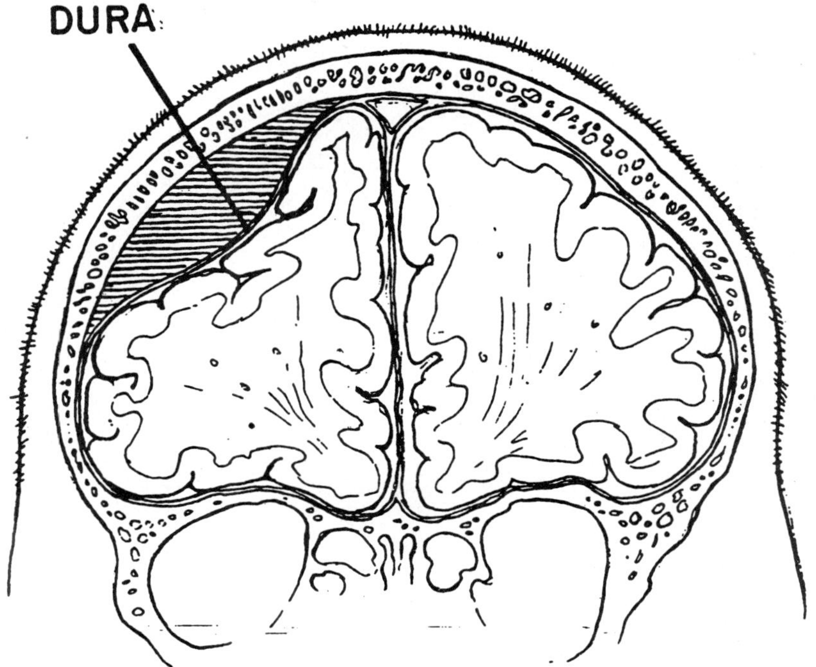

Fig. 9-11. Classic presentation of an epidural (extradural) hematoma.

the patient has no recollection of it. Stretching of the dura may cause headache, and compression of brain tissue from the enlarging hematoma may produce contralateral weakness. Increased intracranial pressure and displacement of brain structures may eventually occur, with potentially fatal herniation of brain tissue if a critical degree of brain displacement occurs.

CT is usually diagnostic, although it can fail to diagnose hematomas of a certain age that have the same density as brain tissue as seen on radiography. Magnetic resonance imaging (MRI) may be necessary for diagnosis in such cases.

Treatment consists of surgical evacuation if the hematoma results in significant mass effect. However, small chronic subdural hematomas that result in only minimal mass effect may be treated conservatively with corticosteroid drugs and their course followed with serial CT (Poirier, 1990; Schochet, 1983; Rowland, 1995a; Adams and Victor, 1993).

Subdural hematomas can occur in battered infants as a result of violent shaking. Child abuse should always be suspected if an infant has a subdural hematoma.

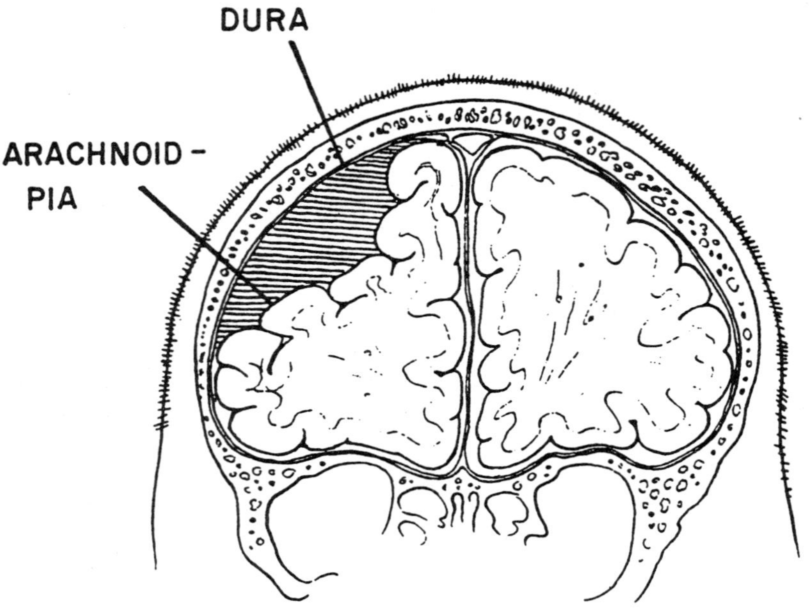

Fig. 9-12. Classic presentation of a subdural hematoma.

[3]   Traumatic Intraparenchymal Hemorrhage

Acute intraparenchymal (within the functional tissue) hemorrhage may result from penetrating or closed head injuries that cause laceration of intraparenchymal intracranial blood vessels. This can cause a rapid rise in intracranial pressure, with compression and displacement of normal brain structures. Such injuries are very often fatal, especially following penetrating injuries. Diagnosis is by computed tomography. Medical management of increased intracranial pressure and surgical hematoma evacuation are of limited value (Poirier, 1990; Schochet, 1983; Rowland, 1995a; Adams and Victor, 1993).

9.20   NONTRAUMATIC CEREBROVASCULAR DISEASE

Stroke and *cerebrovascular accident* (CVA) are terms used to refer to manifestations of nontraumatic cerebrovascular disease. A minority of strokes are caused by hemorrhage, usually either spontaneous subarachnoid hemorrhage or intraparenchymal brain hemorrhage. Most strokes consist of brain infarctions (tissue death) that are either thrombotic or embolic in origin.

9.21   Spontaneous Subarachnoid Hemorrhage

Primary subarachnoid hemorrhage accounts for 3 to 11 percent of strokes in the United States (Sacco, 1995). Approximately 26,000 nontraumatic subarachnoid hemorrhages occur in the United States each year, accounting for about 10 percent of all stroke deaths. Half of those who sustain spontaneous subarachnoid hemorrhage are under the age of 45.

[1]   Etiology

An aneurysm is a sac in the wall of an artery whose underlying pathology involves a defect in the muscular coat and the internal elastic layers of the vessel wall. The weak area allows the arterial wall to bulge outward under pressure in the artery.

Aneurysms typically develop at areas of bifurcation (branching) of arteries. By far the majority of intracranial aneurysms are located in carotid artery territory, and 10 percent are in vertebrobasilar artery territory. Common sites are:

- the vicinity of the anterior communicating artery;
- the origin of the posterior communicating artery from the internal carotid artery;
- the first major bifurcation of the middle cerebral artery;
- the bifurcation of the internal carotid artery into the anterior and middle cerebral arteries;
- the origin of the ophthalmic artery (the first intracranial branch of the internal carotid artery, which supplies the eye with blood);
- the junction of the posterior communicating artery with the posterior cerebral artery;
- the bifurcations of the three pairs of cerebellar arteries; and
- the top of the basilar artery.

The most common type of aneurysm is a "saccular" or "berry" aneurysm. It is commonly accepted that these aneurysms are a result of a congenital defect of the arterial wall. This produces a localized area of arterial dilation, with the aneurysm sac usually connected to the arterial wall by a narrow neck. The wall of the sac consists of elastic tissue that often is very thin.

Saccular aneurysms are rarely seen before puberty, but it is esti-mated that 5 percent of persons age 20 and older have one or more, and that 25 percent of these people have multiple aneurysms. Saccular aneurysms are slightly more prevalent in women than men. They range in size from 2 mm to several cm, with the average size being 7 to 10 mm. Aneurysms greater than 3 cm in diameter are referred to as *giant aneurysms,* and these are at lower risk than smaller aneurysms (7 to 12 mm) of producing massive hemorrhage.

Mycotic aneurysms result from the inflammation of infected arterial walls, most commonly as a result of septic (infected) emboli in people with infective endocarditis (inflammation of the lining of the heart).[6] They usually occur in peripheral branches of the intracranial arteries.

Arteriosclerotic aneurysms are relatively uncommon; when the exist, they are usually cylindrical or fusiform (spindle-shaped; tapering at both ends) in shape. They most commonly involve the proximal (closer to the point of origin) intracranial internal carotid arteries and the basilar artery, and they are often very large. Rupture is uncommon; more often, these aneurysms partially or completely thrombose (clot closed).

Angiomas are congenital malformations of vessels. There are four major types: venous, cavernous and capillary angiomas, and arteriove-nous malformations. Venous angiomas are the most common and consist of anomalous veins. Rupture of this type of angioma is uncommon. Cavernous angiomas are composed of a mass of sinusoidal vessels. Capillary angiomas (telangiectases) are composed of small, capillarylike vessels. Arteriovenous malformations consist of masses of arteries and veins with abnormal direct connections. They vary greatly in size and location, although they most commonly occur in the cerebral hemispheres and are the type of angioma most likely to be symptomatic (Mayberg, et al., 1994; Schochet, 1983).

[2] Pathogenesis

Theories for the pathogenesis of saccular aneurysms include con-genital defects of the arterial media, vestigial remnants of embryonic vessels and arteriosclerosis. None of these explanations is completely satisfactory. Hypertension (high blood pressure) is considered by some to have etiologic significance, but hypertension is less common in patients with aneurysms.

---

[6] *See* 9.37 *infra* for further discussion of endocarditis.

There is also no satisfactory explanation for the cause of rupture of saccular aneurysms. The relationship of physical activity to rupture is not at all clear. The role of trauma in precipitating the rupture of an intracranial aneurysm has long been a matter of controversy. Trauma can only be implicated as a cause by a temporal relationship between the trauma and evidence of aneurysm rupture. It is likely that in many cases, loss of consciousness from a vehicular accident occurred at the time of aneurysm rupture, and that the accident did not cause the rupture. About a third of aneurysmal ruptures occur during sleep.

Angiomas are congenital malformations. Arteriovenous and cavernous angiomas occasionally grow, although most are smaller than 3 cm in size and tend to remain so. Only a minority—perhaps 10 percent—rupture with massive bleeding. No definite cause of angioma rupture has been identified A close association between head trauma and rupture is difficult or impossible to prove (Mayberg, et al., 1994; Schochet, 1983).

[3]   Clinical Presentation

Most aneurysms are asymptomatic until they rupture. Giant aneurysms can compress normal brain structures and have a mass effect on the function of these structures.[7] Occasionally smaller aneurysms enlarge and produce mass effect by compression of normal intracranial structures. The most common example of this phenomenon is compression of the oculomotor nerve by an enlarging posterior communicating artery aneurysm, resulting in ptosis (drooping eyelid), pupillary dilation and impaired extraocular movement (dysfunction of the extraocular muscle, which contributes to excursion of the eye). Retro-orbital pain may result from compression of the ophthalmic division of the trigeminal nerve (the fifth cranial nerve).

About 30 percent of patients with acute aneurysmal rupture report suspicious symptoms a few hours, days or weeks prior to rupture. Symptoms include "sentinel headache," stiff neck, nausea, dizziness, syncope (fainting) and disturbances of vision. These symptoms are often minor or absent but, in retrospect, their presence may signal initial aneurysmal leak (Brust, 1995c).

Arteriovenous malformations more commonly cause symptoms without rupture, including seizures and chronic recurrent headache that

---

[7] *See* 9.10 *supra* for further discussion of mass effect.

is clinically indistinguishable from migraine. A minority of arteriovenous malformations result in subarachnoid hemorrhages, most often in pregnant women.

Subarachnoid hemorrhage is the hallmark of aneurysmal rupture, owing to the arterial saccular aneurysm's rupture into the subarachnoid space. If the aneurysm tip is pointed toward the parenchyma of the brain, blood may rupture into the brain tissue or the ventricular system of the brain. If the arachnoid membrane ruptures, blood can enter the subdural space and form a subdural hematoma.

The first symptom of rupture is usually very sudden onset of excruciating headache, typically described as the worst headache a person has ever experienced. This may be accompanied by neck pain, loss of consciousness and seizure activity. Confusion may be present if consciousness is preserved or regained. There is often moderate fever (102° to 103° F) and elevation of the peripheral white blood cell count (leukocytosis). Many cases have a more subtle presentation (Mayberg, et al., 1994; Adams and Victor, 1993).

[4]   Neurologic Complications

Because the cranium is a rigidly enclosed space, any increase in its contents can raise pressure within the head. With subarachnoid hemorrhage due to aneurysmal rupture, the sudden rush of blood into the subarachnoid space under arterial pressure can cause a sudden, tremendous increase in intracranial pressure. This results in compression and dysfunction of normal brain structures, often with coma and rapidly ensuing death (Plum and Posner, 1980).

Pressure on the hypothalamus can cause impaired body temperature regulation and the inappropriate secretion of antidiuretic hormone (ADH), resulting in excessive fluid retention and hyponatremia (low sodium content in circulating blood). This can cause confusion, stupor and seizures.

[a]   Rebleeding

Without surgical intervention, about 30 percent of patients who survive an initial aneurysmal rupture will rebleed (experience recurrent hemorrhage) within a month. This occurs most commonly between the fifth and ninth day after the initial hemorrhage. Rebleeding has been the cause of death in almost 40 percent of fatal subarachnoid hemorrhages (Sahs, et al., 1981). The use of epsilon aminocaproic acid to reduce rebleeding has been abandoned, owing to complications, its lack of proven effect on outcome and the increasing acceptance of early surgical intervention. After six months, the rate of rebleeding drops to about 3 percent a year (Jane, et al., 1985).

[b]   Vasospasm

Vasospasm is a more common cause of clinical deterioration than rebleeding. The severity of spasm of arteries in the subarachnoid space correlates with the amount of blood that is present. Although the pathogenesis is not entirely clear, there is some evidence that chemical mediators such as histamine, serotonin and angiotensin may be involved. Vasospasm occurs 3 to 21 days after subarachnoid hemorrhage, resulting in ischemia and infarction of brain tissue in the distribution of the arteries in spasm. Brain infarctions can produce a variety of focal neurologic symptoms and signs, including aphasia (difficulty speaking), hemiparesis (paralysis on one side of the body), sensory and visual abnormalities and disturbances of consciousness.

[c]   Hydrocephalus

The presence of clotted blood in the subarachnoid space or the ventricles of the brain can impede the resorption of CSF, resulting in hydrocephalus (ventricular enlargement due to fluid accumulation). This type of hydrocephalus is seen in 5 to 10 percent of persons who sustain nontraumatic subarachnoid hemorrhage. Fibrin (a blood component that is essential to clotting) from the hemorrhage can obstruct the foramina of Luschka and Magendie (openings in the brain stem that connect the fourth ventricle of the brain with the subarachnoid space), or adhesions can develop between the pia mater and arachnoid membrane, blocking the resorption of CSF. This increases intracranial pressure, resulting in generalized brain compression and dysfunction, usually with headache, confusion and a decline in consciousness. Hydrocephalus usually appears two to four weeks after hemorrhage but may present more insidiously (Mayberg, et al., 1994; Adams and Victor, 1993).

[5]   Diagnosis

Definitive diagnosis of an aneurysm or arteriovenous malformation is currently made by conventional cerebral arteriography. Unruptured giant aneurysms and many arteriovenous malformations can be visualized with brain MRI or CT. The technology of intracranial magnetic resonance angiography (MRA) is rapidly evolving. The resolution of intracranial MRA is already adequate for visualizing most saccular aneurysms and arteriovenous malformations, and MRA may eventually replace conventional radiographic arteriography. Some small, asymptomatic aneurysms are identified by MRI, MRA or CT performed for an unrelated indication (Mayberg, et al., 1994; Greenberg, 1995).

Diagnosis of subarachnoid hemorrhage can be difficult and is frequently delayed or missed. Diagnosis begins with a high index of clinical suspicion, especially when patients present to an emergency department with acute headache or other subtle symptoms. The patient may abruptly lose consciousness, remain conscious but confused or remain alert and oriented. Nausea, vomiting, hypertension (high blood pressure) and altered level of consciousness are commonly observed. Seizures and fever are sometimes seen. Neck stiffness is often a prominent complaint, with nuchal (nape) rigidity present on examination. This is due to irritation of the meninges as blood circulates through the CSF into the spinal subarachnoid space. Focal neurologic findings are often absent, unless the aneurysm has ruptured into the parenchyma (functional tissue) of the brain or there is occlusion of an artery distal to the aneurysm, in which case hemiparesis or other focal deficits may be present. Cranial nerve palsies (paralyses), particularly involving the oculomotor (third cranial) nerve, may develop due to sudden compression. Hemorrhage into the retina of the eye may occur; subhyaloid retinal hemorrhage (hemorrhage between the retina of the eye and the hyaloid membrane separating it from the vitreous humor) is virtually diagnostic of subarachnoid hemorrhage (Adams and Victor, 1993; Yatsu, 1995a).

[a] CT Scan

Diagnosis of subarachnoid hemorrhage can usually be confirmed by cranial CT, which is generally superior to MRI for this purpose. CT also allows for the diagnosis of intraparenchymal hemorrhage, subdural hemorrhage and acute obstructive hydrocephalus. If subarachnoid blood is identified on CT, lumbar puncture is usually unnecessary. However, CT will miss a small percentage of cases of subarachnoid hemorrhage. If the CT is nondiagnostic and subarachnoid hemorrhage is still suspected, a lumbar puncture (spinal tap; withdrawal of cerebrospinal fluid through a needle inserted into the low back) should be performed.

[b]   CSF Studies

CSF drawn from a person with subarachnoid hemorrhage is uniformly bloody. Any bloody CSF should be centrifuged. The supernatant (top) layer of the fluid after centrifuging is xanthochromic (yellow), indicating that blood has been present for at least six hours. This differentiates between subarachnoid hemorrhage and the presence of blood from a traumatic lumbar puncture. Spinal fluid pressure is usually elevated, ranging from 200 to 500 mm of water. In addition to red blood cells, excessive white blood cells may be present in the CSF, owing to inflammation of the meninges (chemical meningitis). CSF glucose concentration is often modestly reduced, and CSF protein concentration may be slightly increased (Brust, 1995c; Yatsu, 1995a).

[c]   Arteriography

Following confirmation of subarachnoid hemorrhage by CT or lumbar puncture, complete arteriography of the intracranial vessels is necessary to identify one or more aneurysms. This should typically be done in a timely fashion (within 12 to 48 hours). Arteriography should be complete, because many patients have multiple aneurysms.

The presence of multiple aneurysms can present a challenge regarding diagnosing which aneurysm has ruptured, since clinical symptoms may not accurately reflect the location of the hemorrhage. However, when CT is combined with complete arteriography, the correct site of bleeding can be identified in most cases. If an aneurysm or arteriovenous malformation is not identified, arteriography is commonly repeated after 10 to 14 days.

Arteriography also allows for the identification of vasospasm[8] in cases of subarachnoid hemorrhage (Yatsu, 1995a; Greenberg, 1995; Mayberg, et al., 1994; Brust, 1995c). Vasospasm can also be diagnosed and monitored by transcranial Doppler ultrasonography (Babikian and Wechsler, 1993). Skull radiographs, electroencephalography (which measures the brain's electrical activity) and radionuclide brain scanning (which measures the uptake of radioactive isotopes in the bloodstream as a gauge of pathology) have very limited utility in the diagnosis and evaluation of subarachnoid hemorrhage (Mayberg, et al., 1994).

---

[8] *See* 9.11[4] *supra* for a discussion of vascular spasm.

[6] Treatment

Diagnosis should be made in a timely fashion, and patients should generally be placed in a quiet, dark room. Fluid and electrolyte abnormalities should be corrected, blood sugar levels should be controlled, excessive hypertension should be treated and seizures should be managed with anticonvulsant medications. The administration of oral nimodipine has been demonstrated to reduce the incidence of vasospasm (Pickard, et al., 1989).

Surgery is considered the definitive treatment for saccular aneurysm. In the past, surgery was typically delayed for one or two weeks, due to increased morbidity and mortality associated with vasospasm. However, this introduced a significant risk of rebleeding. Recent technical advances allow neurosurgeons to surgically clip or obliterate most aneurysms soon after rupture (within 24 to 72 hours) and to flush blood from the subarachnoid cisterns (Miyaoka, et al., 1993). Surgery is sometimes still delayed in medically unstable or neurologically devastated patients, in patients with demonstrated severe vasospasm and in patients in whom the source of bleeding cannot be identified.

Three types of surgical failure may necessitate reoperation. During exploration, the surgeon may abandon clipping as dangerous or impractical and choose to wrap the aneurysm with fat or muscle tissue, or to ligate (tie off) the carotid artery. Imperfect placement of a clip can result in slipping. Carotid artery ligation, which is now uncommon, may fail to terminate blood flow to the aneurysm (Drake, et al., 1984).

Surgical evacuation of an intraparenchymal or a subdural hematoma may be necessary to eliminate mass effect. If acute hydrocephalus develops, ventricular drainage by ventriculostomy (surgical opening of the ventricle) may be required (Mayberg, et al., 1994; Adams and Victor, 1993).

Interventional neuroradiology involves the obliteration of some aneurysms, especially giant aneurysms, with balloons, wires and coils introduced via an arterial catheter. These techniques, along with interventional embolization with plastic spheres, are more commonly used to obliterate arteriovenous malformations. Sometimes the obliteration is partial, prior to surgical excision or noninvasive radiosurgical obliteration using a "gamma knife." These treatment modalities are not widely available and are currently experimental (Mayberg, et al., 1994).

[7] Prognosis

Age and condition of the patient, size, location and configuration of the aneurysm, presence of multiple aneurysms, time interval between rupture and surgery, quality of the medical facility and skill of the surgeon are all important variables that influence survival and quality of life following rupture and repair of a saccular aneurysm.

A commonly applied grading system is based on the preoperative neurologic status of the patient:

Grade 1: alert, oriented, with or without headache, with no motor or sensory deficit.

Grade 2: moderate alteration in sensorium or focal deficit; severe headache and meningeal signs.

Grade 3: obtunded (sensorium blunted) and/or major focal deficit.

Grade 4: stuporous or comatose, with or without major lateralizing findings.

The rate of mortality increases progressively with increase in preoperative clinical grade. There is also a close correlation between clinical grade and quality of survival. Patients with grade 3 or 4 clinical status have a much poorer postoperative outcome. Surgery for such patients is sometimes delayed, although this introduces the risk of rebleeding. About 40 percent of patients with ruptured aneurysms die of the initial bleed. At least 40 to 50 percent of patients who rebleed die, and morbidity for survivors of rebleeding is increased (Nishioka, et al., 1984; Ingall, and Wiebers, 1993). Intraventricular hemorrhage is usually fatal.

The results of surgical treatment of saccular aneurysms have improved dramatically over the years. The experience and skill of the surgeon are very important: Operative results tend to be better for neurosurgeons who perform such procedures relatively regularly and frequently (Adams and Victor, 1993).

Restoration of function depends on age of the patient, severity of neurologic damage and absence of rebleeding. With mild to moderate neurologic deficit, full recovery often takes place, especially in the absence of focal neurologic signs indicating intracerebral hemorrhage or infarction from vasospasm. If patients with intraparenchymal bleeding or infarction survive, they often exhibit permanent neurologic sequela, including mental changes, paralysis, aphasia (difficulty speaking), visual field defects and epilepsy.

9.22 Spontaneous Intraparenchymal Brain Hemorrhage

Primary intracerebral hemorrhage accounts for 5 to 10 percent of strokes in the United States (Sacco, 1995).

[1] Etiology

Trauma is the most common cause of intraparenchymal (intracerebral) brain hemorrhage. Acute intraparenchymal hemorrhage may result from penetrating or closed head injuries that cause laceration of intraparenchymal intracranial blood vessels.

Arteriovenous malformation, which can be a source of subarachnoid hemorrhage, usually results in intraparenchymal brain hemorrhage when it ruptures.[9] It is commonly believed that spontaneous intraparenchymal brain hemorrhage with no identifiable cause may be due to a small, "cryptic" arteriovenous malformation that occludes or destroys itself when it ruptures (Schochet, 1983).

Hypertension (high blood pressure) is a common cause of intraparenchymal brain hemorrhage. Hypertensive hemorrhages may be massive, small or petechial (pinpoint size). The most common locations, in descending frequency, are the basal ganglia (a cluster of gray matter at the base of the brain; 50 percent), the cerebral lobes ("lobar hemorrhage"), the thalamus, the cerebellum and the pons of the brain stem (Adams and Victor, 1993; Sacco, 1995; Schochet, 1983). A small number of intraparenchymal hemorrhages arise from a degenerative disorder affecting the media of smaller arteries in elderly people that is referred to as congophilic amyloid angiopathy (Yatsu, 1995b).

Brain tumors typically present subacutely or chronically as they grow, but they may present acutely due to hemorrhage into the tumor. This is especially prevalent with metastatic (traveling from the site of origin to more distant areas) melanoma (a type of skin cancer), renal (kidney) cell carcinoma, choriocarcinoma (a highly malignant tumor with common metastases to the brain) and bronchogenic (related to the lungs) carcinoma (Mohr, 1995b; Schochet, 1983).

Illicit drug use must be considered in the etiology of intraparenchymal brain hemorrhage in a person with drug-induced vasculitis. The two substances most commonly implicated are methamphetamine and crack cocaine.

---

[9] *See* 9.21 *supra* for further discussion of arteriovenous malformations.

Mycotic (septic) aneurysms typically result from endocarditis. These present as intraparenchymal brain hemorrhage more commonly than as subarachnoid hemorrhage (Schochet, 1983).

[2] Pathogenesis

Trauma and arteriovenous malformations both can precipitate intraparenchymal hemorrhage. Hypertensive hemorrhages are believed to result from the rupture of microaneurysms on small intracerebral arteries, and subsequent mechanical distension by arterial hypertension. Referred to as microaneurysms of Charcot and Brouchard, these result in the total replacement of the normal endothelial, muscular and elastic elements of the vessel by a thin layer of connective tissue. This destruction of the normal vascular architecture results in the deposition of lipid (fat) and fibrin (fibrous clotting elements) products (lipohyalinosis), predisposing to fragility of the vessel wall and potentiating rupture and hemorrhage (Poirier, et al., 1990). With congophilic amyloid angiopathy, vascular fragility results from the deposition of amyloid protein in the vessel walls. Drug use can contribute to the development of arteritis (inflammation of the arterial walls), with subsequent vascular fragility.

[3] Clinical Presentation

Neurologic symptoms and signs vary with the site and size of the hemorrhage.The neurologic deficit resulting from intraparenchymal hemorrhage typically begins abruptly, depends on the site of hemorrhage, is usually accompanied by hypertension and may be accompanied by headache, nausea, vomiting and loss of consciousness. Headache may be absent in as much as 50 percent of cases. Seizures occur in about 10 percent of cases of intracerebral hemorrhage. With the advent of CT, many small hemorrhages are now identified that would previously have been clinically diagnosed as cerebral infarctions.

Basal ganglionic hemorrhages tend to involve the internal capsule and result in hemiplegia, with large hemorrhages (greater than 2 to 3 cm in diameter) producing stupor and coma. Similar symptoms are seen with lobar and thalamic hemorrhages. Lobar hemorrhages also commonly produce visual field defects and aphasia. Pontine (referring to the pons; part of the brain stem) hemorrhages are usually devastating, with oculomotor (referring to eye movement) disturbances and deep coma typically developing within minutes. Cerebellar hemorrhage may develop over several hours, with vomiting, headache, vertigo and ataxia (incoordination). Prompt diagnosis of cerebellar hemorrhage is very important if fatal, progressive brain stem compression is to be prevented. Surgical decompression can be lifesaving in such cases (Adams and Victor, 1993; Patten, 1996; Plum and Posner, 1980).

[4] Neurologic Complications

Focal neurologic symptoms and signs vary with the site and size of the hematoma. A zone of edema (swelling due to accumulation of fluid) develops around the hematoma, contributing to the size of the mass. Within the rigidly enclosed space of the cranium, any increase in contents can raise intracranial pressure. This results in compression, brain tissue herniation (protrusion through the foramen magnum, or opening at the base of the skull), ischemia and dysfunction of normal brain structures, often with coma and rapid death. Brain stem hemorrhages have a particularly high mortality. Cerebellar hemorrhages are also extremely dangerous, due to the risk of progressive brain stem compression, which can be rapid and fatal (Plum and Posner, 1980).

[5] Diagnosis

Intraparenchymal and intraventricular intracranial bleeding is very easy to diagnose by CT, which is typically superior to MRI in this situation. The primary purpose of emergent neuroimaging with CT of patients presenting to an emergency department with coma or focal neurologic signs is to diagnose intracranial bleeding (Caplan, et al., 1995; Plum and Posner, 1980; Schochet, 1983).

[6] Treatment

Fluid and electrolyte abnormalities should be corrected; blood sugar levels should be controlled; excessive hypertension (high blood pressure) should be treated and seizures should be treated with anticonvulsants. Ventilatory (respiratory) support may be necessary, as may hyperventilation, which lowers intracranial pressure. A corticosteroid (usually dexamethasone) may be administered to reduce edema, especially in patients with large hemorrhages and poor neurologic condition. However, the value of corticosteroid therapy for improving neurologic deficits is unproved. With acute, massive intracranial pressure and herniation, the administration of mannitol (a hyperosmotic agent) may lower intracranial pressure and be lifesaving (Adams and Victor, 1993).

The goal for treating arterial hypertension after intracerebral hemorrhage is a subject of controversy. Proponents of aggressive treatment favor lowering arterial blood pressure to prevent further bleeding. However, there is evidence that bleeding stops spontaneously within 30 minutes and that excessive lowering of arterial blood pressure can worsen the patient's neurologic status by reducing cerebral blood flow, aggravating ischemia and promoting infarction (Adams and Victor, 1993; Mohr, 1995a).

Cerebellar hemorrhages resulting in brain stem compression and a decline in consciousness should be surgically evacuated. Most other intraparenchymal brain hemorrhages are treated medically, unless there is significant decline in neurologic status resulting from increased intracranial pressure and herniation of brain tissue. Some advocate surgical evacuation of the hematoma at this point, although there is wide variation in the degree of enthusiasm with which neurosurgeons evacuate intracerebral hemorrhages. The outcome is often poor with this type of surgical intervention, because patients for whom it is reserved have typically suffered acute, massive brain injury.

[7] Prognosis

The overall mortality rate is high for patients with intraparenchymal brain hemorrhage, with 30 to 35 percent of patients dying within 30 days (Adams and Victor, 1993). The mortality rate is extremely high for pontine hemorrhages and basal ganglionic hemorrhages that rupture into the ventricular system, regardless of the type of treatment that is rendered. The mortality rate following basal ganglionic, thalamic and lobar hemorrhages depends on the size of the hemorrhage and ranges from 13 percent to 40 percent. With cerebellar hemorrhage, mortality relates to the size of the hemorrhage. Neurosurgical evacuation of the hematoma can be lifesaving in cases of brain stem compression, if it is performed in a timely fashion (Mohr, 1995a; Adams and Victor, 1993; Plum and Posner, 1980; Lampl, et al., 1995).

9.23 Thrombotic Ischemic Brain Infarction

Ischemic infarction accounts for 70 to 80 percent of strokes in the United States.

[1] Etiology

Thrombotic ischemic brain infarction (death of brain tissue caused by a blood clot that blocks a cerebral artery) is the most common type of stroke. Cardioembolism (a blood clot from the heart that travels through the bloodstream) accounts for 15 to 30 percent of strokes,[10] and thrombotic ischemic cerebrovascular infarction makes up the majority of the remainder. Atherosclerosis (deposition of fatty plaques in the arterial wall) is by far the most important underlying pathophysiologic factor for thrombosis of a cerebral artery.

Risk factors for noncardiac cerebral infarction include age, hypertension, diabetes mellitus, cigarette smoking, coronary artery disease, lipid abnormalities and a family history of atherosclerotic disease. Excessive alcohol consumption is a recognized risk factor for stroke. However, there is evidence that light alcohol use may be protective against the development of atherosclerosis (Sacco, 1995; Adams and Victor, 1993; Hachinski, et al., 1996; Whisnant, 1996). Migraine[11] may be an independent risk factor for cerebral infarction (Buring, et al., 1995).

[2] Pathogenesis

The common denominator in the pathogenesis of the most common type of stroke is atherosclerosis, which results from the deposition of lipids, fibrin and platelets on the arterial endothelium and the formation of plaques. Atherosclerosis most commonly affects large arteries, such as the internal carotid, vertebral and basilar, and has a predilection for sites of arterial bifurcation (division). Calcification (hardening due tc calcium deposition), intramural hemorrhage (bleeding in the blood vessel wall) and mural thrombosis (clotting in the blood vessel wall) lead to an increase in plaque size.

Atherosclerotic plaque predisposes to cerebral ischemia, thrombosis and infarction by three mechanisms: ischemia, arterial thrombosis and microembolization. Small vessel occlusion and trauma can also play a role.

[a] Ischemia

Ischemia distal to the site of an atherosclerotic plaque can occur if the lumen of the vessel is sufficiently stenotic (narrowed) to

---

[10] *See* 9.24 *infra* for further discussion of cardioembolic ischemic brain infarction.

[11] *See also* ch. 10.

compromise blood flow in the artery. Arterial stenosis is typically not hemodynamically significant unless the arterial lumen is at least 70 to 80 percent stenotic. In such cases, superimposed arterial hypotension (low blood pressure) can lead to ischemia and infarction without thrombosis.

[b]   Arterial Thrombosis

Arterial thrombosis tends to occur at areas of atherosclerotic plaque. Platelet and fibrin deposition on a plaque results in mural (pertaining to a vessel wall) thrombus formation, with occlusion of the artery. The ensuing ischemia results in infarction of the brain tissue that is supplied by the occluded artery.

[c]   Microembolization

Microembolization probably plays a major role in the pathogenesis of ischemic cerebrovascular symptoms associated with atherosclerosis. Platelet and fibrin deposition on a large-vessel atherosclerotic plaque may result in nonocclusive mural thrombus formation. Small parts of this thrombus (microemboli) may then break off and flow to more distal arterial branches, resulting in transient or permanent occlusion, with transient or permanent focal neurologic symptoms.

[d]   Small Vessel Occlusion

Noncardiac cerebral infarction may also result from small vessel occlusion. This is most commonly due to lipohyalinosis (degeneration of smooth tissue and replacement with fatty tissue) of small arteries associated with arterial hypertension (sometimes referred to as arteriosclerosis). It may also be related to microembolism from atherosclerotic plaques in larger vessels. Small vessel disease is also common in diabetic individuals (Poirier, et al., 1990; Schochet, 1983; Sacco, 1995).

[e]   Trauma

Trauma can play a role in thrombotic infarction. This applies primarily to dissection of the carotid and vertebral arteries (enlargement and extension of a thrombus along the vessel wall) during manipulation of the neck, as well as during other activities associated with sudden neck movement.[12]

----

[12] *See* 9.11[3] *supra* for further discussion of arterial dissection.

[3] Clinical Presentation

Ischemic cerebrovascular disease manifests clinically as one or more focal neurologic symptoms and signs. Subjective symptoms can include having trouble speaking, visual problems, difficulty swallowing, dizziness, imbalance, weakness and numbness. Objective signs can include aphasia (difficulty speaking), visual field defects, loss of ocular motility, ataxia (incoordination), dysarthria (slurred speech), inattention, loss of spatial organization, sensory loss, paresis (partial paralysis) and paralysis. (*See Figure 9-13.*)

Symptoms of ischemic cerebrovascular disease typically begin acutely. They may be transient, evolve and progress, or remain stable. The combination of symptoms and signs depends on the location and size of the ischemic area of the brain. (*See Figure 9-14.*) Cerebral cortical (in the lobes) ischemic lesions produce symptoms experienced on the contralateral (opposite) side of the body and may rarely be accompanied by seizures. Cerebellar ischemic lesions are accompanied by symptoms on the ipsilateral (same) side of the body. Cranial nerve involvement is the hallmark of brain stem ischemic lesions.

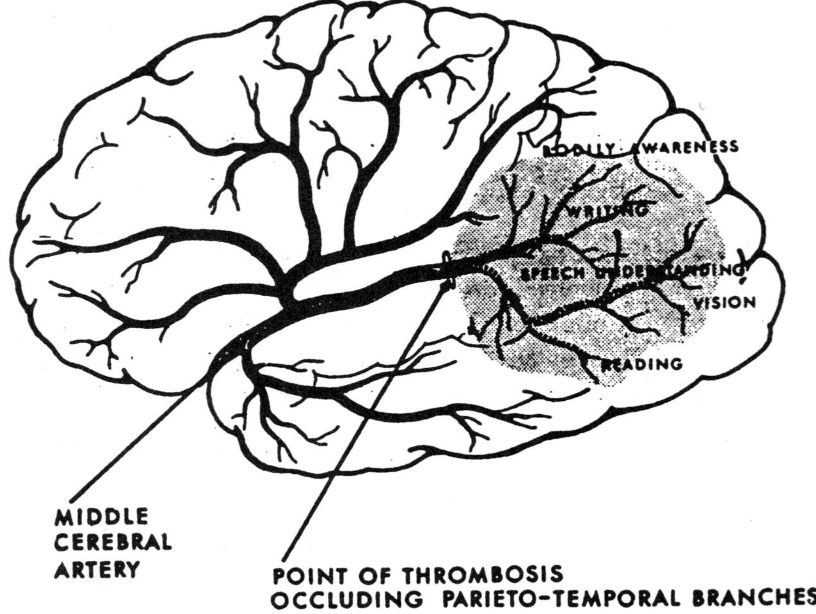

Fig. 9-13. Thrombotic occlusion of a cerebral artery that produces visual field defects, among other problems.

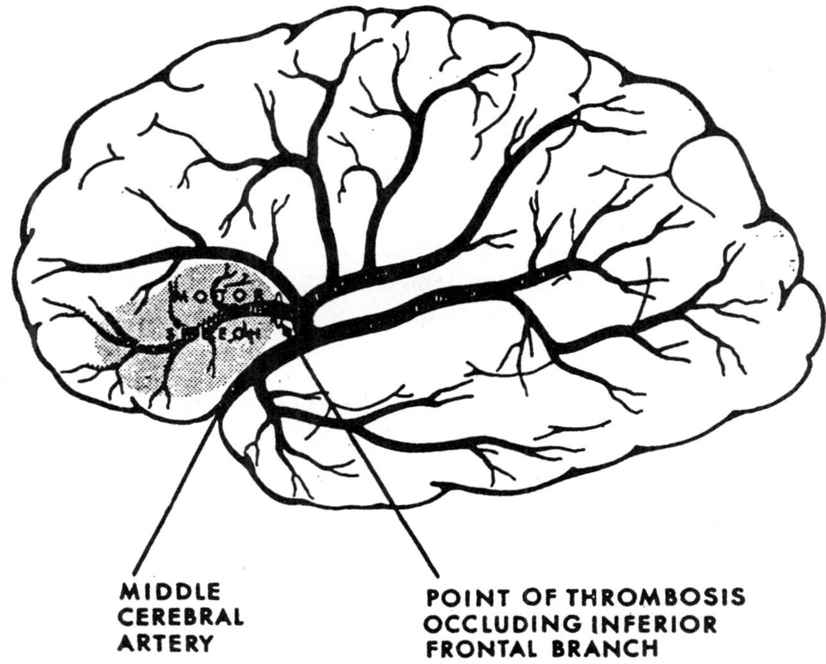

Fig. 9-14. Thrombotic obstruction of a cerebral artery, leading to weakness of the lower part of the right side of the face and tongue that causes disabilities of speech.

A number of common stroke syndromes have been described (Patten, 1996; Poirier, et al., 1990; Adams and Victor, 1993; Brust, 1995b; Kistler, et al., 1994). Stupor and coma may be present with brain stem lesions, bilateral cerebral lesions and large unilateral cerebral lesions with mass effect and increased intracranial pressure (Plum and Posner, 1980).

[a] Lacunar Strokes

Lacunar strokes (characterized by the development of lacunae, or empty spaces in brain tissue) are caused by occlusion of small penetrating arterioles in the subcortical cerebrum and brain stem, resulting in small infarctions that can be clinically silent or devastating, depending on the location. They are most commonly a result of long-standing, untreated hypertension (high blood pressure) that causes arteriosclerosis. As many as 35 percent of lacunar infarctions may be asymptomatic, but most are symptomatic as transient ischemic attacks (TIAs) or sudden, focal neurologic deficit, with a stepwise pattern of deterioration over time as more lacunae develop. Discrete clinical syndromes that have been described include pure motor hemiplegia (motor paralysis on one side of the body), pure hemisensory (loss of sensation on side of the body) stroke, sensorimotor pseudobulbar palsy (paralysis of nerves in the rhombencephalon, or hindbrain, which is comprised of the pons, cerebellum and medulla oblongata), ipsilateral ataxia (incoordination on the same side as the stroke), hemiparesis and dysarthria. Multiple lacunae tend to occur bilaterally in the basal ganglia and brain stem, with dementia, rigidity and gait disturbances developing (Yatsu, 1995b; Adams and Victor, 1993; Critchley, 1983).

[b]   Transient Ischemic Attacks (TIAs)

Transient ischemic attacks (TIAs) are groupings of focal neurologic symptoms resulting from ischemia to the eye (*amaurosis fugax,* a form of temporary blindness) or a part of the brain supplied by the carotid or vertebro-basilar arteries. By definition, such symptoms last less than 24 hours and clinically resolve completely. They typically last a few minutes to a few hours before complete clinical resolution.

Most TIAs probably result from platelet-fibrin microemboli that arise from a more proximal atherosclerotic plaque, although they can result from cardiogenic emboli. Patients who experience TIAs are at increased risk of stroke and myocardial infarction. Improved diagnosis of TIAs in recent years may be partially responsible for an observed reduction of the incidence of strokes. Although clinical resolution is complete within 24 hours, CT and MRI have demonstrated that many patients with clinical TIAs actually experience a small brain infarction. Transient symptoms that resolve after more than 24 hours have often been referred to as reversible ischemic neurologic deficits (rinds), although this is a term with little meaning (Yatsu, 1995b; Brust, 1995a; Adams and Victor, 1993; Kistler, et al., 1994; Waxman, et al., 1983; Hachinski, 1984).

[c]   Ischemic Penumbra

Many patients who have symptoms of brain dysfunction due to ischemic cerebrovascular disease undergo progressive evolution of the neurologic deficit due to complications. However, the concept of the "ischemic penumbra" is of paramount importance. The ischemic penumbra is a zone of viable brain tissue with critically reduced blood flow surrounding an area of ischemic infarction. Factors that further reduce blood flow to this ischemic zone can result in extension of a brain infarction, with evolution of clinical symptoms (Yatsu, 1995a; Adams, 1994; Adams and Victor, 1993).

[d]   Completed Stroke

Many patients with focal neurologic deficits due to ischemic cerebrovascular disease do not experience resolution of their symptoms; neither do they undergo clinical evolution (progression). Such patients, as well as those whose condition has evolved, are said to have a "completed stroke" (Yatsu, 1995a).

[4]   Neurologic Complications

Neurologic deterioration after ischemic brain infarction can occur by several mechanisms, among them evolution of infarction due to loss of viability of the ischemic penumbra. This process is promoted by ischemia-induced collection of neural excitotoxins (products toxic to nerve cells) and calcium in the ischemic, but still viable, neurons of the ischemic penumbra.

Ischemic and infarcted neurons become edematous (swollen due to an influx of water), contributing to the size of the mass. With brain infarctions, maximum edema typically occurs on the third or fourth day after infarction. Brain infarctions can undergo hemorrhagic transformation due to bleeding into the infarcted area of brain tissue. This is more common with infarctions caused by cardiogenic emboli and venous occlusion. Any increase in contents within the rigidly enclosed space of the cranium can raise intracranial pressure. This results in compression, brain tissue herniation, ischemia and dysfunction of normal brain structures, often with coma and rapid death. Distortion of penetrating pontine arteries due to downward herniation of brain tissue can lead to brain stem hemorrhages known as Duret's hemorrhages, which usually lead to death.

There is no convincing evidence that corticosteroid therapy benefits the cerebral edema associated with cerebral infarction. Seizures can occur with acute ischemic brain infarction (Yatsu, 1995a; Adams and Victor, 1993; Plum and Posner, 1980; Poirier, et al., 1990; Schochet, 1983; Kilpatrick, et al., 1990).

[5]   Diagnosis

The initial step in the proper management of patients with cerebral infarction is correct diagnosis in a timely fashion. Diagnosis of brain infarction can usually be made correctly on clinical grounds, although it is important to exclude a diagnosis of intraparenchymal brain hemorrhage, subdural hematoma, neoplasm (tumor) and other causes of focal neurologic deficits. It is also impossible to absolutely differentiate between cardiogenic embolic and thrombotic ischemic infarctions on clinical grounds.

Patients who present with a focal neurologic deficit should undergo a complete medical history and physical examination, as well as an urgent CT scan, primarily to exclude hemorrhage and other pathologic processes.

Acute infarctions may not be visualized initially on early CT. Other routine emergent tests include electrocardiogram (EKG, a measure of the electrical activity of the heart), complete blood count (CBC), platelet count, serum electrolyte levels (measures of substances that facilitate electrical activity in the tissues), blood sugar levels, renal (kidney) function testing, prothrombin time (a measure of the blood's clotting ability), partial thromboplastin time (another measure of the blood's clotting ability) and pulse oxymetry or arterial blood gases. These tests should allow for differentiation of most TIAs and brain infarctions from other causes of acute focal neurologic deficits, often by exclusion, although they do not always allow for the differentiation between cardiogenic embolic and thrombotic ischemic infarctions. In addition, the severity of illness and clinical stability of the patient are simultaneously observed.

If the CT scan is not diagnostic and subarachnoid hemorrhage or meningoencephalitis (inflammation of the brain and meninges) is suspected, a lumbar puncture (spinal tap) should be performed. Additional laboratory tests in selected situations can include blood ethanol (alcohol) level, drug screen and liver function tests. Serum calcium and magnesium levels should be checked if seizures have occurred (Adams, 1994; Adams, 1995; Feinberg, et al., 1994; Mohr, 1995b; Adams and Victor, 1993).

The diagnosis of cardiogenic embolic causes of stroke is sometimes indefinite, but important. The decision that a patient has had a cardiogenic embolus is usually made based on circumstantial evidence provided by the clinical history, physical examination, electrocardiogram, carotid Doppler ultrasound, arteriography and echocardiography.[13]

---

[13] *See* 9.24[5][c] *infra* for further discussion of echocardiography.

All patients with TIAs or acute ischemic cerebral infarction should be evaluated for the presence of significant carotid artery stenosis (narrowing). Technologic advances in carotid Doppler ultrasonography now allow for screening of patients, with high-quality studies eliminating the need for conventional arteriography for many patients. Patients with greater than 50 percent carotid artery stenosis by Doppler should probably undergo conventional arteriography. Technologic advances in the resolution of magnetic resonance angiography may eliminate the need for conventional arteriography (Adams, 1995; von Reutern and von Büdingen, 1993; Greenberg, 1995).

[6] Medical Treatment

Optimally, patients with acute ischemic neurologic events should be admitted to the hospital and undergo continuous cardiac monitoring. There is significant cardiac co-morbidity with ischemic cerebrovascular disease, and as many as 40 percent of patients with symptomatic carotid artery disease have asymptomatic severe coronary artery disease. Cardiac deaths are the major cause of mortality with cerebrovascular disease (Adams, 1995).

Fluid and electrolyte abnormalities should be corrected, hyperglycemia (high blood sugar level) and hypoxemia (low blood oxygen level) managed, and seizures treated with anticonvulsant medications. Airway and ventilatory support should be provided to patients with depressed levels of consciousness.

[a] Antihypertensives

There is general agreement that hypertension (high blood pressure) should not be treated aggressively in the patient with acute focal brain ischemia. This is because aggressive treatment of hypertension can decrease cerebral blood flow to the ischemic penumbra, resulting in extension of infarction with subsequent clinical worsening.[14] It is acceptable to withhold antihypertensive treatment for systolic (while the heart is contracting end ejecting blood) blood pressures lower than 200 to 220 mm Hg and diastolic (while the heart is filling with blood) blood pressures less than 120 to 130 mm Hg (Adams, 1995; Adams, et al., 1994). Some experts advocate aggressive hydration (fluid infusion) and volume expansion in order to enhance cerebral blood flow and decrease blood viscosity.

---

[14] *See* 9.23[3][c] *supra* for further discussion of the ischemic penumbra.

[b] Anticoagulants

Heparin (an anticoagulating agent) binds with intrinsic antithrombin III to inactivate thrombin and the propagation of blood clots. The treatment approach of acute anticoagulation with heparin after TIA and noncardiogenic cerebral infarction is somewhat controversial. Heparin has been recommended and used extensively as an anticoagulant in patients with "crescendo" TIAs and with evolving cerebral infarction (Adams, 1995; Kistler, et al., 1994; Adams and Victor, 1993). However, American Heart Association guidelines conclude that there is no evidence to recommend the routine administration of anticoagulants to patients with TIAs (Feinberg, et al., 1994). These guidelines further conclude that data about the safety and efficacy of using heparin in acute ischemic stroke is insufficient and conflicting. Hemorrhage can be a serious complication of heparin therapy. The use of heparin in this clinical setting remains a matter of preference for the treating physician (Adams, et al., 1994).

[c] Thrombolytic Therapy

There is currently great interest in the application of acute thrombolytic (clot-dissolving) therapy to ischemic stroke victims. The thrombolytic agents streptokinase and urokinase have not yet been demonstrated to be of definite benefit. Intravenous tissue plasminogen activator (tPA) has recently been shown to improve patient outcome following acute ischemic stroke, and it is currently being used at times. However, it has significant limitations, not the least of which is that it must be administered within three hours of the onset of symptoms. In addition, CT of the brain must be obtained prior to administration of tPA to exclude the presence of hemorrhage.

Although the overall outcome is improved, an increased percentage of patients who receive tPA hemorrhage into an ischemic brain infarction, a complication that can be very critical. In addition, use of tPA for acute thrombolytic therapy of stroke has not currently been approved by the FDA; currently stroke is listed as a contraindication to the administration of tPA. Until FDA approval, the use of tPA for acute thrombolytic therapy of stroke is not likely to be widespread (The National Institute of Neurological Disorders and Stroke rt-PA Stroke Study Group, 1995; Adams, et al.,1994).

[d]   Cytoprotective Therapy

There is also currently great interest in the application of cytoprotective therapy to acute ischemic stroke victims. The most commonly used drugs include corticosteroids, barbiturates and calcium channel blockers. However, none of these has been demonstrated to be effective. Current experimental trials are mainly centered around calcium channel blockers, excitatory amino acid inhibitors, 21-aminosteroids (lazaroids), free radical scavengers and antioxidants (Adams, et al., 1994; Yatsu, 1995a).

[e]   Chronic Platelet Antiaggregant Therapy

Additional medical therapy for prevention of recurrent TIA and noncardiogenic ischemic brain infarction involves acute and chronic platelet antiaggregant therapy.

American Heart Association guidelines conclude that there is no evidence to recommend the routine administration of anticoagulants (heparin or warfarin) to patients with TIAs or acute noncardiogenic ischemic brain infarction (Feinberg, et al., 1994; Adams, et al., 1994). Although oral anticoagulants (warfarin) have been used for decades to prevent stroke in TIA patients, there is no conclusive data supporting this use (Feinberg, et al., 1994). The situation is quite different for chronic platelet antiaggregant therapy. There is convincing evidence that aspirin and ticlopidine reduce the risk of primary and recurrent cerebral thrombosis in patients with TIAs or acute noncardiogenic ischemic brain infarction. Aspirin doses ranging from 75 mg to 1,500 mg per day have been shown to be efficacious, although the optimal dosage has not been determined. In the acute phase, a loading dose of 160 mg to 325 mg of aspirin is recommended. In clinical practice, doses of 325 mg to 1500 mg daily are most commonly used for chronic stroke prophylactic therapy (Fuster, et al., 1983; Antiplatelet Trialists' Collaboration, 1994; Antiplatelet Trialists' Collaboration, 1988).

Ticlopidine is a relatively new antiplatelet agent approved in the United States for stroke prevention. It is at least as effective as aspirin, and it may be more effective in certain groups of patients, including women, diabetics and patients with small vessel disease (Feinberg, et al., 1994; Gent, et al., 1989; Hass, et al., 1989).

For patients with TIAs or noncardiogenic ischemic brain infarction, the current recommendation is for the chronic administration of aspirin or ticlopidine. Aspirin should probably be used for most patients, and ticlopidine for selected patients, due to the increased cost and side effects of the latter. Chronic warfarin treatment, although it is unproven, may be used for patients who are allergic or refractory to aspirin or ticlopidine. Persantine and sulfinpyrazone are of unproven value for these patients (Feinberg, et al., 1994; Fuster, et al., 1983; Grotta, et al., 1992; Raps and Galetta, 1995; Kistler, et al., 1994; Adams and Victor, 1993).

[f]   Lowering Risk Factors for Atherosclerosis

After the acute phase, risk factors for atherosclerosis should be modified. Hypertension (high blood pressure) is the most important treatable risk factor for stroke, and it should be treated aggressively on a chronic basis (Whisnant, 1996). Diabetes mellitus should be treated with optimal control of blood sugar levels. Cigarette smoking should be discontinued, and hyperlipidemia (increased blood fat levels) should be treated (Sacco, 1995; Feinberg, 1994). Recent guidelines recommend more aggressive treatment of patients with atherosclerotic disease and hyperlipidemia, as well as of individuals with multiple atherosclerotic risk factors and hyperlipidemia (Hachinski, et al., 1996; Expert Panel, 1993; LaRosa, 1993).

[7]   Surgical Treatment

Atherosclerotic plaque can lead to stenosis (narrowing) of arteries prior to occlusion (blockage). Surgical methods have been devised to open stenosed arteries that supply the brain.

[a]   Carotid Endarterectomy

The carotid arteries are surgically accessible in the neck. Carotid endarterectomy, a surgical technique to re-establish blood flow through the carotid arteries, involves excision of the tunica intima (the innermost layer of the artery) that is thickened with plaque. Carotid endarterectomy with plaque removal has been performed since the 1950s, with minimal evidence of efficacy. However, recent landmark investigations have demonstrated the efficacy of the procedure and clarified acceptable surgical risk for various subgroups of patients.

Carotid endarterectomy definitely reduces the risk of recurrent TIA and noncardiogenic ischemic cerebral infarction in patients with symptomatic carotid artery stenosis greater than 70 percent, and possibly in selected patients with symptomatic carotid artery stenosis greater than 50 percent. Acceptable risk of surgical morbidity and mortality is 3 to 5 percent. For patients with asymptomatic carotid artery stenosis greater than 70 percent, carotid endarterectomy reduces the risk of noncardiogenic ischemic cerebral infarction, and acceptable risk of surgical morbidity and mortality is 3 percent.

Risk of surgical morbidity and mortality up to 10 percent is acceptable for certain patients with symptomatic carotid artery disease. There remains some controversy regarding the appropriate management of patients with asymptomatic carotid artery stenosis (Moore, et al., 1995; Goldstein, et al., 1995; North American Symptomatic Carotid Endarterectomy Trial Collaborators, 1991; European Carotid Surgery Trialists' Collaborative Group, 1991; Mayberg, et al., 1991; The Asymptomatic Carotid Atherosclerosis Study Group, 1989; Clinical Advisory, 1995; National Institute of Neurological Disorders and Stroke, 1995; Barnett, et al., 1996; Barnett, et al., 1995; Brott and Toole, 1995).

Complications of endarterectomy can include stroke, infection, wound hematoma, nerve transection and other general surgical complications.

[b] Bypass Surgery

Extracranial to intracranial (EC-IC) bypass surgery was transiently popular for the treatment of patients with TIAs or acute ischemic cerebral infarction due to surgically inaccessible carotid disease. However, an international randomized trial found EC-IC bypass to be no more efficacious than medical therapy, and the procedure has largely been abandoned (EC-IC Bypass Study Group, 1985). Controversy persists about the possibility that certain groups of patients might benefit from EC-IC bypass, but this remains unproven (Feinberg, et al., 1994).

[8] Prognosis

The 30-day stroke mortality rate after acute ischemic or embolic cerebral infarction is 8 to 15 percent. Mortality after 30 days is more likely to be due to co-morbid disease, particularly cardiovascular disease. Patients with major hemispheric or brain stem infarctions have a cumulative mortality rate of 90 percent at five years. The risk of stroke recurrence is 3 to 8 percent in the first 30 days, with a five-year cumulative recurrence risk of 25 to 40 percent (Sacco, 1995; Sacco, 1982).

9.24 Cardiac Embolic Ischemic Brain Infarction

Ischemic infarction accounts for 70 to 80 percent of strokes in the United States, and cardioembolism results in 15 to 30 percent of these infarctions (Sacco, 1995).

[1] Etiology

Emboli can originate from thrombi in the heart associated with atrial fibrillation (irregular contraction of the atria, or upper chamber of the heart), myocardial infarction (heart attack) and dilated cardiomyopathy (disorder of the heart muscle), infected heart valves (valves that prevent backflow of blood into the chambers of the heart), thrombus on noninfected but diseased heart valves and prosthetic heart valves. Embolism can also occur as a complication of open heart surgery. Intracardiac tumors are rarely a source of cardioembolism (Kistler, et al., 1994; Adams and Victor, 1993; Yatsu, 1995b).

[2] Pathogenesis

Cardioembolism can result from infectious material, tumor or thrombus resident on a heart valve or adherent to the endocardium (inner lining of the heart) breaking loose and migrating through the circulation.

Septic emboli from infected heart valves in persons with bacterial endocarditis is a systemic disease that can present as stroke.[15] In rare instances, tumors called myxomas develop in the heart (most commonly in the left atrium, or upper left chamber of the heart) and embolize to the brain, presenting initially as stroke (Kistler, et al., 1994).

Congenital heart disease, including valvular and septal (referring to the septum, which separates the right and left sides of the heart) defects, can result in an embolic stroke, even in the absence of infection. Cyanotic heart disease, which results from a congenital "right-to-left shunt" (passage of blood from the right to left side of the heart due to higher pressure on the right side of the heart), is one of the most common causes of stroke in children. Mild valvular deformities, in the absence of cardiac arrhythmias, probably do not carry a significant risk of stroke. An example is mild mitral valve prolapse (displacement of the valve separating the left atria, or upper

---

[15] *See* 9.37 *infra.*

chamber of the heart, from the left ventricle, or lower chamber of the heart), which is present in 10 to 15 percent of the normal population (more commonly young women), and probably is asymptomatic most of the time. However, more serious valvular deformities can predispose an individual to an embolic stroke, especially in the presence of significant cardiac arrhythmias, such as atrial fibrillation (Gold, 1995; Yatsu, 1995b; Adams and Victor, 1993).

The role of nonvalvular atrial fibrillation in embolic strokes was not clearly defined until recently. It has now been established that persistent or paroxysmal nonvalvular atrial fibrillation is the most important cause of cerebral embolisms from the heart. Another common source of cerebral embolism from the heart is a left ventricular thrombus forming within the first few weeks after a myocardial infarction. This probably also occurs more commonly than is recognized with dilated cardiomyopathy (Kistler, et al., 1994).

A TIA or embolic stroke is uncommon after cardiac catheterization (threading of a catheter through a blood vessel into the heart for diagnostic purposes). It occurs in fewer than 1 percent of procedures and usually involves the vertebrobasilar circulation. A clinically detectable neurologic deficit is present in as many as 12 percent of people after cardiac bypass surgery. This is most likely a result of microembolization (Heyer and Rowland, 1995). Mitral and aortic valve (the valve between the aorta, or central artery of the body, and the left ventricle) prostheses are associated with embolisms in up to 70 percent of cases (Adams and Victor, 1993). Embolism is more common in persons with metal than with porcine valves.

[3] Clinical Presentation

In general, the clinical presentation of cardioembolic infarction is similar to that of thrombotic infarction or small intraparenchymal hemorrhage. Cardioembolic cerebrovascular disease manifests clinically as one or more focal neurologic symptoms and signs. Subjective symptoms can include trouble speaking, visual problems, difficulty swallowing, dizziness, imbalance, weakness and numbness. Objective signs can include aphasia (difficulty speaking), visual field defects, loss of ocular motility, ataxia (incoordination), dysarthria (slurred speech), inattention, loss of spatial organization, sensory losses, paresis (partial paralysis) and paralysis.

The combination of symptoms and signs depends on the location and size of the ischemic area of the brain. Cerebral cortical embolic lesions are accompanied by symptoms on the contralateral side of the body, and seizures are probably more common than with thrombotic ischemic infarctions.[16] Cerebellar embolic lesions are accompanied by symptoms on the ipsilateral (same) side of the body. Cranial nerve involvement indicates brain stem ischemic lesions.

A number of common stroke syndromes (constellation of findings) have been described (Patten, 1996; Poirier, et al., 1990; Adams, and Victor, 1993; Brust, 1995b; Kistler, et al., 1994). Stupor and coma can be present with brain stem lesions, bilateral cerebral lesions and large unilateral cerebral lesions with mass effect and increased intracranial pressure (Plum and Posner, 1980). Symptoms of embolic cerebrovascular disease typically begin acutely. They may be transient, evolve and progress, or they may remain stable.

Concepts regarding transient ischemic attacks, the ischemic penumbra and completed stroke with regard to thrombotic ischemic brain infarction also pertain to cardioembolic brain infarction.[17]

[4]   Neurologic Complications

Neurologic complications following cardiogenic embolic ischemic brain infarction occur through the same mechanisms as those for thrombotic ischemic brain infarction.[18]

[5]   Diagnosis

The initial step in the proper management of patients with any type of cerebral infarction is correct and timely diagnosis. Diagnosis of brain infarction can usually be made correctly on clinical grounds, although it is important to exclude a diagnosis of intraparenchymal brain hemorrhage, subdural hematoma, neoplasm and other causes of focal neurologic deficits. It is impossible to absolutely differentiate between cardiogenic embolic and thrombotic ischemic infarctions on clinical grounds.

Indications for CT scan and additional laboratory tests in the diagnosis of persons with cardiogenic embolic ischemic brain infarction are the same as those for persons with thrombotic ischemic brain infarction.[19]

---

[16] *See* 9.23[3] *supra.*

[17] *See* 9.23 *supra.*

[18] *See* 9.23[4] *supra.*

[19] *See* 9.23[5] *supra.*

The diagnosis of cardiogenic embolic causes of stroke is sometimes indefinite, but important. The decision that a patient has had a cardiogenic embolism is usually made on circumstantial evidence provided by the clinical history, physical examination, electrocardiogram, carotid Doppler ultrasonography, arteriography and echocardiography. Cardiogenic embolic infarction should be suspected in young patients (under the age of 40) and those with atrial fibrillation, heart valve prostheses or evidence on examination of valvular heart disease, myocardial infarction or endocarditis. Such patients should undergo echocardiography (the use of ultrasound to create an image of the heart on an oscilloscope for diagnostic viewing).

Echocardiography is a low-yield procedure for other patients. However, it is definitely indicated for those at significant risk of cardiogenic embolic brain infarction. Transesophageal echocardiography (in which the ultrasound transducer is inserted into the opening of the throat to place it nearer the heart) is more sensitive than transthoracic (through the chest wall) echocardiography, although both have a significant false-negative rate (incorrectly indicate that pathology is not present) (Yatsu, 1995a; Kistler, et al., 1994; Adams and Victor, 1993).

[6]   Treatment

Patients with acute thrombotic or embolic ischemic neurologic events should be admitted to the hospital and undergo continuous cardiac monitoring. There is significant cardiac co-morbidity with ischemic cerebrovascular disease, with as many as 40 percent of patients who have symptomatic carotid artery disease also having asymptomatic severe coronary artery disease. Cardiac deaths are the major cause of mortality with cerebrovascular disease (Adams, 1995).

Fluid and electrolyte abnormalities should be corrected, hyperglycemia and hypoxemia should be treated, and seizures should be treated with anticonvulsants. Airway and ventilatory support should be provided to patients with depressed levels of consciousness.

[a]   Antihypertensives

There is general agreement that hypertension should not be treated aggressively in the patient with acute focal brain ischemia. This is because aggressive treatment of hypertension can decrease cerebral blood flow to the ischemic penumbra, resulting in extension of infarction with subsequent clinical worsening. It is acceptable to withhold antihypertensive treatment for systolic blood pressures less than 200 to 220 mm Hg and diastolic blood pressures less than 120 to 130 mm Hg (Adams, 1995; Adams, et al., 1994). Some advocate aggressive hydration and volume expansion in order to enhance cerebral blood flow and decrease blood viscosity.

[b]   Anticoagulants

Heparin binds with intrinsic antithrombin III to inactivate thrombin and the propagation of blood clots. Acute anticoagulation with heparin after noninfective cardiogenic TIA and cerebral infarction is somewhat controversial, but accepted by most authorities. After three to five days, patients are generally switched to warfarin (Sherman, et al., 1995; Adams, 1995; Kistler, et al., 1994; Adams and Victor, 1993).

One controversy surrounding anticoagulation of such patients involves the timing of anticoagulation. Because emboli migrate and lyse (dissolve), revascularization (reopening a vessel) is more likely to cause hemorrhagic transformation of an embolic infarction than a thrombotic infarction. Thus, some authorities advocate a delay of three to five days before giving anticoagulants to patients with embolic infarction. However, because there is also a significant risk of re-embolization in this waiting period, with up to 20 percent of patients experiencing recurrent emboli within ten days after the initial embolus, some experts advocate immediate anticoagulation. Whether anti-coagulation is immediate or delayed, brain CT should always be obtained first, to ensure that patients with intracerebral hemorrhage are not anticoagulated (Kistler, et al., 1994; Adams and Victor, 1993). Hemorrhage is the most common complication of anticoagulation. It can involve any part of the body and be very serious if it occurs.

A major recent advance in prevention of cardioembolic stroke has been the recognition that anticoagulation reduces the risk of stroke in patients with nonvalvular atrial fibrillation. Strokes occur in 4.5 percent of untreated atrial fibrillation patients per year. Independent risk factors for stroke in patients with nonrheumatic atrial fibrillation include advanced age, history of prior embolism, hypertension, diabetes mellitus and echocardiographic evidence of left atrial enlarge-ment or left ventricular dysfunction. Warfarin decreases stroke by two thirds and aspirin by one third in these patients. Recommended treatment of patients with nonrheumatic atrial fibrillation at the present time is with warfarin, especially for patients with any of the risk factors noted and patients over the age of 70. For some younger patients with no additional risk factors, persons at risk of falling and persons with significant risk of bleeding, treatment with aspirin is acceptable. The value of persantine and sulfinpyrazone has not been proved for these patients (Laupacis, et al., 1995; Streifler and Katz, 1995; Blackshear, et al., 1996; Ezekowitz, et al., 1992; Connolly, et al., 1991). There is some controversy regarding the optimal level of anticoagulation with nonvalvular atrial fibrillation (The European Atrial Fibrillation Trial Study Group, 1995).

[7] Prognosis

The 30-day stroke mortality rate after acute ischemic or embolic cerebral infarction is 8 to 15 percent. Mortality after 30 days is most likely due to co-morbid disease, particularly cardiovascular disease. Patients with major hemispheric or brain stem infarctions have a cumulative mortality rate of 90 percent at five years. The risk of stroke recurrence is 3 to 8 percent in the first 30 days, with a five-year cumulative recurrence risk of 25 to 40 percent (Sacco, 1995; Sacco, 1982).

9.30 SYSTEMIC DISEASES THAT CAN PRESENT AS STROKE

A variety of systemic diseases can affect the cerebral vasculature and produce symptoms similar to those of stroke.

9.31 Sickle Cell Anemia

Sickle cell disease is an inherited abnormality of hemoglobin (the oxygen-carrying component of blood) that is seen primarily in people of African heritage, but also in Greek and Latin American ethnic groups. Abnormal hemoglobin leads to distortion of the shape of red blood cells, hemolysis (breakdown of the blood cell) and occlusion of vessels in kidney, bone, lung, liver, heart, spleen and brain. Occlusion of vessels in the brain results in ischemic brain infarction.

Neurologic symptoms occur in about a third of people with sickle cell disease and may be the presenting symptoms of the disease. Stroke occurs in 5 to 15 percent of children with sickle cell disease and is the second leading cause of death, after infection. The risk of stroke in children with sickle cell disease is 250 to 400 times that in the general population. The mean age of occurrence of cerebral infarction is 8 years, with about 80 percent of cases occurring before puberty. Hemorrhage occurs in older afflicted individuals, at a mean age of 25 years.

Brain infarctions are more common in the vicinity of large vessels than small vessels. The clinical presentation does not differ from that of infarction or intraparenchymal hemorrhage resulting from other causes.[20] Diagnosis is made on the basis of clinical suspicion for a victim of appropriate ethnic background, especially a child, and confirmation by cranial CT or MRI and hemoglobin electrophoresis. Transfusion reduces the risk of recurrent strokes. Within three years of stroke, there is a 67 percent recurrence rate in patients who are not transfused and a 10 percent recurrence in patients who are transfused (Weksler, 1995; Menkes, et al., 1995; Balmaceda and Fetell, 1995; Schochet, 1983).

9.32 Arteritis

Brain infarctions can result from infective or noninfective inflammatory arteritis of the cerebral arteries. Noninfective inflammatory arteritis of the cerebral arteries is most commonly associated with autoimmune diseases (in which the body mistakenly launches an immune response against its own tissues), especially systemic lupus erythematosus (an autoimmune disease with characteristic skin lesions). It can also be seen with giant cell arteritis, polyarteritis nodosa, Churg-Straus disease and Wegener's granulomatosis, and as an isolated intracranial arteritis. Diagnosis can usually be made with arteriography and appropriate blood studies, although a biopsy is sometimes necessary. Treatment is with corticosteroids and other immunosuppressant drugs (Futrell, 1995; Rowland, 1995b; Moore and Cupps, 1983; Futrell and Millikan, 1989; Harris and Hughes, 1985).

Intracranial arteritis with infarction also occurs with abuse of illicit drugs, most notably heroin. A drug screen should always be performed in young stroke victims, especially if illicit drug use is suspected.

---

[20] *See* 9.20 *supra.*

9.33   Polycythemia Vera

Polycythemia vera is characterized by excessive production of red blood cells. This is believed to increase the viscosity of the blood, resulting in tissue hypoxia (low blood level of oxygen) and ischemia. Alternatively, there is evidence that polycythemia results in infarction as a physiologic response to elevated arterial level of oxygen. Whatever the pathophysiology, brain infarction and, less commonly, hemorrhage can occur with polycythemia. An emergency phlebotomy (cutting into a vein) is indicated in cases with a hematocrit (the volume of blood composed of cells) greater than 60 percent. The presence of hypoglycemia (low blood sugar level) increases the risk of cerebral thrombosis in polycythemic neonates (Weksler, 1995; Menkes, et al., 1995; Balmaceda and Fetell, 1995).

9.34   Hypercoagulable States

Thrombotic thrombocytopenic purpura manifests as thrombocytopenia (low platelet count), purpura (bruising), fever and fluctuating neurologic symptoms due to brain infarction. Diagnosis can be difficult but is crucial, because this is a treatable entity, with recovery in as many of 70 percent of patients.

Protein C deficiency, protein S deficiency and antithrombin III deficiency are rarely recognized entities that can cause a hypercoagulable state and stroke.

Primary antiphospholipid antibody syndrome, an autoimmune disease in which individuals produce autoantibodies to the phospholipid compounds that are embedded in blood vessel walls, is an entity that has been increasingly associated with stroke. Antiphospholipid antibodies are referred to as the lupus anticoagulant and anticardiolipin antibodies (immunoglobulin G and M). They are most commonly associated with spontaneous abortion and venous thrombosis, but they can result in intracranial arterial or venous occlusion. There is some evidence that drug-induced antiphospholipid antibodies may be of little consequence. These entities should be considered in unusual presentations of cerebral thrombosis, especially in young individuals who experience stroke before age 45. They account for about 20 percent of all strokes (Adams and Victor, 1993; Antiphospholipid Antibody Stroke Study Group, 1993; Yatsu, 1995b; Balmaceda and Fetell, 1995).

9.35   Hemophilia

Intracranial hemorrhage can occur with any type of hemophilia, including deficiency of factor VII, factor VIII, factor IX and von Willebrand's disease. Intracranial hemorrhage is the leading cause of death in factor VIII deficiency, with as many as 10 percent of afflicted individuals experiencing intracerebral hemorrhage. Epidural or subdural hematomas develop in about half, often after minor head trauma but sometimes spontaneously. Any hemophiliac who experiences head trauma should undergo cranial CT. The missing factor should be replaced immediately, and surgical evacuation of the clot may be necessary (Weksler, 1995; Menkes, et al., 1995; Balmaceda and Fetell, 1995; Kistler, et al., 1994).

9.36   Polycystic Kidney Disease

Polycystic kidney disease is an inherited renal disorder that can cause flank pain, hematuria (blood in the urine), hypertension (high blood pressure) and chronic renal failure. The incidence rates of intracranial saccular aneurysms and subarachnoid hemorrhages are increased in people with polycystic kidney disease, with reports of subarachnoid hemorrhage in as many as 10 percent of afflicted individuals.[21] Routine screening with cerebral arteriography has not generally been recommended, although this position is being modified with the evolving resolution of noninvasive magnetic resonance angiography (Coe and Kathpalia, 1994; Brust, 1995c; Schochet, 1983).

9.37   Infection

Intracranial mycotic aneurysms develop from septic emboli originating in infected heart valves in persons with bacterial endocarditis (infection of the membranous sac surrounding the heart). These aneurysms are seen most often in people with valvular heart disease and in intravenous drug abusers.[22]

Mycotic aneurysms occur in about 10 percent of individuals with infective endocarditis, and a stroke may be the initial manifestation. They result from dilation and destruction of inflamed and infected

---

[21] *See* 9.21 *supra* for further discussion of saccular aneurysms and their relation to subarachnoid hemorrhage.

[22] *See* 9.21 *supra.*

intracranial peripheral arterial walls. Rupture and hemorrhage are common. Diagnosis is by CT, MRI, MRA and arteriography. Treatment is with antibiotics. Anticoagulation is relatively contraindicated, because septic brain emboli are commonly hemorrhagic. Surgical replacement of the infected cardiac valve with a prosthetic valve is sometimes necessary (Schochet, 1983; Kaye, 1994; Kistler, et al., 1994).

Cerebral infarction can also occur with any type of infectious meningitis, most commonly with bacterial meningitis caused by tuberculosis, syphilis and *Haemophilus*. Brain infarction of this kind results from infective inflammatory arteritis of the cerebral arteries, a condition known as Heubner's arteritis. Any part of the brain can be involved. Individuals with acquired immunodeficiency syndrome (AIDS) resulting from human immunodeficiency virus (HIV) infection are at particular risk for tuberculous meningitis and neurosyphilis (Schochet, 1983; Menkes, 1995; Scheld, 1994; Igarashi, et al., 1984).

9.38   Neoplasm

Stroke can occur as a complication of all forms of leukemia (a disease characterized by excessive production of white blood cells), primarily the acute forms. Three mechanisms may be involved (Weksler, 1995; Balmaceda and Fetell, 1995; Menkes, et al., 1995):

1. With markedly elevated white blood cell counts (greater than 150,000/mm^3), leukostasis (stagnation of white blood cells) can lead to thrombosis of cerebral vessels,with subsequent brain infarction.

2. Leukemic nodules in the brain can predispose to intracerebral hemorrhage.

3. Hemorrhage may also result from thrombocytopenia (low platelet count) caused by chemotherapy.

Brain tumors, both primary and metastatic (spreading from an origin at a distant site), can manifest acutely as stroke. The mechanism is intratumoral hemorrhage, and the clinical presentation is the same as that of any other intracerebral hemorrhage, usually lobar or cerebellar in location. Among primary brain tumors, this is seen most commonly in glioblastoma multiforme. Among metastatic brain tumors, intratumoral hemorrhage is particularly common with melanoma (skin cancer), renal (kidney) cell carcinoma, choriocarcinoma (a highly malignant tumor with common metastases to the brain) and bronchogenic carcinoma (a type of lung cancer). Diagnosis can be difficult at times but is greatly facilitated by MRI (Balmaceda and Fetell, 1995; Kistler, et al., 1994; Adams and Victor, 1993; Schochet, 1983).

Some patients with systemic malignancy develop nonbacterial thrombotic endocarditis, with sterile platelet–fibrin heart valve vegetations resulting in embolization and subsequent brain infarction. Emboli to other organs may also occur (Balmaceda and Fetell, 1995).

9.40 SYSTEMIC COMPLICATIONS OF CEREBROVASCULAR INJURY

A number of systemic complications can occur after any type of stroke. These complications can also occur after traumatic cerebrovascular injury.

9.41 Respiratory Complications

Aspiration pneumonia (inflammation of the lungs caused by the inhalation of food or other substances) is very common in stroke victims with impaired swallowing or cough mechanisms. Many patients should not receive anything by mouth initially. Assessment of the ability to swallow is critical if there is clinical suspicion of impairment. Pneumonia is an important cause of death after strokes, and fever should prompt evaluation by chest x-ray. Pneumonia should be appropriately treated with antibiotics (Adams, et al., 1994; Horner, et al., 1988; Adams, 1993).

Pulmonary embolism (migration of a blood clot to the pulmonary circulation) resulting from deep vein thrombophlebitis (DVT) of the lower extremities accounts for about 10 percent of strokes. Proximal DVT can be identified in up to a third of patients with moderately severe stroke. Prevention includes early mobilization, alternating pressure stockings and anticoagulation if it is not contraindicated (Adams, et al., 1994; Adams, 1993).

Respiratory failure can occur in stroke victims, especially those with pre-existing cardiopulmonary disease, large infarction or hemorrhage and brain stem infarction or hemorrhage. Patients with a predisposing condition have a worse prognosis than those without, and they may require ventilatory support (Adams, 1995).

9.42   Cardiovascular Complications

Cardiac death is the major cause of mortality in patients with cerebrovascular disease. Concurrent brain infarction and myocardial infarction are not uncommon. However, a minority of cerebrovascular disease patients have clear symptoms of coronary artery disease. Forty percent of patients with symptomatic carotid artery disease have asymptomatic coronary artery disease.

Cardiac arrhythmias due to atrial fibrillation and ventricular arrhythmias (uneven, irregular rhythms) are also common among stroke victims.

Minimum cardiovascular evaluation of patients with cerebrovascular disease should include an electrocardiogram (EKG, which measures the heart's electrical activity) and a chest x-ray. Optimally, all patients should undergo continuous cardiac monitoring for the first few days. Hospital stroke units should be utilized when they are available, and patients suspected of having myocardial infarction (heart attack) should be admitted to a coronary care unit. Echocardiography (ultrasonography of the heart) and anticoagulation therapy should be used when indicated, and cardiac arrhythmias (irregular heartbeats) should be treated appropriately. The cardiac evaluation of ischemic stroke patients with severe atherosclerotic disease should probably include stress thallium testing or treadmill stress testing, with coronary arteriography when indicated (Adams, 1995; Adams, et al., 1994).

9.43   Gastrointestinal Complications

Impairment of swallowing ability is a common complication of stroke. Other common gastrointestinal complications include loss of intestinal motility (ileus), constipation and fecal impaction (inability to pass feces). Gastrointestinal bleeding can also occur, particularly in patients who are anticoagulated and have pre-existing peptic ulcer disease (Adams, 1993).

9.44   Genitourinary Complications

In-dwelling urinary catheters are often necessary after a stroke, but their use increases the risk of urinary tract infections, which are common in stroke patients. Secondary septicemia (systemic disease caused by proliferation of microorganisms in the blood) can develop and be fatal. Fever should prompt evaluation of the urine, and infection should be appropriately treated with antibiotics (Adams, et al., 1994; Adams, 1993).

9.45   Endocrine System Complications

Diabetes mellitus is a risk factor for atherosclerosis, and ischemic strokes are common among diabetic individuals. Hyperglycemia (elevated blood sugar level) is common in diabetic stroke victims, and there is suggestive evidence that it may worsen ischemic infarction. Hypoglycemia and hyperglycemia should be controlled after a stroke (Adams, et al., 1994).

Hyponatremia (low blood sodium levels) occurs in up to 34 percent of patients after subarachnoid hemorrhage, usually due to intravascular volume contraction caused by diabetes insipidus (chronic excretion of large amounts of pale urine and excessive thirst). Intravascular volume status may need to be closely monitored. Hyponatremia due to volume contraction should be treated with intravenous isotonic fluids (Mayberg, et al., 1994).

9.46   Dermatologic Complications

Meticulous nursing care, with frequent turning, attention to skin care and early mobilization, is necessary for the prevention of decubitus ulcers (pressure sores). Once they develop, decubitus ulcers can contribute significantly to the morbidity involved in stroke. Treatment is time consuming, expensive and not always effective (Bergstrom, et al., 1994; Adams, 1993).

9.47   Psychiatric Complications

Depression after a stroke is common, occurring in 23 to 63 percent of patients. It is more common with left cerebral lesions than right cerebral lesions. It should be recognized and treated (Kelly-Hayes and Paige, 1995; Adams, 1995; Adams, 1993).

Dementia after multiple large or lacunar strokes is common. Deficiencies are common in orientation, attention, memory, calculation and spatial organization. There is no satisfactory treatment, other than attempts at preventing more strokes.

9.50   REHABILITATION AFTER CEREBROVASCULAR INJURY

A large percentage of survivors of cerebrovascular injury have substantial motor impairment, sensory impairment, difficulty swallowing, cognitive deficit, language deficit, depression and incontinence. Many of these patients will benefit from multidisciplinary rehabilitation if their neurologic deficit is not too severe. Assessment of each patient's individual social support system is important in the decision regarding a patient's potential to achieve the ultimate goal of rehabilitation: to return to the community and be able to perform instrumental activities of daily living. Most patients realize maximal functional recovery in three to six months, but the rehabilitation period is usually much shorter than this. Expectations should be realistic (Agency for Health Care Policy and Research, 1995; Jeffery and Good, 1995; Kelly-Hayes and Paige, 1995; Jorgensen, et al., 1995; Granger, et al., 1992).

9.100   BIBLIOGRAPHY

Text References

Adams, H. P. (Ed.): Handbook of Cerebrovascular Disease. New York: Marcel Dekker, 1993.

Adams, H. P., et al.: Guidelines for the Management of Patients with Acute Ischemic Stroke—A Statement for Healthcare Professionals From a Special Writing Group of the Stroke Council, American Heart Association. Circulation 90(3):1588-1601, Sept. 1994.

Adams, R. D. and Victor, M.: Principles of Neurology, 5th ed. New York: McGraw-Hill, 1993.

Adams, R.J.: Management Issues for Patients with Ischemic Stroke. In: Dobkin, B. (Ed.): Management of the Patient with Stroke. Neurology 45(2, Suppl.1):S15-S18, Feb. 1995.

Agency for Health Care Policy and Research: Post-Stroke Rehabilitation: Assessment, Referral, and Patient Management. Rockville, Md.: U.S. Department of Health and Human Services, 1995.

Antiphospholipid Antibody Stroke Study Group: Anticardiolipin Antibodies are an Independent Risk Factor for First Ischemic Stroke. The Antiphospholipid Antibodies in Stroke Study (APASS). Neurology 43(10):2069-2073, Oct. 1993.

Antiplatelet Trialists' Collaboration: Collaborative Overview of Randomised Trials of Antiplatelet Therapy, I: Prevention of Death, Myocardial Infarction, and Stroke by Prolonged Antiplatelet Therapy in Various Categories of Patients. Br. Med. J. 308(6921):81-106, Jan. 1994.

Antiplatelet Trialists' Collaboration: Secondary Prevention of Vascular Disease by Prolonged Antiplatelet Treatment. Br. Med. J. 296(6618):320-331, Jan. 1988.

The Asymptomatic Carotid Atherosclerosis Study Group: Study Design for Randomized Prospective Trial of Carotid Endarterectomy for Asymptomatic Atherosclerosis. Stroke 20(7):844-849, July 1989.

Babikian, V. L. and Wechsler, L. R. (Eds.): Transcranial Doppler Ultrasonography. St. Louis: Mosby, 1993.

Balmaceda, C. M. and Fetell, M. R.: Hematologic and Related Disorders. In: Rowland, L. P. (Ed.): Merritt's Textbook of Neurology, 9th ed. Baltimore: Williams & Wilkins, 1995.

Barnett, H. J. M., et al.: Do the Facts and Figures Warrant a 10-Fold Increase in the Performance of Carotid Endarterectomy on Asymptomatic Patients? Neurology 46(3):603-608, Mar. 1996.

Barnett, H. J. M., et al.: The Dilemma of Surgical Treatment for Patients with Asymptomatic Carotid Disease. Ann. Intern. Med. 123(9):723-725, Nov. 1995.

Bergstrom, N., et al.: Agency for Health Care Policy and Research: Clinical Practice Guideline Number 15: Treatment of Pressure Ulcers. Rockville Md.: U.S. Dept. of Health and Human Services, Dec. 1994.

Blackshear, J. L., et al.: Management of Atrial Fibrillation in Adults: Prevention of Thromboembolism and Symptomatic Treatment. Mayo Clin. Proc. 71(2):150-160, Feb. 1996.

Brott, T. and Toole, J. F.: Medical Compared with Surgical Treatment of Asymptomatic Carotid Artery Stenosis. Ann. Intern. Med. 123(9):720-722, Nov. 1995.

Brust, J. C. M.: Transient Ischemic Attacks. In: Rowland, L. P. (Ed.): Merritt's Textbook of Neurology, 9th ed. Baltimore: Williams & Wilkins, 1995a.

Brust, J. C. M.: Cerebral Infarction. In: Rowland, L. P. (Ed.): Merritt's Textbook of Neurology, 9th ed. Baltimore: Williams & Wilkins, 1995b.

Brust, J. C. M.: Subarachnoid Hemorrhage. In: Rowland, L. P. (Ed.): Merritt's Textbook of Neurology, 9th ed. Baltimore: Williams & Wilkins, 1995c.

Buring, J. E., et al.: Migraine and Subsequent Risk of Stroke in the Physicians' Health Study. Arch. Neurol. 52(2):129-134, Feb. 1995.

Caplan, L. R., et al.: Neuroimaging in Patients with Cerebrovascular Disease: In: Greenberg, J. O. (Ed.): Neuroimaging. New York: McGraw-Hill, 1995.

Carpenter, M. B.: Core Text of Neuroanatomy, 4th ed. Baltimore: Williams & Wilkins, 1991.

Clinical Advisory: Carotid Endarterectomy for Patients with Asymptomatic Internal Carotid Artery Stenosis. Stroke 25(12):2523-2524, Dec. 1994.

Coe, F. L. and Kathpalia, S.: Polycystic Renal Disease in Adults. In: Isselbacher, K. J., et al. (Eds.): Harrison's Principles of Internal Medicine, 13th ed. New York: McGraw-Hill, 1994.

Connolly, S. J., et al.: Canadian Atrial Fibrillation Anticoagulation (CAFA) Study. J. Am. Coll. Cardiol. 18(2):349-355, Aug. 1991.

Critchley, E. M.: Recognition and Management of Lacunar Strokes [Editorial]. Br. Med. J. [Clin. Res.] 287(6395):777-778, Sept. 1983.

Drake, C. G., et al.: Failed Aneurysm Surgery. Reoperation in 115 Cases. J. Neurosurg. 61(5):848-856, Nov. 1984.

EC/IC Bypass Study Group: Failure of Extracranial-Intracranial Arterial Bypass to Reduce the Risk of Ischemic Stroke: Results of International Randomized Trial. N. Engl. J. Med. 313(19):1191-1200, Nov. 1985.

The European Atrial Fibrillation Trial Study Group: Optimal Oral Anticoagulant Therapy in Patients with Nonrheumatic Atrial Fibrillation and Recent Cerebral Ischemia. N. Engl. J. Med. 333(1):5-10, July 1995.

European Carotid Surgery Trialists' Collaborative Group: MRC European Carotid Surgery Trial: Interim Results for Symptomatic

Patients with Severe (70-99%) or with Mild (0-29%) Carotid Stenosis. Lancet 337(8752):1235-1243, May 1991.

Expert Panel: Summary of the Second Report of the National Cholesterol Education Program (NCEP) Expert Panel on Detection, Evaluation, and Treatment of High Blood Cholesterol in Adults (Adult Treatment Panel II). J.A.M.A. 269(23):3015-3023, June 1993.

Ezekowitz, M. D., et al.: Warfarin in the Prevention of Stroke Associated with Nonrheumatic Atrial Fibrillation. N. Engl. J. Med. 327(20):1406-1412, Nov. 1992.

Feinberg, W. M., et al.: Guidelines for the Management of Transient Ischemic Attacks—From the Ad Hoc Committee for the Management of Transient Ischemic Attacks of the Stroke Council of the American Heart Association. Stroke 25(6):1320-1335, June 1994.

Fuster, V., et al.: Aspirin As a Therapeutic Agent in Cardiovascular Disease. Circulation 87(2):659-675, Feb. 1993.

Futrell, N.: Inflammatory Vascular Disorders: Diagnosis and Treatment in Ischemic Stroke. Curr. Opin. Neurol. 8(1):55-61, Feb. 1995.

Futrell, N. and Millikan, C.: Frequency, Etiology, and Prevention of Stroke in Patients with Systemic Lupus Erythematosus. Stroke 20(5):584-591, July 1989.

Gent, M., et al.: The Canadian American Ticlopidine Study (CATS) in Thromboembolic Stroke. Lancet 1(8649):1215-1220, June 5, 1989.

Gold, A. P.: Stroke in Children. In: Rowland, L. P. (Ed.): Merritt's Textbook of Neurology, 9th ed. Baltimore: Williams & Wilkins, 1995.

Goldstein, L. B., et al.: Comparison and Meta-Analysis of Randomized Trials of Endarterectomy for Symptomatic Carotid Artery Stenosis. Neurology 45(11):1965-1970, Nov. 1995.

Granger, C. V., et al.: Discharge Outcome after Stroke Rehabilitation. Stroke 23(7):978-982, July 1992.

Greenberg, J. O. (Ed.): Neuroimaging. New York: McGraw-Hill, 1995.

Grotta, J. C., et al.: Prevention of Stroke with Ticlopidine: Who Benefits the Most? Neurology. 42(1):111-115, Jan. 1992.

Hachinski, V.: Hypertension in Acute Ischemic Strokes. Arch. Neurol. 42(10):1002, Oct. 1985.

Hachinski, V.: Decreased Incidence and Mortality of Stroke. Stroke 15(2):376-378, Mar.-Apr. 1984.

Hachinski,V., et al.: Lipids and Stroke. Arch. Neurol. 53(4):303-308, Apr. 1996.

Harris, E. N. and Hughes, G. R. V.: Cerebral Disease in Systemic Lupus Erythematosus. Springer Semin. Immunopathol. 8(3):251-266, 1985.

Hass, W. K., et al.: A Randomized Trial Comparing Ticlopidine Hydrochloride with Aspirin for the Prevention of Stroke in High-Risk Patients. N. Engl. J. Med. 321(8):501-507, Aug. 1989.

Heyer, E. J. and Rowland, L. P.: Cerebral Complications of Cardiac Surgery. In: Rowland, L. P. (Ed.): Merritt's Textbook of Neurology, 9th ed. Baltimore: Williams & Wilkins, 1995.

Horner, J., et al.: Aspiration following Stroke. Clinical Correlation and Outcome. Neurology 38(9):1359-1362, Sept. 1988.

Igarashi, M., et al.: Cerebral Arteritis and Bacterial Meningitis. Arch. Neurol. 41(5):531-535, May 1984.

Ingall, T. J. and Wiebers, D. O.: Natural History of Subarachnoid Hemorrhage. In: Whisnant, J. P. (Ed.): Stroke: Populations, Cohorts, and Clinical Trials. Boston: Butterworth-Heinemann, 1993.

Jane, J. A., et al.: The Natural History of Aneurysms and Arteriovenous Malformations. J. Neurosurg. 62(3):321-323, Mar. 1985.

Jeffery, D. R. and Good, D. C.: Rehabilitation of the Stroke Patient. Curr. Opin. Neurol. 8(1):62-68, Feb. 1995.

Jorgensen H. S., et al.: Outcome and Time Course of Recovery in Stroke. Part II: Time Course of Recovery. The Copenhagen Stroke Study. Arch. Phys. Med. Rehabil. 76(5):406-412, May 1995.

Kaye, D.: Infective Endocarditis. In: Isselbacher, K. J., et al. (Eds.): Harrison's Principles of Internal Medicine, 13th ed. New York: McGraw-Hill, 1994.

Kelly-Hayes, M. and Paige, C.: Assessment and Psychologic Factors in Stroke Rehabilitation. In: Dobkin, B. (Ed.): Management of the Patient with Stroke. Neurology 45(2,Suppl.1):S15-S18, Feb. 1995.

Kilpatrick, C. J., et al.: Epileptic Seizures in Acute Stroke. Arch. Neurol. 47(2):157-160, Feb. 1990.

Kistler, J. P., et al.: Cerebrovascular Disease. In: Isselbacher, K. J., et al. (Eds.): Harrison's Principles of Internal Medicine, 13th ed. New York: McGraw-Hill, 1994.

Lampl, Y., et al.: Neurological and Functional Outcome in Patients with Supratentorial Hemorrhages. Stroke 26(12):2249-2253, Dec. 1995.

LaRosa, J.C.: Cholesterol Lowering, Low Cholesterol, and Mortality. Am. J. Cardiol. 72(11):776-786, Oct. 1993.

Laupacis, A., et al.: Antithrombotic Therapy in Atrial Fibrillation. Chest 108(4,Suppl.):352S-359S, Oct. 1995.

Mayberg, M. R., et al.: Guidelines for the Management of Aneurysmal Subarachnoid Hemorrhage—A Statement for Healthcare Professionals From a Special Writing Group of the Stroke Council, American Heart Association. Circulation 90(5):2592-2605, Nov. 1994.

Mayberg, M. R., et al.: Carotid Endarterectomy and Prevention of Cerebral Ischemia in Symptomatic Carotid Stenosis: Veterans Affairs Cooperative Studies 309 Trialist Group. J.A.M.A. 266(23):3289-3294, Dec. 1991.

Menkes, J. H., et al.: Neurologic Manifestations of Systemic Disease. In: Menkes, J. H.(Ed.): Textbook of Child Neurology, 5th ed. Baltimore: Williams & Wilkins, 1995.

Miyaoka, M., et al.: A Clinical Study of the Relationship of Timing to Outcome of Surgery for Ruptured Cerebral Aneurysm—A Retrospective Analysis of 1622 Cases. J. Neurosurg. 79(3):373-378, Sept. 1993.

Mohr, J. P.: Cerebral and Cerebellar Hemorrhage. In: Rowland, L. P. (Ed.): Merritt's Textbook of Neurology, 9th ed. Baltimore: Williams & Wilkins, 1995a.

Mohr, J. P.: Differential Diagnosis of Stroke. In: Rowland, L. P. (Ed.): Merritt's Textbook of Neurology, 9th ed. Baltimore: Williams & Wilkins, 1995b.

Moore, P. M. and Cupps, T. R.: Neurological Complications of Vasculitis. Ann. Neurol. 14(2):155-167, Aug. 1983.

Moore, W. S., et al.: Guidelines for Carotid Endarterectomy—A Multidisciplinary Consensus Statement From the Ad Hoc Committee, American Heart Association. Circulation 91(2):566-579, Jan. 1995.

National Institute of Neurological Disorders and Stroke: Carotid Endarterectomy for Patients with Asymptomatic Internal Carotid Artery Stenosis. J. Neurol. Sci. 129(1):76-77, Mar. 1995.

The National Institute of Neurological Disorders and Stroke rt-PA Stroke Study Group.: Tissue Plasminogen Activator for Acute Ischemic Stroke. N. Engl. J. Med. 333(24):1581-1587, Dec. 1995.

North American Symptomatic Carotid Endarterectomy Trial Collaborators: Beneficial Effect of Carotid Endarterectomy in Symptomatic Patients with High-Grade Carotid Stenosis. N. Engl. J. Med. 325(7):445-453, Aug. 1991.

Nishioka, H., et al.: Cooperative Study of Intracranial Aneurysms and Subarachnoid Hemorrhage: A Long-Term Prognostic Study, II. Ruptured Intracranial Aneurysms Managed Conservatively, III. Subarachnoid Hemorrhage of Undetermined Etiology. Arch. Neurol. 41(11):1142-1146, Nov. 1984.

Patten, J.: Neurological Differential Diagnosis, 2nd ed. London: Springer-Verlag, 1996.

Pickard, J. D., et al.: Effect of Oral Nimodipine on Cerebral Infarction and Outcome after Subarachnoid Hemorrhage. Br. Med. J. 298(3):636-642, Mar. 1989.

Plum, F. and Posner, J. B.: The Diagnosis of Stupor and Coma, 3rd ed. Philadelphia: Davis, 1980.

Poirier, J., et al.: In: Rubenstein, L. J. (Trans.): Manual of Basic Neuropathology, 3rd ed. Philadelphia: Saunders, 1990.

Raps, E. C. and Galetta, S. L.: Stroke Prevention Therapies and Management of Patient Subgroups. In: Dobkin, B. (Ed.): Management of the Patient with Stroke. Neurology 45(2,Suppl.1):S15-S18, Feb. 1995.

Rowland, L. P.: Head Injury. In: Rowland, L. P. (Ed.): Merritt's Textbook of Neurology, 9th ed. Baltimore: Williams & Wilkins, 1995a.

Rowland, L. P.: Vasculitis Syndromes. In: Rowland, L.P. (Ed.): Merritt's Textbook of Neurology, 9th ed. Baltimore: Williams & Wilkins, 1995b.

Sacco, R. L.: Risk Factors and Outcomes for Ischemic Stroke. In: Dobkin, B. (Ed.): Management of the Patient with Stroke. Neurology 45(2,Suppl.1):S10-S14, Feb. 1995.

Sacco, R. L., et al.: Survival and Recurrence Following Stroke: The Framingham Study. Stroke 13(3):290-295, May-June 1982.

Sahs, A. L., et al.: Aneurysmal Subarachnoid Hemorrhage: Report of the Cooperative Study. Baltimore: Urban & Schwartzenberg, 1981.

Scheld, W. M.: Bacterial Meningitis and Brain Abscess. In: Isselbacher, K. J., et al. (Eds.): Harrison's Principles of Internal Medicine, 13th ed. New York: McGraw-Hill, 1994.

Sherman, D. G., et al.: Antithrombotic Therapy for Cerebrovascular Disorders: An Update. Chest 108(4,Suppl.):444S-456S, Oct. 1995.

Schochet, S. S. (Ed.): Neuropathology: In: Rosenberg, R.N. (Ed.): The Clinical Neurosciences. New York: Churchill Livingstone, 1983.

Streifler, J. Y. and Katz, M.: Cardiogenic Cerebral Emboli: Diagnosis and Treatment. Curr. Opin. Neurol.8(1):45-54, Feb. 1995.

von Reutern, G-M. and von Büdingen, H. J.: Ultrasound Diagnosis of Cerebrovascular Disease. New York: Thieme Medical Publishers, 1993.

Waxman, S. G., et al.: Temporal Profile Resembling TIA in the Setting of Cerebral Infarction. Stroke 14(3):433, May-June 1983.

Weksler, B. B.: Hematologic Disorders and Ischemic Stroke. Curr. Opin. Neurol. 8(1):38-44, Feb. 1995.

Whisnant, J. P.: Effectiveness Versus Efficacy of Treatment of Hypertension for Stroke Prevention. Neurology 46(2):301-307, Feb. 1996.

Yatsu, F.: Treatment and Prevention of Stroke. In: Rowland, L. P. (Ed.): Merritt's Textbook of Neurology, 9th ed. Baltimore: Williams & Wilkins, 1995a.

Yatsu, F.: Other Cerebrovascular Syndromes. In: Rowland, L. P. (Ed.): Merritt's Textbook of Neurology, 9th ed. Baltimore: Williams & Wilkins, 1995b.

Additional References

Bullock, R., et al.: Massive Persistent Release of Excitatory Amino Acids Following Human Occlusive Stroke. Stroke 26(11):2187-189, Nov. 1995.

Chimowitz, M. I., et al.: The Warfarin-Aspirin Symptomatic Intracranial Disease Study. Neurology 45(8):1488-1493, Aug. 1995.

Eliasziw, M., et al.: Prognosis for Patients Following a Transient Ischemic Attack With and Without a Cerebral Infarction on Brain CT. North American Symptomatic Carotid Endarterectomy Trial (NASCET) Group. Neurology 45(3Pt.1):428-431, Mar. 1995.

Fisher, M., et al. (Eds.): Current Review of Cerebrovascular Disease, 2nd ed. New York: Churchill Livingstone, 1995.

Gorelick, P. B. (Ed.): Atlas of Cerebrovascular Disease. New York: Churchill Livingstone, 1996.

Gottlieb, L. K. and Salem-Schatz, S.: Anticoagulation in Atrial Fibrillation: Does Efficacy in Clinical Trials Translate into Effectiveness in Practice? Arch. Intern Med. 154(17):1945-1953, Sept. 1994.

Hirsh, J., et al.: Oral Anticoagulants: Mechanism of Action, Clinical Effectiveness, and Optimal Therapeutic Range. Chest 108(4):231S-246S, Oct. 1995.

Holas, M. A., et al.: Aspiration and Relative Risk of Medical Complications Following Stroke. Arch. Neurol. 51(10):1051-1053, Oct. 1994.

Jorgensen, H. S., et al.: Intracerebral Hemorrhage Versus Infarction: Stroke Severity, Risk Factors, and Prognosis. Ann. Neurol. 38(1):45-50, July 1995.

Juvela, S., et al.: Risk Factors for Spontaneous Intracerebral Hemorrhage. Stroke 26(9):1558-1564, Sept. 1995.

Kalra, L. and Eade, J.: Role of Stroke Rehabilitation Units in Managing Severe Disability After Stroke. Stroke 26(11):2031-2034, Nov. 1995.

Kalra, L., et al.: Medical Complications During Stroke Rehabilitation. Stroke 26(6):990-994, June 1995.

Kothari, R. U., et al.: Emergency Physicians. Accuracy in the Diagnosis of Stroke. Stroke 26(12):2238-2241, Dec. 1995.

Lee, K. P., et al.: Neurologic Complications Following Chiropractic Manipulation: A Survey of California Neurologists. Neurology 45(6):1213-1215, June 1995.

Libman, R. B., et al.: Conditions That Mimic Stroke in the Emergency Department. Implications for Acute Stroke Trials. Arch. Neurol. 52(11):1119-1122, Nov. 1995.

Lincoln, N. B., et al.: Comparison of Rehabilitation Practice on Hospital Wards for Stroke Patients. Stroke 27(1):18-23, Jan. 1996.

Mathew, P., et al.: Neurosurgical Management of Cerebellar Haematoma and Infarct. J. Neurol. Neurosurg. Psychiatry 59(3):287-292, Sept. 1995.

Meldrum, B. S.: Cytoprotective Therapies in Stroke. Curr. Opin. Neurol.8(1):15-23, Feb. 1995.

Metzer, W. S., et al.: Anticardiolipin Antibodies in a Sample of Neuroleptic-Treated Chronic Schizophrenics. South. Med. J. 87(2):190-192, Feb. 1994.

Mohr, J. P. and Prohovkik, I.: Neurovascular Imaging. In: Rowland, L. P. (Ed.): Merritt's Textbook of Neurology, 9th ed. Baltimore: Williams & Wilkins, 1995.

Pollock, B. E., et al.: Factors that Predict the Bleeding Risk of Cerebral Arteriovenous Malformations. Stroke 27(1):1-6, Jan. 1996.

Sacco, R. L.: Ischemic Stroke. In: Gorelick, P. A. and Alter, M. A. (Eds): Handbook of Neuroepidemiology. New York: Marcel Dekker, 1994.

Solomon, R. A., et al.: Relationship Between the Volume of Craniotomies for Cerebral Aneurysm Performed at New York State Hospitals and In-Hospital Mortality. Stroke 27(1):13-17, Jan. 1996.

Sotaniemi, K. A.: Long-Term Neurologic Outcome After Cardiac Operation. Ann. Thorac. Surg. 59(5):1336-1339, May 1995.

Sturzenegger, M.: Spontaneous Internal Carotid Artery Dissection: Early Diagnosis and Management in 44 Patients. J. Neurol. 242(4):231-238, Mar. 1995.

Tegeler, C. H.: Ultrasound in Cerebrovascular Disease: In: Greenberg, J.O. (Ed.): Neuroimaging. New York: McGraw-Hill, 1995.

Viktrup, L., et al.: Delayed Onset of Fatal Basilar Thrombotic Embolus After Whiplash Injury. Stroke 26(11):2194-2196, Nov. 1995.

World Health Organization Collaborative Study of Cardiovascular and Steroid Hormone Contraception: A Multinational Case-Control Study of Cardiovascular Disease and Steroid Hormone Contraceptives. Description and Validation of Methods. J. Clin. Epidemiol. 48(12):1513-47, Dec. 1995.

Yatsu, F.: Stroke. St. Louis: Mosby, 1995.

CHAPTER 10

Headache and Migraine

SCOPE

Headaches are divided into three basic kinds—tension type, migraine and cluster. Tension-type headaches are the kind that affect most people and usually respond to a simple analgesic such as aspirin. Migraine, the most common debilitating headache, affects women more than men. It is usually felt on one side of the head and can occur with or without an aura (usually visual symptoms, but sometimes other neurologic symptoms). Migraine without aura can be difficult to distinguish from tension-type headache. Cluster headaches affect many more men than women, and their incidence in the general population is much lower than migraine. In addition, a host of headache types occur secondary to trauma and disease, and miscellaneous headaches occur that are independent of any kind of detectable pathology. Migraines run in families, but the genetic mechanism appears complicated. Newer drugs to treat migraine mimic serotonin by fitting into serotonin subreceptors on the cell surface. However, these drugs do not work for all people with severe headaches.

SYNOPSIS

[b] **Calcium-Channel Blockers**
[c] **Antidepressants**
[d] **Anticonvulsants**
[e] **Steroids**
[f] **Ergotamine**
[3] **Alternative Therapies**
10.43   **Treatment of Chronic Headache Medication Overuse**
10.100   **BIBLIOGRAPHY**

10.00 INTRODUCTION

Forty percent of the world's population reports at least one severe, disabling headache each year. Even small children are not immune. Despite the common impression that headaches are caused by a high-stress urban environment, research shows them to be equally common among city dwellers and rural populations worldwide (Raskin, 1994).

Most people experience what is called a tension-type headache—a bilateral (on both sides) painful sensation in the head that is usually relieved by an over-the-counter analgesic such as aspirin, acetaminophen or ibuprofen.[1]

The next most common form of headache is migraine. Migraine headaches can cause blinding unilateral (on one side) head pain, nausea and many other physical and psychological symptoms. They are usually not relieved by over-the-counter medications.[2]

Cluster headaches, the third major form, are characterized by incapacitating pain and grouped in clusters through the year. Like migraine, cluster headaches are not relieved by simple analgesics.[3]

Secondary headaches, another headache category, are caused by a medical condition, such as a brain tumor, or as an adverse effect of any one of many medications.[4]

10.10 DEFINITIONS AND DIAGNOSIS

Although headaches are easily recognized, they come in different varieties and severities. Head pain can be of a pressing or throbbing

---

[1] *See* 10.11 *infra* for further discussion of tension-type headaches.

[2] *See* 10.12 *infra* for further discussion of migraine headaches.

[3] *See* 10.13 *infra* for further discussion of cluster headaches.

[4] *See* 10.14 *infra* for further discussion of secondary headaches.

nature, act as a minor irritation or leave a person bedridden, involve the entire head or just one side, be preceded by strange visual or neurologic symptoms, cause nausea and vomiting, and last for hours to days.

Until 1988, primary (benign) headache was a diagnosis of exclusion (i.e., every other possible cause, such as brain tumor or cerebral aneurysm, is ruled out first). This "nonsystem" of diagnosis left a great deal of room for individual physician interpretation of tension-type, migraine and cluster headaches, and a good deal of general confusion.

In 1988, the International Headache Society (IHS) released positive criteria for the diagnosis of primary headaches. These criteria were then incorporated into the International Classification of Diseases of the World Health Organization (ICD-10), which standardizes medical diagnoses worldwide. The headache diagnostic criteria incorporated new knowledge of the biochemistry of headache and cleared up what had been at best a cluttered taxonomy (Olesen, 1993).

Headaches are now referred to as *tension type, migraine with aura, migraine without aura, cluster, secondary* and *miscellaneous.* Secondary headaches are those due to another medical condition, such as a brain tumor that has grown to the point that it is pressing or pulling on pain-sensitive structures in the brain, or a medication such as nitroglycerin, which causes headache by dilating cerebral arteries. The category "miscellaneous headaches unassociated with structural lesion" includes the stabbing headache some people get when eating something cold, as well as other kinds of head pain that don't fit easily into the other categories.

Before the introduction of specific criteria for diagnosing headaches, patients suffering from chronic headaches were almost routinely given expensive diagnostic tests such as computed tomography (CT) brain scans or magnetic resonance imaging (MRI) scans to make sure the headaches were not caused by something ominous, such as a malignant brain tumor. Now, however, if the patient fulfills the criteria for migraine with aura, for example, no further testing is required to render a diagnosis.

The introduction of this new diagnostic system does not mean that all headache diagnoses are clear and easy to decide upon. It may be difficult to differentiate migraine without aura from tension-type headache, and sometimes a person can suffer from both simultaneously (Olesen, 1993). It is also true that some clinicians cling to the old classification system with which they and many patients are comfortable (Raskin, 1994).

When a patient complaining of frequent and/or severe headaches comes to a physician for evaluation, a helpful diagnostic tool is a headache calendar, on which the patient keeps track of the timing, severity and treatment outcome of each headache. This allows both the patient and the physician to spot trends and objectively evaluate different medications or other treatment modalities. There are many different kinds of headache calendars, and each physician who deals with headaches usually develops one he or she finds useful.

10.11 Tension-type Headaches

Tension-type headache is the name now used to describe what previously was called either tension headache or muscle-contraction headache. The earlier names for this type of headache connoted a known pathophysiologic process (i.e., that muscle contraction causes the pain) as the cause of these common headaches. Research has raised more questions than it has answered about what causes tension-type headaches, however, so a less definitive name was required (Olesen, 1993).

The criteria for a diagnosis of *episodic tension-type headache* are (Olesen, 1993):

1. At least 10 previous headache episodes fulfilling criteria 2 through 4 below. The number of days with such headaches totals less than 180 per year.

2. Headache lasts from 30 minutes to seven days.

3. At least two of the following pain characteristics are present:

   - pressing/tightening (nonpulsating) quality;
   - mild to moderate intensity;
   - bilateral location; and
   - no aggravation by walking stairs or similar routine activity.

4. Both the following situations exist:

   - There is no nausea or vomiting (but anorexia can occur); and

- Photophobia and phonophobia (sensitivity to light and sound) are absent, or one but not the other is present.

Tension-type headache can become a chronic condition, with frequent episodes.

10.12 Migraines

Migraine is the most common kind of debilitating primary headache. An episodic disorder that is often disabling both during and between attacks, it produces significant headache related disability and economic impact. Migraine is thought to be both underdiagnosed and undertreated, which leaves significant room for cost-effective medical interventions that could lessen the disorder's impact on individuals and its cost to society (Stewart and Lipton, 1994).

[1] Migraines with Aura

A migraine aura consists of one or more sensory, motor or visual symptoms that usually precede the onset of headache by less than an hour. (An aura can also occur without subsequent headache or concurrently with the headache.) Visual symptoms, caused by dysfunction of neurons in the occipital lobe (the visual cortex at the back of the brain), are by far the most common. (*See Figure 10-1.*) These symptoms include:

- shimmering, wavy lines;
- spots similar to those seen after a flashbulb goes off (scotomas);
- areas of blindness within the visual fields (a pie-shaped wedge of black surrounded by normal sight);
- bright flashing lights; and
- blurred vision, similar to having tears in the eyes that won't clear.

Migraine with aura encompasses what previously was most commonly called *classic migraine*. The term also replaces *migraine accompagne, hemiplegic migraine, complicated migraine* and *ophthalmic, hemisensory, aphasic* and *confusional migraine.*

Subtypes of migraine with aura that are recognized under the new system include:

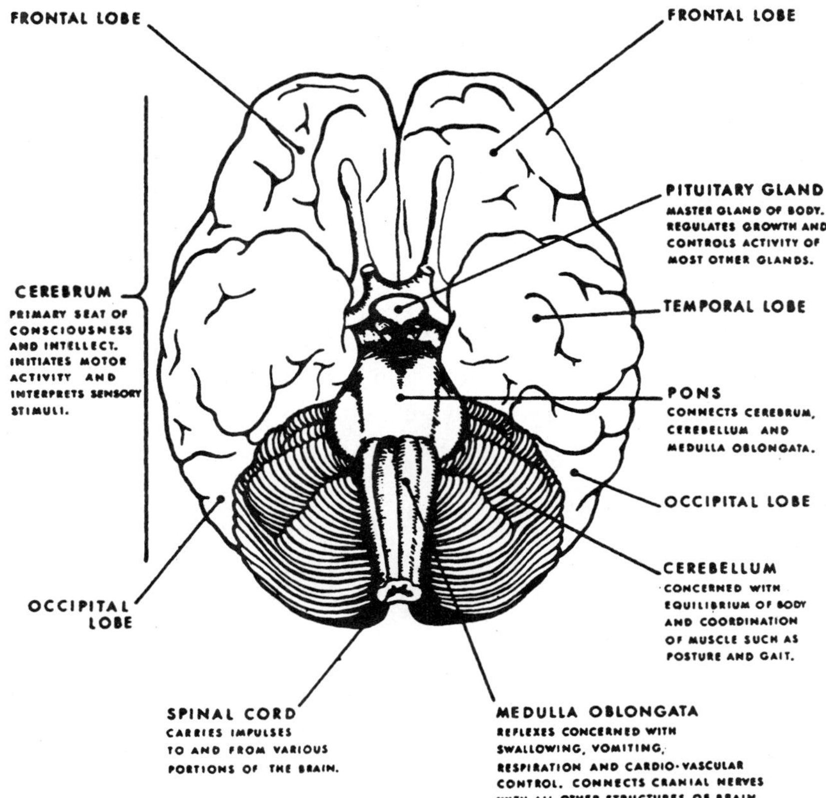

Fig. 10–1. The underside of the brain, showing the relationship of the different lobes to the structures of the brain stem. Visual manifestations of migraine headache are thought to originate in the occipital lobe.

- migraine with typical aura;

- migraine with prolonged aura;

- familial (inherited) hemiplegic migraine (causing temporary partial or total paralysis of one arm and/or one side of the face, as after a one-sided stroke);

- basilar migraine (symptoms caused by migrainous processes in the brain stem, including vertigo, double vision and difficult or defective speech);

- migraine aura without headache; and

- migraine with acute onset aura.

The diagnostic criteria for migraine with aura include at least two attacks with at least three of the four following characteristics:

- one or more fully reversible (with intravenous dihydroergotamine) aura symptoms indicating focal cerebral cortical and/or brain stem dysfunction;

- at least one aura symptom that develops gradually over more than 4 minutes, or two or more symptoms occurring in succession;

- no aura symptom that lasts more than 60 minutes (if more than one aura symptom is present, the accepted duration is proportionally increased); and

- headache follows aura with a free interval of less than 60 minutes (it may also begin before or simultaneously with the aura).

[2] Migraines Without Aura

Migraine without aura replaces the term common migraine. These are by far the most frequently experienced migraine headaches, and they are often difficult to distinguish from tension-type headaches.

The IHS criteria for migraine without aura are (Olesen, 1993):

1. At least five attacks fulfilling the following criteria 2 through 4.

2. Headache attacks lasting 4 to 72 hours (untreated or unsuccessfully treated).

3. Headache has at least two of the following characteristics:

   - unilateral location;

   - pulsating quality;

   - moderate or severe intensity; and

   - aggravated by walking stairs or similar routine physical activity.

4. During headache, the patient experiences at least one of the following:

   - nausea and/or vomiting; and

   - photophobia (sensitivity to light) and phonophobia (sensitivity to sound).

10.13　Cluster Headaches and Related Syndromes

Cluster headache is perhaps the most distinct and easily diagnosed primary headache. Most cluster headache sufferers are young men who describe very similar symptoms of extreme head pain associated with other symptoms in the following list. Cluster headache has traditionally been regarded as a subtype of migraine; however, many researchers now believe it is well documented that cluster headache and migraine are unrelated (Olesen, 1993).

Episodic cluster headache may be defined as severe unilateral head or facial pain lasting from 15 minutes to three hours, commonly associated with ipsilateral (on the same side of the head as the pain) inflammation of the conjunctiva (the tissue that covers the eyeball and lines the interior of the eyelid), blockage of the nostril and lacrimation (tear production; involuntary crying), usually recurring once or more daily for a period of weeks or months, separated by periods of complete freedom from pain (Lance, 1993b).

Chronic paroxysmal hemicrania is an unremitting kind of cluster headache in which the affected person has many episodes during the day that last only briefly. There are many other related head pain syndromes (Lance, 1993b).

IHS criteria for cluster headache are (Olesen, 1993):

1. At least five attacks fulfilling criteria 2 through 4.

2. Severe unilateral orbital, supraorbital and/or temporal pain lasting 15 to 180 minutes untreated.

3. Headache associated with at least one of the following signs, which have to be present on the side with pain:

   - conjunctival injection (inflammation);
   - lacrimation (tears);
   - nasal congestion;
   - rhinorrhea (nasal discharge);
   - forehead and facial sweating;
   - miosis (abnormal contraction of the pupil of the eye); and
   - eyelid edema (swelling).

4. Frequency of attacks: from one every other day to eight per day.

10.14   Secondary Headaches

Secondary headaches are those caused by another medical condition; the headache is a symptom of something else and not a medical entity in and of itself, as in primary headaches. Deciding whether a patient's headaches are primary or secondary requires a careful patient history and physical examination to determine if the patient fulfills the diagnostic criteria for a common form of headache. If the headache has a sudden onset and the person has not had headaches in the past, if it is unremitting, if the patient has nausea and/or vomiting or if the patient has other neurologic symptoms, further evaluation is required. This further evaluation usually involves imaging studies with CT and/or MRI to rule out pathology such as a quickly expanding intracranial bleed[5] or a brain tumor.[6]

10.15   Miscellaneous Headaches Unassociated with Structural Lesions

This class of headache includes various headaches that do not fit into other classifications but that often cause distress and worry for the patient and, occasionally, for the clinician.

Idiopathic (of unknown origin) *stabbing headache,* previously known as ice-pick pain, can be incapacitating. However, this is a benign headache with no worrisome underlying cause, and it responds well to prophylactic treatment with the nonsteroidal anti-inflammatory drug (NSAID) indomethecin (Indocin®).

External compression headache is also an entirely benign headache caused by hats, headbands, tight pulling of the hair (as in pigtails or ponytails) and other things that cause compression of the head. Means for preventing these headaches are obvious, and once a headache is started, it usually responds to simple analgesics.[7]

Cold stimulus headache can be caused by external application of cold (e.g., an ice pack) or by ingestion of a cold substance (usually ice cream). This headache is self-limiting, and although it can be extremely unpleasant, it fades when the cold source is removed or, as in ice cream, melts.

---

[5] *See also* ch. 4.

[6] *See also* ch. 7.

[7] *See* 10.41[1] *infra* for further discussion of analgesics used to treat headache.

Benign cough headache is characterized by transient (seconds to a few minutes), severe head pain brought on by coughing, lifting, bending, sneezing or stooping. Many patients report the onset of the syndrome following a lower respiratory tract pneumonia that was accompanied by severe coughing, or after a strenuous weight-lifting program. This kind of headache afflicts males four times as frequently as it does females, and it is usually diffuse, although it lateralizes (manifests on one side) in about a third of patients. Benign cough headaches may persist for a few years, but they respond well to prophylactic treatment with indomethecin (Indocin®) at dosages ranging from 50 to 200 mg daily.

For about 25 percent of patients, cough headaches are not benign but signal a serious intracranial structural abnormality. The Arnold-Chiari deformity is a common cause in this group. This is a skull defect in which the foramen magnum (the hole at the bottom of the skull through which the spinal cord descends) is abnormally large. Therefore, the lower portion of the cerebellum and the medulla oblongata protrude through the foramen magnum and into the spinal canal (Raskin, 1994).

Benign exertional headache (sometimes called effort migraine) can occur in migraine-prone individuals during sustained physical exertion, building up over hours. These headaches can be completely relieved by a beta-blocker drug, such as propranolol (Inderal®; the oldest and least specific beta-blocker) or atenolol (Tenormin®; newer and less likely to cause respiratory complications in individuals with asthma) (Olesen, 1993).

Headache associated with sexual activity can be dull, explosive or postural in nature. These periorgasmic headaches occur in men by a four-to-one margin over women, and when an organic cause has been ruled out, they can be relieved by a beta-blocker or merely by cessation of sexual activity (Olesen, 1993).

Most headaches associated with sexual activity are sporadic and do not occur with every coitus. Therefore, beta-blockers, which can cause impotence, are better used as an abortive therapy rather than chronically to prevent the headaches. Sex-associated headaches are usually benign, but if a headache persists for hours or is accompanied by vomiting, a subdural hematoma (accumulation of blood beneath the dura mater, or outermost layer of meningeal tissue covering the brain and spinal cord) must be ruled out by cerebrospinal fluid examination (blood in the fluid is considered positive) and a computed tomography scan (CT; computer-enhanced serial x-rays of the skull) (Raskin, 1994).[8]

10.16   Daily Chronic Headaches

Daily chronic headaches (DCHs) represent more than 40 percent of all severe headache cases. They are still a matter of debate, and thus the International Headache Society (IHS) does not include this difficult clinical entity in its 1988 diagnostic criteria. Most cases have a mixture of both migraine and tension-type symptoms, unlike chronic tension headache, which fulfills only the criteria for tension-type headache. Usually the patient develops DCH from previous episodic migraine (Martignoni and Solomon, 1993).

Perhaps the most common factor related to the development of daily chronic headache is overuse of headache relief medications[9] and overuse of caffeine.

Some researchers believe that there are actually two clearly distinguishable syndromes: daily migrainous headache (DMH) and daily tension-type headache (DTH). A 1994 study found that although both groups had a high incidence of caffeine or drug overuse, a family history of headache was more common in the DMH group, and patients with DMH also had a higher incidence of disturbed magnesium metabolism (Mauskop, et al., 1994).

10.20   HEADACHE EPIDEMIOLOGY

Since essentially everyone gets headaches, it is tempting to call headache a normal part of human existence. However, because severe headaches can be disabling and most can be treated, their epidemiology as a disorder is important.

Studies conducted over the years to determine the prevalence of migraine among the general population have varied in their exact results, but women have always been found to be affected more frequently than men.[10] A survey of over 20,000 individuals in the

---

[8] *See also* ch. 4 for further discussion of subdural hematoma.

[9] *See* 10.43 *infra.*

[10] *See* 10.12 *supra* for further discussion of migraine and its characteristics.

United States in 1992 found that 17.6 percent of women and 5.7 percent of men experience severe migraine headaches. The same National Migraine Study found the prevalence of migraine to be more than 60 percent higher in lower income groups than in those with an annual income above $30,000 (Stewart, et al., 1992).

The prevalence of cluster headache is much lower than that of migraine.[11] However, the estimated ratio by which migraine exceeds cluster ranges from 1:6 to 1:50, depending upon the source. Cluster is more common in men than in women and is estimated to affect 0.4 percent of American men and 0.08 percent of American women, though these numbers also vary depending upon who is doing the estimating. A generally agreed upon figure is that roughly 85 percent of cluster headache patients are male (Lance, 1993b).

A study of 215 children 3 to 16 years old who were referred to a neurology clinic for treatment of chronic and/or severe headache found that the most common (27 percent) type of headache was seizure related, and that these headaches responded well to initiating anticonvulsant therapy (Chen, et al., 1994).

An association between migraine and psychiatric disorders has been recognized for over 100 years, but the exact relation between migraines and psychopathology has only recently been investigated systematically (Keck, et al., 1994). Depression and anxiety are common in people who suffer from chronic migraine, but there has always been the "chicken and egg" controversy. Do migraines afflict depressed and anxious people more often than the average person? It seems reasonable that frequent, excruciating headaches could precipitate depression over one's life circumstances and cause anxiety about when the next attack will occur (Lance, 1993b).

Antidepressant drugs often have a positive effect on chronic migraine sufferers, decreasing the number of migraines each month, but the effect is greater than that which would be expected merely by lifting depression; therefore, antidepressant drugs seem to have a headache-preventing function independent of their psychoactive effects.

Migraine sufferers have a reputation for being rigid perfectionists, but research into this area has revealed no clear pattern of a typical

---

[11] *See* 10.13 *supra* for further discussion of cluster headaches and their characteristics.

migraine personality. Studies of migrainous children have found that they have a higher incidence of sleep disturbances, motion sickness, recurrent abdominal pains and temper tantrums than do controls, but there is no difference in intelligence, social class or ambition, or in such symptoms as nervous tics, nail biting or bed-wetting. Migrainous children have been found to be more fearful, tense, sensitive and vulnerable to frustration, and to have less physical endurance than their nonmigrainous cohorts. However, among adults, the Minnesota Multiphasic Personality Inventory (MMPI; a standard psychological test) has repeatedly failed to show any personality abnormalities among migraine sufferers (Lance, 1993b).

10.30   ETIOLOGY

Discovering what is happening inside the head at the start of a headache has proved a great challenge. Many contradictory or never-replicated findings, often derived from very small patient samples, have been published over the years (Ferrari, 1992).

At one time, it was believed that tension-type headaches were caused by tightening of the scalp and neck muscles during stress, while migraines were believed to be a result of constriction followed by hyperdilation (excessive widening) of cerebral blood vessels. Muscle constriction is no longer believed to be the primary cause of tension-type headaches, and many experts think tension-type and migraine headaches are merely at different points on a continuum, with vascular and muscular changes occurring in both kinds of headaches (Marcus, 1993).

The constriction/dilation view of migraine is still considered valid by many. However, evidence also supports a theory of "spreading depression" across the brain. Spreading depression is defined as a slow-moving (2 to 3 millimeters per minute) depression of cortical (referring to the cerebral cortex, or surface of the brain) activity that liberates potassium from the cells. The cortical depression is thought to be preceded by a wave of increased metabolic activity, causing hyperexcitation (Raskin, 1994).[12]

It may be that both neurovascular and spreading depression mechanisms are involved in migraine. Certainly there is evidence for both,

---

[12] *See* 10.35 *infra* for further discussion of the spreading depression theory of headache.

and the expanding headache knowledge base would indicate that an extremely complex migraine biochemistry is at work. As yet, however, there is no unified field theory of headache that knits all these factors together in a coherent whole.

A 1993 study defined migraine as "a neurovascular reaction to sudden changes in the internal or external environment." It promulgated the vascular theory of migraine and proposed that people with migraine have defective pain control pathways in the central nervous system. These defective pathways are thought to fail to block pain impulses coming from the periphery. The fifth cranial nerve (the trigeminal) is thought to cause blood vessel dilation and awareness of pain in the thalamus, a large area in the midportion of the brain that processes sensory stimuli, including pain (Lance, 1993a). (*See Figure 10-2.*)

Most of the academic research into headache mechanisms has involved migraine, the most common disabling headache. Tension-type headaches, although they are very common and often unpleasant, usually respond to simple analgesics and don't require a visit to a doctor or an emergency room. Cluster headaches, although they are usually considerably painful, affect far fewer people than does migraine. Migraine is a complicated mix of genetic predisposition, environmental and food triggers, and biochemical messengers and sensitizers.

10.31 Genetics

Migraine has a strong genetic component, although the exact mechanism by which migraine is inherited and how genetic factors make a person susceptible are far from clear. Some families with migraine, especially familial hemiplegic migraine, appear to inherit the disorder as an autosomal (not sex-linked) dominant (as opposed to recessive) trait. However, in most cases, headache inheritance is not so easily traced to a particular gene but rather appears to involve a complex pattern combining multiple genetic factors.

Despite its complexity, evidence for the genetic inheritance of migraine is strong. When only first-degree relatives (parents and siblings) were considered in one study, 46 percent of migraine patients were found to have a family history of these headaches. In a control group of tension-type headache sufferers, only 18 percent of their first-degree relatives were affected. If grandparents were included in the

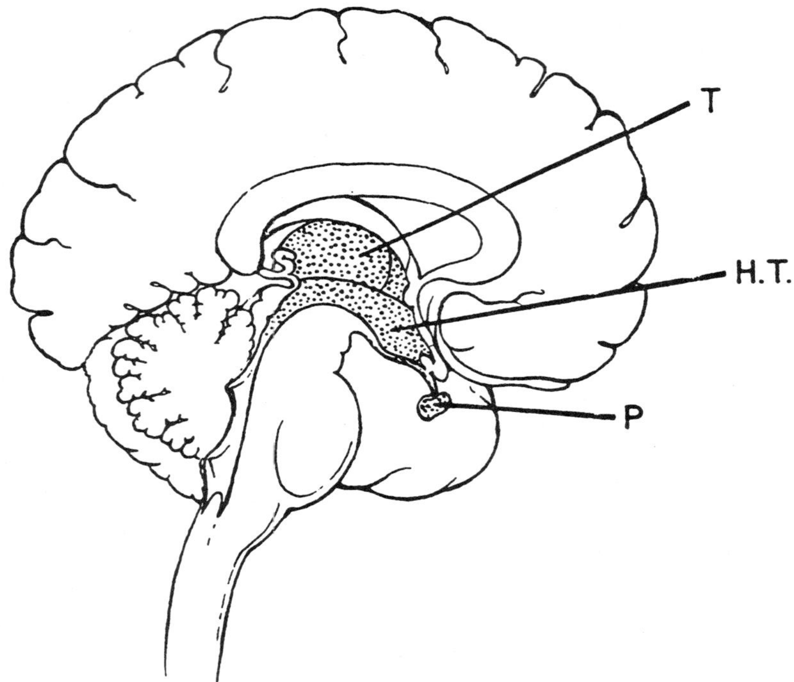

Fig. 10–2. Sagittal section (from front to back) of the brain, showing the thalamus (T), hypothalamus (H.T.) and pituitary gland (P). One theory of migraine headache pain is that the fifth cranial nerve causes dilation of blood vessels and awareness of pain in the thalamus.

survey, the percentage of patients with a family history of migraine jumped to 55 percent (Lance, 1993b).

10.32   Prostaglandins

Prostaglandins have long been postulated to be involved in the etiology of migraine, though no exact mechanism has been discovered and their role remains largely hypothetical. Prostaglandins are a large group of biologically active unsaturated fatty acids that act as local intercellular or intracellular modulators of biological activity. Known to play a significant role in the development of inflammation, prostaglandins sensitize nociceptors (pain-sensing nerves), producing a state called hyperalgesia (excessive pain sensation), and they are involved in platelet (blood elements involved in clotting) aggregation, a process that releases serotonin, the major neurotransmitter believed to be involved in migraine (Hansen, 1994).

Treatment of headache with nonsteroidal anti-inflammatory drugs (NSAIDs) is based on this theorized role of prostaglandins in the initiation and perpetuation of head pain.

10.33 Neurotransmitters

Strong circumstantial evidence exists pointing to serotonin (5-hydroxytryptamine, or 5-HT), a neurotransmitter (a substance that facilitates transmission of impulses between nerve cells) with many functions in the nervous system (sleep, thermoregulation, feeding behavior and sexual behavior), as playing a major role in the initiation of migraine, and perhaps in tension-type and cluster headaches as well.

[1] Serotonin

Studies have shown systemic derangement of 5-HT metabolism in migrainous individuals, during and between headaches (Ferrari, 1992). During attacks, platelet 5-HT levels have been found to decrease, and in some studies, increased levels of 5-HT metabolites have been found, suggesting destruction of the neurotransmitter (Silberstein, 1994).

However, whether serotonin is destroyed during the headache process or whether people with headaches have an inadequate number of serotonin receptors sites—as well as much else about the exact mechanism by which serotonin acts in headache—is not yet clear. It is known that migraine patients have chronically low systemic 5-HT, but it is not known whether it is the 5-HT in the systemic circulating blood or the levels of 5-HT within cells, especially platelets, that are important (Ferrari and Saxena, 1993). A great deal of research is being carried on, and it often produces contradictory results.

Serotonin and other neurotransmitters work by fitting like keys into receptors (the locks) on the cell surface. It is now believed that there are at least seven main families of serotonin receptors, and many have subtypes within the family (Silberstein, 1994). These receptors, which have evolved for bonding with an array of internal hormones and neurotransmitters, also bond with many drugs (sumatriptan reacts most strongly with the 5-HT-1D receptors, while dihydroergotamine reacts most strongly with 5-HT-1A receptors) and other chemicals (the migraine trigger nitric oxide reacts with the 5-HT-2B and -2C receptors) (Fozard and Kalkman, 1994).

A small study of women with tension-type headache found that when they were pain free, the plasma level (plasma is the fluid in which red and white blood cells float within the circulatory system) of serotonin in the headache subjects was no different from that of controls. However, during a headache, there was a significant increase in 5-HT concentration, suggesting that 5-HT may be involved in the pathogenesis of tension-type headache but by a different mechanism than that in migraine (Jensen and Hindberg, 1994). However, this was a small study (15 subjects), and the results must be duplicated before they are taken as absolute fact.

A study that investigated the binding at a peripheral serotonergic (stimulated by serotonin) marker (platelet 3H-imipramine, 3H-IMI) and the activity of the enzyme sulfotransferase (ST), which is involved in the breakdown of catecholamines (epinephrine and norepinephrine), found that both people with migraine and tension-type headache had a lower number of these platelet binding sites than did controls. Levels of the ST enzyme were also reduced in those people with headaches. The reduced number of 3H-IMI binding sites suggests that headache sufferers have dysfunctional peripheral serotonergic receptors. The reduced ST enzyme activity may produce changes in the level of some neurotransmitters (dopamine and tyramine), which may have a role in the pathophysiology of some aspects of primary headache (Marazziti, et al., 1994). The authors were careful to qualify their conclusions, however, pending further study.

Another strong piece of (admittedly circumstantial) evidence for the role of serotonin in headache is the fact that drugs that bond with the serotonin receptor sites (sumatriptan and dihydroergotamine) are effective in relieving migraine in many patients. Also fluoxetine (Prozac®), which does not stimulate serotonergic receptors but blocks reuptake of serotonin into cells, thereby increasing the quantity available for bonding, has proved effective in preventing chronic migraine and tension-type headache.[13]

[2]　Substance P

A study to measure platelet levels of 5-HT and a protein called Substance P (for *pain*) suggests that perhaps Substance P (SP) released from the terminals of the branches of the trigeminal nerve (cranial nerve V) causes migraine, either through direct action on the vessels (SP is known to sensitize nociceptors) or by releasing 5-HT from the platelets. The study found that platelet concentrations of 5-HT and

---

[13] *See* 10.41[2] *infra* for further discussion of the serotonin agonists.

SP were significantly higher in those who suffered from migraine and tension-type headache than in normal controls. Migraineurs had the highest levels of both substances (Nakano, et al., 1993).

10.34 Hormones

Hormonal factors in women often play a considerable role in initiating migraines. These factors include use of birth control pills, menopause, estrogen therapy, pregnancy and especially menstruation.

The two major groups of female sex hormones, the estrogens and progestins, have a profound influence on women who are susceptible to migraine. Women who are prone to menstrual migraine can get the headaches before, during and after their menstrual period, and some also get migraines during ovulation at the middle of their cycle. Menstrual migraines cause an enormous amount of suffering, because they tend to be more severe than nonmenstrually related migraines, and they are also often resistant to treatment strategies that work for most other migraineurs (Robbins, 1994).

The exact mechanism by which the rise and fall of these hormones during the menstrual cycle causes migraine (as well as hormonal changes during menopause) is not understood. However, the role of female hormones in causing migraines probably accounts for the greater number of women who suffer with this kind of headache.

10.35 Magnesium and Excitatory Amino Acids

Magnesium ions (magnesium atoms minus two electrons, which gives them a double-positive charge and thus makes them attracted to ions with a double-negative charge to form a salt, as in magnesium sulfate, $MgSO_4$) play many roles in the body. Magnesium is the second most abundant cation (a positively charged ion) within cells, after potassium. Magnesium is vital to neuromuscular function; severe magnesium depletion (as is seen in many chronic alcoholics) can lead to seizures.

Magnesium helps regulate intracellular metabolism, affects the metabolism of proteins and nucleic acids (the "building blocks" of deoxyribonucleic acid, or DNA) and activates many essential enzyme systems. Magnesium also helps transport sodium and potassium ions across the cell membrane and indirectly influences intracellular calcium levels (Lewis, 1993).

Magnesium is thought to play a central role in establishing a threshold for migraine attacks and in the genetic and pathologic mechanisms involved in headache onset. Magnesium ion concentrations have been found lowered during migraine, especially in those migraineurs who experience an aura. Magnesium depletion is known to cause neuron (nerve cell) hyperexcitability. This condition is believed to precede the neuronal dampening called spreading depression, a process that is theorized to be involved in the initiation of migraine (Lance, 1993b).

However, results from studies of magnesium ion concentrations and metabolism in migraineurs has also been used to enhance the neurovascular view of migraine. A low serum magnesium ion concentration coupled with a high calcium-to-magnesium ion ratio can cause cerebrovasospasm (constriction of the brain's blood vessels), causing reduced blood flow in the brain (Mauskop, et al., 1993). *(See Figure 10-3.)*

Most studies of magnesium levels in migraine patients have involved magnesium levels in the brain and in the circulating blood volume. In comparison with normal subjects, some migraineurs with and without aura have significantly lower levels of red blood cell magnesium, which may be a peripheral expression of the reduced magnesium levels within the brain (Gallai, et al., 1993).

Why migraine sufferers handle magnesium ions in a different manner from the individuals who do not experience migraines is not known. There are some tempting, though not always consistent, hints. The female hormone estrogen has been shown to enhance magnesium utilization and uptake by soft tissues, which could decrease magnesium blood concentrations and presumably initiate migraine when estrogen levels are high around ovulation (Seelig, 1993). This mechanism does not explain, however, the greater incidence of migraine among women during menstruation, when estrogen levels are lowest and, according to this hypothesis, would be interfering less with magnesium metabolism.

Magnesium taken orally has been shown to ameliorate migraine headache for some patients. Taking a magnesium supplement and strictly following dosage recommendations on the package is inexpensive and probably worth a try by all migraineurs. Taking more than the recommended dosage can cause magnesium poisoning and potentially lead to death.

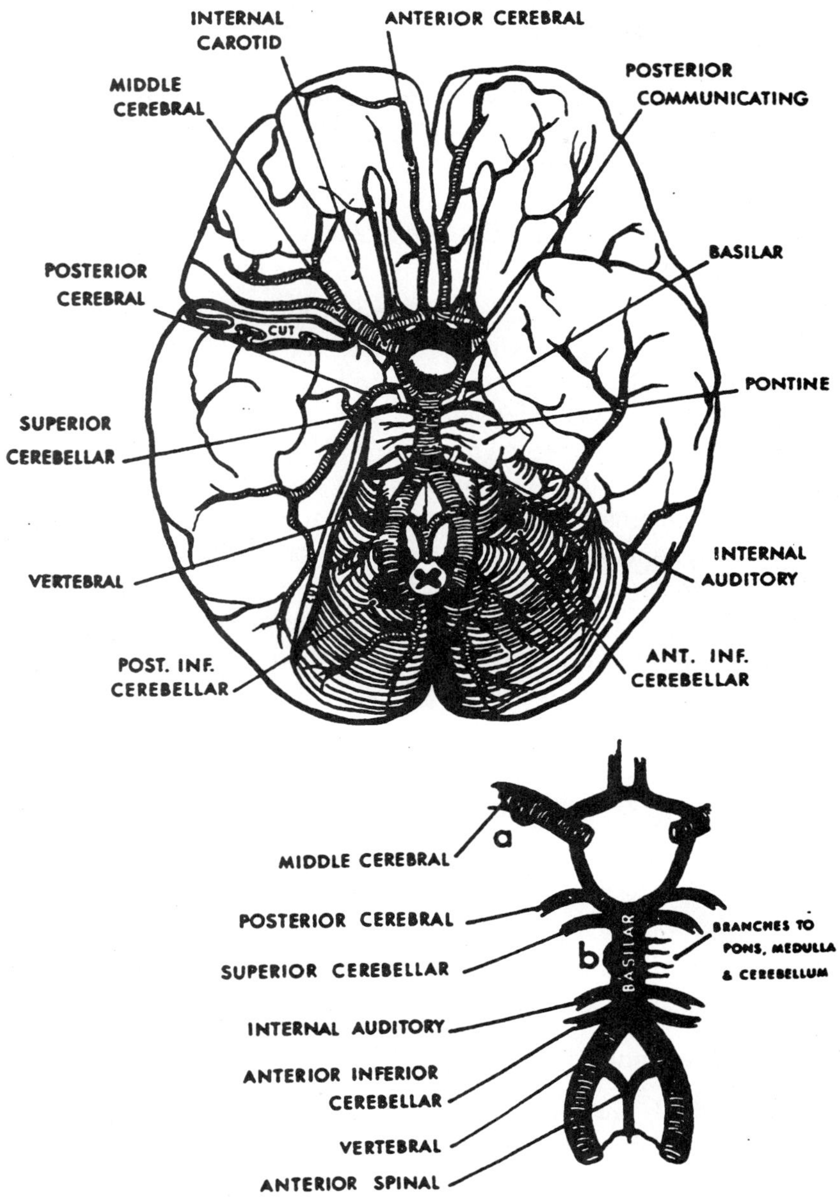

Fig. 10–3. The underside of the brain, showing the arteries that give rise to cerebral blood vessels. Vasospasm caused by upset of serum magnesium levels is thought to play a role in migraine headache pain.

Amino acids are the small units from which proteins are built. Amino acids form a large group of organic compounds constructed with an amino group (NH_2) on one end of the molecule and a carboxyl group (COOH, a carbon atom double-bonded to one oxygen and single-bonded to a hydroxy group, OH) on the other end of the molecule. Some amino acids on their own, not joined together into proteins, act as neuron (nerve cell) stimulators. These are the excitatory amino acids, two of which—glutamate and aspartate—have been associated with migraine.

The glutamate and aspartate content of platelets has been found to be increased in patients who are subject to migraine with aura during headache-free periods, when compared both with normal controls and patients subject to migraine without aura. The platelet glutamate level in patients who experienced migraine with aura was found to rise even further during headache. Similar results were obtained when plasma levels of glutamate were measured in migraine patients. Increased levels of excitatory amino acids in migraine sufferers could lend credence to the spreading depression theory of migraine initiation, since spreading depression is believed to be preceded by a period of hyperexcitation of brain neurons, which could be caused by excitatory amino acids (Lance, 1993a).

10.36 Headache Triggers

Most migraineurs should try to avoid certain common triggers; however, each person must go through a painful process of trial and error to find his or her personal list of triggers. How these particular factors precipitate headaches is not entirely known, and why specific triggers cause headache in some headache-prone people and not in others is also not clear.

[1] Food and Drink

Many foods are common migraine triggers, although the degree of sensitivity to foods varies widely among migraineurs. The common food triggers include:

- monosodium glutamate (MSG);
- red wine, white wine, beer, miscellaneous alcoholic drinks (vodka is least likely to trigger a migraine);
- chocolate;

- citrus fruits;

- aged cheeses (cheddar, bleu, brick, Colby, Roquefort, brie, Gruyére, mozzarella, Parmesan, Romano, boursalt);

- processed cheese;

- hot dogs, pepperoni, sausage, salami, bologna;

- canned or aged meats;

- cured meats (ham, bacon);

- marinated meats;

- cocoa, buttermilk, chocolate milk, acidophilus milk;

- hot homemade yeast breads (once cooled, they are not triggers), yeast extracts;

- sour cream, yogurt; and

- caffeine (usually caffeine, a vasoconstrictor, helps headaches, but too much caffeine can cause rebound headaches, and its sudden cessation can cause withdrawal headaches).

Food-provoked headaches are not a result of food allergy but rather of sensitivity to chemicals in the foods, such as tyramine, nitrates and nitrites (in hot dogs and similar foods), monosodium glutamate and phenylethylamine (in chocolate) (Robbins, 1994). How these foods actually trigger headache on a biochemical level is not known, though nitrates are believed to be converted in the body into nitric oxide, a potent migraine inducer.

Excessive fatigue, lack of sleep and irregular sleeping patterns (commonly seen in people who change work shifts) can affect all migraine patients, but it appears to be especially important that children with migraines keep to a regular sleep schedule. Oversleeping can trigger a migraine in an adult (even sleeping for an extra hour on a weekend is enough to produce a headache in some people) but does not appear to affect children.

Most migraine patients are sensitive to bright light, both artificial and sunlight. Waking up with strong sunlight in the eyes can trigger a migraine. Camera flashes can trigger an aura and/or a headache, and some migraine sufferers have trouble with bright fluorescent lights like those in grocery stores. Bright flashing lights, like those seen in night clubs, on some amusement park rides and even in some aerobic dance classes can also trigger migraines (Robbins, 1994).

[2] Odors

Strong odors, especially those from gasoline, perfume, smoke and organic solvents, can trigger both tension and migraine headaches in susceptible people. Magazines and department store bills that include perfume samples can be hazardous to susceptible individuals, and sensitivity to cigarette smoke can develop at any time in life, even in ex-smokers (Robbins, 1994).

[3] Sexual Activity and Exercise

Sex can trigger a headache in some migraineurs. However, sex has been shown to stop or improve migraine in some people. This effect is thought to be due to the release into the nervous system of narcoticlike endorphins during sex.

In certain people, some kinds of exertion are predictable headache triggers. The headache usually starts within minutes of stopping the exercise. Taking a nonsteroidal anti-inflammatory (NSAID) drug like ibuprofen before sex or exercise is often helpful in preventing these migraines (Robbins, 1994).

[4] Weather

Weather changes (due to changes in barometric pressure) and strong winds can also precipitate migraines. Spring tends to be the worst season for migraine, followed by fall. However, this is not true of everyone who gets migraines; many find the hot and humid days of summer to be the worst time for headaches (Robbins, 1994). For many southern Californians, the strong, dry winds called Santa Anas that blow out of the California desert and are accelerated as they move through the canyons are a major headache trigger. In southern France, the strong winds known as the Mistral have a similar effect.

10.37 Post-traumatic Headaches

Estimates of the incidence of headache after head trauma vary widely—from 12 to 70 percent, depending upon the study. It is possible to develop post-traumatic headache after a relatively minor head injury, and loss of consciousness or amnesia is not a prerequisite. Studies on the heads and necks of trauma victims who had new-onset headaches and then subsequently died (i.e., were not killed immediately in the accident) found subtle disc and facet joint injuries at autopsy that were not detectable before death. Researchers stressed that these results support the view that post-traumatic headache, although it is often without a detectable cause, should not be automatically assumed to be psychogenic (Lance, 1993b).

Post-traumatic headache can be divided into two groups: acute and chronic. Head pain after trauma is also caused by scalp contusions, hematomas and lacerations; this is not strictly considered headache and therefore will not be covered here.[14]

[1] Acute Post-traumatic Headaches

A headache shortly after a bump on the head is a common occurrence. Most of these headaches occur in incidents that do not cause intracranial, scalp or skull injuries, although headache occurs after more serious injuries as well. Therefore, the International Headache Society (IHS) divides acute post-traumatic headache into two subgroups: acute post-traumatic headache with significant head trauma, and acute post-traumatic headache without significant head trauma (by far the more common of the two).

Criteria for acute post-traumatic headache with significant head trauma and/or confirmatory signs are:

1. Significance of head trauma documented by at least one of the following:

   - loss of consciousness;

   - post-traumatic amnesia lasting more than 10 minutes; and

   - at least two of the following showing relevant abnormality: clinical neurologic examination, skull x-ray, neuroimaging, evoked potentials (stimulation of particular nerves to record the electric response in the brain), cerebrospinal fluid examination ("spinal tap"), vestibular function testing (sense of balance), neuropsychological testing.

2. Headache occurs fewer than 14 days after regaining consciousness (or after trauma if there has been no loss of consciousness).

---

[14] *See also* ch. 3 for a discussion of contusions and lacerations of the brain, and ch. 4 for a discussion of intracranial hemorrhage and hematoma.

3. Headache disappears within eight weeks after regaining consciousness or after trauma if consciousness was never lost.

IHS criteria for acute post-traumatic headache without significant head trauma are the same as those for those headaches associated with significant head trauma except that they do not meet any of the requirements for criterion 1.

A review of studies that tracked patients who suffered headaches soon after head trauma found that about half of these patients had headaches one week later or on discharge from the hospital, and about a third of the total group still complained of headache two months after injury (Haas, 1993).

Migraine can be triggered by a mild head injury. This is usually seen in children and adolescents prone to migraine who are stunned or knocked unconscious briefly. The headache usually begins within 1 to 10 minutes of the trauma, but a delay of up to four hours is not rare. The migraine usually presents as headache and vomiting, but visual, hemiparetic (paralysis on one side of the body), stuporous, convulsive and amnestic symptoms are also possible (Haas, 1993).

[2] Chronic Headaches

Chronic post-traumatic headaches can either be acute post-traumatic headaches that just don't go away, therefore extending past the characteristic eight-week period, or they can appear *de novo* weeks or even months after the injury. Chronic post-traumatic headaches can be caused by whiplash-type injuries to the head and neck, as well as by the more typical cranial impact. These headaches can be migraine-like in their pattern of pain and symptoms.

Chronic post-traumatic headaches can be associated with other symptoms (dizziness, irritability and impaired concentration) that, together, are called the postconcussional or post-traumatic syndrome (Haas, 1993).[15]

Like acute post-traumatic headache, the incidence and severity of chronic post-traumatic headache does not correlate with the severity of the head injury or with the degree of brain damage. Chronic headache can be caused by relatively minor trauma. The exact incidence of this kind of headache and how long they last are not known, partly because studies of headaches in head-injured patients

---

[15] *See also* ch. 2 for a discussion of concussion.

are relatively short term (two years is considered a long study). As a result, long-term data just does not exist (Haas, 1993).

The question of whether a relationship exists between the development of chronic post-traumatic headache and the desire for financial compensation is still a matter of dispute. Some studies have shown a strong correlation between chronic post-traumatic headaches and seeking compensation, while others are less conclusive. A major headache text states that these headaches are probably "independent of any effect the trauma had on the brain or other intracranial structures. Instead they seem to arise from psychological disturbances generated by the physical and emotional stresses of the accident and perpetuated by persistent individual concerns regarding the injury suffered, the ability to work, and many other matters" (Haas, 1993).

Chronic post-traumatic headaches are difficult to treat. Most individuals who have headaches that last longer than eight weeks after the trauma continue to suffer with their headaches for another one to two years. The prognosis of some patients can be improved with the use of one of the prophylactic medications that are helpful in treating migraine (beta-blockers and antidepressants), coupled with psychotherapy (Haas, 1993).

10.38　Secondary Headaches

It is hard to find any illness that cannot cause a headache. Headache is a common symptom of the flu, mononucleosis and other viral syndromes. Other illnesses that characteristically cause headache include systemic lupus erythematosus (an inflammatory disease of connective tissue), chronic pulmonary failure (which presents as early morning headache), Hashimoto's thyroiditis, withdrawal from glucocorticoids (steroids such as cortisone and prednisone), inflammatory bowel disease, acute hypertension (high blood pressure) and many illnesses associated with infection with human immunodeficiency virus (HIV) (Raskin, 1994).

It is beyond the scope of this chapter to discuss in depth all the medical conditions that can cause headaches, but brief examination follows of some and the mechanisms by which they are believed to cause head pain.

[1]   Lumbar Puncture Headaches

This type of headache has traditionally been known as spinal tap headache, which many women were affected by in the 1960s, when spinal anesthesia was widely used during childbirth (as opposed to the currently popular epidural anesthesia, which does not puncture the outer membranes of the spinal cord and therefore should not cause headache). Lumbar puncture involves inserting a needle through the dura, the protective membrane that covers the spinal cord. This procedure is done in the lumbar region of the lower back because it is below the level where the spinal cord terminates, where the dura forms essentially a membranous tube filled with cerebrospinal fluid (CSF). The entering needle can do no harm to the spinal cord at this level but still has access to the CSF, and an anesthesiologist can inject anesthetics that will then rise in the column up to the level of the cord itself.

Lumbar puncture headaches have traditionally been thought to be caused by loss of CSF, either during spinal anesthesia or spinal puncture done to remove CSF for examination. This loss of CSF has been thought to decrease the brain's fluid cushion, so that when the patient sits or stands, there is tension on the pain-sensitive supporting structures of the brain (the dural sinuses). The syndrome is not entirely understood, however, because it can occur in the presence of normal CSF levels. Also, the injection of a small amount of the patient's own blood (a homologous blood patch) over the puncture site brings immediate relief, which would be unlikely if the blood were acting merely as a plug to stop CSF leakage (Raskin, 1994).

About 30 percent of lumbar puncture patients experience associated headache. The onset of the headache is usually within 48 hours, but it can be delayed up to 12 days. The head pain is usually dull but can be throbbing and severe. It starts with sitting or standing, and is relieved by reclining or with abdominal compression. The longer the patient is upright, the longer it takes for the headache to resolve when he or she lies down again. Head shaking and pressure on the jugular vein make the pain worse.

The headache is often accompanied by a stiff neck and nausea. Vertigo (sensation of whirling in space), ringing in the ears, blurred vision and photophobia are also possible (Raskin, 1994). After lumbar puncture, the patient is kept flat, with his or her head even with or below the level of the hips, for from 4 to 24 hours in the hope of preventing headache. The patient is also encouraged to drink fluids to help replenish CSF levels (Cahill, 1991).

Without treatment, the symptoms usually resolve in a few days, but they can persist for weeks or months. Treatment is simple and effective. Intravenous caffeine sodium benzoate, 500 mg, given over a few minutes will abort a headache in 75 percent of patients. A second dose given in one hour will relieve another 10 percent of patients. Homologous blood patch brings relief to the final 15 percent of patients with lumbar puncture headache (Raskin, 1994).

[2]   Giant Cell Arteritis

Giant cell arteritis, also known as temporal arteritis, is a chronic inflammation of the large arteries in the brain, accompanied by giant cells (large cells containing one or more nuclei) that are not normally present in the nerves. This condition usually affects the temporal, occipital or ophthalmic arteries and produces thickening of the intima (the smooth interior lining of the arteries), which narrows and eventually entirely occludes the arterial lumen (hollow interior space). (*See Figure 10-4.*)

Giant cell arteritis is a relatively common disorder of the elderly; the incidence is 77 per 100,000 population (much less than the incidence of migraine among the elderly, however). The average age of onset is 70 years, and 65 percent of those affected are women. If the condition is left untreated, roughly 50 percent of patients will become blind. The most common initial symptoms are headache, polymyalgia rheumatica (systemic flulike muscle aches), jaw claudication (pain in the jaw with movement due to impaired blood supply), fever and weight loss (Raskin, 1994).

The headache can be unilateral or bilateral, and in 50 percent of patients, it is located over the temporal regions at the sides of the head. The pain is usually described as dull and drilling, with superimposed periodic "ice-pick-like" shooting pains. The headache is often worse at night, and it is aggravated by cold. Most patients feel that the pain is superficial, beneath the skin, rather than deep within the brain, as in migraine. The scalp is often tender, to the point that laying the head down on a pillow is impossible, and there can be raised, reddened nodules or streaking over the temporal arteries (Raskin, 1994).

Temporal artery biopsy can confirm the inflammatory changes within the arterial wall. Giant cell arteritis is treated with 80 mg of

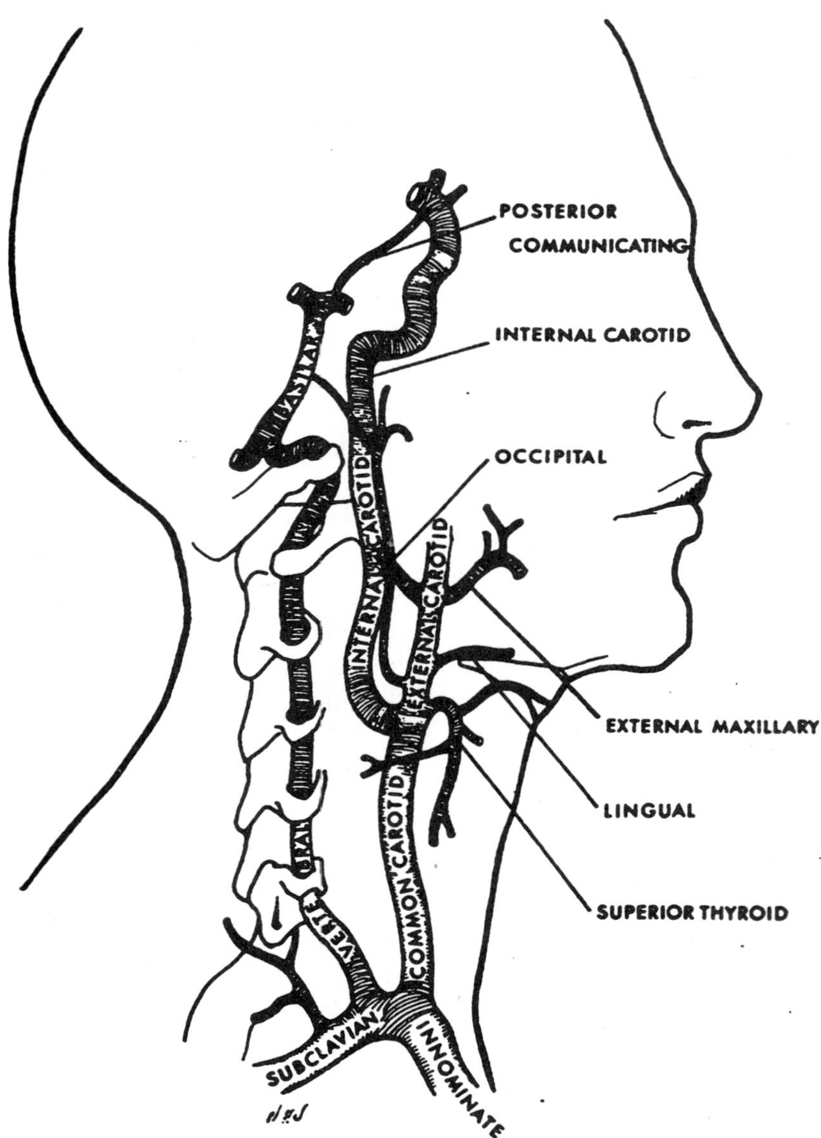

Fig. 10–4. The arteries of the neck passing into the brain. Giant cell arteritis, an inflammatory condition that causes thickening of the intima (internal layer) of the cerebral arteries, including the temporal artery, is a potential cause of secondary headache.

the steroid prednisone by mouth daily for four to six weeks. Because of the potential for serious side effects (diabetes, thinned skin, immune system suppression, high blood pressure and others) as well as interactions with many drugs (especially in the elderly population affected by this disease), it is important to evaluate the patient's response to the prednisone and carefully weigh the risks and benefits of the therapy during and after an initial course.

[3]   Space Occupying Lesions

A space occupying lesion is anything that takes up room in the skull that shouldn't be there; tumors, abscesses and various kinds of hematomas (collections of blood, usually clotted) are most common. Because the skull is a sealed space that is incapable of expanding, it has very little excess space, and therefore a growing tumor, an abscess or especially a rapidly expanding hematoma will make itself known relatively quickly, by headache and other symptoms.

[a]   Brain Tumors

About 30 percent of patients with brain tumors consider headache to be their chief complaint. Ten percent wake up at night with a headache. The headache is usually intermittent, of moderate intensity, dull and deeply aching in character, worsened by exertion or change in position, and associated with nausea and vomiting. Many individuals with bothersome headaches worry that they may actually have a brain tumor. However, headache and nausea and vomiting, as well as neurologic symptoms such as numbness in an arm and blurred vision, are much more likely to be caused by migraine than by brain tumor (Raskin, 1994).

[b]   Brain Abscesses

A brain abscess is a collection of pus (a liquid product of inflammation/infection composed of albumin, a thin fluid, bacteria and white blood cells) within the brain. Brain abscesses have a number of possible etiologies: an infection that spreads from the ear, jaw or sinuses; a blood-borne infection from a distant site, especially chronic pyogenic (pus-producing) lung disease; or as a complication following head trauma or surgery. Headache is present in 70 percent of cases of brain abscess because, like abscesses elsewhere in the body, they tend to expand until they are opened and removed. A bacterial brain abscess is treated with antibiotics, but because an abscess is a closed pocket with little blood circulation (by which the antibiotics are delivered), surgery to drain the site is also required (Scheld, 1994).

[c]   Cerebral Hematomas

Cerebral hematomas are caused by bleeding within the skull and are described by the position they occupy: subdural, epidural, subarachnoid and intracerebral. Cerebral hematomas are dangerous and can quickly cause coma and death; therefore, headache is merely part of the totality and is usually a minor symptom when compared to the dramatic neurologic symptoms an expanding hematoma can produce.[16] (*See Figure 10-5.*)

Subdural hematomas are caused by head trauma and form between the brain and its protective outer meningeal membrane, the dura mater. In acute subdural hematoma, the patient becomes symptomatic within minutes to hours of injury, and if he or she remains conscious (two thirds of patients are drowsy to comatose immediately after injury), he or she will complain of a unilateral headache. A small subdural hematoma caused by a vein that clots off soon after the trauma may not initially cause any problem. However, in a week or two, as the hematoma is breaking up, the small bits of clotted blood increase the osmotic pressure under the dura, pulling water into the space and increasing intracranial pressure, causing headache and potentially coma.

Chronic subdural hematoma often is associated with only a minor injury or no injury at all. A period of weeks or months goes by during which neurologic symptoms emerge as the hematoma slowly expands. Headache is common (but not universal), and it is associated with slowed thinking, confusion, seizures, changes in personality and hemiparesis (paralysis on one side). These hematomas are difficult to diagnose, especially in the elderly (Ropper, 1994).

Epidural (between the dura and the skull) hematomas expand more rapidly than do subdural hematomas and therefore are much more dangerous. Epidural hematomas are usually caused by tearing of the middle meningeal artery, and headache is not a predominant issue because the patient quickly becomes unconscious (Ropper, 1994). (*See Figure 10-6.*)

Subarachnoid (in the space below the arachnoid, or second meningeal membrane, and the pia mater, the innermost membrane covering

---

[16] *See also* ch. 4 for further discussion of cerebral hematoma.

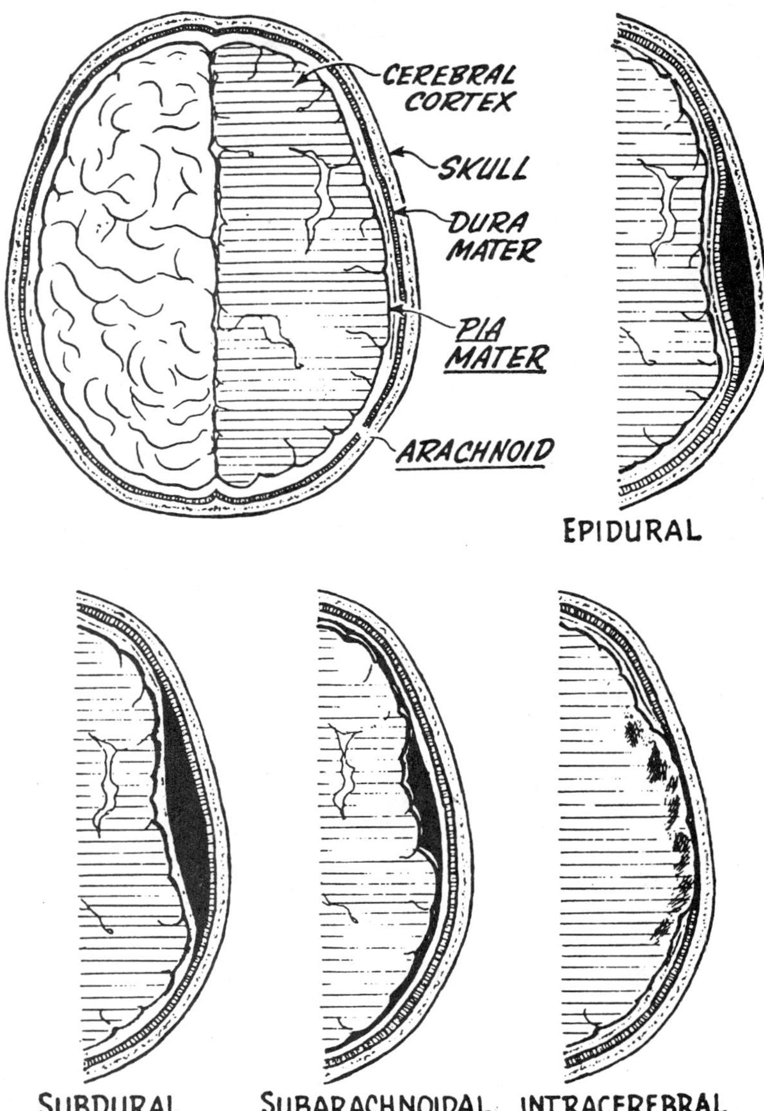

Fig. 10–5. The different types of cerebral hematoma and their relationship to the brain and meningeal tissues.

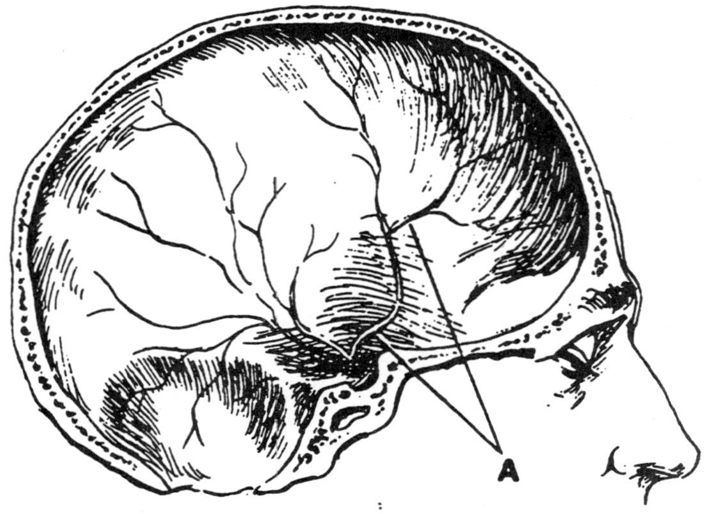

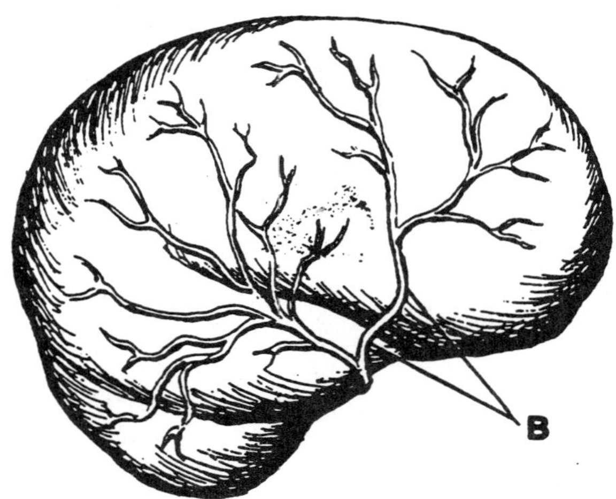

Fig. 10–6. The course of the middle meningeal artery. Tearing of this artery can result in the formation of a space-occupying lesion known as an epidural hematoma.

the brain) hemorrhage is usually caused by rupture of an aneurysm (an abnormal ballooning of the wall of an artery). Sudden, transient loss of consciousness occurs in up to 45 percent of patients, and it may be preceded by excruciating headache. However, these patients usually complain of headache after regaining consciousness. In another 45 percent of patients, the presenting complaint is severe headache associated with exertion, usually not associated with any focal neurologic symptoms. If the hematoma continues to grow, stupor and coma can result. If the patient continues to deteriorate, surgery is required to remove the clot and fix the aneurysm (Kistler, et al., 1994).

Intracranial hematomas occur within the brain and are usually a result of aneurysm rupture or arteriovenous malformation (AVM; a congenital malformation in which a vein and an artery are joined and blood shunts from the artery into the vein) or trauma. Headache resembling migraine can be associated with AVM. When a small AVM ruptures, there may be little or no damage. However, rupture of a large AVM can cause death (Kistler, 1994).

[4]　Temporomandibular Joint Disorder (TMJ)

The temporomandibular joint is formed where the mandible (lower jaw bone) joins the temporal bone of the skull, allowing the jaw to move up and down. The ligaments that hold the bones together can loosen, causing a slipping in the joint, which in turn can cause pain that may extend to the face and head. The joint also is subject to both osteoarthritis and rheumatoid arthritis.

Osteoarthritis (caused by joint wear and tear) generally causes little pain, but rheumatoid arthritis causes pain, swelling and limitation of movement. Heat, rest and anti-inflammatory drugs usually provide good pain relief (Greenspan, 1994).

[5]　Hypertension

Many types of acute and chronic pain can raise blood pressure to a mild degree. Headache is usually not associated with hypertension (high blood pressure), but when it is, it constitutes a medical emergency. Hypertension (often called essential, idiopathic or primary) is defined as sustained diastolic blood pressure (the lower blood pressure number) at or above 95 millimeters of mercury (mm Hg) and/or a systolic (the upper blood pressure number) at or above 160 mm Hg.

When the blood pressure is stable, even if it is high enough to be unhealthy, the affected person does not experience headache

(Strandgaard and Henry, 1993). It is only when there is an acute rise of the diastolic blood pressure of greater than 25 percent that headache becomes a factor in hypertension. Four conditions can cause this sort of rapid and severe rise in blood pressure, and in all of them, the headache is secondary to the dangerous rise in blood pressure. The high blood pressure must be quickly treated to avoid disastrous results, and once the blood pressure is brought down, the attendant headache will resolve.

The first of these conditions in which blood pressure can rise dangerously high in a short time is an acute response of the blood-pressure-regulating system to a toxin or medication (cocaine, for one). The second is pheochromocytoma, a tumor (usually benign) of the sympatho-adrenal system that produces the sympathetic hormones norepinephrine and epinephrine (also called adrenaline). These hormones are part of the fight-or-flight mechanism of the sympathetic nervous system, which causes an increase in blood pressure and heart rate to help the individual cope with a perceived danger. Under normal circumstances, these hormones are secreted for a short period during stress. However, a pheochromocytoma pumps out epinephrine and does not respond to the feedback mechanisms that would normally stop the hormone release. This continuous release of sympathetic hormones can cause an enormous rise in blood pressure, which produces a pounding headache.

The third kind of headache-causing high blood pressure is malignant hypertension, which develops in about 1 percent of hypertensive patients. Its pathogenesis is unknown. In malignant hypertension, the diastolic blood pressure is consistently above 120 mm Hg, and small hemorrhages are visible at the back of the eye (these "cotton wool hemorrhages" look like small puffs of cotton through an ophthalmoscope).

Malignant hypertension is a medical emergency, and along with severe headache, it will often present with nausea, vomiting, visual disturbances, transient paralyses, stupor and even coma. The two body systems most likely to be seriously affected by malignant hypertension are the cardiovascular and the renal (Williams, 1994).

The fourth cause of hypertension-associated headache is pre-eclampsia and eclampsia. These conditions of pregnancy are really the same disorder, along a continuum. If the high blood pressure and increased neurologic irritability of pre-eclampsia are not treated, the pregnant woman will become "eclamptic" and develop seizures, and perhaps a cerebrovascular accident (stroke) and kidney failure, and lose the fetus. The cause of pre-eclampsia/eclampsia is not known, but it is associated with extremes of reproductive age, a first-degree relative who had pre-eclampsia, nulliparity (never having been pregnant before), black race, essential (primary) hypertension, diabetes and multiparity (having had many children) (Day, 1991).

[6]   Headaches As Adverse Effects of Medication

Many medications cause headaches as a side effect. It is beyond the scope of this chapter to examine every drug that could possibly cause headaches, because the list is in the hundreds. Instead, we will touch on several medications that often cause headache. The common-sense course of action if a patient has new-onset headaches coinciding with the initiation of a drug therapy or with a change in dosage of an ongoing medication is to contact the prescribing physician.

Nitroglycerine (and related nitrates such as isosorbide dinitrate) has a long medical history in the treatment of angina pectoris (chest pain caused by insufficient blood supply through fat-clogged coronary arteries to the heart muscle). Nitroglycerine works by relaxing the smooth muscle layer in the wall of the coronary arteries, thus dilating the vessels and allowing more blood to get to the oxygen-starved heart muscle. Unfortunately, nitroglycerine also dilates arteries in the brain (and elsewhere in the body), thereby perhaps producing tension on pain-sensing structures and causing headache. Even nurses administering nitroglycerine in a paste form spread on the patient's skin have been known to develop headaches if they get the paste on their own skin. Fortunately, both patient and nurse usually develop resistance to the headache-producing effects of nitrate-based medications.

Zidovudine, better known as AZT (from azidothymidine), is the first-line antiretroviral agent used in treating acquired immunodeficiency syndrome (AIDS). At the start of AZT therapy, many patients experience headaches. However, headaches lessen in most people and stop altogether in some. Rarely, however, AZT will cause such crashing, unremitting headaches that the drug must be discontinued, and one or both of the antiretrovirals ddI (didanosine) or ddC (zalcitabine) is substituted.

Of special interest to patients with recurring headaches is the fact that the ergot derivatives, simple analgesics such as aspirin and nonsteroidal anti-inflammatories, and the mild stimulant caffeine, used alone and in combination with other medications, can, if overused, cause what is called rebound headache. The mechanism of rebound headache is poorly understood, but for some patients who find themselves caught in the cycle of headache–medication–rebound headache, the number of headaches can be drastically reduced by keeping the use of pain medications to an absolute minimum and substituting a prophylactic medication such as the beta-blocker propranolol or the antidepressant amitryptilene (Solomon and Rose, 1993). Naproxen, now available over the counter in the United States, is the simple analgesic least likely to cause rebound headache (Lance, 1993b).

[7]   Sinus Headaches

Contrary to popular belief, a headache that centers around the nose and face is probably not a sinus headache but most often is a migraine without aura. True sinus headaches are caused by inflamed or blocked sinuses and are relatively rare. The acute phase of many types of headaches, especially cluster headaches, has often been misinterpreted as sinusitis. This misinterpretation is reinforced by the fact that often, tension-type headaches are helped by decongestant medications, which are combined with a mild analgesic (usually aspirin or acetaminophen) in many over-the-counter "sinus headache" preparations (Saunte and Soyka, 1993).

International Headache Society diagnostic criteria for acute sinus headache include (Saunte and Soyka, 1993):

1. Purulent discharge in the nasal passage, apparent either spontaneously or with suction.

2. Pathologic findings in one or more of the following tests: x-ray examination, CT or MRI scan, transillumination (viewing the sinuses from the side opposite a direct light source shone through them).

3. Simultaneous onset of headache and sinusitis.

4. Headache location:

   - In acute frontal sinusitis, headache is located directly over the sinus and may radiate to the top of the head or behind the eyes.

- In acute maxillary sinusitis, headache is located over the antrum (a cavity in the maxillary bone that communicates with the middle meatus of the nasal cavity).

- In acute ethmoiditis (the ethmoid is the bone of the skull that surrounds the eye and nose cavities), headache is located between and behind the eyes, and may radiate to the temporal area on the side of the head.

- In acute sphenoiditis (the sphenoid is the bone at the front of the skull base that articulates with every other cranial bone), headache is located in the occipital area at the back of the head, the vertex (top of the head), the frontal region or behind the eyes.

5. Headache disappears after treatment of sinusitis.

Patients with genuine acute or chronic sinusitis or obstruction of the paranasal sinuses do complain of head and facial pain, usually during the acute phase. Inflammation of the ethmoid and maxillary sinuses usually presents with rhinitis (an inflamed, runny nose). Many people who get sinus inflammation/headache have an inherited allergic condition that makes them prone to sinus problems, or they inherit a tendency to develop nasal and sinus polyps (benign growths) that interfere with air flow and can lead to sinus inflammation (Saunte and Soyka, 1993).

10.40 TREATMENT

Abortive drug therapy is the mainstay of migraine, cluster and tension-type headache treatment. Prophylactic medications are reserved for those patients with frequent or severe attacks (Diener, 1994). Currently there is no complete "cure" for migraine or cluster headache. There are treatments that work to some degree for many headache sufferers, but no drug or therapy can ensure that an individual will never get another headache. The patients for whom nothing works to either adequately prevent or abort headache often get caught in a depressing cycle of headache and analgesic/ergot/caffeine overuse (known as analgesic-rebound headache), requiring specialized treatment.[17]

---

[17] *See* 10.38[6] *supra.*

10.41 Abortive Therapy

The majority of acute headache therapies have been in use for many years. Most headaches respond to treatment with mild over-the-counter analgesics, such as aspirin, acetaminophen and the nonsteroidal anti-inflammatories (NSAIDs) ibuprofen (Motrin® and others) and naproxen. Some products combine aspirin in a mixture with caffeine (a mild stimulant and cerebral vasoconstrictor) to boost the painkilling properties of the aspirin (Anacin®), or with an antacid (Ascriptin®) or a buffer (Bufferin®) to overcome the gastric irritation that is common with aspirin.

More severe headaches (migraines and cluster) usually require intervention with medications stronger than simple analgesics. If aspirin is used, the dosage is generally 1 gm, and it is often paired with metoclopramide. Stronger drugs used to treat migraine include the well-known narcotics (usually codeine in a mixture with acetaminophen or other drugs, or intramuscular meperidine in an emergency department setting), the vasoconstrictor (and serotonin agonist) ergotamine or the newer serotonin agonist sumatriptan (Imitrex®). (In medicine, the word *agonist* stimulates receptors, while an *antagonist* would block receptor stimulation.)

[1] Analgesics

Analgesics are pain medications. Extracts of the oriental poppy (the source of natural opiates) and the willow tree (the source of aspirin) have been used to relieve pain for centuries without a clear understanding of how they work. However, recent research into the neurophysiology of pain has not only led to a better understanding of the actions of existing analgesics but pointed the way to possible new analgesics that may relieve severe pain without many of the side effects of current medications.

[a] Aspirin and NSAIDs

Aspirin and the newer nonsteroidal anti-inflammatory drugs (NSAIDs) interfere with the production of prostaglandins and other substances that sensitize peripheral pain receptors (nociceptors), so that they respond to stimuli that previously would not have been sensed as painful.[18] Aspirin and the related NSAIDs block the aggregation

---

[18] *See* 10.32 *supra* for further discussion of prostaglandins and their method of action.

of platelets, causing an antithrombotic (anti-blood-clotting) effect. Platelets are now thought to play an important role in headache, because several disturbances in platelet function have been reported in both migraine and tension-type headache patients that do not exist in normal controls, and platelets release neurotransmitters believed to be involved in the initiation of migraine (Kitano, et al., 1994).

Aspirin and NSAIDs may also decrease the production of free radicals (highly reactive molecules that damage tissues) and may interact with the enzyme adenylate cyclase to alter cellular concentrations of cyclic adenosine monophosphate (cAMP), a molecule that is involved in a second system of producing pain and inflammation. These drugs also reduce inflammation by decreasing the release of inflammatory mediators from three kinds of white blood cells: granulocytes, basophils and mast cells. The NSAIDs decrease the sensitivity of blood vessels to the dilating effects of histamine and bradykinin (two mediators of inflammation), reversing vasodilatation.

At usual doses, the main adverse effect of aspirin and other NSAIDs is gastric irritation, which can be minimized by taking the drug with food or following it with an antacid. Serious adverse reactions to aspirin include prolonged bleeding time, tinnitus (ringing in the ears) and hearing loss, nausea, vomiting, occult bleeding, abnormal liver function, rash and allergic sensitivity manifested by anaphylaxis and/or asthma. Its use is contraindicated in patients with gastrointestinal ulcer or bleeding, and in those who are allergic to the drug (Loeb, 1991).

Acetaminophen (Tylenol® and many others) is used as an aspirin substitute to relieve mild headaches. It does not cause aspirin's gastric upset and potential bleeding, and it has no effect on platelet aggregation. Acetaminophen is safe to use in children. However, acet—aminophen has no anti-inflammatory action. Acetaminophen produces pain relief probably by inhibiting the synthesis of prostaglandins; however, many substances sensitize pain receptors, and acetaminophen may block production of other pain mediators.

[b] Narcotics

Narcotics, also called opioids, are a group of natural, semisynthetic and synthetic drugs that form a family of pain medications ranging from codeine (moderately weak) to morphine (very strong). Narcotics produce analgesia by fitting (like keys) into the opioid receptors (which act like locks) in the central nervous system. Opioid receptors in the brain are thought to bond normally with the body's own painkillers: the endorphins, enkephalins and dynorphins.

Three types of opioid receptors have been discovered: the mu, kappa and delta receptors. Most narcotics are mu receptor agonists; they bond with and thus stimulate the mu receptors. Some newer synthetic narcotics are active at the kappa receptors. No delta receptor agonists have yet been developed for use in humans.

In headache, a narcotic does not actually relieve the pain but produces a mental or emotional state in which the patient knows the pain is there but is less aware of it and less concerned about it. It is possible to give enough narcotics to cause a migraine or cluster headache sufferer to lose consciousness without truly eliminating the pain. Narcotics have a role in the acute treatment of severe headache, but because of the problems of both rebound headache and potential addiction, patients receiving narcotics require good physician follow-up.

Codeine (methylmorphine) is a component of opium and is closely related to morphine. It is the standard weak narcotic analgesic to which all others are compared. It is used to treat headaches, primarily when mixed with other drugs—either acetaminophen or the combination drug Fiorinal® (aspirin, butalbital and caffeine) in oral form. It is thought possible that the analgesic effect is caused by a partial transformation of codeine to morphine within the body. Codeine can cause all the usual narcotic side effects, although its abuse potential is much lower than that for stronger narcotics (Loeb, 1991).

Meperidine (Demerol®) is a strong analgesic and is the most familiar of its class of semisynthetic narcotics, the phenylpiperidines. Until the release of subcutaneous sumatriptan, intramuscular meperidine (usually paired with the antihistamine hydroxyzine to potentiate the painkilling effect and decrease the risk of nausea and vomiting) was often used in emergency rooms to treat patients with extreme migraine or cluster headaches.

Meperidine is still used in this setting to treat headaches in those for whom sumatriptan does not work. It has all the usual narcotic side effects: somnolence (sleepiness), euphoria, nausea and vomiting, constipation, urinary retention and respiratory depression. It must not be given with the monoamine oxidase (MAO) inhibitor antidepressants, barbiturates or the antitubercular drug isoniazid. The anticonvulsant medication phenytoin (Dilantin®) can decrease blood levels of meperidine and thus reduce its analgesic power (Loeb, 1991).

Butorphanol (Stadol®) is a strong analgesic with mixed kappa agonist/mu antagonist activities at opioid receptors in the central nervous system. Butorphanol has been used for years intramuscularly in the hospital setting as a preoperative sedative or postoperative pain medication; however, it was approved in 1992 for intranasal administration to relieve migraine headaches. This mu antagonism contraindicates butorphanol's use in mu-narcotic-dependent patients, as it can precipitate withdrawal symptoms. The most frequent adverse reactions include sedation, headache, vertigo, nausea, excessive sweating and respiratory depression. Respiratory depression does not seem to increase as the dose increases (Loeb, 1991).

[c] Combination Drugs

In treating headache, combination drugs often work better than single medications on their own.

Midrin® is a combination drug often used to treat migraine in children and adolescents. It includes isometheptene (a milder vasoconstrictor than ergotamine), chloralphenazone (a mild sedative) and acetaminophen (a mild analgesic). Many physicians prefer Midrin® because it has fewer side effects than ergotamines,[19] and especially if it is taken early in the course of a migraine, when the pain is dull and there is reactive muscle contraction, it can be as effective as stronger medications (Gallagher, 1990). The dosage should not exceed five capsules in a 12-hour period. Side effects include fatigue and gastrointestinal upset. Contraindications for treatment with Midrin® are the same as those for other vasoconstrictors such as ergotamine.

Fiorinal® combines aspirin, butalbital and caffeine, which is often used alone or in combination with codeine to provide acute relief in migraine. Butalbital is a short-acting, mild but highly addictive barbiturate that in the above combination can be highly effective in aborting migraine in some people. However, problems of habituation (the need for ever-increasing doses to achieve the same effect) can develop, and rebound headache is also a threat with Fiorinal®.

---

[19] *See* 10.42[2][f] *infra.*

[2] Sumatriptan and Other Serotonin Agonists

Sumatriptan (Imitrex®) is a serotonin (chemically known as 5-hydroxytryptamine or 5-HT) agonist. Therefore, sumatriptan stimulates 5-HT receptors (an antagonist would block receptor stimulation).

Sumatriptan was developed under the hypothesis (not yet confirmed by research) that stimulation of 5-HT receptors in the central nervous system would interrupt a migraine headache.[20] Sumatriptan stimulates serotonin subreceptors designated 5-HT1B and 5-HT1D.

Newer serotonin agonists that stimulate other serotonin subreceptor types (a 5-HTD1 agonist is showing promise) are in clinical trials, because sumatriptan does not work for every migraineur. Sumatriptan can cause chest pain in patients with cardiovascular disease by initiating vasospasm of the coronary arteries, and most people who take the drug experience a sense of heaviness or other symptoms like tingling, a worse headache, numbness, "feeling strange" and others. Beyond the unpleasant side effects, sumatriptan's two major drawbacks, up until very recently, have been cost ($30 to $40 per injection dose, often not covered by insurance) and route of administration (many people find giving themselves a subcutaneous injection, even with an autoinjector, worse than the headache).

Oral sumatriptan, which was recently released in the United States, is available in 25 mg and 50 mg pills. The oral form of sumatriptan is not as effective as the injectable (even though the injectable dose is only 6 mg), because it is not well absorbed from the gastrointestinal tract and degrades in the stomach. However, a study comparing oral sumatriptan with oral aspirin plus oral metoclopramide (Reglan®) found that oral sumatriptan produced a faster improvement and resolution of migraine attacks than did aspirin plus metoclopramide (The Oral Sumatriptan and Aspirin Plus Metoclopramide Comparative Study Group, 1992). The difficulties encountered with oral sumatriptan may soon be moot, as an intranasal form of the drug is in clinical trials. This route would bypass both the unpleasantness of self-injection as well as the decreased efficacy found in the oral preparation.

[3] Ergot Derivatives

Ergot has been known for centuries as a vasoconstrictor. The product of a mold that infects rye as it grows in the field, it historically

---

[20] *See* 10.33 *supra.*

caused epidemics of miscarriages if the rye on which it grew was harvested and then baked into bread.

Until the release of sumatriptan, ergotamine was one of the primary drugs used to abort migraine and cluster headaches, and it is still much in use. Ergotamine has traditionally been assumed to relieve migraines by constricting the blood vessels in the head, though new biochemical evidence suggests that ergot alkaloids stop headaches in a manner similar to that of sumatriptan: by activation of 5-HT1 sub-receptors on the primary afferent (going toward the brain from the periphery) trigeminovascular fibers (fibers of the trigeminal, or fifth, cranial nerve, which affects blood vessels) (Moskowitz and Macfarlane, 1993).

Ergot derivatives are contraindicated in pregnancy and in the presence of any vascular disease in which the vasoconstricting effect could worsen the condition, such as peripheral vascular disease, coronary artery disease, hypertension (high blood pressure) and impaired kidney or liver function.

Frequent use of ergotamine can cause rebound headaches, trapping the patient in a downward spiral of pain and ineffective medication use, so it should not be taken more frequently than every four to five days (Gallagher, 1990). Overuse of ergot derivatives can also affect the circulation in the fingers and toes by overconstricting the arteries in the extremities. Therefore, tingling in fingers or toes is a significant symptom that should be reported to the physician.

Ergotamine (Ergomar®, Wigrettes®) directly stimulates the smooth muscle of blood vessels in the periphery and the brain to contract by blocking alpha-adrenergic binding sites. It also produces depression of central vasomotor centers and interferes with the action of the neurotransmitter (and nociceptor sensitizing agent) serotonin. Adverse reactions include numbness in fingers or toes, transient tachycardia (rapid heartbeat) or bradycardia (slow heartbeat), angina pectoris (heart pain due to decreased blood supply), nausea, vomiting, weakness in legs, muscle pains in extremities and localized swelling.

Dihydroergotamine (D.H.E. 45®) is an injectable form of ergotamine that has nearly identical chemical actions to the oral form. Dihydroergotamine is given intravenously or intramuscularly to abort or prevent vascular headaches when rapid control is needed or when other routes of administration are not feasible. The intranasal form of DHE should be available in the near future.

Dihydroergotamine is more pronounced an alpha-adrenergic blocker than is ergotamine, but its vasoconstricting properties are somewhat less strong. This injectable form of the drug is also less likely to cause nausea and vomiting than is oral or inhaled ergotamine. Dosages for vascular headache are 1 mg intramuscularly at the first warning sign of headache, repeated at one-hour intervals up to a total of 3 mg. The drug may also be given intravenously when an even more rapid onset of effect is desired, to a maximum of 2 mg. The total weekly dosage should not exceed 6 mg. Adverse reactions to dihydroergotamine are identical to those for ergotamine, except that there have been reports of pleural (the tissue that covers the lungs) and retroperitoneal (behind the peritoneum in the abdomen) fibrosis (abnormal growth of fibrous tissue) in patients who have taken dihydroergotamine for an extended period.

Cafergot® is a combination of ergotamine tartrate 1 mg and caffeine 100 mg in an oral form, and 2 mg ergotamine with 100 mg caffeine in suppositories. Cafergot® is frequently prescribed to abort or prevent migraine or cluster headaches. Caffeine is added to the vasoconstrictor ergotamine because caffeine is also a cranial vasoconstrictor. The addition of caffeine enhances the effect of ergotamine while keeping its dosage as low as possible.

Serious adverse reactions and contraindications to Cafergot® are related to the ergotamine in the preparation. However, the caffeine can cause transient tachycardia (high heart rate), nervousness, nausea and vomiting. Patients who overuse Cafergot® can experience rebound headaches, which lead to increased drug use and virtually continuous headaches (Gallagher, 1990).

Bellergal-S® is a combination drug containing phenobarbital (40 mg), ergotamine tartrate (0.6 mg) and alkaloids of belladonna (0.2 mg). It is used in the intermittent treatment of recurrent, throbbing headache. The ingredients in Bellergal-S® are meant, according to the manufacturer, to correct imbalance of the sympathetic (controls the "fight or flight" reaction) and parasympathetic (constricts pupils, slows heart rate and other effects) nervous systems, which together make up the autonomic nervous system. Ergotamine inhibits the sympathetic nervous system; belladonna inhibits the parasympathetic nervous system; and both work synergistically with phenobarbital to dampen cortical centers. The recommended dosage is one tablet, morning and evening, as a prophylactic treatment for vascular headaches.

Bellergal-S® has all the potential side effects, interactions and contraindications of its component parts. Therefore, it has an addiction potential due to the phenobarbital, which is a barbiturate. The belladonna component has anticholinergic effects; it can cause dry mouth and other symptoms, and can cause exacerbation in patients with asthma or obstructive uropathy.

Methylsergide (Sansert®) is a vasoconstrictor structurally related to methylergonovine, a drug used in obstetrics to stimulate uterine contractions. Methylsergide has been shown to inhibit or block the effects of serotonin, 5-HT. Methylsergide is considered by many the drug of choice for cluster headaches (Gallagher, 1990). It is used for the prevention or reduction of intensity and frequency of vascular headaches in patients suffering one or more severe headaches per week, and for patients suffering from vascular headaches that are uncontrollable or so severe that preventive therapy is indicated regardless of the frequency of the attack. However, retroperitoneal fibrosis (growth of fibrous tissue behind the peritoneum near the kidneys), pleuropulmonary fibrosis (growth of fibrous tissue in and around the lungs) and fibrotic thickening of the valves of the heart may occur in patients receiving long-term methylsergide therapy. Therefore, methylsergide should be used only in patients for whom nothing else has worked and whose headaches seriously interfere with their functioning. Patients taking this drug must be kept under close medical supervision, and there must be a medication-free interval of three to four weeks after every four-month interval of therapy. The usual adult dosage is 4 to 8 mg daily.

[4] Other Drugs

Metoclopramide (Reglan® and others), a derivative of para-aminobenzoic acid, has long been used to help promote gastric motility and relieve nausea. However, since the mid-1980s, metoclopramide has been used alone and in combination with other drugs to treat migraine. At first, it was thought a good idea to precede oral migraine abortive medications with metoclopramide, because during pain, the gastrointestinal tract often stops moving or even moves in the wrong direction, resulting in vomiting. Subsequently, however, metoclopramide has been found to have headache-relieving qualities of its own, separate and distinct from those of the ergotamine and aspirin with which it has been traditionally paired (Ellis, et al., 1993).

Metoclopramide (10 mg) is effective in intravenous form when it is paired with intravenous dihydroergotamine (1 mg) to treat severe migraine in the emergency setting, and some researchers believe it should replace the standard intramuscular (IM) narcotic and antiemetic as the parenteral (through a means other than the digestive tract) treatment of choice after sumatriptan for severe migraine headache (Klapper and Stanton, 1993).

It may seem odd to consider oxygen a drug, but it is one. Nine liters of oxygen per minute delivered to a tight face mask or 100 percent oxygen via face mask is considered an effective abortive treatment for a cluster headache in progress (Raskin, 1994). The mechanism by which it works remains unclear. Drawbacks to oxygen therapy for cluster headaches include the expense of the equipment and its relative lack of portability compared to pills, especially when considering the fact that although they are hideously painful, cluster headaches are often very brief. This would mean that by the time the patient got to the oxygen supplies, his or her headache could well be over.

Topical or viscous lidocaine (a local anesthetic that has replaced Novocaine® in medical and dental applications) can be self-administered through the nose during a cluster headache to reach a group of nerves called the sphenopalatine ganglion. The deadening of those nerves with the lidocaine can be remarkably effective in aborting an attack (Raskin, 1994). The number of people willing and able to swab the upper reaches of their nasal passages during terrific pain could well limit the widespread use of this therapy, however.

Tolfenamic acid, a drug in clinical trials in Europe, inhibits prostaglandin biosynthesis and inhibits platelet aggregation in a manner similar to aspirin. Clinical trials have shown this drug to be better than aspirin and as effective as ergotamine in treating acute migraine attacks. Tolfenamic acid has fewer side effects than ergotamine and is as effective as propranolol (Inderal®) in preventing migraines (Hansen, 1994).

10.42   Prophylaxis

Headache prophylaxis involves two main elements: avoidance of triggers and chronic medication therapy.

[1]   Trigger Avoidance

Most people who have migraine headaches get to know the specific triggers that can give them a headache, e.g., foods including preserved meats and red wine. General life-style considerations are also often helpful in avoiding headache, though this advice may be hard to follow. Strategies include trying to spread work evenly at home and on the job, in order to avoid peaks and troughs of stress; getting up at the same time every morning, including weekends, to avoid "let-down" headache; avoiding excessive fatigue; eating at regular times and not skipping meals; limiting intake of tea, coffee, ergotamine and analgesics, because they can cause "rebound headache"; avoiding craning the neck forward; sitting with a straight back; keeping muscles as relaxed as possible when not active; avoiding frowning and jaw clenching; avoiding exercise on a hot day and avoiding glare and exposure to flickering light (Lance, 1993b).

Certain factors can increase the frequency and/or severity of migraines, the treatment of which can lead to better control of headaches. These exacerbating states include anxiety or depression, the onset of systemic hypertension (high blood pressure) and the use of oral contraceptives or vasodilating drugs (Lance, 1993b).

[2]   Medications

A number of classes of medications have proven helpful in preventing headaches, especially migraine. However, because of side effects and the general risks involved in taking any prescription drug on a chronic basis, headache specialists prefer to reserve preventive medications for patients with particularly severe and/or frequent headaches.

[a]   Beta-Adrenergic Blockers

Beta-adrenergic blockers (propranolol, naldolol, antenolol, timolol, metoprolol) have proved to be relatively safe and effective migraine preventatives, though they have no pain-relieving actions. It is thought that they interact with central noradrenergic pathways from the locus ceruleus (a dark-colored depression on the floor of the brain's fourth ventricle) that may play a part in control of nociception (pain sensation) (Goadsby, 1993).

[b]   Calcium-Channel Blockers

Calcium-channel-blocking drugs (such as verapamil and diltiazem) have also proven to be safe migraine and cluster headache preventatives, with few side effects. They also have no pain-relieving capability. The mechanism was thought to involve prevention of extreme changes in blood vessel size, though with recent advances in the knowledge of headache mechanisms, this theorized mechanism seems less likely. It can take from two to eight weeks of therapy before there is any effect.

[c]   Antidepressants

The tricyclic antidepressants, such as amitriptyline (Elavil®), have proven effective in preventing migraine and chronic tension-type headaches. The tricyclics apparently have primary analgesic capabilities that are unrelated to their antidepressant actions, through their actions on CNS neurotransmitters, though the mechanism remains unclear.

The antidepressant fluoxetine (Prozac®) is also used to prevent migraine. Fluoxetine is a serotonin uptake inhibitor that blocks the neurotransmitter's normal uptake into platelets (cells primarily involved in blood clotting) and neurons but does not interfere with the uptake of the neurotransmitter norepinephrine. Neurotransmitters like serotonin work by attaching to receptor sites on the exterior of central nervous system cells. Once the neurotransmitter has been transported into the platelet interior, it can no longer react with its receptor sites and is therefore not active. By blocking serotonin's uptake into platelets, fluoxetine increases the amount of serotonin available for bonding with (and therefore stimulating) serotonergic receptor sites. The exact mechanism by which serotonin, or the lack of it, is involved in the initiation of migraine in susceptible people is not entirely understood, but it has been found that increasing the amount of serotonin in the central nervous system can prevent headaches in some migraineurs.[21]

Lithium is best known for treating manic-depressive disorder (now called bipolar disorder), a psychiatric condition for which it can be very effective. In the early 1970s, lithium was tried to prevent and treat cluster headaches, the rationale being that manic-depression and cluster headaches are both cyclical brain disorders. Lithium was found to be effective in treating cluster headaches and to have analgesic properties, thought to be due to its complex actions on central nervous

---

[21] *See* 10.33 *supra* for further discussion of the role of neurotransmitters in headache.

system catecholamines (noradrenaline and adrenaline) and, of course, serotonin. However, lithium can be quite toxic, and the therapeutic dose is often dangerously close to the toxic dose. Serious adverse effects include seizures, a drop in the number of white blood cells and cardiac arrhythmias (irregular heartbeat) (Loeb, 1991).

[d]   Anticonvulsants

Anticonvulsant drugs, particularly valproate, which normally are used to prevent seizures in various kinds of epilepsy, have been helpful in preventing migraines in some patients for whom more traditional prophylactic drugs have failed. The exact mechanism by which these drugs prevent headache is not known, but since anticonvulsants prevent seizures by depressing neuronal electrical function, it is possible that these drugs prevent the hyperexcitation believed to precede "spreading depression," theorized by many to cause migraine.[22]

[e]   Steroids

The anti-inflammatory steroid drug prednisone is an effective cluster headache preventative. Because cluster headaches occur at regular intervals, it is possible to prevent the headaches with a short course of this strong steroid drug, which should not be given on an open-ended basis. A 10-day course of prednisone, beginning at 60 mg daily (a moderately high dose) for 7 days and then tapering quickly to nothing over the last 3 days can abort the cluster cycle in many patients. The mechanism of action is unclear (Raskin, 1994).

[f]   Ergotamine

Ergotamine is another drug that should not be used on a chronic basis, but again, because cluster headaches are predictable, 1 mg of ergotamine taken one to two hours before the expected attack can successfully abort the headache. If the patient tends to wake up with an attack in the middle of the night, a 1-mg ergotamine suppository can prevent the headache (Raskin, 1994).[23]

---

[22] *See* 10.35 supra for further discussion of the "spreading depression" theory of headache.

[23] *See* 10.41[3] *supra* for further discussion of ergotamine and other ergot derivatives.

[3]   Alternative Therapies

Many "alternative" therapies are used by individuals with persistent headache problems and by people who do not believe in standard medical treatment. The range of these therapies is great: from acupuncture, to herbal treatments, biofeedback, homeopathy, hypnosis, meditation and prayer. It is not unusual for a headache specialist to suggest (or at least not oppose) that a patient try one of these treatments when everything else has given no relief.

Acupuncture and Chinese herbal remedies have proven helpful for some people. The mechanism by which acupuncture works is believed to involve stimulating the release of endorphins and related internal narcotics. Minute doses of herbs and minerals administered by homeopaths are also helpful for some people. The relaxed state that can be achieved during meditation, self-hypnosis and with the help of biofeedback are also helpful to some headache sufferers in getting a headache under control and to better cope with stress generally so that fewer headaches are started. Obviously these techniques are most helpful to those whose headaches are triggered by stress rather than by hormones or a chemical in food.

Many herbalists recommend feverfew, a composite flower of the daisy family that grows wild in the eastern United States. The feverfew is administered in capsule form daily as a headache preventative. Feverfew has a long medicinal history (Ulrich, 1990).

Because these therapies exist outside the realm of academic Western medicine, virtually no studies have been undertaken to determine if they are really effective. However, the placebo effect, in which up to 30 percent of patients will get better using a particular treatment simply because they believe it will work, cannot be ignored as a valid source of relief.

10.43   Treatment of Chronic Headache Medication Overuse

Medication overuse is a constant concern in treating patients with frequent headaches. Although controlled drugs used to abort migraines (such as codeine and butalbital contained in the combination drug Fiorinal®) can be addictive, in these patients, so can aspirin, caffeine and ergot derivatives. Headache patients do not take the drugs for a high, and they are not dependent upon them in the way we tend to think of drug addicts on the street, but as their headaches become more frequent, they take more of their headache medications, which, in turn, causes more rebound headaches; therefore the name *analgesic rebound headaches.* Such patients occasionally require in-patient hospital care to safely wean them from their medications with repetitive intravenous infusions of dihydroergotamine to stop the headache cycle. Then the patients are started on a prophylactic medication, depending upon their previous experience with prophylaxis (Primavera and Kaiser, 1994).

10.100 BIBLIOGRAPHY

Text References

Cahill, M. (Ed.): Illustrated Manual of Nursing Practice. Springhouse, Penna.: Springhouse Publications, 1991.

Chen, J., et al.: Etiological Classification of Chronic Headache in Children and Their Electroencephalographic Features. Acta Paediatr. Sin. 35(5):397-406, Sept.-Oct. 1994.

Day, L.: Hypertension in Pregnancy. In: Frederickson, H. and Wilkins-Haug, L. (Eds.): Ob/Gyn Secrets. Philadelphia: Hanley and Belfus, 1991.

Diener, H.: A Review of Current Treatments for Migraine. Eur. Neurol. 34(Suppl.2):18–25, 1994.

Ellis, G., et al.: The Efficacy of Metoclopramide in the Treatment of Migraine Headache. Ann. Emerg. Med. 22(2):191–195, Feb. 1993.

Ferrari, M.: Biochemistry of Migraine. Pathol. Biol. (Paris) 40(4):287–289, Apr. 1992.

Ferrari, M. and Saxena, P.: On Serotonin and Migraine: A Clinical and Pharmacological Review. Cephalgia 13(3):151–165, June 1993.

Fozard, J. and Kalkman, H.: 5-Hydroxytryptamine (5-HT) and the Initiation of Migraine: New Perspectives. Naunyn. Schmiedebergs Arch. Pharmacol. 350(3):225–229, Sept. 1994.

Gallagher, M.: Headaches: Muscle Contraction, Migraine and Cluster. In: Weiner, R. (Ed.): Innovations in Pain Management: A Practical Guide for Clinicians. Orlando, Fla.: Paul M. Deutsch Press, 1990.

Goadsby, P.: The Anatomy and Physiology of the Cerebral Circulation in Relationship to the Assessment and Management of Headache. In: International Association for the Study of Pain: Refresher Course Syllabus. Seattle: IASP Publications, 1993.

Gallai, V., et al.: Red Blood Cell Magnesium Levels in Migraine Patients. Cephalalgia 13(2):74-81, Apr. 1993.

Greenspan, J.: Oral Manifestations of Disease. In: Isselbacher, K., et al. (Eds.): Harrison's Principles of Internal Medicine, 13th ed. New York: McGraw-Hill, 1994.

Haas, D.: Acute and Chronic Posttraumatic Headache. In: Olsen, J., et al. (Eds.): The Headaches. New York: Raven Press, 1993.

Hansen, P.: Tolfenamic Acid in Acute and Prophylactic Treatment of Migraine: A Review. Pharmacol. Toxicol. 75(Suppl. 2):81-82, 1994.

Jensen, R. and Hindberg, I.: Plasma Serotonin Increase During Episodes of Tension-Type Headache. Cephalgia 14(3):219–222, June 1994.

Keck, P., Jr., et al.: Diagnostic and Treatment Implications of Psychiatric Comorbidity with Migraine. Ann. Clin. Psychiatr. 6(3):165–171, Sept. 1994.

Kistler, J., et al.: Cerebrovascular Diseases. In: Isselbacher, K., et al. (Eds.): Harrison's Principles of Internal Medicine, 13th ed. New York: McGraw-Hill, 1994.

Kitano, A., et al.: Increased 11-Dehydroxythromboxane B2 in Migraine: Platelet Hyperfunction in Patients with Migraine During Headache-Free Period. Headache 34(9):515–518, Oct. 1994.

Klapper, J. and Stanton, J.: Current Emergency Treatment of Severe Migraine Headaches. Headache 33(10):560–562, Nov.-Dec. 1993.

Lance, J.: Current Concepts in Migraine Pathogenesis. Neurology 43(6 Suppl. 3):S11–S15, June 1993a.

Lance, J.: Mechanism and Management of Headache, 5th ed. Oxford, England: Butterworth-Heinemann, 1993b.

Lewis, J. (Ed.): Illustrated Guide to Diagnostic Tests. Springhouse, Penna.: Springhouse Books, 1993.

Loeb, S. (Ed.): Physician's 1991 Drug Handbook. Springhouse, Penna.: Springhouse Books, 1991.

Marazziti, D., et al.: Platelet 3H-imipramine Binding and Sulphotransferase Activity in Primary Headache. Cephalgia 14(3):210–214, June 1994.

Marcus, D.: Serotonin and Its Role in Headache Pathogenesis and Treatment. Clin. J. Pain 9(3):159–167, Sept. 1993.

Martignoni, H. and Solomon, S.: Chronic Daily Headache. Cephalalgia 12(13 Suppl.):72-77, Apr. 1993.

Mauskop, A., et al.: Chronic Daily Headache — One Disease or Two? Diagnostic Role of Serum Ionized Magnesium. Cephalgia 14(1):24–28, Feb. 1994.

Mauskop, A., et al.: Deficiencies in Serum Ionized Magnesium But Not Total Magnesium in Patients With Migraines. Possible Role of ICa2 + /IMg2 + Ratio. Headache 33(3):135–138, Mar. 1993.

Moskowitz, M. and Macfarlane, R.: Neurovascular and Molecular Mechanisms in Migraine Headaches. Cerebrovasc. Brain Metab. Rev. 5(3):159–177, Fall 1993.

Nakano, T., et al.: Platelet Substance P and 5-Hydroxytryptamine in Migraine and Tension-Type Headache. Headache 33(10):528–532, Nov.–Dec. 1993.

Olesen, J.: The Classification and Diagnosis of Headache Disorders. In: International Association for the Study of Pain: Refresher Course Syllabus. Seattle: IASP Publications, 1993.

The Oral Sumatriptan and Aspirin Plus Metoclopramide Comparative Study Group. Eur. Neurol. 32(3):177–184, 1992.

Primavera, J., 3rd and Kaiser, R.: The Relationship Between Locus of Control, Amount of Pre-Admission Analgesic/Ergot Overuse, and Length of Stay for Patients Admitted for Inpatient Treatment of Chronic Headache. Headache 34(4):204–208, Apr. 1994.

Raskin, N.: Headache. In: Isselbacher, K., et al. (Eds.): Harrison's Principles of Internal Medicine, 13th ed. New York: McGraw-Hill, 1994.

Robbins, L.: Management of Headache and Headache Medications. New York: Springer-Verlag, 1994.

Ropper, A.: Trauma of the Head and Spine. In: Isselbacher, K., et al. (Eds.): Harrison's Principles of Internal Medicine, 13th ed. New York: McGraw-Hill, 1994.

Saunte, H. and Soyka, M.: How Many Different Headaches Do You Have? Cephalalgia 13(2):136-137, Apr. 1993.

Scheld, W.: Bacterial Meningitis and Brain Abscess. In: Isselbacher, K., et al. (Eds.): Harrison's Principles of Internal Medicine, 13th ed. New York: McGraw-Hill, 1994.

Seelig, C. B., et al.: Physician Recognition of Magnesium Status in Patients with Coronary Artery Disease Admitted to a Regional Medical Center. Am. J. Cardiol. 72(2):226-227, July 15, 1993.

Silberstein, S.: Serotonin (5-HT) and Migraine. Headache 34(7):408–417, July-Aug. 1994.

Solomon, S. and Rose, F.: General Principles of Management. In: Olesen, J., et al. (Eds.): The Headaches. New York: Raven Press, 1993.

Stewart, W. and Lipton, R.: The Economic and Social Impact of Migraine. Eur. Neurol. 34(Suppl. 2):12–17, 1994.

Stewart, W., et al.: Prevalence of Migraine Headache in the United States. Relation to Age, Income, Race and Other Socioeconomic Factors. J.A.M.A. 267:64–69, 1992.

Strandgaard, S. and Henry, P.: Arterial Hypertension. In: Olsen, J., et al., (Eds.): The Headaches. New York: Raven Press, 1993.

Ulrich, L.: A Midwife's Tale: The Life of Martha Ballard, Based on Her Diary, 1785–1812. New York: Vintage Books, 1990.

Williams, G.: Hypertensive Vascular Disease. In: Isselbacher, K., et al. (Eds.): Harrison's Principles of Internal Medicine, 13th ed. New York: McGraw-Hill, 1994.

Additional References

Klapper, J.: Toward a Standard Drug Formulary for the Treatment of Headache. Headache 35(4):225–227, Apr. 1995.

Launay, J. et al.: Serotonin Receptors and Therapeutics. Cell Mol. Biol. (Noisy-le-grand) 40(3):327–336, May 1994.

Sandyk, R. and Awerbuch, G.: The Co-Occurrence of Multiple Sclerosis and Migraine Headache: The Serotonergic Link. Int. J. Neurosci. 76(3–4):249–257, June 1994.

Trotsky, M.: Neurogenic Vascular Headaches, Food and Chemical Triggers. Ear Nose Throat J. 73(4):228–230, Apr. 1994.

CHAPTER 11

Post-traumatic Epilepsy

SCOPE

It is well established that post-traumatic epilepsy may develop months or years after brain trauma. The risk of developing epilepsy following head injury varies, largely dependent on the severity of the injury. Epilepsy may be primary, secondary or cryptogenic. The seizure may assume a wide spectrum of diverse clinical features, including aura, motor or sensory loss, unconsciousness, affective (such as déjà vu and jamais vu) and autonomic nervous system symptoms, among others. A number of medications are available to treat the condition, with varying degrees of success, and rarely, surgical intervention is the method of treatment.

SYNOPSIS

11.00   INTRODUCTION

There is a well-established association between head trauma and the possibility of developing epilepsy some months or even years after the trauma. However, the exact mechanisms responsible for the development of epilepsy are still not well understood and have been a subject of intense debate.

One percent of the United States population suffer from epilepsy (Devinsky, 1990). Although many patients experience the first epileptic symptoms within a year of the injury, the latency period between head injury and development of epilepsy varies (Willmore, 1992). Studies of military populations surviving missile injury have shown that in this group, an increased risk of epilepsy can be identified as long as 15 years or more after the injury (Salazar, et al., 1985).

The risk of acquiring post-traumatic epilepsy depends to a great extent on the type and severity of injury that was incurred and the duration of the seizure-free period following trauma. An early seizure, occurring during the first week after injury, increases the likelihood of incidence of late epilepsy (Jennett, 1981).

In general, 10 to 15 percent of the survivors of severe head injury are at substantial risk for later epilepsy (Hauser, 1990). Moderate trauma is associated with a much lower rate—under 2 percent. Adults have a higher risk than children (Kurtzke and Kurland, 1986).

Epilepsy is not a single disease but rather a spectrum of paroxysmal (occurring in short spasms) disorders marked by wide variations in manifestation, severity and etiology (Devinsky, 1990). Epilepsy may be idiopathic, with no known neurologic etiology (sometimes referred to as genetic, essential or primary), or symptomatic, when it is acquired as a result of brain injury or disease (sometimes referred to as secondary epilepsy).

A third category, cryptogenic epilepsies, applies to syndromes that are similar to symptomatic epilepsies, except that the underlying cause is not known. As it becomes known, a cryptogenic epilepsy is reclassified as symptomatic (Thadani and Williamson, 1990).

The fundamental symptom in epilepsy is the seizure, which may assume a diverse spectrum of clinical features, including hallucinations and illusions, psychic phenomena such as déjà vu and jamais vu,[1] affective (mood) and autonomic (the part of the nervous system that controls involuntary actions such as respiration) symptoms, impairment of consciousness and involuntary movements (Devinsky, 1990). It is important to emphasize that epilepsy refers to patterns of recurrent attacks that occur when the brain is presumably under normal physiologic circumstances. Isolated convulsions occurring during the period immediately after head trauma, during high fevers or during the course of drug therapy do not necessarily establish a clinical diagnosis of epilepsy.

Although most of the large studies concerning post-traumatic epilepsy pertain to war injuries, accidents are a major public health problem in the United States. Automobile and motorcycle accidents are among the most common sources of head trauma. Other causes of head trauma include sports injuries as well as work-related accidents. It is important to note that many of these causes of head injuries are for the most part preventable; therefore, any preventive measures taken would decrease the incidence of acquired epilepsy.

Another area to consider is head injury among children. This can result from accidental causes or from child abuse. Infants are at special

---

[1] *See* 11.12[1][b] *infra.*

risk because their skull bones are not yet fully fused, and the resulting open fontanelles (the so-called soft spots) fail to provide the protection against head and brain trauma offered by an adult cranium. Head injury is the second most common identifiable cause of seizures in children under the age of seven (febrile, or fever-related, seizures being the first).

There is also a small, though unavoidable, risk of post-traumatic epilepsy developing as a complication of neurosurgery; this would be an iatrogenic (treatment-induced) trauma. One figure that is still commonly quoted today is that the risk of epilepsy following cranio-tomy (surgical cutting into the skull, or cranium) is 20 percent (Jennett, 1983). The risk obviously varies, depending on the site and extent of the surgery as well as on the specific procedure.

Advances in medical treatment have resulted in long seizure-free periods for the majority of individuals with epilepsy. Indeed, in some cases, the complete discontinuation of medication remains a real possibility. For others with more intractable seizures, surgical proce-dures hold promise.

11.10 CLASSIFICATION OF EPILEPSY

Various criteria have been used to categorize epilepsy. These include seizure type, electroencephalographic (EEG) findings, age at onset of symptoms, factors that may precipitate epileptic attacks, natural history, cause and anatomic location of seizures (Farrell, 1993). Complete agreement on the details, terminology and classification is still lacking. Confusion exists because some experts classify epilepsy strictly according to clinical symptoms, while others base certain categories (psychomotor variant, for example) strictly on the features of the electroencephalogram.

The International League Against Epilepsy (ILAE) has developed and modified several classification systems that have gained wide usage. The latest of these modifications (Commission on Classification and Terminology of ILAE, 1989) emphasizes that the natural history and response to treatment of a particular seizure are often influenced by the setting in which the seizure occurred. Therefore, the response of seizure types to antiepileptic drugs and the prognosis for remission need to be included among the criteria used to classify epilepsy (Farrell, 1993). Despite the numerous revisions, however, the original structure of the ILAE classification stays the same.

The ILAE classification first makes a distinction between partial and generalized seizures, and then considers all the various factors just mentioned.

11.11   Stages of an Epilepsy Episode

Distinct clinical stages are associated with epilepsy. In some forms of epilepsy, the individual may first experience what is known as an *aura,* characterized by premonitory signs and symptoms that indicate the onset of the seizure. Auras may manifest as ringing in the ears, seeing spots or generalized sensory disturbances, such as chest tightness or an uncomfortable stomach feeling. Convulsions or a psychomotor seizure (in which the patient suffers impairment of consciousness and performs semipurposeful movements, with loss of memory for the entire episode) usually begin shortly after the aura in grand mal or psychomotor epilepsy. Auras are not present in all types of seizures, however. For example, individuals suffering a petit mal seizure do not experience an aura.

Next the individual experiences the seizure proper, commonly known as a convulsion. The neurologic term for this stage is *ictus.* The ictal stage varies greatly in its manifestations; a loss of consciousness and convulsions are typical in grand mal seizures, while a brief "staring spell" known as an absence seizure is common in petit mal.

Following the actual seizure, the *postictal* phase takes effect. This is the interval between the seizure and the return to normal consciousness. The seizure-free period between the end of one episode and the onset of the next seizure is termed the *interictal* period.

Another important term in the understanding of seizure disorders is *status epilepticus.* This refers to persistent and recurrent seizure activity lasting for extremely long periods of time, during which the patient does not return to the usual level of functioning between seizure episodes. This type of seizure is only injurious to the brain if there is inadequate cerebral oxygenation and blood flow. Emergency treatment for respiratory control is often necessary.

11.12   Seizure Types

A complete description of each seizure type, within the classification of partial and generalized seizures and status epilepticus, appears in this section.

[1] Partial Seizures

Partial seizures are characterized by clinical and electroencephalographic (EEG) abnormalities that suggest the involvement of only one location in the brain (Thadani and Williamson, 1990). Partial seizures are divided into two major categories: (1) simple (also called elementary or focal), without impairment of consciousness, and (2) complex, with altered or impaired consciousness.

[a] Simple Partial Seizures

Simple partial seizures may be further subclassified because of the different kinds of symptoms that can be experienced during the seizure. Simple partial seizures with motor symptoms are characterized by *clonic* movements (rapid succession of alternating contraction and relaxation) of individual muscles or group of muscles. The site of the muscle activity reflects the site of abnormality in the brain, and the extremities are more frequently involved than the trunk. For example, in seizures determined by neuronal changes in the frontal part of the brain, contraversive head and eye deviation is typical, with posturing of the arm so that it is externally rotated (a clockwise movement for the right arm) and flexed (bent) at elbow (Thadani and Williamson, 1990).

Simple partial seizures with somatosensory (pertaining to the body and senses, as opposed to the mind) symptoms involve a wide variety of symptoms, including paresthesia (abnormal sensations such as tingling), burning or pain beginning in an extremity and then spreading to involve the face or other portions of the same site of the body. Visual or auditory hallucinations may occur. These include seeing spots, balls or stars, which may be static or whirl around, as well as hearing loud noises or hissing sounds.

Both visual as well as auditory hallucinations seem to be associated with neuronal changes in the temporal region of the brain (Thadani and Williamson, 1990). (The temporal lobe is located at the base of the cortex of the brain.) *(See Figure 11–1.)* Olfactory hallucinations may also occur and include unpleasant odors, such as the smell of burning rubber or metal. Autonomic symptoms, such as dilation of pupils and sweating, are unusual but do occur.

Simple partial seizures may be associated with several other epileptic syndromes, such as the benign epileptic syndrome, which occurs between the ages of 3 and 13 years (Thadani and Williamson,

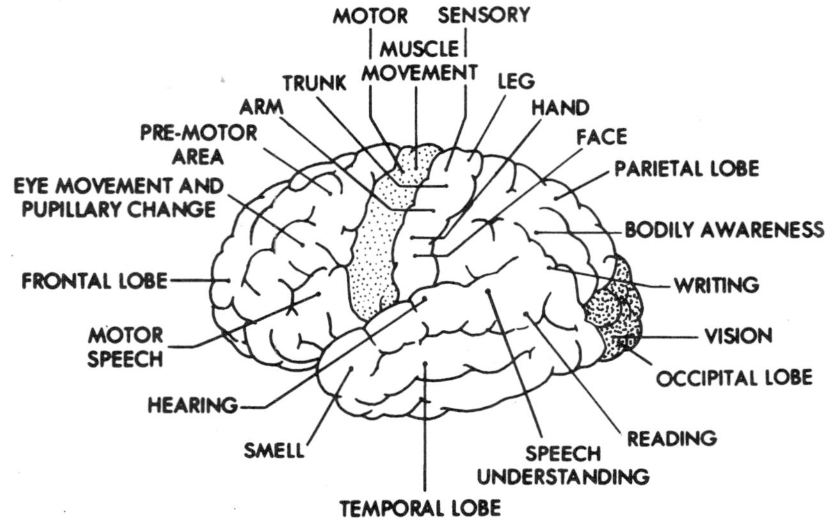

Fig. 11–1. The temporal lobe is located at the base of the cortex of the brain. Note the localization of specific motor and psychological functions to specific portions of the cerebral cortex.

1990), some forms of childhood epilepsy and Jacksonian or focal epilepsy (in which the convulsion starts with twitches in a certain part of the body and then proceeds distally to other parts, usually with loss of consciousness).

[b] Complex Partial Seizures

Complex partial seizures are also known as psychomotor or temporal lobe seizures (temporal lobe epilepsy). This disorder is very common in adults and is characterized by focal (localized) onset as well as alteration of consciousness.

Typically a seizure in temporal lobe epilepsy begins with an aura. Auras with a gastric sensation, emotional content, feeling of déjà vu and visual disturbances are the most common, but other sensory and autonomic symptoms may also be present. The seizure itself may begin with a motor arrest or motionless stare, often followed by lip smacking and swallowing (Thadani and Williamson, 1990). In déjà vu, the patient experiences either visual manifestations or thoughts that seem strangely familiar and that he feels he has lived through or observed before. In jamais vu, the patient is not aware of the fact that a particular experience or place should be familiar.

The aura is usually remembered by the patient, who experiences a progressive impairment of consciousness when the seizure spreads. Ictus lasts several seconds or minutes. Later in the seizure, complex automatisms (performance of acts that normally require volition, without an apparent exercise of the will), such as walking, drinking and undressing, may occur (Thadani and Williamson, 1990). The postictal period lasts from two to ten minutes and is marked by disorientation, irritability and confusion. Patients in this state have often been considered by police or passersby to be severely intoxicated.

[c]   Tonic-Clonic Seizures

Both simple and complex partial seizures can progress to generalized, tonic-clonic episodes. Therefore, a psychomotor seizure may develop into a grand mal seizure.

During the psychomotor seizure, the patient appears to be conscious, but her or his movements are automatic and not under voluntary control. There is a limited awareness of the environment; patients have been known to fall or otherwise injure themselves during this period.

[2]   Generalized Seizures

Generalized seizures are defined as those in which the clinical manifestations and the EEG patterns suggest a bilateral (affecting both sides) involvement of the brain (Thadani and Williamson, 1990). They are usually bilaterally symmetric and without focal onset. They are generally assumed to be caused by genetic factors and are not usually associated with trauma.

It is important to distinguish primary generalized seizures from secondary generalized seizures, which originally have a focal onset and later spread to involve the whole brain (Thadani and Williamson, 1990). In some cases, however, secondary generalization is so rapid that it cannot be distinguished clearly from a primary generalized syndrome (Thadani and Williamson, 1990).

Seizures of the primary generalized variety may take many forms. The maximal epileptic response of the brain is represented by the tonic-clonic, or grand mal, seizure. The absence attack, also known as petit mal, causes a brief lapse of consciousness and is less severe in character than the tonic-clonic episode.

[a] Absence (Petit Mal) Seizures

The second most common type of generalized seizure (after complex partial seizure) is the absence or petit mal seizure. It may occur alone or in combination with other forms of seizures. In general, absence epilepsy, which may be an inherited disease, begins in patients at 6 to 7 years of age (Thadani and Williamson, 1990). It is relatively common in childhood, less common in adolescence and quite rare in adults.

Seizures are brief, typically lasting from 30 seconds to 1 minute, and are characterized by sudden loss of contact and staring into space. There is no warning or aura associated with this type of seizure. Extremely rarely, motor symptoms such as falling and retropulsion may be experienced by the patient (Thadani and Williamson, 1990). Blinking is common, and oral automatism may occur (Thadani and Williamson, 1990).

In the majority of patients, there is no postictal stage following absence. After the seizure, the individual resumes the same task he was engaged in or completes the sentence he was speaking.

Although the patient stares and is unresponsive during the petit mal attack, this change may not be identified readily, particularly in children by casual observers. These attacks can occur several times a day and may, in certain cases, account for poor school performance.

Spontaneous remission of absence seizures is common, although patients with childhood absence epilepsy may also develop generalized tonic-clonic seizures in adolescence (Thadani and Williamson, 1990).

[b] Myoclonic Seizures

This category includes a heterogeneous group of seizures that are difficult to classify and may be either epileptic or nonepileptic. Myoclonic seizures occur most frequently during childhood, and most of the types are fortunately relatively uncommon. They are marked by rapid, involuntary muscle contractions that may generalize or be limited to certain muscle groups. The upper extremities are more affected than the lower limbs, and the flexor muscle groups are most often involved.

Myoclonic seizures are characteristic of childhood benign myoclonic epilepsy and several more severe types of epilepsies in infancy. Benign myoclonic epilepsy is characterized by brief bursts of myoclonus that usually start in children between the ages of one and two years and resolve spontaneously in the majority of cases (Thadani and Williamson, 1990). Other childhood myoclonic epilepsies are often associated with mental retardation that suggests an underlying brain disease (Thadani and Williamson, 1990).

[c]   Tonic-Clonic Seizures (Grand Mal)

The tonic-clonic, or grand mal, attack is the most common—and dramatic—type of generalized seizure. It produces a profound and abrupt loss of consciousness. Motor activity can be divided into two phases: the tonic (muscle contraction) phase and the clonic (convulsive) phase.

The tonic phase is marked by persistent contractions of large muscle groups, with the arms and legs extended and the back arched. The clonic phase is marked by violent spasms or jerks of the whole body alternating with periods of relaxation. The typical clonic-tonic attack lasts from a few seconds to a few minutes and is associated with tongue biting, loss of urinary or bowel control, labored breathing or prolonged periods of apnea (cessation of breathing). Although most individuals with tonic-clonic seizures escape serious injury, trauma may be sustained either from the initial fall (especially from heights), when driving a car or from hitting objects during jerking movements. Among the elderly, osteoporotic spinal fractures have occurred from the force of muscle contractions.

The postictal period is variable. The patient is usually drowsy and poorly responsive for minutes to hours, and may require extended sleep. Muscle aches and headache are often experienced during the recovery phase.

[d]   Atonic and Akinetic Seizures

Atonic seizures (sometimes referred to as astatic) are more often seen in children and are relatively rare. This type of seizure is sometimes associated with absence epilepsy but more commonly with Lennox-Gastaut syndrome, a congenital disorder characterized by multiple seizure types (Thadani and Williamson, 1990).

Atonic seizures are associated with a sudden loss of tone in various muscle groups, which frequently results in falling (drop attacks).

Traumatic consequences may be severe, particularly if the head is injured. Drop attacks may be precipitated by auditory, photic (light) or touch stimulation, and are sometimes associated with stress or fever. Attacks last from a second to a few seconds. Consciousness is lost briefly or not at all (Thadani and Williamson, 1990).

Akinetic seizures involve a temporary and transient paralysis. Many feel that these convulsions are a type of atonic epilepsy.

[3]　Status Epilepticus

Status epilepticus is defined as prolonged or recurrent seizure activity without the regaining of consciousness. These seizures can last 30 minutes or longer.

[a]　Generalized Status Epilepticus

Generalized status epilepticus can be either primary or secondary in nature. It often results from an organic process, such as a brain tumor or a late sequel of head trauma. It is also associated with precipitous drops in anticonvulsant medication levels. Generalized status epilepticus is relatively common and significantly associated with mortality.

Correct and prompt seizure diagnosis is essential,[2] because most patients can control their seizures well with medication or by eliminating precipitating factors, such as alcohol (Devinsky, 1990). Failure to recognize and treat seizures can lead to accidental death from impaired consciousness while driving, missed therapeutic opportunities (e.g., early surgery for tumors), education and employment handicaps, and psychosocial devastation.

Seizures are diagnosed most commonly by neurologists, primarily by the patient history. A complete description by the patient and any observer who may have been present of what was experienced and witnessed is fundamental to a correct diagnosis. When the initial history is vague, it is important to instruct both patient and witness to observe carefully and immediately record their findings after future episodes (Devinsky, 1990).

Clinical testing is also necessary to complete the diagnosis of status epilepticus. Cardiac tests are important for both pediatric and adult populations. Monitoring of an epileptic episode through EEG and alternative diagnostic systems is also very helpful.

---

[2] *See* 11.30 *infra.*

[b]   Other Forms of Status Epilepticus

Other types of status epilepticus are not as common or as dangerous as the generalized form. Status epilepticus is infrequently associated with complex partial seizures or absence status.

11.13   Staging of the Onset of Post-traumatic Epilepsy

Post-traumatic epilepsy can be classified into three groups: immediate, early and late, according to the time of occurrence of seizures after trauma. The risk for development of post-traumatic epilepsy is generally related to the severity of injury and brain trauma.

[1]   Immediate Post-traumatic Epilepsy

Immediate post-traumatic epilepsy, also called impact seizures, refers to seizures occurring within the first 24 hours after a trauma, with most occurring within the first few hours (Temkin, et al., 1991). In general, these kinds of seizures are considered to be an acute reaction to trauma that will not necessarily lead to post-traumatic epilepsy (Temkin, et al., 1991).

[2]   Early Post-traumatic Epilepsy

Early post-traumatic epilepsy refers to the development of seizures within the first week following head injury. Overall, early post-traumatic seizures occur in about 1.9 percent of civilian head trauma patients receiving any medical attention and in about 4.6 percent of consecutive admissions to a trauma unit (Temkin, et al., 1991). This complication is more common in children than in adults. The incidence is also higher in patients with intracranial hematoma (collection of blood within the cranium, or skull) and/or depressed skull fractures.

The occurrence of early post-traumatic seizures can complicate the management of the head trauma patient by causing several different complications (Willmore, 1992). A series of seizures may also develop into post-traumatic status epilepticus, a serious complication especially in patients who may have multiple trauma to other areas of the body as well.

Early seizures increase the likelihood of incidence of late epilepsy (Willmore, 1992). Guidelines identifying patients at risk for late epilepsy include early epilepsy. Twenty-five percent of patients suffering early epilepsy may develop late epilepsy (Willmore, 1993).

[3] Late Post-traumatic Epilepsy

Late post-traumatic epilepsy refers to the development of seizures more than one week after the trauma. Unlike immediate and early seizures, which are often viewed as an acute reaction to trauma, late seizures are considered unprovoked occurrences that are in fact epileptic (Temkin, et al., 1991). Also in contrast to early seizures, late post-traumatic epilepsy usually involves a loss of consciousness.

The risk for development of late seizures is generally related to the severity of injury or brain trauma (Willmore, 1993). Within the first year after head trauma, the incidence of post-traumatic seizures exceeds 12 times the population risk for the expected development of epilepsy (Willmore, 1993).

Several factors have been associated with the risk of developing late post-traumatic epilepsy. They include occurrence of an early seizure, presence of an intracerebral hematoma, prolonged post-traumatic amnesia, history of injury from a missile and presence of cortical laceration occurring with a depressed skull fracture (Willmore, 1993). Of course, all these factors indicate a relatively severe degree of brain trauma.

11.20 ETIOLOGY AND GENETIC ASPECTS

From an etiologic point of view, epilepsy can be divided into two main types. The first, *idiopathic* or *primary* epilepsy, includes cases in which no underlying cause is found, and usually the patient does not experience symptoms other than seizures. A hereditary predisposition often exists, and different syndromes are defined by the age of the patient at onset, the clinical characteristics and EEG abnormalities (Thadani and Williamson, 1990).

The second type of epilepsy is referred to as *symptomatic* or *secondary*. It is acquired and can be directly attributed to an underlying brain disorder. This may be a congenital malformation, trauma such as head injury, an inborn error of metabolism, tumor or any of the other causes that have been proved to determine epilepsy (Thadani and Williamson, 1990). Those epilepsies that are similar to symptomatic epilepsies, except that the underlying cause is not known, are defined by some authors as *cryptogenic* epilepsies (Thadani and Williamson, 1990). As the cause becomes known, a cryptogenic epilepsy is reclassified as symptomatic.

It is important to emphasize that a single etiology is not implied for each syndrome or type of epilepsy. Both the genetic makeup and the various traumatic and otherwise injurious events that happen during fetal development and in subsequent life play roles in establishing the thresholds for paroxysmal brain disorder. Some epilepsies have a biochemical basis (with grossly normal brain structure) and others are caused by structural lesions. Within each of these two groups, there will be some epilepsies that are inherited and others that are acquired (Thadani and Williamson, 1990).

11.21   Idiopathic or Primary Epilepsy

As previously discussed, idiopathic or primary epilepsy seems to be associated with a hereditary predisposition. The exact mechanism of heredity is not clear.

11.22   Symptomatic or Secondary Epilepsy

Although specific etiologies are involved in symptomatic or secondary epilepsy, hereditary influences may play some role. Research has pointed to a link between patients with seizures resulting from brain damage and the development of seizures in their relatives. Other studies have shown that severe trauma with laceration of the brain may lead to post-traumatic seizures in one individual and not in another, again suggesting a possible genetic link. It is postulated that a single gene or a group of genes may denote a predisposition for specific seizure disorders. Thus, head trauma may unmask this tendency and result in symptomatic epilepsy.

Although trauma, especially head injury, may be the cause of the onset of epilepsy, it is important to realize that the epilepsy may be due to some other concomitant disease or condition. As scientific understanding advances, etiologies may be discovered that produce more than one syndrome in varying circumstances, as well as single syndromes that would have more than one etiology (Thadani and Williamson, 1990). Following are some of the major underlying causes of symptomatic or secondary epilepsy.

[1]   Head Injury

A well-established association exists between head trauma and the possibility of developing epilepsy some months or even years following injury. The latency period between head injury and development of epilepsy varies, although 57 percent of patients have onset of seizure within one year of injury (Willmore, 1992). Common causes of traumatic brain injuries include vehicular accidents, falls, gunshot wounds and complications of neurosurgery.

[2] Birth Trauma

Birth trauma and inadequate fetal presentation (especially breech) that result in a lack of sufficient oxygen (anoxia) to the newborn are important perinatal factors that can contribute to seizures. Anoxia produces diffuse symmetric lesions that can lead to generalized seizures.

Convulsion in the newborn can have many etiologies, including perinatal trauma, anoxia, intracranial hemorrhage, congenital anomalies, infections and metabolic disorders. Convulsions in the newborn rarely take the generalized (grand mal) form. Rather, they are usually irregular, jerky movements, tonic spasms, tremors or slight movements of fingers or toes.

Convulsions are very variable and may be difficult to diagnose. They may be associated with slowing of the respiration, occasional apneic (cessation of breathing) spells, drooling and feeble cry. Early assessment of the trauma may be critical for treatment success.

[3] Congenital Anomalies and Hereditary Diseases

Some hereditary diseases and congenital defects may predispose an individual to seizures. These include tuberous sclerosis (a familial disease involving the nervous system and the skin), neurofibromatosis (a condition marked by the presence of numerous tumors arising from the cells of nerve fibers), Lesch-Nyan disease (which occurs only in male children and is marked by mental retardation, spastic paralysis, abnormal movements and self-mutilation by biting; the condition is due to an enzyme deficiency), phenylketonuria (a hereditary metabolic disorder) and an extensive list of other rare disorders. Certain congenital (present at birth) infections, such as toxoplasmosis and cytomegalic viral diseases, have also been associated with seizures in infancy. The specific role that these anomalies play in the development of acquired epilepsy remains unknown (Willmore, 1992).

[4] Metabolic Disorders

Several metabolic disorders may produce seizures, particularly in the neonatal period, including hypoglycemia (low blood sugar level), hypocalcemia (low blood calcium level) and acute intermittent porphyria, an inborn error of metabolism.

Older children and adults can also have seizures secondary to a metabolic disorder. These include severe hypoglycemia, such as that associated with insulin overdose or insulin-secreting tumors; hypochloremia (low sodium level, as is seen in Addison's disease); and acute renal failure, occurring in approximately a third of patients. The lack of certain trace elements may also be linked with epilepsy in adults.

These seizures only occur during the period of altered metabolism. They abate when the disorder is corrected.

[5] Cerebral Infections

Meningitis (inflammation of the membrane enveloping the brain and spinal cord), encephalitis (inflammation of the brain), tetanus and congenital infections can all cause seizures. In addition, seizures have also been noted in patients with acquired immunodeficiency syndrome (AIDS) who display the AIDS-dementia complex, a common disorder seen in advanced stages of the disease.[3]

[6] Systemic Toxins, Drugs and Alcohol

Metallic toxins, such as mercury or lead, and withdrawal from the chronic consumption of alcohol or central nervous system depressants (especially barbiturates, tranquilizers and sedatives) can induce seizures. Certain medications may also induce the development of seizures, generally as a manifestation of drug overdose. These include certain antidepressants and stimulants, aminophylline (an asthma medication), isoniazid (an antituberculosis drug) and penicillin derivatives.

[7] Degenerative Diseases

Some degenerative diseases have been associated with seizures. These include the Sturge-Weber syndrome (a congenital disease that is also associated with a type of brain tumor) and, rarely, multiple sclerosis.

---

[3] *See also* ch. 13.

[8] Brain Tumors

Seizures are frequently associated with brain tumors. The location and type of tumor are two important factors in seizure development.

[9] Cerebrovascular Diseases

Compromised blood flow, as is evident in cerebrovascular disease, can be responsible for seizure episodes. Seizures can occur before, during or after a stroke.[4] Epilepsy is fairly frequent in post-stroke victims, and a number of other cerebrovascular disorders have been associated with seizures.

[10] Miscellaneous Disorders

Inoculation against smallpox, pertussis and typhoid has been indicated as a rare cause of seizures, most likely due to allergic reactions.

11.30 DIAGNOSIS

When a patient seeks medical attention because he or she is experiencing symptoms that can suggest a diagnosis of epilepsy and also has a history of head trauma, the physician is faced with a difficult task in sorting out the possible relationship between the two. As previously discussed, epilepsies may be caused by many different factors. In determining the etiologic role of head injury in post-traumatic epilepsy, the examiner must fully assess the medical history of the patient to determine whether epilepsy has been a problem in the past and to rule out primary epilepsy.

The next important issue to be addressed is the history of the head trauma, with regard to the type, location and severity of the head injury. Earlier medical records should be obtained if possible.

Generally minor head trauma without impairment of consciousness or scalp laceration is highly unlikely to lead to epilepsy. In contrast, open wounds in which the scalp, skull and dura mater (the outermost and toughest of the three membranes enveloping the brain and spinal cord) have been penetrated, with subsequent direct traumatic injury to the brain, result in an incidence of epilepsy much greater than in patients with closed head injuries. The risk of development of seizures is also increased by trauma-induced hemorrhage, which may be an important etiologic factor (Willmore, 1992). *(See Figure 11–2.)*

---

[4] *See also* ch. 9.

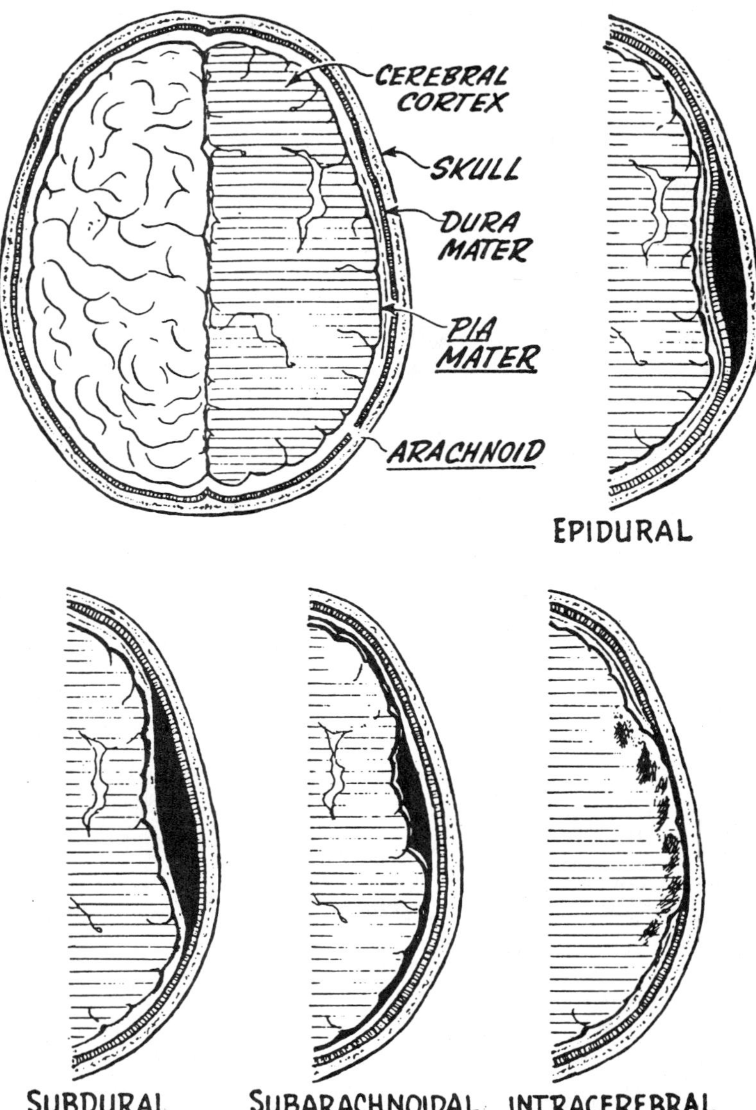

Fig. 11–2. Open wounds that penetrate the dura mater (top left) and trauma-induced hemorrhage (top right and bottom) greatly increase the risk of developing seizures.

The causal relationship between trauma and epilepsy can also be elucidated by an attempt to correlate the clinical pattern of epileptic attacks with the site of injury. In other words, if a patient experienced trauma to a particular area of the brain, one would expect any subsequent seizure disorder to reflect epileptic activity from this injured region. The severity and location of the cerebral injury is particularly important in penetrating wounds of the brain; it is relevant to the risk of developing post-traumatic epilepsy and it shapes the type of epileptic seizure.

Another important factor in assessing the risk of seizure development is the duration of the period between the head injury and the onset of epileptic symptoms. Approximately 80 percent of severely head injured patients who have developed seizures have their first attack within two years following injury. In one study, veterans who survived penetrating brain wounds were at risk for epilepsy from 10 to 15 years postinjury (Weiss, et al., 1986). Even after 10 or 15 years, this risk is still 25 times higher than in the general age-matched population (Salazar, et al., 1985).

The frequency of post-traumatic seizures is variable, ranging from one or two seizures per year to one or more attacks per day. Post-traumatic epilepsy can occur in virtually any degree of severity as well, with the more serious cases resulting in complete disability.

From 25 to 50 percent of patients with post-traumatic epilepsy begin to have less frequent and less severe attacks approximately two to three years after the traumatic injury. This regressive pattern is more common in patients whose attacks began relatively soon after injury, as compared with those in whom there was a delay of a year or more in the onset of seizures.

In general, the diagnosis of epilepsy may be difficult to make, because it is based on clinical observation of an attack plus knowledge of the patient's medical history. Key to the diagnosis are the history, the physical examination, laboratory studies, x-rays and electroencephalogram (EEG) results.

Susceptibility to seizures does not necessarily indicate brain damage that is severe enough to affect mental ability. When they are adequately treated, individuals with post-traumatic epilepsy may have no clinically significant symptoms at all other than a heightened tendency to develop paroxysmal electrical brain activity, for which they must receive medication.

11.31   History and Physical Exam

Seizures are diagnosed primarily by history. Ideally but rarely, the seizure is witnessed by the examiner. When this is not possible, a complete description is fundamental to the diagnosis. In an outpatient setting, it may be helpful to contact the patient prior to the initial evaluation and ask for observations made by witnesses during the attack. If possible, the observer should accompany the patient for the office visit.

The goal of the history is to obtain a precise description of the episode. If the initial history is vague because the patient tends to be forgetful, the examiner should ask the patient and witness to observe carefully and to immediately record their findings after future episodes. Precise instructions should be given by the physician. These include asking the observer to test the patient's responsiveness (for example, "Show me your left thumb") and memory (for example, "Remember the color yellow") if there is uncertainty about the integrity of these functions during the episode (Devinsky, 1990).

Physical examination, especially a complete neurologic examination, is essential and may provide important etiologic clues. A family history should also be elicited, including, of course, any occurrences of epilepsy.

11.32   Electroencephalography (EEG)

The electroencephalogram (EEG) is a recording of the electrical activity of the brain obtained from electrodes attached to the surface of the scalp. It should be noted that the EEG most accurately depicts the superficial areas of the brain and thus has the disadvantage of providing a relatively inadequate look at any deeper structural abnormalities.

EEG is harmless and noninvasive and remains the most important of the laboratory tests in the study of seizure patients. A different spectrum of usefulness exists for each EEG technique to be discussed.

The routine laboratory EEG is usually the first electrographic test ordered in the evaluation of patients with presumed epilepsy. Relative to other types of EEG, it is easy to perform, can be accomplished quickly, provides data that are easily and rapidly interpreted, is readily available and is relatively inexpensive.

Unfortunately, the relatively short duration of a standard EEG is not well suited to detecting infrequent paroxysmal abnormalities. Studies of a population of known epileptics have revealed that only about 50 percent of them will show epileptiform abnormalities on an initial routine EEG. This percentage is higher among those with primary generalized epilepsy and lower among those with secondary partial seizure disorders (Ebersole, 1990). Repeated routine EEGs increase the possibility of identifying epileptiform features. However, misleading results occur frequently enough to suggest that EEG findings be considered only as one component in the overall assessment of the patient.

Misleading results may be due to technical problems, such as loose electrodes and poor electrode-skin contact; eye and eyelid movement and muscle twitches may also produce false results.

In order to optimize the detection of abnormalities on the EEG recording, several procedures may be used to enhance epileptic activity. Chief among these techniques are hyperventilation, photic (light) stimulation and sleep deprivation.

Hyperventilation is particularly useful in precipitating some seizures, especially those characteristic of absence epilepsy, in patients with primary epilepsy. It is less useful in generalized and focal convulsive epilepsies (Ebersole, 1990).

Photic stimulation is useful in a smaller group of patients whose seizures are photosensitive. In these patients, a strobe light is used to enhance the recording.

Lack of sleep is a general activator of epileptiform discharges in most, but not all, epilepsies. Depriving the patient of sleep the night before the test not only increases the chance of the patient falling asleep in the lab (an advantage, as movement of the patient distorts the results) but may additionally enhance epileptiformic activity.

11.33   EEG Findings in Head-Injured Patients

Patients with recent head injuries present special problems in recording satisfactory EEG tracings. Because the patient may be restless, disoriented or unable to lie still, the EEG may be adversely affected. Scalp injuries may make electrode placement difficult, and swelling in the injured area may also interfere.

However, the electroencephalogram is helpful in many phases of the evaluation of the head-injured patient. In the acute phase, specific EEG patterns are found. These include partial or complete suppression of the usual (alpha) rhythm in a focal region of the head, even after only mild injury. Bilateral disturbances of this rhythm occur with more severe head trauma. Recovery of the normal pattern may take weeks or months.

The EEG can also be helpful in monitoring the process of head-injured patients in the recovery period. Clinical signs of a fluctuating course with increasing degrees of coma, or failure of the expected recovery to take place, raise the possibility that a subdural hematoma (collection of blood, or clot, under the outermost membrane covering the brain) is developing. The EEG can be helpful in clarifying this situation.

In the 1930s, when the EEG was first introduced into clinical practice, it was hoped that this method would offer a reliable guide in predicting which patients would develop late post-traumatic epilepsy. This hope has not been fulfilled. Although, as a general rule, EEG tracings do show initial changes after head injury, the findings tend to normalize within a few weeks or months. In some patients, the EEG does not completely normalize, but this residual abnormality does not correlate with the development of late post-traumatic epilepsy. Thus EEG findings are of little or no use in predicting the development of late post-traumatic epilepsy.

11.34 X-rays and Computed Tomography (CT)

The use of x-rays to determine the presence and extent of lesions such as skull fractures that may be responsible for seizures has gradually been superseded by computed tomography (CT). CT scanning, which creates a series of x-ray pictures along many planes that is then integrated by a computer, is rapid and painless, and it exposes the patient to much less radiation than contrast studies, involving the injection of a dye to identify lesions on x-ray. As with PET scanning,[5] CT visualizes the image in slices and thus can locate an abnormality precisely.

____

[5] *See* 11.36[3] *infra.*

11.35 Laboratory Studies

Laboratory studies are directed at specific diagnostic considerations. Blood chemistries and cell counts are routinely performed but rarely helpful (Devinsky, 1990). If a metabolic or toxic cause is suspected, blood and urine studies at or near the time of the episode provide the most information (Devinsky, 1990).

The examination of cerebrospinal fluid (CSF) was at one time routinely performed upon suspicion of epilepsy. However, it was found not to be helpful and is generally not done anymore.

11.36 Other Diagnostic Techniques

Several techniques that go beyond routine laboratory recording and classic encephalogram have been developed in the last few years. The majority of them provide a more precise localization of epileptic foci. Therefore, their use is contributing to the understanding and treatment of seizure disorders.

[1] Twenty-four-hour EEG and Videotape Recording

Individually, both 24-hour ambulatory EEG (AEEG) and videotape monitoring of patient behavior add significantly to epilepsy diagnosis. Combining the two can be even more productive (Ebersole, 1990). New video technologies and inexpensive portable cameras and recorders have made this combination of AEEG and videotape recording an attractive and easily accomplished method of diagnosis.

To the extent that patients are willing or able to stay within view of the camera, valuable information can be gathered. The only technical necessity is that the cassette EEG tape and the videotape of patient behavior must be synchronized so that temporal correlations can be made. A videotape record of the patient allows a more accurate classification of seizure types and may help differentiate pseudoseizures (psychologically induced epilepsy)[6] (Ebersole, 1990; Leroy, et al., 1988).

[2] Intracranial Electroencephalography

Intracranial electroencephalography, also known as depth electroencephalography, entails inserting fine wires with multiple electrodes

---

[6] *See* 11.37[8]*infra.*

into the brain for monitoring, in conjunction with 24-hour videotaping of seizure activity. Electrographic sophistication reaches its zenith in these endeavors. Much progress has been made over the past few years. At one time, 16-channel recordings were the rule; now 64-channel EEG is the standard (Ebersole, 1990).

Depth electrodes have the advantages of being able to record from structures beneath the surface of the cortex (the outer layer of the brain) that otherwise are relatively inaccessible. Their disadvantages include limited spatial coverage, unless many are inserted in parallel, and the possibility of causing brain damage, such as hemorrhage or infection, during or as a consequence of the electrode insertion (Ebersole, 1990).

Intracranial EEG helps minimize the recording deficiencies of other methods. Several centers are now using this approach routinely.

[3]   Positron Emission Tomography (PET)

Positron emission tomography (PET) imaging is another new diagnostic technique that has facilitated the localization of epileptic foci. It is based on the fact that seizures increase metabolism and blood flow in the involved area of the brain. This change in activity can be detected by using radioactive tracers, much like the traditional brain scan.

The advantage over the brain scan is that with PET, the image can be visualized in slices, much like a computed tomography (CT) scan, and thus can more precisely locate an abnormality. This technique also has the advantage of sampling a wide area of the brain, including deeper areas that are not usually shown by the superficial EEG. Although results are most impressive if scanning is done during a seizure (an impractical test requirement), interictal (between seizures) PET scans do show depressed activity at seizure foci.

This technique is especially useful for the evaluation of patients who are surgical candidates, mainly those with severe partial seizures. Indeed, the use of PET imaging for the confirmation of lesion sites has increased the number of patients who can be considered for corrective surgical treatment.[7]

---

[7] *See* 11.43 *infra.*

[4]   Magnetic Resonance Imaging (MRI)

Magnetic resonance imaging (MRI) can provide a map of human brain function with high spatial and temporal resolution. At this time, it is the test of choice for anatomically surveying the brain for a seizure workup. A noninvasive imaging technique, MR measures the response of atoms in different tissues when they are pulsed with radio waves while under the influence of a strong magnet. Each type of tissue responds differently, emitting characteristic signals from the nuclei of their atoms. The signals are transmitted to a computer that translates them into a composite picture of the scanned area. Imaging of brain activity by MR depends on the detection of the different changes and dynamics occurring in the brain.

This noninvasive technique has been used to map the cortical activation that occurs during focal seizures (Jackson, et al., 1994). In a four-year-old boy suffering from frequent partial motor seizures of his right side, MRI studies revealed sequential activation associated with specific regions in the left hemisphere of the brain. These activated regions were partially abnormal structurally (Jackson, et al., 1993).

11.37   Conditions That Mimic Epilepsy

A number of conditions, both neurologic and non-neurologic, can be mistaken for epilepsy. Included in this category are syncope, migraine headache and sleep disorders. Various other conditions can be added to this group, such as paroxysmal (epilepsylike) symptoms and isolated seizures, as well as the phenomenon of pseudoseizures, or psychologically induced epilepsy.

Because of the consequences determined by late diagnosis or misdiagnosis of epilepsy, it is extremely important to carefully evaluate patients with suspected epilepsy in order to exclude other possible diagnoses.

[1]   Syncope

Differentiation of syncope from seizure can be difficult; both are common and occur in all age groups. Syncope, also known as fainting, is a transient loss of consciousness resulting from an acute decrease in cerebral blood flow. The condition is often caused by bradycardia (slow heartbeat) or by another irregularity of cardiac rhythm.

The diagnosis of syncope is supported if episodes (1) exclusively occur while the individual is standing or sitting, (2) are precipitated by anxiety or pain, (3) are associated with facial pallor and sweating and (4) are not associated with tonic-clonic movements and tongue biting or postepisode confusion, lethargy and headache (Devinsky, 1990). Although the patient history is usually sufficient to distinguish syncope from seizures, routine as well as ambulatory 24-hour EEG and regular EEG studies may be required for diagnosis.

[2] Migraine Headache

Migraine is a hereditary disorder manifested by predominantly unilateral headaches usually beginning before age 35 years. Classic migraine occurs in 1 percent, and common migraine in up to 10 percent, of the population (Devinsky, 1990).

Classic migraine and the less frequent migraine variants may be misdiagnosed as epilepsy, since both are episodic, paroxysmal disorders with overlapping neurologic symptoms. Migraine, like some forms of epilepsy, is characterized by an aura that is commonly present during the postictal stage of some epileptic attacks. Both migraine and epilepsy may appear in the same patient, especially following head trauma.

The symptoms of basal artery migraine are very similar to those of certain types of epilepsy. They include alterations of consciousness and speech disturbances, and may also include syncope (fainting). In general, the symptoms of unilateral throbbing headache associated with nausea and vomiting strongly suggest migraine, especially when they are supported by a positive family history (Devinsky, 1990).[8]

[3] Sleep Disorders

Certain sleep disorders, such as narcolepsy (sudden, uncontrollable onset of sleep) and cataplexy (sudden onset of muscle weakness), apparently represent rapid-onset, short-lasting abnormal brain activity. Adequate history and sometimes nighttime EEG recording, formal sleep study or overnight ambulatory EEG may be essential to rule out these common sleep disorders.

Seizures may occur only during sleep (Devinsky, 1990). Most generalized epilepsies are enhanced by non–rapid-eye-movement

---

[8] *See also* ch. 10.

(NREM) or slow-wave sleep. Generalized seizures occur predominantly during the first or last hour of sleep, most often during stage 2 NREM sleep, during a transitional stage or upon waking spontaneously.

Drowsiness and induction of NREM sleep is the most useful activator of epileptiform activity in the case of complex partial seizures (Degen and Niedermeyer, 1984). Sleep deprivation undoubtedly precipitates seizures (Gunderson and Dunne, 1973).

[4] Hyperventilation Syndrome

The onset of rapid, irregular breathing often has an emotional etiology. It may lead to syncopal loss of consciousness as well as tachycardia (rapid heartbeat), paresthesia ("pin-prick" and other abnormal sensations), dizziness, blurred vision and precardiac pain.

Rebreathing expired air (carbon dioxide) from a paper bag sometimes helps relieve these symptoms promptly. They are usually self-limiting and terminate spontaneously.

[5] Hypoglycemia

A sudden change in body chemistry resulting in hypoglycemia (low blood sugar level) may produce symptoms that appear superficially similar to epilepsy. Hypoglycemia causes episodic dizziness, tremulousness, stupor, coma, confusion, bizarre behavior, seizures and sudden hemiparesis (paralysis on one side of the body).

A typical hypoglycemic episode involves a feeling of nervousness and hunger, accompanied by sweating. In exceptional cases, unconsciousness and seizures occur, marked by gradual and insidious onset.

[6] Other Paroxysmal Symptoms

Paroxysmal (resembling epilepsy) symptoms include periodic attacks of spasms or seizures that manifest as convulsions. Certain neurologic disorders, such as parkinsonism,[9] multiple sclerosis and dissociative disorders, exhibit paroxysmal symptoms.

[7] Isolated Seizures

The first occurrence of a single seizure in the absence of injury or other known possible cause should be evaluated carefully as a possible

---

[9] *See also* ch. 12.

symptom of a serious disorder. However, a single seizure (or even two or three) following head injury does not necessarily suggest that epilepsy will persist. The transient pathophysiologic disturbance may account for the seizure episode; later seizures may reflect a scarring process that will usually give rise to traumatic epilepsy.

[8]   Pseudoseizures (Psychologically Induced Seizures)

Malingering is the term applied to a conscious effort to deceive the physician by contending that illness is present. Individuals may fake an attack of epilepsy in order to manipulate the outcome of unpleasant interpersonal situations or to attract attention or sympathy. Another reason for such behavior may be financial gain as a result of pending litigation. A minority of patients with pseudoseizures have real epileptic seizures.

In general, these pseudoattacks very closely resemble authentic epileptiform episodes. The clue to malingering can be seen when the patient gently lowers himself or herself to the floor, an action that is not at all typical of a true tonic-clonic episode. In addition, the autonomic symptoms of true motor seizures—sweating, salivation and pupillary changes—cannot be feigned, and the classic EEG findings of true epilepsy are absent in the malingerer.

Pseudoseizures are also characteristic of Münchausen syndrome, a chronic form of factitious illness in which the motive is obscure (Devinsky, 1990). Patients present for treatment with severe and emergent illnesses. Self-mutilation is common, and scars from multiple abdominal or even cranial operations may be present (Devinsky, 1990; Ireland, et al., 1967). Pseudoseizures and other neurologic disorders occur in both childhood and adult cases of Münchausen's syndrome.

11.40   TREATMENT

The ultimate goal of treatment is to eliminate or reduce the frequency and severity of seizures. Anticonvulsant medications remain the treatment of choice for most forms of epilepsy. Neurosurgery, designed to eliminate the epileptogenic brain tissue, has been helpful in some cases of refractory seizures. There has also been an attempt to prevent the onset of seizures in patients with head injury by giving them anticonvulsant medications prophylactically, that is, before symptoms appear.

11.41   Prophylaxis in Patients with Head Injury

Prophylaxis is the process of guarding against the development of a specific disease by an action or treatment that affects its pathogenesis. Anticonvulsant drugs have been widely used in the hope of preventing the development of persistent seizures following head trauma.

A 1972 survey of neurosurgeons indicated that more than 60 percent were recommending anticonvulsant medication as prophylaxis for epilepsy after head trauma (Hauser, 1990; Rapport and Penry, 1972), and the percentage is likely to be higher now (Hauser, 1990). However, although prevention of acute seizures that occur after head injury is a practical goal, such treatment is not likely to have a prophylactic effect against later development of epilepsy (Willmore, 1993). For example, phenytoin, the most used prophylactic medication, exerts a beneficial action by reducing seizures only during the first week after severe head injury (Temkin, et al., 1990).

11.42   Anticonvulsant Medications

Most available antiepileptic drugs are used for the purpose of preventing recurrent seizures rather than having a specific effect on the course of epilepsy. They also have some degree of side effects. The selection of a drug frequently is made by assessing the best balance between adequate seizure control and an acceptable degree of side effects.

Although serious systemic or life-threatening side effects would, of course, be unacceptable to all patients, those of lesser severity may have differing importance to specific individuals (Mattson, 1990). For example, fatigue may be tolerable to one person and unacceptable to another, whereas mild cognitive disturbances may be a major problem for the first person and of little importance to the second. It is important to recognize all these variable issues in selecting a drug that corresponds to individual needs.

The choice of medication is also dependent on other factors, including the patient's age, prior experience with medication and any drug allergies. Some medications are contraindicated during pregnancy. Concomitant non-neurologic pathology, such as liver disease, may also affect the choice of medication, as most anticonvulsants are metabolized by the liver and may be poorly tolerated in the presence of liver disease.

In most cases, generic forms of anticonvulsant medications should be avoided, as these drug forms have not been studied in drug trials. Seizure breakthroughs may occur more often with generic anticonvulsants, due to differing bioavailabilities, absorption and drug interactions (Gilman, et al., 1993; Hartley, et al., 1990).

[1] Establishing a Drug Regimen

There are varied approaches to initiating drug therapy. The older view that polytherapy (starting off with more than one anticonvulsant drug) was best is now being replaced by a preference for monotherapy (single drug treatment), adding a second medication only after going to the maximum limit of the first without evidence of adequate response. The rationale behind monotherapy is the increasing awareness of drug interactions as well as considerations of patient compliance (factoring in problems such as the well-known difficulty of taking more than one medication according to directions).

In addition, side effects are more likely to develop as the number of medications increases. However, in some cases, two anticonvulsants may act synergistically, thus producing a greater overall therapeutic effect than either medicine would if taken alone.

An important distinction needs to be made about the effectiveness of monotherapy in patients suffering from idiopathic epilepsy versus those who are affected by symptomatic epilepsy. Approximately 80 to 85 percent of patients having seizures associated with idiopathic epilepsy can be controlled with monotherapy based on the administration of valproate or ethosuximide (Mattson, 1990). In contrast, complete control is less commonly achieved in the treatment of partial and secondary generalized seizures due to symptomatic epilepsy (Mattson, 1990). For these patients, when optimal trials of single drugs provide inadequate control, unacceptable side effects or both, a combination of two drugs should be attempted.

[2] Dosage

Another aspect of anticonvulsant therapy is the amount of medication. In general, it is best to start at a low (subtherapeutic) dosage and gradually increase to the effective (maintenance) dosage. This minimizes the side effects, so that the patient gradually becomes increasingly tolerant to the medication.

This approach is also important because the plasma clearance (elimination) rate of some of these medications is initially lower in patients who have never been on the medication before. It can take time for a patient's liver to build up the enzymes necessary to adequately eliminate the medication and thus not reach toxic levels. This approach is not appropriate in the emergency treatment of status epilepticus, in which large loading doses are necessary.

Fortunately, there is no need to continually increase the dosage once an effective treatment regimen is obtained, as most patients do not develop a tolerance for these medications. There is a crucial need for patients to be monitored by a physician, however, particularly during the initial phase of treatment. The physician should inquire about seizure frequency, any complaints of drug side effects and the effect of the illness on the patient's psyche, life-style and relationships. Physical examination and appropriate laboratory tests are essential, including, in some cases, blood count and liver or kidney function tests, which may reveal adverse consequences of medication.

In addition, monitoring of anticonvulsant drug levels can be extremely helpful for the following reasons:

- to adjust dosage to therapeutic range;
- to determine baseline level in well-controlled patients;
- to adjust to fluctuations due to metabolic changes, as during pregnancy or a disease state;
- to determine possible interactions with other medications; and
- to assure compliance with the prescribed regimen.

The timing of drug level tests is crucial and depends on the way the body metabolizes the specific medication. For some, an accurate test can be performed one or two days after initiation of the medication or new dosage. For drugs with slower rates of metabolism, it takes much longer for the drug to reach a steady level; in these instances, optimal timing for checking a drug level may be one or two weeks after initiation of a new dosage.

[3] Specific Medications

Many anticonvulsants, with the notable exception of valproic acid, are chemically related to either phenobarbital or phenytoin.

[a] Phenobarbital

Phenobarbital has been used to control seizures since 1912. It has a broad spectrum of efficacy, and it is particularly appropriate in treating neonatal seizures; its use is limited in adults because of its sedative qualities and its potential for triggering dependence. It is no longer a drug of first choice but is still considered effective, relatively safe and inexpensive (Mattson, 1990). The drug is also commonly used for febrile seizure prophylaxis.

As it is absorbed, metabolized and eliminated very slowly, phenobarbital has the longest half-life of any of the anticonvulsants, averaging four to five days. This long half-life permits once-a-day dosing and minimizes the effect of an occasional missed dose (Scheyer and Cramer, 1990).

The drug is metabolized primarily in the liver, so caution is required with patients suffering from liver disease. Side effects are usually dose related and include irritability, loss of concentration, sedation and sleep disturbances.

Children may respond with hyperactivity. Children with absence seizures who are given phenobarbital inadvertently may experience an increase in the frequency of seizures. The elderly are more susceptible to side effects at lower dosages, which may appear as confusion, depression or restlessness. At higher dosages, symptoms of toxicity include slurred speech, staggered gait and nystagmus (involuntary movements of the eye).

Respiration must be monitored when using high dosages, such as in the treatment of status epilepticus. Long-term side effects are uncommon but may include impotence or rashes. As with all anticonvulsants, drug interactions are prominent.

Phenobarbital is also used as a recreational drug; therefore, if a patient keeps returning for frequent medication refills, the provider should consider the possibility of abuse. The drug is also often an attractive vehicle for suicide. These considerations must be kept in mind whenever it is prescribed.

[b] Phenytoin

Phenytoin (Dilantin®) was developed in the 1930s and is still a very widely prescribed anticonvulsant medication. Chemically related to the barbiturates, it is one of the drugs of choice for generalized tonic-clonic seizures as well as for the treatment of status epilepticus. It is usually not helpful in petit mal seizures, however. When other first-line medications fail, phenytoin is frequently prescribed as an alternative choice in the treatment of other seizure types.

Phenytoin has been widely used in the past few years for seizure prophylaxis in post-trauma cases. In fact, the drug reduces the occurrence of seizures in patients at risk during the first week after severe head injury (Temkin, et al., 1990). However, phenytoin doesn't seem to interfere with the process through which unprovoked seizures develop after the acute effects of brain trauma have worn off (Temkin, et al., 1990). Although early administration of loading doses of intravenous phenytoin to patients with severe head injury may be warranted to prevent early seizures and their complications, prolonged therapy after stabilization does not seem justified (Hauser, 1990).

The body's metabolism of phenytoin is complex, involving elimination through both a hepatic (liver) and a renal (kidney) component. Thus caution must be used when treating patients with either liver or kidney disease. The time required for elimination of half the drug accumulated in the body (half-life) will depend on the concentration of drug in the body. The half-life of this drug, nominally 24 hours, may actually range from 8 hours to 3 days in a young, healthy patient and longer in an elderly patient or one with significant hepatic disease (Scheyer and Cramer, 1990).

The side effects of phenytoin are numerous and may be divided in two categories: dose-related and allergic. Dose-related effects include nystagmus (abnormal eye movements), slurred speech, dizziness, delirium, ataxia (muscular incoordination, resulting in irregularity of muscular movements) and lethargy. Allergic side effects are more unusual and may include an acute reaction (with such signs as rash, fever, swollen lymph glands and, at times, abnormal white blood cell count, or leukopenia) approximately one week after initiation of the medication. More unusual reactions can include severe hepatitis (liver infection) or lupus erythematosus (inflammation of skin); the outcome may be fatal.

Long-term side effects are often very bothersome. Cosmetic ones include darkening and increased amount of facial hair and coarsened facial features, which can be especially troubling to women. Acne also occurs. Gingival hyperplasia (overgrowth of the gums) is common. In its mild form, it can be managed solely with good oral hygiene;

more severe forms may result in loss of teeth, requiring oral surgery. Other side effects include peripheral neuropathy (nerve disorder) and folate (a B vitamin) deficiency, which may result in a serious form of anemia. Glucose and thyroid hormone metabolism may be impaired.

[c]　Primidone

Also known by the brand name Mysoline®, primidone is a type of barbiturate. It has the same indications for use as phenobarbital, that is, as an alternative drug for generalized tonic-clonic seizures. Primidone is not used for status epilepticus. In addition, it is thought by many to be a drug of choice for treating complex partial seizures (in the same rank as carbamazepine).

Primidone's anticonvulsant effect is due both to the drug itself and to its active metabolites (by-products created as it is metabolized by the body): phenyl-ethyl-malonamide (PEMA) and phenobarbital. Its metabolism is thus complex, with each of the three components having a different half-life.

Side effects include drowsiness, loss of concentration and irritability. Decreased libido and potency are most reported with use of primidone and often improve with a change to other anticonvulsants (Mattson, 1990). The use of primidone has also been associated with a variety of connective tissue disorders, such as generalized aches and pains and frozen shoulder (Mattson, 1990). Toxic reactions with high dosages include dizziness, vertigo (sensation of spinning), diplopia (double vision), nystagmus, ataxia (lack of muscular coordination) and nausea.

[d]　Ethosuximide

Ethosuximide (Zarontin®) was introduced in 1958 and is a drug of choice, side by side with valproate, for absence epilepsy. It has no other uses.

Ethosuximide metabolism is linear: The rate of elimination decreases markedly with age (Scheyer and Cramer, 1990). The half-life is 30 hours in children and 60 hours in adults (Scheyer and Cramer, 1990). The dosage may need to be decreased as patients age, and once-daily dosing is possible for adults. However, this drug is seldom used to treat adults, as they rarely experience absence seizures.

Side effects are numerous and include headache, sedation, dizziness, nausea, vomiting and hiccups. Some children manifest psychiatric symptoms, including lack of initiative, euphoria, agitation, nightmares and paranoid delusions, the latter being more common in those with mental retardation. Rarer reactions include hematologic changes, such as thrombocytopenia (abnormally low number of platelets in the circulating blood) and leukopenia (abnormally low number of white blood cells), lupuslike syndromes and rashes, each of which may necessitate discontinuation of the medication.

[e] Carbamazepine

Carbamazepine (Tegretol® and others) is recommended for treatment of generalized tonic-clonic seizures and for partial seizures. Intolerance to the drug can often be avoided by starting at a low dosage and increasing the amount taken at weekly intervals until reaching the usual maintenance dosage.

Carbamazepine can cause drowsiness, blurred vision, nausea, vomiting and several kinds of rashes. Mild transient leukopenia, which does not necessarily require stopping treatment, is fairly common. Aplastic anemia (low red blood cell count) may also occur. Carbamazepine is carcinogenic and teratogenic (causes birth defects) in rats and may be teratogenic in humans.

[f] Valproate

Valproate (Depakene®) is currently approved by the U.S. Food and Drug Administration (FDA) only for the treatment of absence seizures, but because it is effective and usually well tolerated, it is also widely used for many other types of seizures, including primary generalized tonic-clonic, myoclonic and atonic seizures, and for patients with more than one form of generalized seizures (Abramowicz, 1991). The drug may also be useful for the treatment of partial seizures.

Drowsiness due to valproate alone is usually slight and temporary, and cognitive effects are minimal. Serious adverse effects of the drug are uncommon, but fatal liver failure has occurred rarely, particularly in children less than two years old who were taking valproate in addition to another anticonvulsant. Pancreatitis (inflammation of the pancreas) can also occur.

More common side effects include nausea and vomiting, which may be minimized by using the enteric-coated formulation, divalproate sodium (Depakote®), or by taking the drug with food. Other side effects include hair loss, insomnia, weight gain, rash, tremor, leukopenia, red blood cell aplasia (malformation) and thrombocytopenia.

Congenital malformations have been reported in children born to women who took the drug during pregnancy (Abramowicz, 1991).

[g]   Benzodiazepines

Used primarily in the field of psychiatry for the treatment of anxiety disorders, this class of drugs does play a small role in the treatment of epilepsy. The three drugs in this class are diazepam, clonazepam and lorazepam.

Diazepam (Valium®) is excellent for the treatment of status epilepticus, especially of the generalized type but also for other forms as well, including myoclonus and absence epilepsy; long-term oral use is generally not helpful for epilepsy.

The response to intravenous (IV) administration is rapid and occurs in less than one minute. Diazepam is metabolized into two by-products. Its half-life is complex, dependent on the half-life of each of the metabolites: the first is 7 to 10 hours; the second, two to six days.

The most common side effects are fatigue and drowsiness. Less common side effects include nausea, constipation, hematologic (pertaining to blood) and hepatic (liver) toxicity, hypotension (low blood pressure), decreased libido and impotence, rashes, muscular spasticity and urinary retention. Neurologic adverse reactions are numerous and include ataxia, headache, tremor, depression, diplopia (double vision), vertigo, confusion, slurred speech, insomnia, hallucinations and anxiety. Excessively rapid intravenous infusion can cause respiratory arrest.

Clonazepam (Clonopin® and Klonopin®) is indicated for absence epilepsy when other drugs fail. It is also used for myoclonic and atonic epilepsy and infantile spasms. Clonazepam has a side effect profile similar to that of diazepam. Lorazepam (Ativan®) has not received FDA approval, but most academic epilepsy programs advocate its use for status epilepticus.

[h]   Felbamate

Felbamate was approved in 1993 for monotherapy and adjunctive therapy for the treatment of partial seizures in adults and for these seizure types in children with Lennox-Gastaut syndrome (an epilepsy type that occurs only in children) (Harden, 1994). Based on preliminary data, the drug may be useful for other seizure types.

Felbamate was synthesized as a potential sedative in the context of an extensive program that also produced therapeutic treatment of anxiety disorders (Harden, 1994). Felbamate seems safe and effective. Although the drug does not cause serious toxicity, in some patients, it may cause headache, nausea, insomnia and anorexia (loss of appetite) with weight loss. A few cases of aplastic anemia have been reported. Its side effects may be managed by decreasing co-medication when it is used in adjunctive therapy.

[i]   Gabapentin

A recently developed antiepileptic drug, gabapentin was first marketed in January 1994 as adjunctive therapy for the treatment of partial and secondary generalized seizures in adults (Harden, 1994). A monotherapy trial is currently underway.

Although it is still being evaluated, scientific evidence suggests that the best use of gabapentin will be in partial seizure disorders (Harden, 1994). The drug is generally well tolerated but requires multiple daily doses. A major advantage of gabapentin is its lack of interaction with other antiepileptic drugs, which permits easier use and eliminates the unwanted additive side effects commonly associated with the administration of multiple antiepileptic medications.

[j]   Lamotrigine

Lamotrigine (Lamictal®) is the most recent of the new antiepileptic agents to be released in the United States. Lamotrigine is unrelated chemically to currently marketed antiepileptic medications. It inhibits the release of glutamate and blocks activation of voltage-sensitive sodium channels (Matsu, et al., 1993).

Lamotrigine is an add-on therapy for adult patients who have breakthrough or refractory partial seizures (Schapel, et al., 1993). A third of patients who receive 500 mg per day of lamotrigine had a 50 percent reduction in seizure frequency. The drug is well tolerated, and patient compliance is improved with the twice-daily regimen. The adverse effects with Lamictal® include dizziness, diplopia (double vision), blurred vision, nausea, vomiting and fatigue. Advantages include the lack of association with adverse effects as demonstrated in blood chemistry assays, electrocardiograms, hematology workups, or when used with other anticonvulsant medications.

[4] Drug Interactions

When two or more drugs are administered concurrently or within a short amount of time, they may interact in numerous ways. Possible results include an increase or a decrease in the clinical effects of the drugs, or an unexpected reaction.

In addition, a very abbreviated list of drugs that interact with phenytoin would include oral contraceptives, many antibiotics, steroids, oral anticoagulants, theophylline (an asthma medication), cimetidine (an ulcer drug), folic acid (a vitamin) and lithium (a psychiatric medication). Similar side effect reactions of the other anticonvulsants are being discovered each day; the prudent practitioner will consult the literature prior to prescribing any new regimen.

[5] Compliance

As in all chronic diseases, the issue of compliance (the extent to which a patient follows the regimen prescribed by the physician) comes into play with treatment of epilepsy. Patients with generalized epilepsy are less likely to comply with treatment than are those with partial seizures. The reasons for poor compliance are numerous. People with epilepsy have varied responses to their illness, which include denial and self-destructive behavior. Some patients feel that they can conquer it on their own, without medication; for some, the mere taking of anticonvulsants seems a sign of weakness.

The numerous bothersome side effects associated with anticonvulsant medications decreases patient compliance. Common side effects such as drowsiness and lack of concentration may interfere with the patient's ability to take medication as prescribed. Cosmetic effects of phenytoin, such as growth of excessive facial hair or gingival hyperplasia, can lead patients to discontinue the medication on their own or decrease the dosage to a subtherapeutic level.

[6] Discontinuation of Medication

In treating patients with epilepsy who have been seizure-free for some time while taking antiepileptic medications, the question of whether to discontinue medications inevitably arises. Several studies have reported on the outcome of discontinuing therapy in children and adults after a seizure-free period. There is a general agreement that most children who are seizure-free for several years while they are on antiepileptic drug therapy will remain so when medications are withdrawn, but there is less agreement about the risk of relapse for adults (Berg and Shinnar, 1994), with recurrence rates ranging from 20 percent to 70 percent in various population studies. Whether one can successfully identify risk factors, such as etiology, age at onset and electroencephalogram (EEG) findings, that would reliably distinguish patients with a favorable prognosis for remaining seizure-free from those with a high probability of relapse is still a matter of controversy.

[7] Issues in Pediatric Therapy

Anticonvulsant medication poses many problems for children. Because of their rapid growth rate and changing metabolism, drug dosages need to be monitored carefully and adjusted accordingly. Some drugs have a paradoxic or opposite effect in children. For example, as opposed to its usual side effect of drowsiness, phenobarbital can cause a hyperactive, restless state in some children.

Adolescence often presents a different treatment problem. Some teenagers, in an effort to strive for independence and to rebel against authority figures, stop taking their medication. Rarely, some abuse their medication, overusing it in an attempt to get high or to commit suicide. Others sell their medication on the street. In addition, the teen years often coincide with the onset of problems with alcohol abuse, which can affect the metabolism of anticonvulsant medication. In addition, the relationship with the physician needs to be redefined at this time, through the adolescent and not through the parent.

11.43 Surgical Treatment Modalities

Surgical procedures are most commonly indicated for individuals with partial epilepsy. When seizures arise because of space-occupying brain lesions, such as brain tumors or hematomas, these masses can be removed.

[1] Indications for Surgery

Among the specific indications for surgery are: (1) recalcitrant cases of epilepsy that do not respond to optimal anticonvulsant medication; (2) seizure frequency that is intolerable; (3) strictly or predominantly unilateral focal lesions; and (4) lesions in surgically accessible areas, where removal will not result in significant neurologic deficits.

Other factors to be considered in selecting a surgery candidate include a normal intelligence level (IQ) and lack of psychiatric illness, diffuse brain damage, generalized seizures or other systemic illnesses.

[2] Location of Seizure Focus

Prior to surgery, it is important to clearly delineate the seizure focus area through some of the available diagnostic methods. Advanced techniques such as simultaneous EEG monitoring and video recording, intracranial electroencephalography and PET (positron emission tomography) scanning[10] are useful in determining the location of the seizure focus. If intracranial EEG is the diagnostic method of choice, the surgery is performed at least one month after this diagnostic session, in order to allow the brain to recover from the trauma of the implanted electrodes.

[3] Surgical Procedure

The most common surgical procedure performed in the treatment of post-traumatic epilepsy is the removal of scar tissue formed on the brain after the injury, commonly called the epileptogenic scar. In the case of psychomotor epilepsy, a standardized surgical removal of the anterior portion of the temporal lobe on one side may be performed. This procedure should be done only in major medical centers with experienced neurosurgeons.

Several complications may occur as a result of the surgery. Profound memory defects, resulting in the need for permanent institutional care, have been reported in some patients. However, the risk of such complications may currently be less, because of advances in diagnostic tools to secure preoperative information.

[4] Results of Surgery

It is expected that any scar tissue formed after surgery will be less epileptogenic than the scar tissue that was created by the head injury or brain disease. However, many surgically treated patients experience a recurrence of epilepsy within a few years of the surgery, with most of the recurrences developing 6 to 12 months postoperatively. Recurrence may be due to reformation of epileptogenic scar tissue or because not all centers of epileptic activity in the brain were excised.

---

[10] *See* 11.36 *supra.*

11.50 PROGNOSIS

It is difficult to make a generalized statement about the prognosis of patients with post-traumatic epilepsy. Each case must be considered individually, since the development and prognosis of the condition depend on the severity of the brain injury. In many cases, the outlook is hopeful, with frequent spontaneous remissions or therapeutic success in controlling symptoms. In the last few years, new medications and some improvement in surgical technique have had a positive impact on the disorder prognosis.

11.51 Long-term Effects of Post-traumatic Epilepsy

Epileptic patients usually face many challenges in managing the symptoms associated with the disorder as well as the consequences that epilepsy may have on their lives. Many patients are often confronted with social and employment obstacles.

Popular and medical opinion about epilepsy has swung from the ancient belief that it was a manifestation of the supernatural to the modern view that it is a disease with natural causes. The ancient Greeks thought of epilepsy as the entry of evil spirits into the body. Indeed, the term *epilepsy* is derived from Greek words meaning "to seize upon, lay hold of, overtake." Early in the eighteenth century, ideas about seizures were especially confused; it was common medical opinion that "hysterical convulsions were simulated epilepsy" (Goldblatt, 1990).

Only when epilepsy became the subject of intensive medical inquiry and its etiology became known did misconceptions regarding the disease began to abate. Yet even today, the sight of an apparently normal, healthy individual suddenly losing consciousness and having violent convulsions may fill the bystander with fear. One commonly held misconception is that people with epilepsy become violent during or after a seizure. In reality, unprovoked aggressive acts are extremely rare during seizures. In addition, seizure activity is usually brief, random and undirected.

Another issue that affects individuals suffering from epilepsy is related to the lack of understanding of the disorder. Epileptic patients are often subjected to discrimination that leads to occupational difficulties and social isolation. Fortunately, in the last few years, some of these misconceptions have been corrected.

11.52   Fertility and Pregnancy Outcome

Epilepsy itself, as well as the medications that are used in its treatment, have a significant impact on reproductive patterns and pregnancy outcome. Individuals suffering from epilepsy, especially those with partial seizures, have a marked reduction in fertility rates.

In addition, maternal epilepsy has been associated with higher rates of malformation in offspring than in the general population (Scolnick, et al., 1994). Another difficulty is that although it is generally agreed that women at risk of seizures during pregnancy should continue to be treated with effective antiepileptic therapy, several of the drugs that are commonly used to treat epilepsy have been documented to be human teratogens.

11.100   Bibliography

Text References

Abramowicz, M. (Ed): Drugs for Epilepsy. In: Drugs of Choice. New York: The Medical Letter, 1991.

Berg, A. T. and Shinnar, S.: Relapse Following Discontinuation of Antiepileptic Drugs: A Meta-Analysis. Neurology 44(4):601–608, 1994.

Caveness, W. F.: Epilepsy, A Product of Trauma in Our Time. Epilepsia 17:207–215, 1976.

Commission on Classification and Terminology of the International League Against Epilepsy: Proposal for Revised Classification of Epilepsies and Epileptic Syndromes. Epilepsia 30:389–399, 1989.

Degen, R. and Niedermeyer, E. (Eds.): Epilepsy, Sleep and Sleep Deprivation. Amsterdam: Elsevier, 1984.

Devinsky, O.: The Differential Diagnosis of Epilepsy. Semin. Neurol. 10(4):321–327, 1990.

Ebersole, J.: Electrophysiologic Methods of Evaluating Epilepsy. Semin. Neurol. 10(4):339–348, 1990.

Farrell, K.: Classifying Epileptic Syndromes: Problems and a Neuro-biologic Solution. Neurology 43(5S):S8-S11, 1993.

Gilman, J. T., et al.: Carbamazapine Toxicity Resulting from Generic Substitution. Neurology 43(12):2435–2436, Dec. 1993.

Goldblatt, D.: The Fooling Sickness—Fictitious, Factitious, or Faked? Semin. Neurol. 10:(4):431-433, 1990.

Gunderson, C. H., et al.: Sleep Deprivation Seizures. Neurology 23:678–686, 1973.

Harden, C. L.: New Antiepileptic Drugs. Neurology 44(5):787–795, 1994.

Hartley, R., et al.: Breakthrough Seizures with Generic Carbamazapine. Dev. Med. Child. Neurol. (Eng.) 32(5)460–462, May 1990.

Hauser, A. W.: Prevention of Post-Traumatic Epilepsy. N. Engl. J. Med. 323(8):540–542, 1990.

Ireland, P., et al.: Münchausen's Syndrome. Am. J. Med. 43:579, 1967.

Jackson, G. D., et al.: Functional Magnetic Resonance Imaging of Focal Seizures. Neurology 44:850–856, 1994.

Jennett, B.: Epilepsy after Head Injury and Craniotomy. In: Godwin-Austen, R. B. and Espir, M. L. E. (Eds.): Driving and Epilepsy. Royal Society of Medicine International Congress and Symposium Series, no. 60. London: Academic Press, 1983.

Jennett, B. and Teasdale, G.: Management of Head Injuries. Philadelphia: Davis, 1981.

Kurtzke, J. F. and Kurland, L. T.: The Epidemiology of Neurologic Disease. In: Baker, A. B. and Joynt, R. J. (Eds): Clinical Neurology. Philadelphia: Harper and Row, 1986.

Leroy, R. F., et al.: Intensive Neurodiagnostic Monitoring in Epilepsy Using Ambulatory Cassette EEG with Simultaneous Video Recording. In: Ebersole J. S. (Ed): Ambulatory EEG Monitoring. New York: Raven Press, 1988.

Luders, H. O., et al.: Expanding the International Classification of Seizures to Provide Localization Information. Neurology 43:1650–1655, 1993.

Mattson, R. H.: Selection of Drugs for the Treatment of Epilepsy. Semin. Neurol. 10(4):406-413, 1990.

Matsuo, F., et al.: Placebo-controlled Study of the Efficacy and Safety of Lamotrigine in Patients with Partial Seizures. Neurology 43:2284–2291, 1993.

Rapport, R. L. and Penry, J. K.: A Survey of Attitudes Toward the Pharmacological Prophylaxis of Post-Traumatic Epilepsy. J. Neurosurg. 38:159–166, 1973.

Salazar, A. M., et al.: Epilepsy after Penetrating Head Injury. I. A Report of the Vietnam Head Injury Study. Neurology 35:1406–1414, 1985.

Scheyer, R. D. and Cramer, J. A.: Pharmacokinetics of Antiepileptic Drugs. Semin. Neurol. 10(4):414–430, 1990.

Schapel, et al.: Double-blind, Placebo-controlled, Crossover Study of Lamotrigine in Treatment Resistant Partial Seizures. J. Neurol. Neurosurg. Psychiatry 56:448-453, 1993.

Scolnick, D., et al.: Neurodevelopment of Children Exposed in Utero to Phenytoin and Carbamazepine Therapy. J.A.M.A. 271(10):767–770, 1994.

Temkin, N. R., et al.: Posttraumatic Seizures. Neurosurg. Clin. N. Am. 2(2):425–435, 1991.

Temkin, N. R., et al.: A Randomized, Double-Blind Study of Phenytoin for the Prevention of Post-Traumatic Seizures. N. Engl. J. Med. 323(8):497–502, 1990.

Thadani, V. M. and Williamson, P. D.: Classification of Epileptic Seizures and Syndromes. Semin. Neurol. 10(4):328-338, 1990.

Weiss, G. H., et al: Predicting Post-Traumatic Epilepsy in Penetrating Head Injury. Arch. Neurol. 43(8):771–773, 1986.

Willmore, J. L.: Post-Traumatic Seizures. Neurol. Clin. 11(4):823–833, 1993.

Willmore, J. L.: Posttraumatic Epilepsy. Neurol. Clin. 10(4):869–878, 1992.

Additional References

Schaumann, B. A., et al.: Family History of Seizures in Post-Traumatic and Alcohol-Associated Seizure disorders. Epilepsia 35(1):48–52, 1994.

Wolff, D. L. and Graves, N. M.: Update on Epilepsy: The LP/VN's Perspective. J. Practical Nurs. 43(4):47–58, 1993.

CHAPTER 12

Parkinson's Disease

SCOPE

Parkinson's disease is a group of neurologic disorders characterized by a gradual decrease and slowing of movement, tremor, muscle rigidity and postural instability. It can be caused by cerebral infarcts, reactions to therapeutic drugs and exposure to toxins, or, among the largest group of patients, arise from an unknown etiology. Risk factors include genetic differences that may affect susceptibility, coupled with exposure to either causative or protective factors. The clinical course varies among affected individuals but most often includes tremor, slowness of voluntary movement, abnormal gait and posture, and rigidity; decrease in cognitive functioning is also common. The most common assessment vehicle is the Hoehn-Yahr scale, which charts patients in five stages from mild to advanced. Diagnosis is based on motor signs. Therapy includes administration of drugs, e.g., levodopa, carbidopa and selegiline, that restore the balance among neurotransmitters, thereby alleviating symptoms but without retarding or preventing the progression of the disease. Adverse drug effects are common. Other therapies include cerebral and adrenal medullary transplantation and fetal tissue transplantation, an issue surrounded by political and ethical controversy in this country.

SYNOPSIS

12.00   INTRODUCTION

Parkinson's disease is a degenerative brain disorder that affects cells needed for normal movement; these cells are located in a part of the brain called the substantia nigra. During the course of the disease, the patient progressively loses the capabilities of appropriate movement and balance. The manifestations vary in type and severity among Parkinson's patients, as does the degree to which cognitive, sensory and autonomic functions are affected.

Despite considerable research and some promising leads, the etiology of Parkinson's disease remains unknown, and to date, there is no cure or any preventive strategy. Treatment focuses on relief of symptoms and attempts to slow or halt the progression of the disease. Treatment is primarily pharmacologic, though a small number of patients have undergone surgical tissue implantation procedures designed to replace lost brain cells.

12.01   Definition

Parkinson's disease is classified as a movement disorder. It is one variety of parkinsonism, a term applied to a group of neurologic disorders characterized by a gradual decrease and slowing of movement as well as by tremor, muscle rigidity and postural instability. Parkinsonian syndrome occurs in association with a number of primary degenerative disorders of unknown etiology.[1] It may also result from a number of known causes (Bannister, 1992).

---

[1] *See* 12.53 *infra.*

One form of parkinsonism of known etiology—arteriosclerotic parkinsonism—is caused by multiple cerebral infarcts (regions of dead or dying tissue as a result of sudden obstruction of blood circulation supplying that part). In the past, parkinsonism frequently developed in people who had had encephalitis lethargica, a viral disease. This form is also known as postencephalitic parkinsonism[2] (Greenberg, 1993). Therapeutic drugs are currently the most common cause of secondary parkinsonism (Bannister, 1992). Exposure to toxins such as manganese and carbon disulfide is another cause (Greenberg, 1993).

Classic Parkinson's disease develops without an obvious cause. Also known as idiopathic parkinsonism or paralysis agitans (Bannister, 1992), this form of the disease affects the largest subgroup of people who have parkinsonism (Uitti and Calne, 1993). Two clinical categories have been described. *Tremor dominant* Parkinson's disease involves earlier onset, slower progression and less cognitive impairment. *Postural instability and gait disturbance* (PIGD) Parkinson's disease develops at a later age, progresses more rapidly and frequently involves dementia (Stacy and Jankovic, 1993).

12.02 History

The specific group of symptoms now called Parkinson's disease was first described by the English physician and geologist James Parkinson in 1817. He described six individuals with tremor, stooped posture and abnormal gait (Coleman, 1992). The word *palsy,* or *paralysis,* refers to the slowness of movement characteristic of this syndrome, which we now call bradykinesia (Lieberman, et al., 1993). The disease was named after Parkinson by the French physician Jean-Martin Charcot in 1861–1862 (Duvoisin, 1992). Although the disease had been defined, its cause remained unknown.

In the early twentieth century, the same group of symptoms was found to afflict survivors of an epidemic of encephalitis lethargica (a viral disease causing inflammation of the brain) that appeared in Europe in 1915 and recurred around the world until 1926. The mortality rate was around 40 percent. Within three to five years, the survivors developed a syndrome involving bradykinesia (abnormal slowness of movement) and muscle rigidity. The similarities between these patients and those with idiopathic Parkinson's disease were so

---

[2] *See* 12.31 *infra.*

great that it became clear that parkinsonism could have more than one etiology.

Postencephalitic parkinsonism was the most common type seen during the 1930s and 1940s. By the 1940s, however, most survivors of the epidemic had died, and cases of postencephalitic parkinsonism are no longer found (Duvoisin, 1992).

By the 1960s, developments in neurologic research enabled investigators to identify the defining lesion of Parkinson's disease as a loss of neurons (nerve cells) in the substantia nigra and to determine that the presence of a sphere called a Lewy body[3] within the dying neurons was a marker for the disease. It was during this time that the most effective drug to date, levodopa, was introduced for treatment (Duvoisin, 1992).

A major breakthrough in Parkinson's disease research occurred in the late 1970s, when some young narcotics addicts injected themselves with a homemade drug intended to be a form of meperidine (Demerol®). This drug contained a substance called MPTP (1-methyl–4-phenyl–1,2,3,6–tetrahydropyridine), which induced all the clinical and neuropathologic features of idiopathic (of unknown cause) Parkinson's disease. Unlike idiopathic parkinsonism, this syndrome was reversible (Lieberman, et al., 1993).

Not only did MPTP-induced parkinsonism suggest that a neurotoxin might be the cause of the idiopathic disease, but it made possible an animal model for research that led to further insights about the pathogenesis of Parkinson's disease (Greenberg, 1993).

12.03 Anatomy and Neurophysiology

Parkinson's disease results from a degenerative process affecting a specific small area of the basal ganglia—the substantia nigra—and resulting in a deficiency of the neurotransmitter (chemical substance that transmits nerve impulses) dopamine.

[1] Basal Ganglia

The principal brain structures involved in movement disorders are the basal ganglia (gray masses of neurons located deep in the cerebral hemispheres and the upper brain stem). The structures comprising the

---

[3] *See* 12.40 *infra.*

basal ganglia include the caudate nucleus and the putamen, which together are referred to as the corpus striatum, and the globus pallidus.

One of four smaller masses of the basal ganglia that lie beneath the corpus striatum in the midbrain is the substantia nigra, so called because the neurons of which it consists are darkly pigmented. An interconnecting neuronal pathway called the nigrostriatal tract links the substantia nigra to the striatum. The nigrostriatal tract depends on the neurotransmitter dopamine for transmission of nerve impulses.

The basal ganglia are part of the extrapyramidal motor system, which also includes the cerebellum, reticular formation and cerebrum. In this system, which regulates reflex movements such as balance and walking, the striatum functions as a motor control center, receiving information about the body's position from different areas in the brain and preparing the motor system to accomplish voluntary movements such as lifting the foot to begin walking. Disturbance of the basal ganglia and nigrostriatal tract therefore leads to movement disorders (Bannister, 1992; Lieberman, et al., 1993).

[2]   Neurotransmission in the Basal Ganglia

Transmission of nerve impulses depends upon the presence of neurotransmitters, chemicals that enable electrical impulses to pass across the synapses (gaps between nerve cells across which transmission occurs). The pigmented cells of the substantia nigra project to the striatum and release the neurotransmitter dopamine, which enables the movement-regulating neuronal activity of the striatum to occur (Ahlskog, 1993). In all types of parkinsonism, degeneration of the nigral cells results in dopamine deficiency.

Another neurotransmitter, acetylcholine, is also found in the corpus striatum. Acetylcholine has an excitatory effect on the neural output from the striatum—that is, it increases the rate of transmission—whereas dopamine has an inhibitory effect. Normally a balance exists between these antagonistic neurotransmitters (Greenberg, 1993).

Dopamine is synthesized in the body from the amino acid tyrosine. An enzyme, tyrosine hydroxylase, converts tyrosine into a precursor substance, levodopa, which then is converted into dopamine by the enzyme dopa decarboxylase. Dopamine is also synthesized by the adrenal glands.

After neural transmission by means of dopamine has occurred, metabolic breakdown of dopamine takes place by means of the enzyme monoamine oxidase B, which is present at the synapse (Lieberman, et al., 1993).

12.10　EPIDEMIOLOGY

Epidemiologic studies indicate that the prevalence of Parkinson's disease may be related to risk factors, including genetic differences that may affect susceptibility, and exposure to either causative or protective factors.

12.11　Prevalence

No matter what methodology is used to estimate it, the prevalence of Parkinson's disease varies considerably across geographic areas, from 31 cases per 100,000 individuals in Libya to 328 per 100,000 in the Parsi community in Bombay (Tanner, 1992a). In the United States, the prevalence is between 1 and 2 cases per 100,000 (Greenberg, 1993). A study in Baltimore found a prevalence of 128 per 100,000, and one in Rochester, Minnesota, found a prevalence of 187 per 100,000. It has been suggested that a different distribution of risk factors—including genetic differences affecting susceptibility and exposure to either causative or protective factors—among different populations may explain this geographic variation (Tanner, 1992a).

12.12　Risk Factors

Parkinson's disease rarely occurs in individuals under the age of 30, and its incidence increases after that age. Most cases begin in people who are between 50 and 60. The disease only rarely develops in individuals older than 65 (Tanner, 1992a; Bannister, 1992).

Slightly more males than females develop the disease. It affects all racial groups, with the highest rates occurring in Europe and North America; the rates are far lower in China, Japan and Africa. In the United States, the rate is much lower among blacks than whites. These figures have been interpreted to mean that whites are more at risk (Tanner, 1992a).

Genetic predisposition appears to be a factor only in some families, although studies of twins have indicated that it is not a prominent factor. The geographic variations in prevalence have suggested the possibility of environmental toxins present in some locations as a risk factor. Finally, it has also been suggested that emotional stress causes changes in dopamine systems in the brain that could be a factor in the development of parkinsonism, though such a relationship would be difficult to establish (Tanner, 1992a).

12.13 Protective Factors

The pathogenesis of Parkinson's disease is thought to involve oxidative mechanisms in the substantia nigra. Hence it is possible that eating foods or supplements containing antioxidative factors prevents the disorder. Two case-control studies found that intake of food rich in tocopherol (an alcohol that has the properties of vitamin E) or of vitamin E, multivitamins or cod liver oil was associated with decreased risk of developing Parkinson's disease (Tanner, 1992a).

Numerous studies have found an inverse relationship between smoking and Parkinson's disease. However, instead of reflecting a biological factor that protects against Parkinson's, decreased smoking may simply be an accompaniment of the more conservative personality type that may develop with the disease (Tanner, 1992a).

12.20 CLINICAL MANIFESTATIONS

The clinical features of the disease have not changed since Parkinson's time. However, its clinical course varies among individuals.

12.21 Symptoms

The person with Parkinson's disease presents a characteristic appearance. The muscles of the face are unnaturally immobile, with staring eyes that move spontaneously only infrequently. The trunk and limbs are somewhat flexed, giving the body a typical stooped posture. As a rule, the limbs are adducted (turned inward) and the fingers flexed (bent) (Bannister, 1993). Four characteristic movement abnormalities are recognized.

[1] Tremor

Tremor occurs in 70 percent of patients who have Parkinson's. It has a frequency of 4 to 6 Hertz (Hz) and is typically greatest at rest, often diminishing or disappearing during voluntary movement. Most often, tremor appears initially in an upper limb, then extends to the lower limb on the same side. The tremor may be confined to one or both of these limbs for months or years before affecting all the limbs.

In the hand or foot, the tremor involves rhythmic flexing and extending. It may also take the form of rhythmic turning of the forearm so that the palm faces up, then down. Additionally, it may involve the area of the face around the mouth (Coleman, 1992; Greenberg, 1993; Bannister, 1992).

[2] Bradykinesia

Also called hypokinesia or akinesia, bradykinesia is the classic and most disabling symptom of Parkinson's disease. It involves a slowness of voluntary movement and a decrease in automatic movements such as swinging the arms while walking. In general, the small muscles are most affected.

Bradykinesia is responsible for the masklike facies (facial appearance) and poverty of gesture of Parkinson's patients. The patient's arms are clumsy, and he or she has trouble performing rapid or repetitive motions and accomplishing tasks that require fine movements, such as handwriting. Speech is slurred, and the voice becomes low in volume and monotonous. The patient has difficulty walking, getting into and out of chairs, and performing two movements at once. Even simple motor tasks require intense concentration. At its worst, bradykinesia results in a total "freezing," in which the patient gets stuck and is unable to move at all (Bannister, 1992; Glendinning and Enoka, 1994; Coleman, 1992; Greenberg, 1993).

[3] Rigidity

Muscular rigidity is a result of increased tone or stiffness, and causes the flexed posture of Parkinson's patients. (*See Figure 12–1.*) Because the muscles resist being passively moved through the entire range of motion of a given joint, this symptom has been called *lead pipe* rigidity. When there are repeated stops as the limb is passively moved, it is described as *cogwheel* rigidity. (*See Figure 12–2.*) This type of interrupted motion is thought to be caused by an underlying tremor that is masked by the rigidity (Greenberg, 1993; Glendinning and Enoka, 1994).

During the early stages of the illness, rigidity may occur only in an upper limb and be evident only when the limb is moved passively.

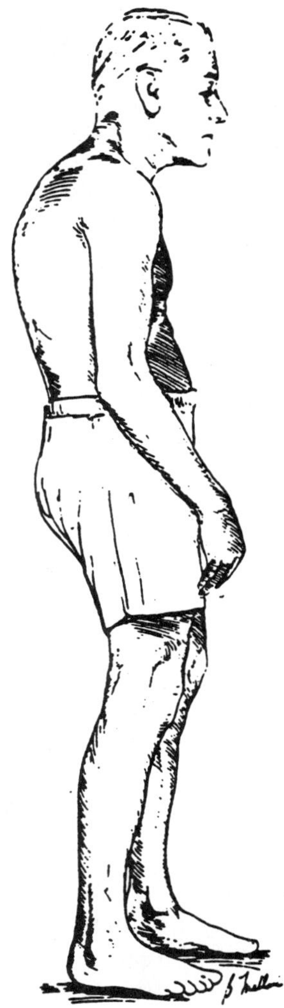

Fig. 12-1 A patient with Parkinson's disease. Note the characteristic flexed position of the arms, legs and trunk.

By the advanced stage, all joints show considerable resistance to passive movement (Bannister, 1992).

[4]   Abnormal Gait and Posture

Often the patient has difficulty beginning to walk and starts by leaning forward and walking in place before actually moving forward. The patient takes short, shuffling steps and tends to speed up, as though trying to catch up to his or her center of gravity to prevent a fall. This

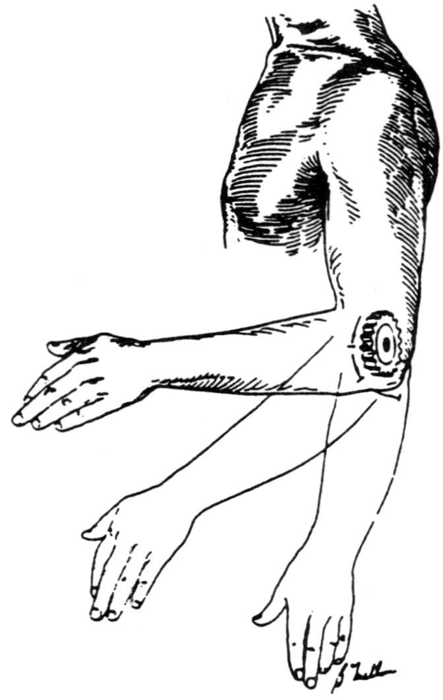

Fig. 12-2 A schematic representation of the "cogwheel" sensation that is felt on extension and flexion of the arm in Parkinson's disease.

is the classic "festinating gait" described by Parkinson (Bannister, 1992; Greenberg, 1993).

Patients may further experience instability when turning during walking as well as difficulty in stopping. This postural instability, along with periodic episodes of freezing, leads to frequent falls in the advanced stages of this illness. Nevertheless, even patients who have considerable difficulty walking can often run very fast (Stacy and Jankovic, 1993; Bannister, 1992; Greenberg, 1993).

[5]　Other Symptoms

Commonly patients at advanced stages experience pains in the spine and limbs and extreme restlessness. Aches and pains result from soreness of the muscles due to rigidity and to holding the body in abnormal postures. Excessive sweating, urinary incontinence and constipation, flushing of the skin, greasiness of the face and drooling (possibly because swallowing is affected) are also seen. Sleep disturbances may be due to rigidity that makes it difficult to relax, or to tremors (Bannister, 1992; Greenberg, 1993; Lieberman, et al., 1993).

12.22   Cognitive Impairment and Dementia

Individuals with Parkinson's disease frequently experience some decrease in cognitive functioning during the illness, although there is controversy as to whether these changes can be categorized as cortical, as in Alzheimer's type dementia, or as subcortical, as in Huntington's disease and progressive supranuclear palsy (Levin, et al., 1992).

Parkinson's disease patients have an increased incidence of dementia, most often caused by co-existing Alzheimer's disease (Coleman, 1992). It has been estimated conservatively that about 15 percent of Parkinson's patients meet the American Psychiatric Association's *Diagnostic and Statistical Manual* (DSM) criteria for dementia. A larger number do not meet these criteria but exhibit milder forms of cognitive impairment (Levin, et al., 1992). These mild impairments can be made much worse by a co-existing disease or the effects of therapeutic drugs (Coleman, 1992).

Cognitive impairment is directly related to the patient's age at onset of the disease. Patients who were over 65 when the disease developed consistently show greater impairment on memory, intellectual and executive functions than younger patients. At the same time, a long duration of the disease does not itself appear to impair cognitive functioning. Studies of the relation of motor symptoms to cognitive function have found consistently that when the major clinical feature is tremor, the mental status is usually normal or close to normal, whereas when bradykinesia and rigidity predominate, they are associated with cognitive decline (Levin, et al., 1992).

Studies of patients with Parkinson's disease have found some deficits in language functions, such as sentence forming, as well as impairment in visuospatial skills, such as facial recognition and judgment of distance. However, there is controversy as to whether the findings related to visuospatial impairment actually represent methodologic problems of the studies (Levin, et al., 1992).

Impairment of memory and of executive function (planning, initiating and overseeing goal-directed behavior) have also been documented in patients with Parkinson's disease (Levin, et al., 1992).

12.23   Depression

Depression is seen in about half of people with Parkinson's disease but may be overlooked unless the patient is asked specific questions to elicit the diagnosis (Coleman, 1992). Since the incidence of depression in Parkinson's disease is higher than in other chronic disabling illnesses, it has been suggested that in addition to the psychological effects of confronting the reality of chronic illness, the changes in brain chemistry associated with the disease may contribute to the development of depression in these patients (Lieberman, et al., 1993).

The majority of cases are mild to moderate in severity. Depression in Parkinson's patientsinvolves loss of appetite, sleep disturbances, impaired concentration and psychomotor retardation. It may take the form of major depression, which is chronic, or dysthymic depression, which is relieved by periods in which the mood is normal (Levin, et al., 1992).

Depression is treated with antidepressant drugs, particularly tricyclics, which include imipramine, nortriptyline and amitriptyline. In some cases, when drug therapy is ineffective, electroconvulsive therapy (ECT) may be considered. ECT has been reported to have antiparkinsonian as well as antidepressant effects (Coleman, 1992).

12.24   Clinical Course

Parkinson's disease begins insidiously, and the initial, subtle signs may not be noticed (Coleman, 1992). Its course is highly unpredictable, varying both in severity and in the rate of progression. At one extreme, mild symptoms are present on one side of the body only, with progression occurring slowly over as long a period as 30 years. At the other, there are cases whose rapid progression over a period as brief as 3 years leaves the patient almost totally incapacitated (Bannister, 1992). In most cases, however, advances in drug treatment have enabled patients to live active, fairly normal lives, although the symptoms will inevitably worsen over time (Lieberman, et al., 1993).

Despite the unpredictability of the course of Parkinson's disease, several rating scales have been devised. Although they cannot completely describe a particular individual's condition, they do sketch the general chronologic course and, by predicting to some extent its progression, help physicians make treatment decisions. The most widely used is the Hoehn-Yahr scale, which describes five stages (Carroll, 1992; Lieberman, et al., 1993). (*See Table 12–1.*) Stages 0 to 2 are considered mild parkinsonism; stage 3 is moderate; and stages 4 and 5 are advanced. As a rule, each stage lasts for years.

Table 12–1

The Hoehn-Yahr Scale of Parkinson's Progression

STAGE	CHARACTERISTICS
Stage 0	No visible symptoms.
Stage 1	Symptoms are present but affect one side of the body only.
Stage 2	Symptoms affect both sides of the body and rigidity becomes more general, but balance is not affected and the patient does not experience immobility. With medication, the patient can lead a normal life.
Stage 3	Balance and walking are affected, festinating gait develops, falls occur. The patient needs some assistance in activities of daily living, and some memory deficits appear.
Stage 4	Balance and walking are seriously impaired, so that the patient needs assistance to rise from a chair and perform such activities as cutting food with a knife. Mobility is considerably restricted.
Stage 5	Rigidity and bradykinesia dominate the clinical picture. The patient is completely immobile, needing a wheelchair and round-the-clock help with daily activities.

12.30 ETIOLOGY

Although a number of causes of secondary parkinsonism are known, the cause of idiopathic Parkinson's disease remains obscure.

12.31 Postencephalitic Parkinsonism

In the case of survivors of encephalitis lethargica,[4] the death of cells in the substantia nigra was secondary to inflammation resulting from the viral infection (Bannister, 1992). Attempts to identify other infectious agents that might cause idiopathic Parkinson's disease have not been successful, although some investigators have raised the possibility that rural residence constitutes a risk factor by exposing people to a virus species called coronavirus (Tanner, 1992a).[5]

12.32 Drug- and Toxin-Induced Parkinsonism

Exposure to various toxic substances can cause parkinsonian syndromes.

[1] Therapeutic Drugs

Many therapeutic drugs, particularly the powerful tranquilizers, have been found to produce a reversible parkinsonian syndrome in some people who take them. Symptoms appear after several weeks of therapy and disappear either weeks or months after the patient stops taking the drug. Medications that have this effect include the phenothiazines (major tranquilizers, including chlorpromazine (Thorazine®)), reserpine (a sedative and blood pressure medication), metoclopramide (an antiemetic) and the butyrophenones (another class of major tranquilizers). These agents either deplete the level of dopamine in the brain or block dopamine receptors in the striatum (Greenberg, 1993; Lieberman, et al., 1993).

[2] MPTP

In one report, the chemical MPTP mistakenly contaminated a "designer drug" produced by addicts trying to create an analogue of meperidine. Within a few days, the addicts developed a severe form of parkinsonism with all the clinical signs of Parkinson's disease and that responded to levodopa treatment. MPTP in itself is not a neurotoxin. Once introduced into the body, however, it is metabolized to 1-methyl–4-phenyl-pyridinium ion (MPP+), a neurotoxin that destroys dopamine-containing neurons in the substantia nigra. The enzyme that catalyzes the conversion is monoamine oxidase B. MPP+

---

[4] *See* 12.02 *supra.*

[5] *See* 12.33[3] *infra.*

is taken up into dopaminergic neurons, where it poisons mitochondria (cell structures involved in the generation of energy from the oxidation of food). The result is death of these pigmented dopaminergic neurons (Bannister, 1992).

Injection of MPTP into primate brains caused the same severe parkinsonism, leading to the hypothesis that an environmental toxin might be a cause of the idiopathic disease. In addition, MPTP provided an animal model that could be used to develop new drugs for treating it (Greenberg, 1993; Bannister, 1992).

[3] Toxins

Parkinson's disease is known to be caused by many types of chemical exposures, including exposure to manganese dust, carbon disulfide and organic solvents. It has also followed severe carbon monoxide poisoning (Tanner, 1992a; Tanner, 1992b; Greenberg, 1993).

12.33 Idiopathic Parkinson's Disease

Genetic factors, normal aging and environmental factors have all been proposed as causes of Parkinson's disease. A number of investigators now hypothesize that causation involves one or more environmental factors acting on a genetic predisposition[6] (Uitti and Calne, 1993).

[1] Aging

It has been suggested that the loss of brain cells during the aging process contributes to the development of Parkinson's disease, possibly as a result of an interaction between depletion of dopamine due to aging and some acute event that causes damage to nigrostriatal cells. However, studies of the rate of dopamine receptor loss in young and old patients, and of the rate of striatal dopamine uptake in normal individuals, have not supported this theory. The results of one study, which found that both those without Parkinson's and those with Parkinson's had the same rate of reduction in dopamine uptake over time, suggest that Parkinson's results from a sudden insult that caused damage in the past rather than from a gradual decrease in dopamine. In general, studies indicate that aging is not a significant factor in the development of Parkinson's disease (Riederer and Lange, 1992).

---

[6] *See* 12.40 *infra* for a description of propounded pathologic processes.

[2]　Genetic Factors

Research has shown that Parkinson's disease can be transmitted through families and that this familial disease is clinically the same as nonfamilial Parkinson's. It appears, however, that heredity is only important in a few families, or that inheritance of Parkinson's disease involves multiple factors, with the actual symptoms depending on the influence of environmental factors.

Studies have not found that identical twins of patients with the disease also develop it, but since familial Parkinson's has been shown to exist, the genetic hypothesis requires further investigation. Because age of onset and clinical manifestations vary considerably within families, it is possible that asymptomatic twins of patients with Parkinson's would show symptoms if they are examined over a long time period. Further, sophisticated diagnostic techniques such as positron emission tomography (PET) may be able to detect a preclinical stage of the disease in clinically unaffected siblings of patients with Parkinson's (Tanner, 1992a; Riederer and Lange, 1992).

[3]　Environmental Toxins

The fact that MPTP and certain other toxins are known to cause parkinsonism suggests that environmental influences may be a factor in the etiology of idiopathic Parkinson's disease. Many pesticides and herbicides are chemically similar to MPTP, and studies indicate that Parkinson's disease is less prevalent in countries that have undergone industrialization more recently. Geographic areas with the highest prevalences are those in which vegetable farming, wood pulp mills and steel alloy industries are present.

Some studies have revealed an association between increased risk of Parkinson's disease and rural residence, well-water drinking and exposure to pesticides and herbicides. It has been suggested that the rural living risk factor may involve exposure to coronaviruses, which affect farm animals such as pigs. Antibodies to these viruses have been found in the cerebrospinal fluid of persons with Parkinson's (Tanner, 1992a; Riederer and Lange, 1992).

Other studies, however, have not shown increased prevalence associated with these risk factors in different geographic areas that have an equal presence of the same chemical-using industries. It is possible that the etiology may involve a toxic agent or a virus affecting a genetically susceptible individual, and that different factors cause

Parkinson's in different people (Riederer and Lange, 1992; Lieberman, et al., 1993).

[4] Trauma

Head injury has been considered a possible cause of Parkinson's disease. However, although retrospective studies show an association between Parkinson's and head trauma, prospective studies—which use data obtained before the disease appears—do not show this association. This indicates that the association may be a result of recall bias, since people who have a chronic illness are more likely to think about the possible relevance of traumatic events in the past (Tanner, 1992a; Riederer and Lange, 1992).

12.40 PATHOLOGY

In all forms of parkinsonism, a dopamine deficiency of approximately 25 percent is present in the putamen, caudate nucleus and substantia nigra (portions of the brain) (Bannister, 1992). In idiopathic Parkinson's disease, pathology examination reveals cell loss and depigmentation in the substantia nigra, cell loss in the putamen and globus pallidus, and the presence of round structures known as Lewy bodies in the basal ganglia, brain stem, spinal cord and sympathetic ganglia. Lewy bodies are considered a marker of Parkinson's disease (Greenberg, 1993). Cell loss increases as the disease progresses (Coleman, 1992).

Research on the neurotoxicity of MPTP[7] has identified several biochemical changes occurring in the brain in patient's with Parkinson's disease that point to a pathogenic mechanism involving selective destruction of dopaminergic neurons and consequent disturbance of the balance between excitatory and inhibitory neurotransmitter systems.

12.41 Defects in Mitochondrial Respiration

MPP+, the toxic product of oxidation of MPTP, is concentrated in mitochondria (cell structures involved in the generation of energy from the oxidation of food), where it poisons an enzyme known as complex I that is important in the process of energy metabolism.

------

[7] *See* 12.32[2] *supra.*

Complex I deficiency has been found in the substantia nigra in patients with idiopathic Parkinson's disease, suggesting a similar pathogenic mechanism to parkinsonism induced by MPTP. It is also possible, however, that complex I deficiency is caused by a genetic defect (Riederer and Lange, 1992).

12.42 Oxidative Stress

Oxidative processes within neurons generate free radicals—groups of atoms that are extremely reactive because they carry an unpaired electron. It is thought that free radicals are produced from the oxidation of MPTP by monoamine oxidase B, the process that synthesizes MPP+, and that monoamine oxidase B may be responsible for the formation of other free radicals as well (Coleman, 1992).

Free radicals can destroy neurons by reacting with the lipids (fats) in cell membranes, thereby damaging the membranes. The free radicals produced by oxidation reactions within the neurons of the substantia nigra may contribute to the development of Parkinson's disease by causing neuronal death. An increase in the level of iron found in the substantia nigra of patients with Parkinson's disease may also contribute to oxidative stress by contributing to the generation of free radicals.

The discovery of disturbed mitochondrial function and free radical formation as possible pathogenetic mechanisms for Parkinson's disease is the basis for the use of neuroprotective treatments, such as the drug selegiline, which inhibits monoamine oxidase B, as well as other antioxidants. These agents may be able to slow the progression of the disease[8] (Riederer and Lange, 1992; Coleman, 1992).

12.43 Changes in Excitatory and Inhibitory Systems

It appears that in idiopathic parkinsonism, the degeneration of dopaminergic neurons and resulting depletion of dopamine disturbs the normal balance in the corpus striatum between inhibitory dopamine and excitatory acetylcholine. As a result, there is a considerable change in neuronal activity, the net result of which is an increased inhibitory output from the basal ganglia to the thalamus. This increased inhibition in turn decreases activation of the cortex, accounting for rigidity and bradykinesia (Riederer and Lange, 1992).

---

[8] *See* 12.65 and 12.66 *infra.*

12.44   Mechanisms Producing Motor Symptoms

Several mechanisms have been proposed to explain the motor symptoms of Parkinson's disease. It appears that the disease alters motor unit behavior. A motor unit consists of one motor neuron (nerve cell) and the muscle fibers it innervates. In people with Parkinson's disease, motor units have inconsistent discharge rates, more motor units are activated at lower contraction forces than in normal subjects and there is more coactivation of motor units.

These changes may be caused by abnormal commands sent to the motor neurons from the motor cortex or from other higher brain centers that received input from the basal ganglia. Another possible mechanism involves disturbance in the normal balance between excitatory and inhibitory stimulation of motor neurons due to degeneration of neurons in the locus ceruleus, thalamus, brain stem, spinal cord and autonomic nuclei, all of which can also be affected by Parkinson's disease. Third, it is possible that abnormal motor unit behavior represents a variation on the process of cell death that is part of normal aging (Glendinning and Enoka, 1994).

12.50   DIAGNOSIS

Since no marker specific to Parkinson's disease has been found, diagnosis is based on motor signs. The cardinal signs are (Stacy and Jankovic, 1993):

- rigidity;
- bradykinesia;
- resting tremor;
- loss of postural reflexes; and
- freezing.

To an experienced clinician, the diagnosis may be apparent from simple observation of a patient. Nevertheless, a complete history and physical, neurologic and motor examination should be performed. Diagnostic imaging may also be used to rule out other conditions that can produce similar symptoms (Lieberman, 1992).

12.51 History and Examination

An important function of the history taking is to elicit early symptoms the patient may have dismissed but that are significant to the clinician (Carroll, 1992). As one expert puts it, statements such as "my hand only begins to shake when I sit down" or "my handwriting has gotten so small that the bank won't cash my check" are almost as diagnostic as finding Lewy bodies (Lieberman, 1992).

In addition to a description of symptoms, the patient history covers general health and medical issues, occupational history (to detect possible exposure to toxic substances) and physical trauma (Carroll, 1992).

Part of the history is a review of the patient's experience with activities of daily living such as speech, turning in bed, swallowing, salivating, falling, walking, cutting food and handling utensils. Parkinson's disease involves changes in personality, perception and behavior that may prevent the patient from recognizing that motor abnormalities exist. In addition, patients who know someone who is extremely disabled due to Parkinson's disease will require reassurance that his or her own case will not necessarily develop the same way.

Thorough and perceptive questioning is important to bring out symptoms the patient may not have recognized as being part of the disease process. One example is turning over in bed; another is salivating from the corner of the mouth at night so that the pillow is wet. Similarly, the patient's ability to write, cut food and carry out personal hygiene depends on whether the disease has affected the dominant hand. To determine whether the nondominant side is affected, the clinician can ask about tasks performed with that hand, such as buttoning the right shirtsleeve for a right-handed person.

The clinician also performs a complete physical and neurologic examination, which includes testing blood pressure while the patient is lying or sitting and then while standing, and testing for tremor, bradykinesia, muscle tone and rigidity, abnormal reflexes and sensory function, and postural stability. For example, in a common test for bradykinesia, the patient is asked to tap the fingers rapidly one after another against the thumb. People with Parkinson's are likely to get stuck on the third or fourth tap. Gait difficulties may be detected by asking the patient to turn while walking (Lieberman, 1992; Carroll, 1992).

Finally, since Parkinson's disease can induce subtle personality, perceptual and behavioral changes, the clinician may also perform a mental status exam. The patient may be asked to count to 30 by threes, be questioned about current events or asked to spell a word backward andforward. It may also become apparent during the history that the patient does not realize that he or she has certain motor difficulties, because of an inability to sense them or because of denial (Carroll, 1992; Lieberman, 1992; Lieberman, et al., 1993).

12.52   Use of Imaging Techniques

Imaging techniques are generally used to rule out other conditions, but one, the PET scan, is capable of detecting dopamine deficiency.

[1]   Magnetic Resonance Imaging (MRI)

Magnetic resonance imaging (MRI; a nonradiographic diagnostic modality that uses magnetic fields, radio waves and atomic nuclei to produce detailed cross-sectional images) is replacing computed tomography (CT) as the preferred modality for ruling out mass lesions, unsuspected strokes or normal-pressure hydrocephalus (Lieberman, 1992).[9] MRI is also capable of detecting the presence of increased iron in the substantia nigra and striatum in nonidiopathic forms of parkinsonism, although it is not currently able to recognize the level of deposition occurring in idiopathic Parkinson's (Lieberman, 1992; Olanow, 1992).

[2]   Positron Emission Tomography (PET)

Positron emission tomography, or the PET scan, is a brain-imaging technique that uses a gamma-ray detector to pick up the radiation emitted by (18F)6-fluoro-L-dopa (levodopa to which a radioactive isotope has been attached), which is introduced into the brain. The resulting image is a picture of the level of uptake of fluorodopa into the striatum.

Studies have found that people with Parkinson's disease have decreased uptake of fluorodopa into the striatum, in comparison with control subjects. However, scanning units are extremely expensive and available at only a few research centers (Shults, 1992).

---

[9] *See* 12.53[8] *infra.*

12.53 Differential Diagnosis

Differentiating idiopathic Parkinson's disease from other parkinsonian syndromes can be difficult. In fact, neuropathologic examination has shown that the clinical diagnosis is correct only about 75 percent of the time. This is partly because the clinical picture of the idiopathic disease can be so variable (Poewe, 1993). In addition, the symptoms of a number of other conditions can be mistaken for parkinsonism.

[1] Essential (Benign) Tremor

This type of tremor occurs in otherwise normal individuals and is often inherited. It may develop as early as the teenage years. Typically it is more rapid than the tremor of Parkinson's, affects the head (causing nodding or shaking) rather than the face and lips as in Parkinson's, but not the legs, and is briefly relieved by drinking a small amount of alcohol (Greenberg, 1993; Stacy and Jankovic, 1993).

[2] Wilson's Disease

Also known as hepatolenticular degeneration, this rare progressive disease is caused by a defect in copper metabolism and can cause a parkinsonian syndrome. Wilson's disease is distinguished, however, by a pigmented ring (the Kayser-Fleischer ring) at the outer edge of the cornea of the eye as well as by abnormalities in levels of serum and urinary copper, and abnormal movements other than those of parkinsonism (Greenberg, 1993).

[3] Huntington's Disease

This progressive hereditary disorder involves abnormal involuntary movements that may resemble parkinsonism if there is rigidity and bradykinesia. However, the true diagnosis is indicated by a family history of the disease or by dementia (Greenberg, 1993).

[4] Shy-Drager Syndrome

Also known as multisystem atrophy, Shy-Drager syndrome is a degenerative condition characterized initially by a disturbance of the autonomic nervous system. It results in postural hypotension (low blood pressure and dizziness when rising to an upright position), impotence and incontinence, followed by parkinsonian symptoms such as rigidity, tremor and bradykinesia, and more general neurologic deficits involving the lower motor neurons (Greenberg, 1993; Lieberman, et al., 1993).

[5] Striatonigral Degeneration

Striatonigral degeneration is a rare condition involving loss of neurons mostly in the putamen, globus pallidus and caudate nucleus of the brain rather than in the substantia nigra. Patients experience rigidity and bradykinesia, though usually not tremor, and this condition can be clinically indistinguishable from Parkinson's disease. However, it does not respond to treatment with levodopa or other antiparkinsonian medications. MRI may detect an increased level of iron in the putamen (Greenberg, 1993; Bannister, 1992; Lieberman, et al., 1993).

[6] Progressive Supranuclear Palsy

This is a degenerative disorder that mostly affects subcortical areas of the brain, resulting in inability to control eye movements, dementia, co-existing pseudobulbar palsy (a condition occurring in individuals with arteriosclerosis that involves small strokes that damage the brain center that controls balance and walking), difficulty speaking, rigidity, bradykinesia and axial (pertaining to the vertebra of the neck) rigidity. Progressive supranuclear palsy responds not at all or poorly to antiparkinsonian drugs (Greenberg, 1993; Lieberman, et al., 1993).

[7] Creutzfeldt-Jakob Disease

Creutzfeldt-Jakob disease is a viral encephalopathy causing degeneration of the pyramidal and extrapyramidal systems (bundles of nerves that move voluntary muscles). There may be some parkinsonian symptoms, but progressive dementia, ataxia (loss of muscle coordination) and jerking muscle contractions are also seen. Electroencephalography (EEG) shows characteristic findings (Greenberg, 1993).

[8] Normal-pressure Hydrocephalus

Normal-pressure hydrocephalus is caused by enlargement of the fluid-containing cerebral ventricles (cavities) of the brain, often after head injury. This condition leads to difficulty in walking that is frequently mistaken for parkinsonism, to dementia and to urinary incontinence. ACT scan can detect the dilation of the ventricles (Lieberman, et al., 1993; Greenberg, 1993).[10]

---

[10] *See also* ch. 5 for further discussion of hydrocephalus, including normal-pressure hydrocephalus.

12.60 DRUG THERAPY

The treatment of Parkinson's disease is pharmacologic. Although some surgical therapies, especially cerebral transplantation techniques,[11] have been performed on a small scale, these procedures are controversial and in any case not generally available. The goal of drug treatment is to restore the balance between dopamine and acetylcholine in the striatum, either by blocking the action of acetylcholine or by enhancing the action of dopamine.

Breakthroughs in our understanding of neurotransmitters have led to great advances in drug therapy for Parkinson's disease, enabling most patients to lead functional lives for many years. For the most part, however, all that drug treatment can accomplish is relief of symptoms. With few exceptions, drugs do not retard or prevent the progression of the disease. Further, these agents cause side effects ranging from annoying to severe; and because their effectiveness decreases with long-term therapy, necessitating an increase in the dosage, the adverse effects frequently also increase in severity.

Several classes of drugs are used in treating Parkinson's disease.

12.61 Anticholinergic Drugs

Anticholinergic drugs relax the smooth muscles and reduce stomach, intestinal, salivary gland and bronchial tube secretions by blocking the excitatory effect of acetylcholine on these organs. The earliest drugs used to treat Parkinson's disease, in the nineteenth century, were extracts of the plant belladonna, whose active ingredients were natural anticholinergics. These agents were originally administered to improve drooling of saliva experienced by Parkinson's patients, and it was noticed that they relieved other disease symptoms somewhat. Subsequently, synthetic anticholinergic drugs were developed (Coleman, 1992).

[1] Types of Drugs Used

Many anticholinergics have been used to treat Parkinson's disease, and different patients are likely to prefer different ones. Commonly prescribed drugs include trihexyphenidyl (benzhexol; Artane®), orphenadrine (Disipal®; Norflex®), benztropine (Cogentin®), biperiden,

---

[11] *See* 12.70 *infra.*

methixene and procyclidine (Kemadrin®). These drugs are more effective for rigidity and tremor than for bradykinesia, and in general, they are less effective than dopaminergic drugs. However, they are often prescribed for patients with mild symptoms, making it possible to put off the time at which levodopa is started (Coleman, 1992; Greenberg, 1993; Lieberman, 1992).

[2] Side Effects

Frequent side effects of anticholinergic therapy are dry mouth, constipation, urinary retention in men with prostatitis and blurred vision caused by dilation of the pupils. These drugs can also delay gastric emptying, thereby decreasing the effectiveness of other anti-parkinsonian medications.

The most serious side effect, however, is mental status changes, resulting in confusion and memory impairment. These changes occur particularly in elderly patients, who may have co-existing Alzheimer's disease that makes them more vulnerable to anticholinergic-related cognitive impairment.

Side effects may be severe enough to require withdrawal of the drug, which must be carried out gradually in order to avoid the possibility of symptoms increasing beyond their original level. If one anticholinergic drug is ineffective, another may be tried (Greenberg, 1993; Coleman, 1992).

12.62 Amantadine

Amantadine is an antiviral drug that was found by accident to have antiparkinsonian properties. About half of patients find it effective either alone or combined with an anticholinergic agent. It is thought to work by promoting the release of dopamine from substantia nigra cells. Amantadine improves all parkinsonian symptoms, although the degree of benefit obtained is much less than that from levodopa and dopamine agonists.

Side effects include confusion, restlessness, livedo reticularis (reddish-blue rash on the legs with swelling of the ankles) and disturbed heartbeat. Amantadine is often given in the early stages of Parkinson's disease (Coleman, 1992; Greenberg, 1993).

12.63   Levodopa

The introduction of levodopa therapy in the 1960s changed the prognosis for patients with Parkinson's disease by both reducing disability and prolonging life expectancy (Coleman, 1992). Levodopa is now the drug of choice for treating patients whose disease is progressing, with bradykinesia and rigidity more prominent than tremor (Bannister, 1992). However, it does not stop the underlying pathology of the disease, and after a time, its effectiveness diminishes and extremely troublesome side effects appear.

The discovery that Parkinson's disease was caused by a dopamine deficiency led to attempts to develop a treatment that would replace the dopamine from another source. It was found that dopamine taken by mouth could not cross the blood-brain barrier but instead had to be administered as its precursor levodopa, which is then converted into dopamine by the enzyme dopa decarboxylase. However, the patients who initially took levodopa experienced acute side effects, including severe nausea and vomiting, postural hypotension and cardiac arrhythmias. These reactions were due to the effects of dopamine synthesized outside the blood-brain barrier.

This difficulty was resolved by combining levodopa with carbidopa, a drug that inhibits the action of dopa decarboxylase but does not cross the blood-brain barrier. Carbidopa has the effect of reducing the amount of levodopa converted to dopamine outside the central nervous system, not only eliminating the acute side effects but also increasing the amount of levodopa that can enter the brain. Carbidopa thereby makes levodopa more effective, so that a smaller amount can be used.

As a result, levodopa is almost always prescribed together with carbidopa in a fixed combination known as Sinemet®. Treatment starts with a small dose, Sinemet® 10/100 (10 mg carbidopa to 100 mg levodopa) or Sinemet® 25/100, taken three times a day. As time passes, the dosage is increased, depending on the patient's response to the drug. Most patients eventually need to take Sinemet® 25/250 three to four times a day (Coleman, 1992; Greenberg, 1993). About 15 percent of people with Parkinson's disease have no therapeutic response to levodopa (Bannister, 1992).

Although levodopa improves all the major symptoms of Parkinson's disease, particularly bradykinesia, eventually the disease progresses to a point that the drug is no longer fully effective. Initially most patients receive a prolonged beneficial effect from a dose of levodopa. After about two to five years, however, about 50 percent of patients find that the therapeutic effect from one dose wears off before the next dose is to be taken. Eventually this wearing-off effect occurs several times a day and develops into a phenomenon known as response fluctuations (Lieberman, 1992). Other extremely troublesome complications of levodopa therapy are dyskinesia (difficulty performing voluntary movements) and psychiatric problems.

For these reasons, most experts consider it desirable to delay giving the Parkinson's patient levodopa as long as possible. This is especially true since oxidation of the dopamine produced from levodopa increases the formation of free radicals that hasten the death of neurons in the substantia nigra (Stacy and Jankovic, 1993).

[1] Response Fluctuations

After prolonged treatment with levodopa, the patient's motor response to the drug starts to fluctuate. The time period varies, but by five years, about half of patients notice these effects (Stacy and Jankovic, 1993). As mentioned, at first the effects of one dose wears off before the next is due. As time passes, the wearing off occurs more rapidly, until the patient becomes subject to sudden switches from functioning well to having severe symptoms. This is known as the on-off phenomenon. At the advanced stage of the disease, the fluctuations appear to be random, with no relationship to when the previous dose was taken.

Response fluctuations can be "smoothed out" by continuous intravenous or duodenal infusions of levodopa, which keep the plasma level of the drug stable. However, these techniques are impractical for chronic treatment and can only be used for brief periods under medical supervision. For this reason, oral controlled-release preparations have been developed, in particular Sinemet CR®. Although these formulations have been shown to produce longer "on" periods with fewer "off" periods, they have not resolved the problem. Patients who have only begun to experience the "on-off" phenomenon are helped most by controlled-release preparations, while they are of limited benefit for those at a more advanced stage whose fluctuations are unpredictable (Coleman, 1992; Stacy and Jankovic, 1993; Greenberg, 1993).

Other ways of controlling response fluctuations include adding a dopamine agonist to levodopa, adding selegiline, fractionating the levodopa regimen into smaller doses taken more frequently, and restricting intake of dietary protein, which in excess is thought to interfere with transport of levodopa to the brain. None of these approaches, however, is fully effective, especially once fluctuations have become unpredictable (Coleman, 1992; Greenberg, 1993; Lieberman, et al., 1993).

[2] Dyskinesias

Many patients with response fluctuations also develop dyskinesias—involuntary chorea-type (rapid, complex and jerky) movements—that usually occur during "on" periods. They can be exhausting and may affect any part of the body. Examples are clasping of the hands, twisting of the trunk, bobbing of the head and thrusting of the tongue (Coleman, 1992; Lieberman, et al., 1993).

Dyskinesias are of two categories. The first results from deterioration occurring at the end of the dose and is caused by inadequate levels of dopamine. It is managed by making the doses more frequent or adding a longer-acting dopamine agonist. The second type occurs at the peak of the dose and is caused by high plasma concentrations of levodopa. It is managed by reducing individual doses (Bannister, 1992).

Response fluctuations and drug-induced dyskinesias appear to be related to the duration of the disease, so that they are often most severe in patients with early-onset Parkinson's disease (Coleman, 1992).

[3] Psychiatric Complications

Psychiatric side effects also occur in patients taking levodopa. These disturbances, which include visual hallucinations, confusion, nightmares, paranoia and personality changes, are more likely to occur in demented patients and in those also taking dopamine agonists (Lieberman, 1992). Between 30 percent and 60 percent of patients in the late stages of the disease experience these drug-induced psychoses (Danielczyk, 1992).

Older patients are more likely to experience confusion, agitation, delusions and hallucinations; 17.6 percent of patients over the age of 60 have been reported to experience them (Saint-Cyr, et al., 1993). Younger patients receiving higher doses may develop hypomania (a moderate level of mania). About 10 percent of patients experience psychotic or confusional states or hallucinations serious enough to require reduction or discontinuance of the drug. In one group of 775 patients, about a third had hallucinations. Risk factors were age, taking anticholinergics and multimodal therapy (Saint-Cyr, et al, 1993).

Hallucinations are usually visual rather than aural or tactile and occur at night. Patients also usually have vivid dreams and sleep disturbances. Nightmares and night terrors, involving calling out at night without remembering it the next morning, also occur.

Delusions are generally paranoid beliefs about persecution and are associated with older age and dementia. Levodopa may also lead to elevation of mood, which may simply manifest as a sense of well-being but may also reach an extreme form of manic and life-threatening behavior. Two thirds of patients who experience the "on-off" phenomenon have increased anxiety, sometimes severe, when "off." Between 1 percent and 10 percent of patients taking levodopa experience increased libido (Saint-Cyr, et al., 1993).

Decreasing the dosage of the drug generally results in improvement of the psychiatric symptoms, but most often, the parkinsonian symptoms worsen (Stacy and Jankovic, 1993). For some patients, it may be necessary to temporarily discontinue levodopa in a brief "drug holiday." This must be done in a hospital, since levodopa withdrawal entails serious risks. First, the patient may develop a severe parkinsonian syndrome with the potential for aspiration (inhalation of stomach contents, leading to respiratory distress) and phlebitis (vein inflammation). Second, there is a risk of a malignant neuroleptic syndrome, involving fever, autonomic nervous system instability, severe rigidity, obtundation (mental dulling), stupor and coma. Because of these risks, which can be life threatening, drug holidays are seldom recommended (Lieberman, 1992; Saint-Cyr, et al., 1993; Coleman, 1992).

If these interventions fail to improve the psychiatric symptoms, the patient may be given thioridazine, a low-potency neuroleptic (antipsychotic) agent, or clozapine, an atypical neuroleptic that selectively inhibits one type of dopamine receptor and has been found to improve psychiatric symptoms without exacerbating motor symptoms (Stacy and Jankovic, 1993; Saint-Cyr, et al., 1993).

Finally, electroconvulsive therapy (ECT) may reduce psychiatric symptoms such as hallucinations, but at the cost of inducing or increasing confusion (Saint-Cyr, et al., 1993).

12.64   Dopamine Agonists

Dopamine agonists act directly on the dopamine receptors in the brain, eliminating dependence on the dying neurons of the substantia nigra. Consequently a smaller dose of levodopa is required to produce a clinical effect. However, dopamine agonists cannot entirely replace levodopa, because they stimulate only one of the two major classes of dopamine receptors, whereas the greatest efficacy requires stimulation of both types (Lieberman, 1992).

There are two types of dopamine agonists: ergot derivatives and apomorphine. Dopamine agonists are generally given in combination with levodopa when the patient's response to levodopa begins to fail. They are also used in the earlier stages together with levodopa to delay the appearance of dyskinesias.[12]

For younger patients, fairly high doses of ergot derivatives may be given alone as the initial treatment for Parkinson's disease. These patients should understand that they are exchanging the greater symptomatic improvement afforded by levodopa for the lesser relief of dopamine agonists in order to gain the benefits of delaying the introduction of levodopa. The effectiveness of dopamine agonist monotherapy generally diminishes in one to three years, and these drugs are then combined with levodopa (Bannister, 1992; Lieberman, 1992; Montastruc, et al., 1993).

Patients' responses to a given dose of a dopamine agonist vary considerably, requiring closeindividual attention in order to adjust the dosage properly. Although dopamine agonists result in less dyskinesia than levodopa, they are likely to induce especially terrifying hallucinations (Bannister, 1992).

[1]   Bromocriptine

Bromocriptine (Parlodel®) is an ergot derivative that was originally used in combination with levodopa for patients with advanced Parkinson's. Subsequently given as the initial treatment when patients were first diagnosed, it seemed to prevent the development of response fluctuations and dyskinesias. Most patients eventually require the addition of levodopa, and this combination may result in a much lower incidence of later complications (Coleman, 1992). Because delusions and hallucinations are especially frequent with bromocriptine, it is

---

[12] *See* 12.63[2] *supra.*

contraindicated for patients with a history of mental illness (Greenberg, 1993).

[2] Lisuride

Lisuride (Dopergin®) is an ergot derivative that has effects comparable to bromocriptine. It is given early in the disease, alone or together with levodopa, to reduce the incidence of later complications, or at a later stage, it is added to levodopa. Lisuride is water soluble and thus can be given as intravenous and subcutaneous infusions, which is useful for patients who are temporarily unable to take medications orally (Coleman, 1992).

[3] Pergolide

Pergolide (Permax®), a relatively new drug, is an ergot derivative that stimulates both types of receptors. Studies have shown both that its effectiveness is the same as that of bromocriptine and that it is slightly more effective. If the latter is true, this may be because of its ability to stimulate both types of dopamine receptors. Its value for newly diagnosed patients is as yet unknown. Pergolide's side effects are similar to those of bromocriptine (Coleman, 1992; Greenberg, 1993).

[4] Apomorphine

Apomorphine is a dopamine agonist that is chemically unrelated to the ergot derivatives. Because it is not effective when taken by mouth, it must be administered parentally (other than through the digestive system); it produces a brief but powerful antiparkinsonian effect. Originally it caused vomiting to an extent that limited its use. However, the development of domperidone, a peripheral dopamine receptor antagonist that counteracts apomorphine's adverse effects, as well as drug delivery systems such as ambulatory minipumps, has brought renewed interest in apomorphine.

Apomorphine has been found to be extremely useful in treating patients with refractory on-off fluctuations; it may also diminish the severity of dyskinesias. It relieves pain, bladder dysfunction, dystonia and gastrointestinal symptoms. Patients can self-administer a single subcutaneous injection when necessary. Those with frequent unpredictable on-off fluctuations can receive a continuous infusion by means of a portable pump. Apomorphine's psychiatric side effects are reported to be less severe than those of the ergot derivatives (Lees, 1993; Coleman, 1992).

12.65   Selegiline

Selegiline (deprenyl; Eldepryl®) is a monoamine oxidase B (MAO-B) inhibitor. By inhibiting this enzyme, selegiline interferes with the metabolic breakdown of dopamine, thus potentiating the effect of levodopa. For many years, selegiline was used as an adjunct to levodopa that made it possible to obtain the same benefit from a 20 percent smaller dose of levodopa (Bannister, 1992; Coleman, 1992).

Then, in the mid–1980s, it was reported that patients who received selegiline with levodopa had a greater life expectancy than those who took levodopa alone, although the mechanism was unknown (Coleman, 1992). Subsequently it was found that the destruction of nigral neurons by MPTP in primates could be blocked by administering selegiline. This led to the hypothesis that selegiline has a neuroprotective effect against damage to dopaminergic cells caused by free radicals produced either by the oxidation of MPTP or from the natural metabolism of dopamine by MAO-B. Two studies of patients with early untreated Parkinson's disease, one including 801 patients, found that selegiline appeared to slow the progression of the disease, as indicated by the fact that patients given selegiline needed to start levodopa approximately 1.8 times later than did controls (Coleman, 1992; Lieberman, 1992; Maier Hoehn, 1992).

These results have led many experts to conclude that all newly diagnosed patients should be placed on selegiline and should continue to take it. It has been estimated that if selegiline is also able to slow the progression of the disease in patients who are already on levodopa, serious levodopa-related complications would be delayed long enough for most patients to live out their natural life span without severe functional disability (Lieberman, 1992).

Selegiline may potentiate the psychiatric side effects of levodopa, but it does not usually cause such effects when it is given alone. It seems to have few other side effects (Saint-Cyr, et al., 1993).

12.66   Other Neuroprotective Strategies

The theory that decreasing oxidative stress in the substantia nigra by reducing the generation of free radicals may slow the progression of Parkinson's disease has led to interest in the possibility of using antioxidants other than selegiline, including tocopherol (vitamin E), vitamins C and D, selective calcium channel blockers and iron chelators as neuroprotective agents (Maier Hoehn, 1992; Riederer and Lange, 1992).

12.67 Contraindicated Drugs

The benefits of levodopa and dopamine agonists will be counteracted by drugs that act as dopamine antagonists within the central nervous system. These agents, therefore, should not be given to Parkinson's patients unless absolutely necessary. They include neuroleptics such as chlorpromazine and haloperidol, and antiemetics such as prochlorperazine and metoclopramide. In addition, methyldopa, an antihypertensive, should not be given, because it is converted in the body into a substance with antidopaminergic properties. Finally, vitamin B_6 (pyridoxine) can counteract the action of carbidopa, thus decreasing the amount of levodopa that crosses the blood-brain barrier (Coleman, 1992).

12.70 SURGICAL THERAPIES

Surgical therapy for Parkinson's disease has taken two forms. The first approach attempts to restore dopamine-producing cells to the caudate nucleus through transplantation of autologous (from the individual himself or herself) adrenal medullary tissue or of fetal substantia nigra tissue. The second is the use of stereotactic thalamotomy to relieve tremor.

12.71 Cerebral Transplantation

The nature of the lesion in Parkinson's disease seems particularly appropriate for treatment by cerebral transplantation, since the motor symptoms result from the death of one small, localized group of cells. If dopaminergic cells transplanted to the patient's caudate nucleus were able to continue synthesizing and releasing dopamine, they might replace the patient's own substantia nigra cells and provide a more consistent delivery of dopamine to the striatum than drugs, thus smoothing out response fluctuations (Ahlskog, 1993).

The two types of transplant tissue employed in these procedures have been fetal neural cells and autologous (from the same individual) cells from the medulla of the adrenal gland. Transplantation of dopaminergic neurons from fetal brains was first performed to reverse the effects of dopamine deficiency in adult animals. The transplanted cells produced dopamine and formed synapses with striatal neurons in the host. Then it was recognized that the chromaffin cells of the adrenal medulla produce dopamine and could be used as a source for grafts (Ahlskog, 1993; Shults, 1992).

To date, however, the clinical success of these procedures has been limited, and fetal tissue transplants are highly controversial.

[1] Adrenal Medullary Transplantation

The first attempts at cerebral transplantation for Parkinson's disease in humans were performed using adrenal medullary autografts. Using tissue from the patient's own body has the advantage of avoiding the need for immunosuppressive therapy to prevent the host from rejecting the graft.

Although some striking successes were reported in Mexico and China (one patient confined to a wheelchair was said to have achieved normal functioning without medication), later attempts by many centers to replicate these results largely failed to achieve the same level of improvement. Some patients did show marked improvement, but in most cases, improvements were only mild to moderate and often reversed within 18 months after surgery. Patients also experienced considerable morbidity and mortality as a result of the surgical procedures required first to obtain the adrenal tissue from the abdomen and then to implant it in the brain. For these reasons, adrenal medullary transplantation has not been performed in the United States since 1990.

It appears that this procedure failed primarily because the graft did not survive. Current work using trophic (growth) factors, which enhance survival of the graft, may lead to more successful use of this procedure (Ahlskog, 1993; Shults, 1992).[13]

[2] Fetal Tissue Transplantation

The failure of adrenal transplants led investigators to turn to transplantation of dopamine-producing brain cells from human fetuses

---

[13] *See* 12.102 *infra.*

of between 6 and 10 weeks gestation (Stacy and Jankovic, 1993). Fetal neural cells could be considered the best type of tissue for this procedure, in the sense that they are precursor cells with the genetic capacity to develop into dopamine-producing neurons (Redmond, et al., 1993). They are also more viable and have greater potential to create synaptic connections with host cells than mature cells. To date, over 100 patients with Parkinson's disease have had fetal tissue transplant procedures (Ahlskog, 1993).

Aside from medical questions related to unresolved technical issues in performing these procedures, however, the question of using material from aborted fetuses has raised profound ethical questions and generated heated political controversy in this country. This has resulted in a limitation in the number of procedures that could be performed (Lieberman, et al., 1993; Stacy and Jankovic, 1993).

[a]　Outcomes

Comparisons of published reports are difficult because of differences among patients, rating systems and the extent of patient scrutiny at each center. Generally speaking, however, the improvements (in motor control and activities of daily living) shown by patients who received fetal tissue transplants, as reported in seven different clinical series from around the world, ranged from none to marked, although in no case were the symptoms completely reversed. Excluding one series in Cuba, in which 28 of 30 patients showed marked improvement, a roughly equal number of patients in all the other series experienced no or mild improvement, moderate improvement and marked improvement (Ahlskog, 1993).

Markedly improved patients had less disability and better control of symptoms than they had when they were only taking medications. Improvements generally involved decreases in "off" time and in response fluctuations. A few patients who had been unable to work resumed their jobs. All patients except one, however, still needed to take levodopa, although in much smaller doses. Generally the improvements were seen in some parkinsonian symptoms but not in others, and the affected symptoms varied among patients and medical centers. Complications from the procedure were reported to be minimal (Ahlskog, 1993).

[b]　Technical Issues

The procedures employed for transplantation vary considerably, since a number of technical questions remain unresolved. One is whether immunosuppressive therapy, consisting of cyclosporine with or without prednisone, should be given. It is not clear from reported outcomes of transplant procedures whether immunosuppression is necessary to prevent rejection of the graft. Immunosuppression is extremely expensive and carries a 1 percent to 10 percent yearly risk of serious infection or malignancy and a 1 percent annual risk of mortality.

Another question is how long the interval can be between abortion of the fetus and implantation of the cells into the Parkinson's patient's brain. Some investigators claim this period must be extremely brief (e.g., little over an hour), while others report that cryopreservation (freezing) can maintain the graft's viability for a longer interval. It is difficult to compare outcomes in patients given cryopreserved tissue to those in patients who received fresh tissue.

A third issue involves the volume of fetal tissue required for graft survival. Some workers believe that since only 5 percent to 10 percent of the grafted fetal neurons survive, several fetuses are required to produce a large enough volume of tissue for one implantation.

Finally, there is debate over the most appropriate site within the striatum in which to place the graft, whether it should be unilateral or placed on both sides of the brain (incurring greater risk of complications such as strokes and hemorrhage) and whether the graft cells should be implanted in a single site or distributed uniformly through the striatum (Ahlskog, 1993).

12.72 Thalamotomy

Before the introduction of levodopa, ablative surgery (which removes tissue by cutting) was performed more frequently than today in an attempt to reduce tremor by selectively cutting the motor pathways. Today these procedures have been largely replaced by drug therapy, but they still have a use in certain cases. One example would be a relatively young patient with a mostly unilateral tremor and rigidity that are unresponsive to drugs. Another example would be a patient over the age of 70 with tremor as the major symptom, who cannot take anticholinergics because of the risk of mental impairment (Greenberg, 1993; Lieberman, 1992).

The development of stereotactic surgery has made neurosurgical procedures more effective and less dangerous than in the past. This technique uses x-rays or computed tomography (CT) to locate discrete brain structures according to three-dimensional coordinates. The coordinates are set by computer, and a circular frame called a stereotactic halo holds the patient's head in a fixed position while guiding the surgeon's needle to the precise location of the target tissue through a small hole.

Stereotactic thalamotomy, which destroys specific cells within the thalamus (an area at the base of the brain, the chief relay center of sensation), has been found to be highly effective in relieving tremor and rigidity (Stacy and Jankovic, 1993). Another neurosurgical procedure used to treat parkinsonism is pallidotomy (ablation of the lateral globus pallidus), which has had encouraging results in decreasing bradykinesia and rigidity (Stacy and Jankovic, 1993; Widner and Rehncrona, 1993).

12.80   PATIENT MANAGEMENT

Since there is no cure for Parkinson's disease, the goals of management are improving symptoms and slowing the pathologic process (Stacy and Jankovic, 1993). An important element in treating Parkinson's disease is establishing a successful relationship with the patient, for the medication regimen needs to be customized to each patient, and good rapport will enhance the process of deciding among the various treatment options. Management goals differ, depending on the patient's age; thus an employed person under 50 would be managed differently from a retired person over 70, even though both may be at the same disease stage (Lieberman, 1992).

12.81   Early Stage

The discovery of the neuroprotective effect of selegiline has led many experts to advocate starting all newly diagnosed patients on this drug and having them continue to take it, even though in most cases, it has little therapeutic effect if the patient is not taking levodopa (Siemers, 1992; Lieberman, 1992).

The question of when to start levodopa and/or a dopamine agonist generates more controversy. Some writers advocate that because levodopa may increase the formation of free radicals, its use should be delayed as long as possible by using an anticholinergic or amantadine when the patient gets to the point of needing treatment for symptoms (Stacy and Jankovic, 1993). Another option is early symptomatic treatment with dopamine agonists, especially for younger patients (Lieberman, 1992).[14]

Still other experts believe that starting dopaminergic treatment in the early stage will eventuate fewer response fluctuations and dyskinesias in the future. This may be done with a combination of selegiline, levodopa and a dopamine agonist; with a dopamine agonist initially, then adding selegiline and levodopa when necessary to control symptoms; or with selegiline alone to start, next adding a dopamine agonist and finally levodopa when clinically necessary (Rinne, 1993).

12.82 Moderate Stage

In many cases, levodopa is started at this stage. This decision should be thoroughly reviewed with the patient, who may be upset by the implication that the disease has progressed and may fear becoming an invalid. The physician must weigh the possibility that levodopa accelerates disease progression by generating free radicals against the possibility that levodopa may promote survival by improving symptoms and delaying complications related to immobility. It is also necessary to weigh the symptomatic improvement produced by levodopa against the possibility of future response fluctuations and dyskinesias (Lieberman, 1992).

Eventually the wearing-off effect appears and begins to occur several times a day. Response fluctuations are managed by keeping the dose of levodopa as low as possible, and adding selegiline and a dopamine agonist if the patient is not already taking them. Sinemet CR® also usually increases "on" periods and reduces "off" periods (Lieberman, 1992).

12.83 Advanced Stage

Before the advent of levodopa, patients at advanced stages of Parkinson's disease were rigid; they had bradykinesia, tremor and difficulty walking. Today drug therapy has enabled advanced-stage patients to walk (although they do fall); they are not rigid, and their bradykinesia may be only moderate. Some, however, do have severe tremors, and others are demented.

---

[14] *See* 12.64 *supra.*

Falling at this stage is due to impairment of structures in the brain stem that do not involve dopamine, and levodopa may exacerbate postural instability. Management becomes extremely complex, for in some cases, falling, freezing and festination improve when levodopa is reduced, while in others, these symptoms improve when the dosage is increased or combined with a dopamine agonist (Lieberman, 1992). A precursor of norepinephrine called threo-dihydroxy-phenyl-serine (threo-DOPS) was reported by Japanese researchers to be effective in treating freezing, but others were unable to replicate this effect (Coleman, 1992).

Patients who have disabling postural instability should have an MRI scan to rule out other causes, such as subdural hematoma caused by frequent falling. To avoid serious complications such as hip or skull fractures, the patient may need to use a wheelchair and walk only when supported.

Mental changes may occur, including confusion or dementia. Sometimes patients progress from sleep disturbances to visual hallucinations to psychosis; sometimes psychosis appears full-blown. Since mild cognitive impairment can be seriously worsened by dehydration or infection (e.g., urinary or respiratory), such a condition should first be ruled out or treated if it is present.

If antiparkinsonian medications are suspected of causing cognitive impairment, the next step is to withdraw them. Use of anticholinergic drugs or amantadine should be gradually discontinued first. For patients taking selegiline, that drug should be discontinued next, since it potentiates the effects of dopaminergic agents. Next dopaminergic drugs should be reduced or withdrawn, and finally levodopa can be reduced with care, since doing so is likely to increase the motor symptoms.

Some patients may need a drug holiday from levodopa. If side effects continue, antidepressant therapy or electroconvulsive therapy (ECT) for underlying depression, or a neuroleptic such as clozapine can be tried (Lieberman, 1992; Coleman, 1992; Saint-Cyr, et al., 1993).

12.84 Management of Other Symptoms

Another common symptom in Parkinson's patients is sleep disturbance, which is often related to depression.[15] Sleep disturbance may

---

[15] *See* 12.23 *supra.*

also be related to the use of certain drugs, particularly levodopa and selegiline, which tend to promote alertness. In that case, doses should not be taken in the evening.

Sleep problems may also arise because of difficulty turning over in bed, in which case, Sinemet CR® may help; or because of anxiety, which may respond to benzodiazepine, a tranquilizer, or to a soporific (sleep-inducing) antidepressant such as nortriptyline (Lieberman, 1992).

Dysarthria (difficulty speaking due to impaired muscle control), urinary incontinence, constipation, impotence, dizziness on standing, headaches and palpitations are other drug-or disease-related adverse effects that are, unfortunately, difficult to control. Nausea and vomiting, which used to be common before the use of carbidopa, rarely occur today. If dopamine agonists do lead to vomiting, the antiemetic domperidone can be given (Lieberman, 1992; Coleman, 1992).

12.85 Other Aspects of Management

Aside from drug treatment, managing Parkinson's disease requires attention to physical health and fitness, since the increasing difficulty of movement means that patients will need more strength and energy to perform even ordinary tasks. Some assistance can be provided by aids to daily living such as rails or banisters placed at appropriate locations in the home, tableware with large handles, voice amplifiers, speaker phones and electric chairs that help the occupant rise. But patients also need to maximize their own physical abilities through appropriate diet, exercise and often physical or speech therapy (Greenberg, 1993).

[1] Diet

Eating a healthful diet is important to maintain fitness in general. In addition, Parkinson's disease requires attention to specific aspects of diet. First, because protein tends to interfere with levodopa absorption, it may be necessary to redistribute protein intake so that protein-rich foods are eaten in the evening, when the wearing-off effect will cause the least disruption. Second, in the later stages, patients often lose weight because of difficulty chewing, swallowing and handling utensils, as well as from tremor and bradykinesia that burn up calories.

These difficulties may be dealt with through tactics such as eating during "on" periods, eating several small meals instead of a few large ones or taking small bites. In addition, a physician may prescribe supplements or calorie-rich foods (Lieberman, et al., 1993).

[2] Exercise

Exercise to keep muscles strong and flexible is an important component of management, for exercise both maintains fitness and alleviates some symptoms. Exercise programs designed specifically for the Parkinson's patient focus on cardiovascular health and on muscular flexibility and strength. They include aerobic exercise as well as a variety of routines geared to stretch the muscle groups most affected by Parkinson's disease. Many patients find it beneficial to consult a physical therapist to obtain an individualized exercise program (Lieberman, et al., 1993).

[3] Physical and Speech Therapy

The goal of physical therapy is to maximize the patient's ability to function independently. It aims to prevent musculoskeletal deformities (such as stooped posture or a twisted trunk) and to enable the patient to balance while walking and carry out activities of daily living for as long as possible. The therapy focuses on motor control, preventing unwanted movements and developing muscle strength.

The physical therapist provides strengthening and stretching exercises individualized to a patient's particular needs, in a program that ensures that every muscle gets a workout. In addition, the therapist teaches the patient the most effective ways to get out of bed, cook, eat, dress and perform other tasks. By improving function, physical therapy helps prevent falls and the resulting fractures (Glendinning and Enoka, 1994; Lieberman, et al., 1993).

About half of Parkinson's disease patients develop speech difficulties caused by the disease's effect on muscles related to respiration, voice production, facial expression and articulation. The speech therapist teaches the patient how to compensate for these deficits and facilitates communication skills for the family as well (Lieberman, et al., 1993).

12.86 Psychosocial Considerations

Aside from the effects of physical symptoms, the overall condition of patients with Parkinson's disease is considerably affected by psychological factors. Psychological difficulties include depression, bradyphrenia (easily fatigued interest, motivation and psychomotor activity), lack of affect, anxiety in social situations and lack of motivation. The patient's tendency to be emotionally inexpressive, as well as his or her slower cognitive functioning, can seriously affect family relationships. In addition, patients fear negative comments when their motor deficits become evident in public places, and therefore they often tend to withdraw socially.

The stress resulting from all these factors, as well as from the need to adjust to having a chronic illness, in its turn can cause a worsening of motor symptoms. Stress-induced increase in motor symptoms is common among Parkinson's patients. For example, a patient may feel well until remembering that he or she must leave the house soon, and then all at once be unable to move.

Psychological interventions have been developed to help patients learn to maintain their emotional balance as well as to provide problem-solving strategies for specific situations. Cognitive restructuring helps change negative thoughts. Training in social skills and relaxation aids in coping with stressful social situations (Ellgring, et al., 1993).

Family members or other caretakers also experience high levels of stress and require psychological support themselves in order to continue taking care of the person with Parkinson's. Physical symptoms, depression and uncommunicativeness on the part of the patient take a high toll on the caregiver.

Underlying problems within a marriage or family may be exacerbated by the patient's diagnosis, which may also strain family finances, especially if the patient becomes unable to work. To prevent burnout, some form of respite such as home care or adult day care can provide a period of relief for the caregiver. The American Parkinson's Disease Association and other organizations offer educational materials and support groups (Ellgring, et al., 1993; Lieberman, et al., 1993).

12.90   PROGNOSIS

Before levodopa came into use, Parkinson's disease shortened life expectancy. Although even in the nineteenth century, some patients lived 20 to 30 years after symptoms appeared, on average, patients lived only 10 years after onset; less than 25 percent of people with

Parkinson's disease were over 75 at the time of their death (Maier Hoehn, 1992).

Today, however, although the disease is always progressive, levodopa has not only reduced disability but increased life expectancy. Whereas in the prelevodopa period, the estimated mortality rate (the ratio of observed to expected deaths) was 3 to 1, today it is 1.5 to 1 in all patients receiving treatment and 1 to 1 (that is, normal) in patients who are able to take levodopa over a long term (Coleman, 1992). Furthermore, the rate at which disability progresses varies considerably, so that symptoms may remain stable—for example, affecting only one side of the body—for longer periods (Bannister, 1992).

12.100 FUTURE THERAPIES

Research is underway into treatments for Parkinson's disease that can provide a cure by attacking the cause: the death of dopaminergic neurons in the substantia nigra of the brain. Two strategies are being developed. The first involves protecting the remaining dopaminergic neurons, either by interfering with the process by which they are damaged or by providing factors that help them survive. To be as effective as possible, this protective strategy in turn depends on the capability of detecting individuals at risk of Parkinson's disease before symptoms develop. Thus, some investigators are working on presymptomatic diagnosis.

The second strategy focuses on restoring dopaminergic innervation to the striatum. An example of such restorative therapy is cerebral transplantation of fetal or adrenal medullary tissue.[16]

Other therapies being developed involve the use of trophic (growth) factors and the transplantation of genetically engineered cells (Ahlskog, 1993).

12.101 Presymptomatic Diagnosis

The value of presymptomatic diagnosis of Parkinson's disease is highlighted by the fact that at the time symptoms appear, between 20 percent and 40 percent of dopaminergic neurons are still functioning. Investigators have been seeking a specific marker that could detect

---

[16] *See* 12.71 *supra.*

the early stages of deterioration of the nigral neurons and thereby identify people at risk (Stacy and Jankovic, 1993). Several types of biochemical, physiologic and radiologic markers have been suggested, but to date, none has been shown to be either sensitive or specific enough to be useful.

[1] Biochemical Markers

Some researchers are looking for possible biochemical markers in the cerebrospinal fluid (CSF) of Parkinson's patients. Although the levels of the dopamine metabolites homovanillic acid and 3,4-dihydroxyphenylacetic acid are decreased in the CSF of these patients, these levels were not sufficiently different from those in control subjects (Shults, 1992). Another biochemical marker, mitochondrial complex I activity, which is reduced in the substantia nigra in Parkinson's patients, was reported to be also considerably reduced in these patients' blood platelets, but this difference may be too small to be useful for diagnosis (Jenner, 1993).

Another possible marker is a reduced level in the substantia nigra of glutathione, a substance that acts as the respiratory carrier of oxygen and is involved in clearing hydrogen peroxide from the brain. Decreased glutathione activity has been reported in the substantia nigra of Parkinson's patients, apparently contributing to oxidative stress (Riederer and Lange, 1992). Development of a peripheral indicator of altered glutathione function could be useful for early detection of Parkinson's disease pathology (Jenner, 1993).

[2] Physiologic Markers

It is possible that simple tests of bradykinesia may be developed to identify presymptomatic Parkinson's disease. One early manifestation of bradykinesia is a decrease in the rate of eye blinking. In one study, patients with Parkinson's disease who were not taking medication blinked fewer times per minute than control subjects who did not have the disease. Thus, counting blinks might be used as a screening test.

Another physiologic function that has been investigated is identification of odors, which is impaired in Parkinson's. However, this impairment does not correspond to the stage of the disease, and it also appears in Alzheimer's disease. Therefore, testing olfactory function might be useful for detecting some types of degenerative neurologic disease but is not specific to Parkinson's (Shults, 1992).

[3] Radiologic Markers

Reduced striatal uptake of fluorodopa in patients with Parkinson's disease has been demonstrated by PET scan. However, there is controversy as to whether this reduction is also a function of normal aging. If so, there will be too much overlap between presymptomatic and normal individuals for this test to be reliable. In addition, PET scans are difficult to use on a routine basis due to limited availability of the equipment, the extent of radiation exposure entailed and the need to puncture an artery to introduce the isotope (Shults, 1992).

The ability of MRI to detect iron accumulation in the substantia nigra[17] makes it possible that with some refinements in technique, this modality may become capable of detecting nigral abnormalities with enough sensitivity to identify individuals at risk of developing Parkinson's disease (Olanow, 1992).

12.102 Neurotrophic Factors

Substances known as neurotrophic or growth factors function to promote the survival of developing neurons during maturation and later to maintain the normal function of mature nerve cells and their regeneration after injury (Lindsay, et al., 1993). It appears that neurotrophic factors may be useful in treating Parkinson's disease in three ways.

First, studies of cerebral transplantation in animals found that neurotrophic factors could promote survival of transplanted adrenal medullary cells as well as induce these cells to assume a more neuronal form. In these studies, the grafts were either treated with an infusion of nerve growth factor (NGF), or other types of cells that produced NGF were co-grafted along with the adrenal tissue (Shults, 1992).

Second, some studies have indicated that neurotrophic factors may induce residual dopaminergic neurons and their axons to sprout collateral axons that reinnervated the striatum and improved parkinsonian symptoms in animals. However, it has not been confirmed that the sprouting was the cause of the functional improvement.

Third, it seems that by administering neurotrophic factors to patients with Parkinson's disease, it may be possible to retard or stop the degeneration in the neurons of the substantia nigra. Studies have

---

[17] *See* 12.42 *supra.*

demonstrated that three neurotrophic factors—brain-derived neurotrophic factor, basic fibroblast growth factor and acidic fibroblast growth factor—could promote the survival of dopaminergic neurons (Shults, 1992).

Interestingly, in the studies just described, survival of the grafts and sprouting of dopaminergic neurons occurred even when the adrenal graft did not survive or when the graft consisted of adipose or sciatic nerve tissue treated with nerve growth factor. In some instances, it seemed that the process of grafting itself, together with infusion of nerve growth factor, stimulated production of endogenous (produced by the body itself) neurotrophic factors leading to sprouting and functional improvement.

These findings have led to reconsideration of the concept that the graft tissue must contain cells that can synthesize and release dopamine. It is possible that stimulation of reinnervation by neurotrophic factors is the essential component in treating Parkinson's disease through cerebral transplantation. In that case, fetal tissue would not be necessary, since other types of tissues could be used for grafting. It is also possible that Parkinson's disease symptoms such as dementia, which are not related to dopamine deficiency, could also be addressed by neurotrophic-factor-secreting grafts that replenish neurotransmitters other than dopamine (Ahlskog, 1993).

12.103　Genetic Engineering

Another solution for replenishing dopamine that would avoid relying on fetal tissue involves genetic engineering. This technique would involve transplanting cells that have been genetically engineered to produce dopamine or neurotrophic factors into the patient's brain. Three approaches are under investigation.

The first involves use of a virus (retrovirus or herpes simplex virus type 1) as a gene-carrying vector injected into the brain, which would genetically modify the host brain cells. The second approach would use an immortalized line of dopaminergic fetal brain cells that could provide an unending supply of transplant material. The third approach involves genetic manipulation of the patient's own extracerebral tissue, such as skin fibroblasts (connective tissue cells), which is then transplanted into the brain.

All these techniques have potential drawbacks and hazards, especially the possibility of development of tumors or viral infection, triggering of an immune response and uncontrolled growth of the modified cells. It is also not clear whether the goal should be synthesis of dopamine or production of neurotrophic factors. Although this work is still in its early stages, it holds promise for the future (Ahlskog, 1993).

12.104 Other Treatments

Another new treatment approach under investigation involves surgical implantation into the brain of polymer capsules containing dopaminergic drugs or cells that secrete dopamine or neurotrophic factors. The use of the capsule prevents an immune system reaction (Stacy and Jankovic, 1993; Lieberman, et al., 1993).

Glutamate is a neurotransmitter that inhibits neural excitation; loss of dopamine leads to glutamatergic overactivity in the basal ganglia. NBQX (6-nitro–7-sulphamobenzo(f)quinoxaline–2,3-dione), a glutamate antagonist, has been reported to improve bradykinesia, postural instability, tremor and motor function in monkeys when co-administered with levodopa. It may prove effective for treating Parkinson's disease in humans (Stacy and Jankovic, 1993; Riederer and Lange, 1992).

12.110 EVALUATION OF PERMANENT IMPAIRMENT

The American Medical Association (AMA) system for evaluating permanent impairment describes several categories of impairment resulting from disorders of the forebrain or cerebrum, such as Parkinson's disease. These include motor and movement disorders, mental status disturbances, emotional or behavioral disturbances and sleep disorders. The AMA criteria for impairment are defined not by diagnosis but in terms of the degree to which the patient's ability to perform activities of daily living is affected. The grading system assigns a specific percentage value to each level of impairment within each category.

Many patients with Parkinson's disease suffer dysfunction in more than one of the seven categories of impairment resulting from cerebral disorders. In such a case, the most severe of the five categories relating to mental functioning is used to represent the cerebral impairment. This value may be combined with the values of any of four other categories relating to physical functioning (movement, sleep, etc.) to calculate a value representing the total cerebral impairment.

An impairment evaluation includes three components. The medical examination covers history, diagnosis and current clinical status. The analysis of the findings documents the effect of the impairments on the patient's ability to perform activities of daily living. Comparison of thisanalysis with the impairment criteria shows how the clinical findings relate to specific criteria and concludes with an overall estimate of the patient's impairment (American Medical Association, 1993).

Specific criteria relating to major impairments resulting from Parkinson's disease are described next. Percentages represent impairment of the whole person.

12.111   Mental Status Disturbances

Criteria for mental status impairment range from some impairment, with ability to perform most daily activities satisfactorily (1 percent to 14 percent), to severe impairment to the extent that the patient requires supervision to care for self and remain safe (50 percent to 70 percent).

12.112   Emotional or Behavioral Disturbances

Criteria range from mild limitation of social and interpersonal functioning (0 percent to 14 percent) to severe limitation of all daily functions with total dependence on another person (50 to 70 percent).

12.113   Sleep Disorders

Criteria range from reduced daytime alertness with ability to perform most daily functions (0 percent to 9 percent) to severely reduced alertness that makes the patient unable to care for self at all (40 percent to 60 percent).

12.114   Dysarthria

The criteria for difficulty swallowing and speaking range from mild dysarthria, dystonia or dysphagia with choking on liquids or semisolid food (1 percent to 14 percent) to severe inability to swallow with choking on oral secretions and need for assistance and suctioning (40 percent to 60 percent).

12.115   Disturbance of Station and Gait

These criteria range from being able to stand up and to walk, although having difficulty negotiating elevations, grades, stairs, deep chairs and long distances (1 percent to 9 percent), to inability to stand without assistance from another, need for mechanical support and a prosthesis (40 percent to 60 percent).

12.116   Impairment of the Upper Extremities

The criteria for impairment of the arms and hands depend on whether the preferred or nonpreferred extremity is affected. Impairment of the preferred extremity usually results in greater impairment. This impairment should be re-evaluated periodically, however, since over time, the nonpreferred limb may develop the ability to function as well as the preferred one. The percentages assigned for impairment of both upper limbs are greater than for impairments of the preferred and nonpreferred extremities added together.

[1]   One Impaired Upper Extremity

Criteria range from being able to use the affected limb, although having difficulty with digital dexterity (1 percent to 9 percent for preferred extremity; 1 percent to 4 percent for nonpreferred), to inability to use the limb at all (40 percent to 60 percent; 30 percent to 45 percent).

[2]   Two Impaired Upper Extremities

Criteria range from being able to use both limbs, although having difficulty with digital dexterity (1 percent to 19 percent), to inability to use the limbs at all (less than 80 percent).

12.200   BIBLIOGRAPHY

Text References

Ahlskog, J. E.: Cerebral Transplantation for Parkinson's Disease: Current Progress and Future Prospects. Mayo Clin. Proc. 68(6):578–591, June 1993.

American Medical Association: Guides to the Evaluation of Permanent Impairment, 4th ed. Chicago: American Medical Association, 1993.

Bannister, R.: Brain and Bannister's Clinical Neurology, 7th ed. New York: Oxford University Press, 1992.

Carroll, D. L.: Living with Parkinson's: A Guide for the Patient and Caregiver. New York: HarperCollins, 1992.

Coleman, R. J.: Current Drug Therapy for Parkinson's Disease. A Review. Drugs Aging (2):112–124, Mar.-Apr. 1992.

Danielczyk, W: Mental Disorders in Parkinson's Disease. J. Neural Transmis. 38(Suppl.):115–127, 1992.

Duvoisin, R. C.: A Brief History of Parkinsonism. Neurol. Clin. 10(2):301–316, May 1992.

Ellgring, H., et al.: Psychosocial Aspects of Parkinson's Disease. Neurology 43(Suppl.67):S41–S44, Dec. 1993.

Glendinning, D. S. and Enoka, R. M.: Motor Unit Behavior in Parkinson's Disease. Physical Therapy 74:61–71, Jan. 1994.

Greenberg, D. A., et al.: Clinical Neurology, 2nd ed. Norwalk, Conn.: Appleton and Lange, 1993.

Jenner, P.: Presymptomatic Detection of Parkinson's Disease. J. Neural Transmis. 40(Suppl.):23–36, 1993.

Lees, A. J.: Dopamine Agonists in Parkinson's Disease: A Look at Apomorphine. Fund. Clin. Pharmacol. 7(3–4):121–128, 1993.

Levin, B. E., et al.: Cognitive Impairments in Parkinson's Disease. Neurol. Clin 10(2):471–485, May 1992.

Lieberman, A.: An Integrated Approach to Patient Management in Parkinson's Disease. Neurol. Clin. 10(2):553–565, May 1992.

Lieberman A. N., et al.: Parkinson's Disease: The Complete Guide for Patients and Caregivers. New York: Simon & Schuster, 1993.

Lindsay, R. M., et al.: The Therapeutic Potential of Neurotrophic Factors in the Treatment of Parkinson's Disease. Experim. Neurol. 124(1):103–118, Nov. 1993.

Maier Hoehn, C.: The Natural History of Parkinson's Disease in the Pre-Levodopa and Post-Levodopa Eras. Neurol. Clin. 10(2):331–339, May 1992.

Montastruc, J. L., et al.: Current Status of Dopamine Agonists in Parkinson's Disease Management. Drugs 46(3):384–393, Sept. 1993.

Olanow, C. W.: Magnetic Resonance Imaging in Parkinsonism. Neurol. Clin. 10(2):405–420, May 1992.

Poewe, W.: Clinical Features, Diagnosis, and Imaging of Parkinsonian Syndromes. Curr. Opin. Neurol. Neurosurg. 6(3):333–338, June 1993.

Redmond, D. E., Jr., et al.: Neural Transplantation for Neurodegenerative Diseases: Past, Present, and Future. Ann. N.Y. Acad. Sci. 695:258–266, Sept. 24, 1993.

Riederer, P., and Lange, K. W.: Pathogenesis of Parkinson's Disease. Curr. Opin. Neurol. Neurosurg. 5(3):295–300, 1992.

Rinne, U. K.: Strategies in the Treatment of Early Parkinson's Disease. Acta Neurol. Scand. 146(Suppl.):50–53, 1993.

Saint-Cyr, J. A., et al.: Neuropsychological and Psychiatric Side Effects in the Treatment of Parkinson's Disease. Neurology 43(12 Suppl. 6):S47–S52, Dec. 1993.

Shults, C. W.: Presymptomatic Diagnosis, Neural Transplantation, and Trophic Factors. Neurol. Clin. 10(2):567–593, May 1992.

Siemers, E.: Recent Progress in the Treatment of Parkinson's Disease. Compr. Ther. 18(9):20–24, Sept. 1992.

Stacy, M., and Jankovic, J.: Current Approaches in the Treatment of Parkinson's Disease. Ann. Rev. Medicine 44:431–440, 1993.

Tanner, C. M.: Epidemiology of Parkinson's Disease. Neurol. Clin. 10(2):317–329, May 1992a.

Tanner, C. M.: Occupational and Environmental Causes of Parkinsonism. Occup. Med. State of the Art Reviews 7(3):503–513, July-Sept. 1992b.

Uitti, J. R. and Calne, D. B.: Pathogenesis of Idiopathic Parkinsonism. Eur. Neurol. 33(Suppl. 1):6–23, 1993.

Widner, H. and Rehncrona, S.: Transplantation and Surgical Treatment of Parkinsonian Syndromes. Curr. Opin. Neurol. Neurosurg. 6(3):344–349, June 1993.

CHAPTER 13

HIV-1-Associated Dementia

SCOPE

Over 20 viral and nonviral organisms can affect the brain of a person with AIDS. Most of these are opportunistic infections caused by organisms that attack the central nervous system while the immune defenses are hobbled by the human immunodeficiency virus (HIV). It has been found, however, that HIV itself is indirectly involved in a process that damages the brain and produces a progressive deterioration of cognitive, behavioral and/or motor function. About 10 percent of AIDS patients have this HIV-1-associated dementia as their AIDS-defining illness. Diagnosis of HIV-1-associated dementia is by exclusion: ruling out lymphoma and infections that can produce similar signs and symptoms. Treatment of dementia in AIDS patients depends upon the condition producing the dementia. Toxoplasmosis, neurosyphilis and depression, which can produce symptoms similar to dementia, are readily treatable. Even with high-dose chemotherapy, the prognosis for primary central nervous system lymphoma is poor. The incidence of HIV-1-associated dementia has decreased since the introduction of the anti-retroviral drug zidovudine (AZT) in 1987, but it still presents a difficult treatment challenge.

SYNOPSIS

13.00   INTRODUCTION: BACKGROUND AND EPIDEMIOLOGY

As we approach the year 2000, few Americans have not been touched in some way by the acquired immunodeficiency syndrome (AIDS) epidemic. Brothers, sisters, children, lovers, friends, movie stars, dancers . . . the list is distressingly long. In the United States, an estimated 1 million individuals are infected (1 in every 250 adults) with the human immunodeficiency virus (HIV), the agent that is generally accepted as the cause of AIDS. There have been 339,250 cases of full-blown AIDS in this country, and 57 percent of this group has died. The numbers on a global scale are even more unsettling; 12.9 million people are infected with HIV, and there have been more than 2.6 million AIDS cases so far (Carmichael, et al., 1995).

AIDS was first recognized in Los Angeles and New York in 1981, when an abnormally high incidence of two previously rare diseases (*Pneumocystis carinii* pneumonia and Kaposi's sarcoma, a type of cancer) was noted in a group of young homosexual men. However, the current epidemic in this country actually began earlier, in the late 1970s. Research in the United States and in France led to the identification of the human immunodeficiency virus in the early 1980s. The disease by this time had begun its spread to blood product recipients, injection drug users, their sexual partners and, during pregnancy, from infected mother to child.

Tests were developed to identify antibodies to the virus in blood, thus allowing screening of the blood supply to re-establish its safety and testing of individuals for infection with the virus. Next, the behavior of the virus was elucidated. It was found to attack a kind of white blood cell called the CD4 lymphocyte, making AIDS patients vulnerable to infections and cancers that are normally suppressed by those particular immune system cells.

In 1992, just over half of the reported new AIDS cases were among men with homosexual/bisexual contacts. However, from 1992 to 1994, the number of cases from this group declined. Heterosexual transmission of the virus among young Americans is now rapidly increasing. From 1992 to 1994, the number of Americans 13 to 21 years old infected with HIV jumped 77 percent. From 1991 to 1992, cases attributed to heterosexual contact increased 17.1 percent, with 59.4 percent of those affected being women. Overall, women accounted for 14.1 percent of reported AIDS cases in 1992 (Carmichael, et al., 1995). Worldwide, 75 percent of HIV infections are transmitted by heterosexual contact (Catalan, et al., 1995).

Early in the epidemic, many people died quickly of Kaposi's sarcoma, *Pneumocystis* pneumonia and other opportunistic infections (infections that seize the opportunity to take hold when a host's defenses are impaired). It was also noted that some people with AIDS developed a progressive mental/emotional/motor deterioration that was distinct from opportunistic infection of the brain (such as that associated with toxoplasmosis[1]) or AIDS-related brain cancer (lymphoma).[2] This HIV-associated psychoneurologic condition began to be known as AIDS dementia. Dementia is now the initial AIDS-defining illness in approximately 10 percent of HIV-infected people (Fauci and Lane, 1994).

As a result of the development of antiretroviral drugs such as zidovudine (AZT) and didanosine (DDI), which interfere with virus replication but do not kill HIV, and improved treatments and preventive medications to combat opportunistic infections, people with AIDS

---

[1] *See* 13.32[1] *infra.*

[2] *See* 13.33 *infra.*

are now living longer and healthier lives. Antiretroviral therapy also appears to have had a positive impact on the incidence of HIV-associated dementia, though it remains a difficult and distressing treatment challenge.

13.10 DEFINITIONS AND SEMANTICS

The dementia seen in AIDS has been described as a decline in cognitive ability (intellectual functioning, problem-solving etc.) from a previously attained level. The patient may present for treatment with impaired concentration, forgetfulness and difficulty performing complex tasks. This progresses to an inability to work, take care of basic daily needs and understand news or personal events, and can lead to a vegetative state before death.

AIDS dementia also usually involves behavioral and/or motor components. Behavioral problems include apathy and lack of initiative, usually with no change in alertness. Early in the course of AIDS dementia, the cognitive and behavioral changes can be almost impossible to differentiate from symptoms of situational depression or fatigue. The motor component of AIDS dementia starts with an unsteady gait, poor balance and difficulty performing rapid alternating movements. As motor problems become more severe, bowel and bladder incontinence can develop (Fauci and Lane, 1994).

As with many factors in the AIDS epidemic, the terminology surrounding the psychoneurologic symptoms associated with HIV disease can be both confusing and emotionally charged. The group of cognitive, behavioral and motor impairments that can be seen in people with AIDS has variously been termed AIDS encephalopathy, AIDS dementia complex, HIV-1-associated dementia (there are two strains of HIV; HIV-1 is found in Western countries, HIV-2 is primarily seen in Africa), HIV-1-associated cognitive motor complex and at least eight other less commonly used terms (Catalan, et al., 1995).

The term AIDS dementia complex (ADC) was first introduced in the late 1980s and is still in use in the literature and as a MeSH term for searching the National Library of Medicine's MedLine on-line database. However, the term ADC is controversial, because the word *complex* implies that the triad of impairments in cognitive, motor and behavioral functioning always go together. Research has clearly shown, however, that all three psychoneurologic impairments do not always exist in each patient.

Also, the term dementia itself is controversial. Under the *International Classification of Diseases,* tenth edition (ICD-10, the World Health Organization's diagnostic manual), the term dementia applies only in cases of profound amnesia. Under the AIDS dementia complex terminology, however, the term dementia can apply to people with only mild cognitive problems. In the American Psychiatric Association's *Diagnostic and Statistical Manual,* fourth edition (DSM-IV, which is more recent than the ICD-10 and is known as the diagnostic bible of American psychiatry), AIDS dementia has its own listing ("Dementia Due to HIV Disease") and specific definition, thereby avoiding the problem of making the condition fit the standard definition of dementia.

So what should this collection of psychoneurologic symptoms be called? The World Health Association (WHO) and the American Academy of Neurology (AAN) AIDS Task Forces have both tried to render order from this nomenclature chaos. The WHO has opted for the simple "HIV-1-associated dementia." The WHO has now also proposed an additional diagnosis of "HIV-1-associated minor cognitive/motor disorder," which covers those individuals with cognitive impairment that is not serious enough to be called a dementia (Catalan, et al., 1995).

The AAN system is similar to that of the WHO. It calls the condition "HIV-1-associated cognitive motor complex" and then divides that into two main categories to highlight whether the person's symptoms are primarily cognitive/behavioral ("HIV-1-associated dementia complex") or motor ("HIV-1-associated myelopathy") (Catalan, et al., 1995).

The AAN terms, the older AIDS dementia complex and other nomenclature will continue to be used for some time to come. However, in the end, the World Health Organization's system may achieve the widest acceptance, as this epidemic's global proportions become increasingly pronounced. For the purposes of simplicity in this chapter, we will refer to the condition by the WHO term or simply as *dementia.*

13.20   EPIDEMIOLOGY

The early lack of agreement over what exactly constitutes HIV-1-associated dementia produced wildly fluctuating estimates as to the prevalence of the condition. Along with the problems caused by different diagnostic criteria, early prevalence figures were skewed by the fact that they were not representative of the entire population of people with AIDS. Instead, early statistics were drawn from samples of patients at major neurologic centers. Estimates of the percentage of AIDS patients who developed dementia ranged as high as 40 percent.

Subsequent large controlled studies confirmed an annual incidence of dementia in people with AIDS of about 7 percent. In the large Multicenter AIDS Cohort Study (MACS), when patients were followed through to death, a total of 15 percent became demented. The true prevalence of dementia in AIDS may actually be fluctuating. Improved treatment protocols may decrease the incidence of dementia for a time; then the development of resistance to current therapies could lead to an increase (Catalan, et al., 1995).

The risk of developing dementia is not equal in all groups. A study in Scotland comparing the risk among injection drug users (IDUs) with that of homosexual men of developing HIV-1-associated dementia found that dementia developed in 59 percent of IDUs versus 15 percent of homosexuals. The development of dementia was not related to whether the patient developed opportunistic infections or lymphomas (Bell, et al., 1996). The authors did not speculate on the cause of these differences in risk, though it is generally recognized that the two groups tend to differ substantially in motivation, economic and education levels, pre-AIDS health status and compliance with treatment protocols.

Other risk factors for dementia include low body mass, low level of hemoglobin (the red pigment of blood, which gives the blood its oxygen-carrying power), more constitutional symptoms, being at the extremes of age (either a child or an older adult) and longer infection time (Catalan, et al., 1995). A large European study confirmed these risk factors for developing dementia and added female gender (the risk for women was almost double that of men) and decreased CD4 cell count (Chiesi, et al., 1996).

13.30 ETIOLOGIES OF DEMENTIA IN HIV DISEASE

This chapter chiefly covers dementia associated with the human immunodeficiency virus itself. However, other conditions in AIDS can precipitate neurologic symptoms similar to HIV-1-associated dementia. Because some of these conditions can be successfully treated—or at least palliated—it is important to be positive of the diagnosis when a person with AIDS has cognitive/behavioral and/or motor changes (Price, 1996).

13.31 Human Immunodeficiency Virus (HIV)

All viruses have a similar basic structure: a strand of raw genetic material—deoxyribonucleic acid (DNA) or ribonucleic acid (RNA)—surrounded by a protective protein coat. The viral DNA or RNA contains complete instructions for making identical copies of itself. The human immunodeficiency virus belongs to a group of RNA viruses called retroviruses. Retroviruses are characterized by their unique replication process: They possess a special enzyme, called reverse transcriptase, that reverses the normal direction of transcription (transfer of genetic code information) and produces DNA copies of the viral RNA that are then inserted into the DNA of the host cell. *(See Figure 13-1.)*

How HIV produces dementia remains unclear, though some interesting clues offer the promise of a definitive answer in the near future. Infection of brain cells with the virus does not appear to be the direct cause, because postmortem studies have shown that the brains of nondemented people with AIDS are just as likely to contain large quantities of the virus as are the brains of people who died with serious mental deterioration (Worley and Price, 1994).

A Johns Hopkins study confirmed the statistical lack of importance of the presence of HIV in the central nervous system (brain and spinal cord) and the development of dementia. This study did find, however, a significant correlation between the number of macrophages (large immune system cells that engulf and dissolve invading foreign cells) in the frontal lobes and basal ganglia of the brain of people who died of AIDS and the degree of dementia; the more macrophages, the more serious the dementia. This points to an indirect process mediated by macrophages, but the exact mechanism is still not clear (Glass, et al., 1995).

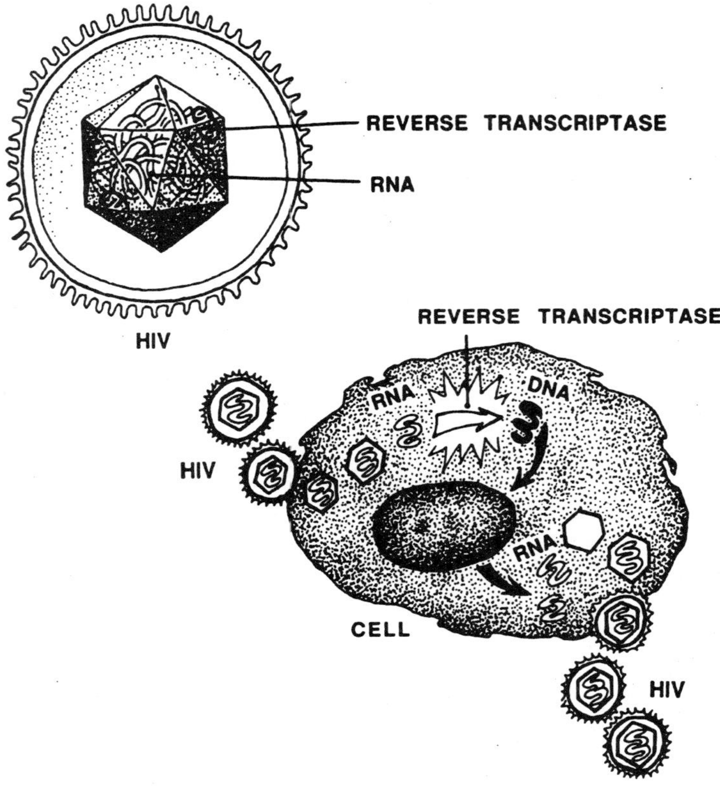

Fig. 13-1. The human immunodeficiency virus (HIV) is a retrovirus that uses a special enzyme, reverse transcriptase, to make DNA copies of the viral RNA.

One pathway that has been suggested is that HIV-1 enters developing macrophages, which then become immune activated and secrete high levels of neurotoxins that, over time, break down brain control mechanisms (Nottet and Gendelman, 1995). Research is continuing into discovering exactly how HIV infection indirectly leads to mental and motor deterioration.

13.32　Opportunistic Infections

Over 20 viral and nonviral opportunistic infections can affect the brain of someone with HIV disease (National Hospice Organization,

1996). The most common of these opportunistic infections, in descending order of frequency, are toxoplasmosis, cryptococcal meningitis, progressive multifocal leukoencephalopathy, neurosyphilis and tuberculosis meningitis. It is important for the physician to sort out the patient's neurologic symptoms and arrive at the correct diagnosis, so that appropriate therapy can be started promptly.

[1]   Toxoplasmosis

Infection with the protozoan (a microscopic animal that is neither bacterium nor virus) *Toxoplasma gondii* is the most common opportunistic infection in AIDS that affects the brain. Toxoplasmosis (the condition of being infected with the *Toxoplasma* organism) is a common, latent infection in many Americans (the organism is frequently found in cat stool, so anyone who cleans a litter box is at risk), but it normally causes the infected person no major problems because it is kept in check by the immune system. However, when the immune system is compromised, serious symptoms can result.

Toxoplasmosis is seen in approximately 15 percent of all patients with AIDS. It is usually a late complication of HIV disease and primarily occurs in patients with a CD4 (helper-inducer) lymphocyte count of less than 100 cells per microliter (a CD4 count of less than 200 cells per microliter is considered diagnostic of AIDS) (Fauci and Lane, 1994).

The most common symptoms of toxoplasmosis in AIDS patients include fever, headache and focal (localized) neurologic deficits. The patient may also have seizures and the strokelike symptoms of hemiparesis (paralysis on one side of the body) and aphasia (inability to speak and/or understand speech). If the brain becomes edematous (swells), the patient may be confused, lethargic, demented or even comatose. These last symptoms are similar to those of HIV-1-associated dementia, and radiologic evidence is required to confirm the diagnosis of toxoplasmosis. On contrast-enhanced computed tomography (CT) and magnetic resonance imaging (MRI, the more sensitive test), toxoplasmosis produces bright, easily visible rings within the brain tissue (Fauci and Lane, 1994).

[2]   Cryptococcal Meningitis

Cryptococcus neoformans is a yeastlike fungus that exists everywhere and that our immune systems normally easily keep in check.

However, cryptococcus is a major threat to people living with AIDS. Six to 12 percent of people with AIDS develop a cryptococcus-caused life-threatening infection of the brain and/or the membranes that cover it and spinal cord: meningitis.

Patients with central nervous system (CNS) cryptococcal infection can have symptoms for weeks or months before the condition is diagnosed. Patients with CNS cryptococcal infection almost always have a fever. Forty percent of patients experience nausea and vomiting, and 25 percent have headache and altered mental status and show typical signs of meningitis (stiff neck, contracted pupils, intolerance to light and sound, delirium). Few patients will have seizures or focal neurologic deficits (Fauci and Lane, 1994).

A presumptive diagnosis can be made by identifying cryptococcus organisms in a stained slide of cerebrospinal fluid (CSF), by measuring the blood or CSF level of cryptococcal antigen or by identifying the organism on a slide made of a biopsy specimen. The definitive diagnosis is made by growing the organism in culture from the CSF or a brain biopsy (Fauci and Lane, 1994).

[3] Progressive Multifocal Leukoencephalopathy

Myelin is the insulating fatty sheath on nerve cells. Progressive multifocal leukoencephalopathy (PML) is a demyelinating (in which the myelin sheath is dissolved) central nervous system disorder caused by a papovavirus (the virus associated with cervical cancer is also a papovavirus) called JC virus. The infection starts as small, discrete areas of demyelination in the white matter under the cerebral cortex (outer portion of the brain). These small areas then join one another, and eventually the cortex, the cerebellum and the brain stem can become affected (Fauci and Lane, 1994).

Approximately 70 percent of the adult general population has antibodies against the JV virus, but only 10 percent shows signs of current JC viral replication. However, close to 33 percent of HIV-infected individuals show signs of active JC viral activity, and 4 percent of AIDS patients become afflicted with PML, the only known clinical manifestation of JC viral infection (Fauci and Lane, 1994).

The clinical course of PML is long, and the presentation can resemble the motor symptoms seen in HIV-1-associated dementia, though mental status usually does not change. Symptoms of PML include:

- ataxia (lack of muscle coordination);

- hemiparesis (paralysis on one side);

- aphasia (impaired or absent ability to talk and/or understand speech);

- sensory deficits; and

- visual field cuts (areas of blindness within the intact visual field).

Diagnosis is usually made via magnetic resonance (MR) scanning, which reveals multiple lesions in the white matter (Fauci and Lane, 1994).

[4] Neurosyphilis

Syphilis is a venereal disease caused by the bacterium *Treponema pallidum,* an organism native to Europe brought to the Americas by explorers in the sixteenth century. Until the mid-1980s, syphilis had long been under control, because it is sensitive to penicillin. However, the AIDS epidemic has produced a resurgence of this sexually transmitted disease. In people with AIDS, syphilis has an unpredictable course and may proceed faster than it does in people who are not infected with HIV. Neurosyphilis involves spread of the bacterium to the nervous system. People with AIDS who contract syphilis are more at risk for the development of neurosyphilis than are non-HIV-infected individuals (Jacobs, 1994).

Neurosyphilis has four stages: It initially has no symptoms and is merely characterized by a positive cerebrospinal fluid (CSF) antibody (serology) test for the spirochete, increased cells and occasionally increased protein level in the CSF.

The second phase is meningovascular syphilis, in which the meninges (membranes that cover the brain and spinal cord) and/or blood vessels in the brain become inflamed. Symptoms of this phase include headache, irritability, cranial nerve palsies (with different symptoms depending upon which nerve is affected), unequal reflexes and irregular pupils with slow reaction to light. If a large blood vessel becomes involved, a cerebrovascular accident (stroke) can occur.[3]

The third stage is called tabes dorsalis, which is a chronic, progressive degeneration of the parts of the brain that control balance and

---

[3] *See also* ch. 9.

vibration sense. The patient develops a wide-based gait and cannot walk in the dark. This is accompanied by lack of muscle tone and reduced reflexes. The legs can be affected with numbness, tingling, lack of sensation or sharp, recurrent, shooting pains.

The final stage of neurosyphilis (which can co-exist with stage 3) is general paresis (paralysis), reflecting involvement of the cerebral cortex. As in HIV-1-associated dementia, there is an insidious onset of memory loss and impaired concentration. The person may be irritable; the joints may ache, and the fingers and lips may tremble. This stage is usually associated with a significant personality change, with the person becoming confused, untidy, irresponsible and, finally, psychotic (Jacobs, 1994).

Laboratory diagnosis of syphilis in persons with AIDS can be difficult because the immune system response to the infection can be blunted, and the antibodies usually detected in a syphilis blood test may not exist in large enough quantities to produce a positive result. Diagnosis of neurosyphilis in HIV-infected patients involves examination of the cerebrospinal fluid (CSF) for evidence of the syphilis bacterium. However, it is complicated by the fact that CSF abnormalities can be caused by either syphilis or HIV itself.

The prevalence of neurosyphilis in AIDS patients is not known. Retrospective studies have shown that in asymptomatic patients with a positive blood test for the syphilis organism, 10 to 50 percent showed signs of infection in the cerebrospinal fluid (Jacobs, 1994).

[5] Tuberculosis Meningitis

Tuberculosis (TB) is caused by a bacillus called *Myobacterium tuberculosis,* and until the mid-1980s, this illness was thought to be in decline, a relic preserved only in nineteenth-century opera. However, with the spread of HIV disease and homelessness, tuberculosis has come roaring back. Tuberculosis is estimated to occur in 4 percent of people with AIDS, and in New York, Miami and other large cities, strains of the organism have appeared that are resistant to the normal regimen of drugs.

Tuberculosis is generally thought of as a respiratory disease. However, the tuberculosis organism can spread from the lungs to many parts of the body, the nervous system among them. In the nervous system, the tuberculosis bacillus causes meningitis, an infection/ inflammation of the membranes that cover the brain and spinal cord.

The infection causes a gradual onset of listlessness, irritability, fever and loss of appetite—nonspecific symptoms that are commonly seen in AIDS patients and can be due to HIV itself, treatment of antiretroviral drugs or a host of AIDS-associated infections. As the condition progresses, the patient develops headache, vomiting, seizures and coma.

Seventy-five percent of patients with TB meningitis have either evidence of active tuberculosis elsewhere in the body or a history of TB in the past. Examination of the cerebrospinal fluid reveals that the fluid is yellowish, with increased amounts of protein, decreased glucose levels and a somewhat elevated pressure. Even though there are 100 to 500 white blood cells per microliter, staining the fluid and looking under the microscope for tuberculosis organisms rarely finds any. Inoculating a culture medium with CSF and allowing cells to grow for several days will produce a positive culture in up to 75 percent of cases. Chest x-ray may show signs of respiratory TB, but it may also appear normal (Chambers, 1994).

13.33   Primary Central Nervous System Lymphoma

Primary lymphoma of the central nervous system (CNS) is the second most common space-occupying brain lesion seen in AIDS (toxoplasmosis is the most common). Lymphoma is a cancer of lymph tissues, and lymphomas in AIDS patients are usually very aggressive. Central nervous system lymphoma is usually a late condition in AIDS, which may account for its aggressiveness and poor prognosis. In immune compromised patients, such as those with AIDS, CNS lymphoma is associated with Epstein-Barr virus infection in 80 to 100 percent of cases. Primary CNS lymphoma is uncommon in people with a normal immune system (Hochberg and Pruitt, 1994).

The signs and symptoms of CNS lymphoma are similar to those of toxoplasmosis. Commonly seen symptoms include personality changes, focal deficits (distinct neurologic problems caused by damage to a particular part of the brain) and/or seizures that evolve over several weeks. Headaches are also frequent.

Magnetic resonance (MR) or computed tomography (CT) generally shows one to three lesions that are 3 to 5 centimeters in size. If contrast material is injected to enhance the CT or MR image, the lesions will appear ringlike; they are difficult to differentiate from the images seen in toxoplasmosis of the brain. Brain biopsy (in which specimens of brain tissue are obtained for laboratory examination) and removal of cerebrospinal fluid from the spinal canal for detection of cancer cells provide definitive diagnosis.

13.40 DIAGNOSIS

A diagnosis of HIV-1-associated dementia is what is known as a diagnosis of exclusion. This means there is no specific test for the condition, and every other possible cause must first be ruled out before the diagnosis can be made.[4] However, several situations are unclear, and aids to diagnosis are discussed here.

13.41 Dementia Versus Depression

Determining whether a patient is suffering from AIDS-related depression and the withdrawal it engenders or HIV-1-associated dementia requires time and continuity of care. It is probably not possible to tell early dementia from depression, especially in a single visit when the patient and clinician are strangers. However, once the patient and clinician have a relationship, and especially if the clinician can get input from the patient's loved ones, it may be easier to determine what is happening to the patient emotionally and mentally.

A trial of an antidepressant drug may be the only objective tool to distinguish early dementia from depression (keeping in mind that these medications often have no effect upon mood for three to four weeks). If the patient's mood and behavior begin to return to baseline after she or he has been taking the antidepressant medication for a few weeks, then the patient was probably depressed and not demented. Dementia is a progressive condition that does not respond to antidepressants. Ultimately dementia will differentiate itself from depression by further deterioration in the patient's psychoneurologic status.

13.42 Psychological Testing

Many psychological tests can detect changes in cognitive and psychomotor function, and it is beyond the scope of this chapter to

---

[4] *See* 13.32 *supra* for a discussion of specific diagnostic test results for opportunistic diseases.

examine these tests in any detail. However, relatively simple tests that evaluate the speed of information processing (e.g., asking a person to follow a trail with a pencil on a piece of paper) have been found to reliably identify the early stages of dementia (Goodwin, et al., 1996).

The Folstein Mini-Mental Status Examination is a widely used, easily administered test that can objectively evaluate declines in cognitive ability. The test asks the patient to complete 12 tasks, each with a range of possible scores adding up to a maximum of 32 points for the entire test. The tasks range from saying where the individual is and giving the date to counting backward by sevens, drawing two intersecting pentagons and saying the words *No ifs, ands or buts.* The test has been validated over the years as a sensitive gauge of cognitive ability, but it is most useful if there is an initial baseline test score with which to compare the results of a person with suspected early dementia (Fauci and Lane, 1994).

Psychological testing in HIV-1-associated dementia may provide not only diagnostic but also prognostic information. In one study, patients who were psychoneurologically impaired at the time of AIDS diagnosis survived for a significantly shorter period of time than did patients who were not initially so impaired (Karlsen, et al., 1995).

13.43   Computed Tomography (CT) and Magnetic Resonance (MR) Scanning

Computed tomography (CT) scanning is performed by a computer-enhanced x-ray machine that produces serial images of the brain (and other portions of the body) like slices of bread. CT scanning is widely available, and when contrast materials are injected into the patient's bloodstream before the scan is performed, subtle changes in brain anatomy are easily seen. CT is helpful when an AIDS patient develops cognitive or motor deterioration, because lymphoma and toxoplasmosis are easily seen on CT, and thus a diagnosis of HIV-1-associated dementia can be ruled out.

Magnetic resonance imagery (MRI) scanning is even more sensitive at finding brain lesions than is CT scanning. In this method, the brain is exposed to a strong magnetic field, and when the field is turned off, a computer constructs an image based on how the molecules realign themselves. The MR scan shows different parts of the brain in color, and although it is more expensive and less widely available than CT scanning, MR scans are frequently used to detect toxoplasmosis, brain lymphoma and progressive multifocal leukoencephalopathy.

13.50 THERAPY

Treatment of psychoneurologic symptoms in people with HIV disease depends upon the cause of the dementia. Many causes of cognitive/behavioral changes in people with AIDS can be treated, thereby both improving the patient's quality of life and perhaps also extending the length of his or her life.[5] Therefore, after a diagnosis has been reached, it is vital that a vigorous plan of therapy be implemented.

13.51 Antiretroviral Medications

Since the introduction in 1987 of the antiretroviral drug AZT (zidovudine; the first and still most widely used anti-AIDS drug), the incidence of HIV-1-associated dementia among AIDS patients has fallen significantly, and it has generally been thought that there is a causal relationship between these two facts (Goebel, 1995). A study comparing the incidence of HIV-1-associated dementia in homosexual men versus intravenous drug users found that within both groups, prolonged treatment with zidovudine was associated with a lower incidence of dementia (Bell, et al., 1996).

However, the literature is not entirely in agreement on the subject. An Italian study also confirmed that treatment with AZT decreases dementia risk, but it found that the effect was time-limited, and after 18 months of therapy, the rate of dementia rose to levels equal to that of individuals who had not been treated with the antiretroviral drug (Chiesi, et al., 1996). The Multicenter AIDS Cohort Study (MACS) has reported conflicting data suggesting that antiretroviral therapy is not protective against HIV-1-associated dementia. However, other researchers have found methodologic weaknesses in the MACS that may limit the general applicability of the results. Studies to track the relationship between AZT therapy and the development and treatment of dementia continue (Portegies, 1995).

---

[5] *See* 13.20 *supra.*

Dideoxyinosine (DDI; didanosine), another antiretroviral medication, has been found to be less effective than AZT in preventing and treating HIV-1-associated dementia. Studies have shown that four hours after administration of the drug, the concentration of DDI in the cerebrospinal fluid (CSF) is approximately half that of AZT, though it remains to be proved that this lower CSF concentration of DDI is the cause of its lower efficacy in AIDS dementia (Burger, et al., 1995).

13.52　Neurologic Opportunistic Infections

Toxoplasmosis, the most common central nervous system opportunistic infection, can be successfully treated in 90 percent of patients with a combination therapy of sulfadiazine (a sulfa drug), given in doses of 1 to 2 grams by mouth (PO) four times a day and pyrimethamine 25 to 100 milligrams PO once a day. Clindamycin in doses of 200 to 400 mg given intravenously (IV) every six hours, followed by clindamycin 300 to 900 mg orally every eight hours, can be substituted for the sulfadiazine. Allergies to sulfa drugs are very common. AIDS patients who are allergic are often still treated with sulfadiazine after being premedicated with acetaminophen and an antihistamine to block the allergic manifestations.

Cryptococcal meningitis and brain abscess can be treated with amphotericin B, 0.3 mg/kg/day given intravenously, with or without flucytosine, 150 mg/kg/day orally for six weeks, followed by fluconazole, 200 mg orally daily, indefinitely.

Progressive multifocal leukoencephalopathy (PML) can be experimentally treated by infusing cytarabine (cytosine arabinoside), a drug that inhibits DNA synthesis and is usually used to fight leukemia, into the spinal canal. Unfortunately, death usually occurs within three to six months (Fauci and Lane, 1994). Some case reports in the literature show AIDS patients with PML responding to high-dose therapy (1,200 mg/day) with zidovudine (AZT) (Singer, et al., 1994).

Neurosyphilis is treated with intravenous (IV) aqueous penicillin G, 2 million to 4 million units daily for 10 to 14 days, or intramuscular (IM) procaine penicillin G, 2.4 million units daily for 10 to 14 days, plus 1 gram daily of probenecid for 10 days. Patients who are allergic to penicillin can be treated with the cephalosporin ceftriaxone in doses of 1 to 2 grams given intramuscularly or intravenously daily.

Tuberculosis meningitis is treated with the same drugs that are used to treat respiratory TB. Often it is necessary to add additional drugs because of the risk of mult-drug-resistant TB in certain communities. Patients with a decreased level of consciousness may require intravenous rather than oral administration of antitubercular drugs (Fauci and Lane, 1994).

13.53 Lymphoma Therapy

In HIV-infected patients, the symptoms and radiologic evidence of central nervous system (CNS) lymphoma and toxoplasmosis are often virtually the same. Therefore, patients are frequently initially treated presumptively for toxoplasmosis, with a two-week course of sulfadiazine and pyrimethamine. If there is no improvement, clinically and radiologically, a brain biopsy is usually performed. If the biopsy is consistent with lymphoma, recommended treatment is radiation, with or without chemotherapy.

However, many patients cannot tolerate even moderate doses of chemotherapy, because the chemotherapeutic agents kill normal white blood cells called neutrophils, producing neutropenia. The bone marrow can be encouraged to produce neutrophils by the hematopoietic (pertaining to blood cell production) growth factor granulocyte-macrophage colony stimulating factor (GM-CSF or GC-CSF). This growth factor can allow an escalation of chemotherapy dose, but not always to a level that ensures remission (Freedman and Nadler, 1994).

13.54 Psychotropic Drugs

Psychotropic drugs have been found useful in treating AIDS patients who develop delirium (confusion, excitement, disorientation to time and place, and often hallucinations), cognitive decline, depression or anxiety. Symptoms of mania, delirium, agitation and aggressive behavior need early, decisive intervention by a psychiatrist experienced in treating patients with HIV-1-associated dementia (National Hospice Organization, 1996).

A 1994 case report suggests that patients with HIV-1-associated dementia have an increased risk of developing acute-onset parkinsonism (tremors and rigidity)[6] and dystonia (impaired muscle tone) when

---

[6] *See also* ch. 12.

they are treated with antipsychotic drugs, such as haloperidol (Haldol®) and chlorpromazine (Thorazine®), which interfere with the neurotransmitter dopamine in the brain (Factor, et al., 1994).

However, a 1996 controlled double-blind study (this type of study is considered a better test of a hypothesis than observations of a single case) compared the efficacy and side effects of the phenothiazine antipsychotics haloperidol and chlorpromazine and the benzodiazepine antianxiety drug lorazepam (Ativan®, a short-acting relative of Valium®) in treating delirium symptoms in AIDS patients. This controlled study found no increased risk of serious side effects from the antipsychotic drugs. The study found that treatment with either haloperidol (which is often used to treat delirium in the elderly) or chlorpromazine (once the mainstay of schizophrenia therapy) in relatively low doses caused significant improvement in delirium symptoms. Patients who were treated with these two drugs had a very low incidence of extrapyramidal side effects (sedation, Parkinson's-disease-like tremors and slow, rhythmic, automatic, local or generalized movements called tardive dyskinesia). No improvement in delirium symptoms was found in the patients treated with lorazepam, and all patients in this group developed treatment-limiting adverse effects (Breitbart, et al., 1996).

Clinical experience in men with AIDS who complained of decreased memory, concentration and attention span, as well as of apathy and slowing, has shown that the stimulant drug methylphenidate (Ritalin®, which is often used to treat hyperactivity in children) can produce improvement. However, placebo-controlled studies and studies with women have not been published (Brown, 1995).

Antidepressant drugs such as the tricyclics (amitriptyline; Elavil® and others) and the newer serotonin reuptake inhibitors (fluoxetine; Prozac® and others) have a role in treating the depression and withdrawal that are often encountered in the AIDS population. Early in the course of HIV-1-associated dementia, symptoms can be indistinguishable from depression, and a trial of therapy using an antidepressant drug may be indicated. It is important to remember that these drugs often take three to four weeks to begin to show a clinical effect, so they should not be discontinued too soon. Antianxiety drugs such as the benzodiazepines (lorazepam, clonazepam and others) can successfully treat anxiety symptoms but will not affect the cognitive decline associated with dementia.

13.60 AIDS DEMENTIA IN CHILDREN

The incidence of HIV-1-associated dementia is much higher in the pediatric population than it is among adults. Roughly half of all children with HIV disease develop neurologic manifestations (Lipton, 1994). Pediatric AIDS and HIV infection will soon be the primary infectious cause of perinatally acquired (acquired before, during or just after birth) developmental disabilities in this country (other perinatal infections that affect the nervous system are rubella and gonorrhea), which means that the number of neurologically impaired children with AIDS will continue to climb (Armstrong, et al., 1993).

The human immunodeficiency virus affects a child's nervous system differently from the way it affects an adult's, because the virus interferes with the actual growth and development of the child's brain rather than merely impacting what is already there, as it does in an adult. Children who develop HIV-1-associated dementia typically show developmental delay (for example, not walking or talking within the normal time frame for a child of that age), hypertonia (increased muscle tone), microcephaly (abnormally small head circumference) and calcification of the basal ganglia of the brain (American Psychiatric Association, 1994). Behavior in these children can suddenly become impulsive, hyperactive and aggressive (Cesena, et al., 1995).

A National Institutes of Health study comparing language development between children suffering with AIDS, with and without evidence of dementia, and uninfected siblings found that all children with HIV disease had impaired expressive language functioning (talking), and the impairment was most severe in children with dementia (Wolters, et al., 1995).

13.70 CONCERNS OF LOVED ONES

It is beyond the scope of this chapter to examine in great detail the concerns of people dealing with an individual who is suffering with HIV-1-associated dementia. However, it cannot be stressed enough that when an AIDS patient becomes demented, the situation for those around him or her becomes even more poignant. Dementia kills the person's identity before it kills the body. Caring for a person with dementia can be physically, emotionally and financially exhausting. There are worries that the patient may wander off and get lost, and eventually the person cannot be left alone. At the end, the opportunity for a meaningful farewell is lost because the patient can no longer understand what is happening.

Health professionals and counselors can help a patient's loved ones by educating them about the progression of the disease. Knowing what to expect, how to prepare for care as it becomes necessary, how to communicate and what their loved one is actually capable of can improve coping (Harvath, et al., 1995). Referral to a support group, respite care services and just empathic listening can all be of great help.

13.100   BIBLIOGRAPHY

Text References

American Psychiatric Association: Diagnostic and Statistical Manual of Mental Disorders, 4th ed. Washington, D.C.: American Psychiatric Association, 1994.

Armstrong, F., et al.: Pediatric HIV Infection: A Neuropsychological and Educational Challenge. J. Learn. Disabil. 26(2):92-103, Feb. 1993.

Bell, J., et al.: Influence of Risk Group and Zidovudine Therapy on the Development of HIV Encephalitis and Cognitive Impairment in AIDS Patients. AIDS 10(5):493-499, May 1996.

Breitbart, W., et al.: A Double-Blind Trial of Haloperidol, Chlorpromazine, and Lorazepam in the Treatment of Delirium in Hospitalized AIDS Patients. Am. J. Psychiatry 153(2):231-237, Feb. 1996.

Brown, G.: The Use of Methylphenidate for Cognitive Decline Associated with HIV Disease. Int. J. Psychiatry Med. 25(1):21-37, 1995.

Burger, D., et al.: Study on Didanosine Concentrations in Cerebrospinal Fluid. Implications for the Treatment and Prevention of AIDS Dementia Complex. Pharm. World Sci. 17(6):218-221, Nov. 24, 1995.

Carmichael, C., et al.: HIV/AIDS Primary Care Handbook. Norwalk, Conn.: Appleton and Lange, 1995.

Catalan, J., et al.: Psychological Medicine of HIV Infection. Oxford, England: Oxford University Press, 1995.

Cesena, M., et al.: Case Study: Behavioral Symptoms of Pediatric HIV-1 Associated Encephalopathy Successfully Treated With Clonidine. J. Am. Acad. Child Adolesc. Psychiatry 34(3):302-306, Mar. 1995.

Chambers, H.: Infectious Diseases: Bacterial and Chlamydial. In: Tierney, L., Jr., et al.: Current Medical Diagnoses and Treatment, 33rd annual revision. Norwalk, Conn.: Appleton & Lange, 1994.

Chiesi, A., et al.: Epidemiology of AIDS Dementia Complex in Europe. AIDS in Europe Study Group. J. Acquir. Immune Defic. Syndr. Hum. Retrovirol. 11(1):39-44, Jan. 1, 1996.

Factor, S., et al.: Persistent Neuroleptic-Induced Rigidity and Dystonia in AIDS Dementia Complex: A Clinico-Pathological Case Report. J. Neurol. Sci. 127(1):114-120, Dec. 1, 1994.

Fauci, A. and Lane, H.: Human Immunodeficiency Virus (HIV) Disease: AIDS and Related Disorders. In: Isselbacher, K., et al. (Eds.): Harrison's Principles of Internal Medicine, 13th ed. New York: McGraw-Hill, 1994.

Freedman, A. and Nadler, L.: Malignant Lymphomas. In: Isselbacher, K., et al. (Eds.): Harrison's Principles of Internal Medicine, 13th ed. New York: McGraw-Hill, 1994.

Glass, J., et al.: Immunocytochemical Quantitation of Human Immunodeficiency Virus in the Brain: Correlations with Dementia. Ann. Neurol. 38(5):755-762, Nov. 1995.

Goebel, F.: Combination Therapy from a Clinician's Perspective. J. Acquir. Immune Defic. Syndr. Hum. Retrovirol. 10(Suppl. 1):S62-S68, 1995.

Goodwin, G., et al.: The Edinburgh Cohort of HIV-Positive Injecting Drug Users at 10 Years After Infection: A Case-Control Study of the Evolution of Dementia. AIDS 10(4):431-440, Apr. 1996.

Harvath, T., et al.: Dementia-Related Behaviors in Alzheimer's Disease and AIDS. J. Psychosoc. Nurs. Ment. Health Serv. 33(1):35-39, Jan. 1995.

Hochberg, F. and Pruitt, A.: Neoplastic Diseases of the Central Nervous System. In: Isselbacher, K., et al. (Eds.): Harrison's Principles of Internal Medicine, 13th ed. New York: McGraw-Hill, 1994.

Jacobs, R.: Infectious Diseases: Spirochetal. In: Tierney, L., Jr., et al. (Eds.): Current Medical Diagnosis and Treatment, 33rd Annual Revision. Norwalk, Conn.: Appleton and Lange, 1994.

Karlsen, N., et al.: A Follow-Up Study of Neuropsychological Functioning in AIDS Patients. Prognostic Significance and Effect of Zidovudine Therapy. Acta Neurol. Scand. 91(3):215-221, Mar. 1995.

Lipton, S.: Neuronal Injury Associated with HIV-1 and Potential Treatment with Calcium-Channel and NMDA Antagonists. Dev. Neurosci. 16(3-4):145-151, 1994.

National Hospice Organization: Resource Manual for Providing Hospice Care to People Living with AIDS. Arlington, Vir.: National Hospice Organization, 1996.

Nottet, H. and Gendelman, H.: Unraveling the Neuroimmune Mechanisms for the HIV-1 Associated Cognitive/Motor Complex. Immunol. Today 16(9):441-448, Sept. 1995.

Portegies, P.: Review of Antiretroviral Therapy in the Prevention of HIV-Related AIDS Dementia Complex (ADC). Drugs 49(Suppl. 1):25-31, 1995.

Price, R.: Neurological Complications of HIV Infection. Lancet 348(9025):445-452, Aug. 17, 1996.

Singer, E., et al.: AIDS Presenting as Progressive Multifocal Leukoencephalopathy with Clinical Response to Zidovudine. Acta Neurol. Scand. 90(6):443-447, Dec. 1994.

Wolters, P., et al.: Differential Receptive and Expressive Language Functioning of Children with Symptomatic HIV Disease and Relation to CT Scan Brain Abnormalities. Pediatrics 95(1):112-119, Jan. 1995.

Worley, J. and Price, R.: HIV-1 and the Nervous System. In: McKendall, R. and Stroop, W.: Handbook of Neurovirology. New York: Marcel Decker, 1994.

Additional References

Bluestine, S. and Lesko, L.: Psychotropic Medications in Oncology and in AIDS Patients. Adv. Psychosom. Med. 21:107-137, 1994.

Brady, M., et al.: Randomized Study of the Tolerance and Efficacy of High– versus Low-Dose Zidovudine in Human Immunodeficiency Virus-Infected Children with Mild to Moderate Symptoms. J. Infect. Dis. 173(5):1097-1106, May 1996.

Buhrich, N. and Judd, F.: HIV and Psychiatric Disorders. Med. J. Aust. 164(7):422-424, Apr. 1, 1996.

Dursun, S. and Reveley, M.: Serotonin Hypothesis of Psychiatric Disorders During HIV Infection. Med. Hypotheses. 44(4):263-267, Apr. 1995.

Jay, C.: Neurology of Human Immunodeficiency Virus Infection—Past, Present, and Future. West. J. Med. 163(5):470-471, Nov. 1995.

Lennox, S. and Ward, G.: Assessing Patients with HIV-Associated Dementia. Prof. Nurse 10(9):588-589, June 1995.

McKeogh, M.: Dementia in HIV Disease—A Challenge for Palliative Care? J. Palliat. Care 11(2):30-33, Summer 1995.

Price, N.: The Role of the Consultation-Liaison Nurse. Caring for Patients with AIDS Dementia Complex. J. Psychosoc. Nurs. Ment. Health Serv. 33(12):31-34, Dec. 1995.

Price, R.: AIDS Dementia Complex and HIV-1 Brain Infection: A Pathogenic Framework for Treatment and Evaluation. Curr. Top. Microbiol. Immunol. 202:33-54, 1995.

Vigliano, P., et al.: Subacute Measles Encephalitis in a Boy with Perinatal HIV-1 Infection. Dev. Med. Child Neurol. 37(12):1117-1119, Dec. 1995.

Whipple, B. and Scura, K.: The Overlooked Epidemic: HIV in Older Adults. Am. J. Nurs. 96(5):18, May 1996.

Wright, E., et al.: HIV-Induced Neurological Disease. Med. J. Aust. 164(7):414-417, Apr. 1, 1996.

Wyness, M.: AIDS Dementia Complex: Guidelines for Nursing Care. Axone. 16(2):37-46, Dec. 1994.

INDEX

[References are to sections.]

[References are to sections.]

[References are to sections.]

[References are to sections.]

[References are to sections.]

[References are to sections.]

[References are to sections.]

[References are to sections.]

[References are to sections.]

[References are to sections.]

[References are to sections.]

[References are to sections.]

[References are to sections.]

[References are to sections.]

[References are to sections.]

[References are to sections.]

[References are to sections.]

[References are to sections.]

[References are to sections.]

[References are to sections.]

[References are to sections.]

[References are to sections.]

[References are to sections.]

[References are to sections.]

[References are to sections.]

[References are to sections.]

[References are to sections.]

[References are to sections.]

[References are to sections.]

[References are to sections.]

[References are to sections.]

[References are to sections.]

[References are to sections.]

[References are to sections.]

[References are to sections.]

[References are to sections.]

[References are to sections.]

[References are to sections.]

[References are to sections.]

[References are to sections.]

[References are to sections.]

[References are to sections.]

[References are to sections.]

[References are to sections.]

[References are to sections.]

[References are to sections.]

[References are to sections.]

[References are to sections.]

[References are to sections.]